HurstReviews

Pathophysiology Review

HurstReviews

Pathophysiology Review

Marlene Hurst, RN, MSN, FNP-R, CCRN-R

President
Hurst Review Services
Brookhaven, Mississippi

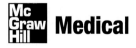 **Medical**

New York   Chicago   San Francisco   Lisbon   London   Madrid   Mexico City
Milan   New Delhi   San Juan   Seoul   Singapore   Sydney   Toronto

HurstReviews: Pathophysiology Review

1 2 3 4 5 6 7 8 9 0   CTP/CTP   0 9 8

Set ISBN 978-0-07-148986-7
Set MHID 0-07-148986-X
Book ISBN 978-0-07-154573-0
Book MHID 0-07-154573-5
CD ISBN 978-0-07-154574-7
CD MHID 0-07-154574-3

This book was set in Minion Roman by International Typesetting and Composition.
The editors were Quincy McDonald and Karen Davis.
The production supervisor was Catherine H. Saggese.
Project management was provided by Madhu Bhardwaj, International Typesetting and Composition.
The designer was Alan Barnett; the cover designer was David Dell'Accio; the cover photo is from Veer.
The index was prepared by Kevin Broccoli.
China Translation & Printing Services was printer and binder.

This book is printed on acid-free paper.

Library of Congress Cataloging-in-Publication Data

Hurst, Marlene.
   Pathophysiology review / Marlene Hurst.
      p. ; cm. — (Hurst reviews)
   Includes bibliographical references and index.
   ISBN-13 978-0-07-148986-7 (pbk. : alk. paper)
   ISBN-10   0-07-148986-X (pbk. : alk. paper)
   1. Physiology, Pathological—Examinations, questions, etc.   2. Nursing—Examinations,
questions, etc.   I. Title.   II. Series.
   [DNLM: 1. Nursing Care—Examination Questions.   2. Pathology—
Examination Questions.   WY 18.2 H966p 2008]
   RB113.H83 2008
   616.07076—dc22   2007041499

To my parents—Marceline and Garland Coldiron

CONTENTS

CONTRIBUTORS

Linda L. Altizer, RN, MSN, ONC, FNE-A
Armed Forces Medical Examiner's Office
Rockville, Maryland
Child Advocacy Center
Hagerstown, Maryland
Chapter 11: Musculoskeletal system

Sherri Bailey Barstis, RN, MSN
Performance Improvement
St. Dominic Hospital
Jackson, Mississippi
Chapter 5: Respiratory system

Shawn L. Boyd, CCRN, MSN
Faculty, University of Texas at Austin,
School of Nursing
Austin, Texas
Chapter 6: Cardiovascular system

Patricia Clutter, RN, MEd, CEN, FAEN
St. John's Hospital Emergency Department
Springfield and Lebanon, Missouri
Med-Ed, Inc.
Holland America Cruise Lines
Stafford, Missouri
Chapter 8: Hematology

Kimberly A. Gordon, RN, MSN
Instructor, Department of Associate Degree Nursing
Copiah-Lincoln Community College
Wesson, Mississippi
Chapter 13: Nutritional abnormalities

Allison P. Hale, MSN, BA, RN
Cain, Hale & Associates, Inc.
Wilmington, North Carolina
Chapter 9: Nervous system

Cynthia K. Halvorson, RN, MSN, CR
Peri-operative Clinical Nurse Specialist/Educator
Zurich, Switzerland
Chapter 12: Gastrointestinal system

James F. Holtvoight, BSN, MPA, RN
Clinical Education Specialist
Emergency Department
New Hanover Regional Medical Center
Wilmington, North Carolina
Chapter 18: Environmental emergencies

Mary F. King, RN, MS
Adjunct Faculty
Delta State University
Cleveland, Mississippi
Education & ICU Consultant, NWMRMC
Clarksdale, Mississippi;
ICU Staff Nurse, HRMC
Helena, Arkansas
Chapter 7: Shock; Chapter 16: Reproductive system

Autumn Langford RN, BSN, CCRN
Hurst Review Services
Brookhaven, Mississippi
Illustrations Manager

Lisa Lathem, RN, BSN, CIC
Infection Control Nurse
St. Dominic-Jackson Memorial Hospital
Jackson, Mississippi
Chapter 20. Infectious diseases

Debbie McDonough MSN, RN
Professor of Nursing
Alcorn State University
Natchez, Mississippi
Chapter 10: Sensory system

Wendy S. Meares, MSN, RN
Associate
Cain, Hale & Associates, Inc.
Wilmington, North Carolina
Chapter 17: Integument system

Mary Renquist, MSN, RN, CDE, CMSRN
Cain, Hale & Associates
Wilmington, North Carolina
Chapter 14: Endocrine system

Tamela J. Sill, MSN, RN
Medical University of South Carolina
Charleston, South Carolina
Chapter 15: Renal system

Cory Yingling, RN, MSN, BC
Clinical Education Specialist
Emergency Department
New Hanover Regional Medical Center
Wilmington, North Carolina
Chapter 18: Environmental emergencies

REVIEWERS

Kim Gordon, RN, MSN
Copiah-Lincoln Community College
Wesson, Mississippi

Autumn Langford RN, BSN, CCRN
Hurst Review Services
Brookhaven, Mississippi

Jena Smith, RN, MSN, NP-C
Hurst Review Services
Brookhaven, Mississippi

Carole D. Thompson, RN, CMC
Kings Daughters Medical Center
Brookhaven, Mississippi

ACKNOWLEDGMENTS

A very special thank you to Dr. Paul Johnson, Ann Stephens, Marcia Smith, Joey Johnson, Autumn Langford, Michaelan Bailey, and my husband Malcolm Cupit, for your help and patience during the completion of this project.

To Jena Smith: Thank you so much for all of the long hours of research, reading, writing, and fun! You are a joy!

PREFACE

Hello, nursing students! My name is Marlene Hurst, President and owner of Hurst Review Services and author of this book. Hurst Review Services, which is based in Brookhaven, Mississippi, opened its doors in 1988 when I began my new teaching job at a major university. As I began to teach nursing students, I quickly realized how much additional help they needed while in nursing school. Actually, I figured that out during my days as a nursing student, but at that time I just assumed that I was the only one struggling to survive nursing school! Today, my passion to help nursing students is just as strong as it ever was. Every time a struggling nursing student calls, emails, or visits me in my office, I still get just as fired up to help them as I did when I first started teaching! There is no better feeling than to help someone achieve their goal of becoming a nurse! I pray that every single person I help will go and help another nursing student. I certainly have had my share of help! When you become an experienced nurse, I hope you will help another new nurse and answer their endless questions happily! I'll never forget my first preceptor, Mrs. Ann Hilton. I know she got so tired of me saying, "Miss Ann"! If it were not for somebody like Miss Ann, I know I would have not stayed in nursing and certainly would not be writing a Pathophysiology book!

I love to make difficult nursing concepts fun and easy to understand! I believe that if students are relaxed, they will learn and retain more information. I've always said that nursing isn't meant to be difficult: it's meant to be understood! My specialty is guiding students to a true understanding of the "why" behind nursing content. The more "why's" you understand, the more your application and critical thinking skills will improve and then your test scores are going to go up! YES! Knowing "why" is the key! You will see as you read different content areas what I mean. I hope you find this book easy and fun to read. At the same time, I hope your study time is significantly decreased.

I hope that this book helps you to achieve your dream and makes your life a little easier in the process. If I can point out what you need to focus on as you go through Med-Surg; help you develop a true understanding; save some time; and decrease some of your stress . . . then my goal has been met!

I would love to hear from you. You may visit me at www.hurstreview.com to say "hello" or to learn more about what we have available to help you. I hope you like my work because I'm already working on many more items to come. Spread the word!

Best of Luck,
Marlene Hurst
President, Hurst Review Services

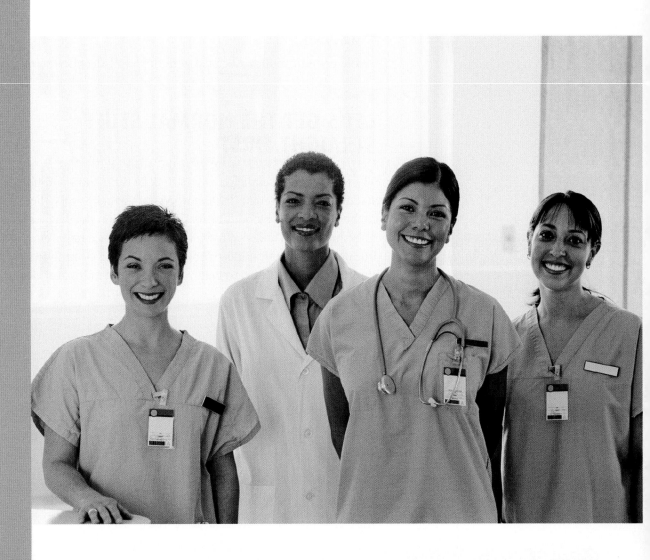

CHAPTER

1

Fluids and Electrolytes

OBJECTIVES

In this chapter, you'll review:

* The key concepts associated with fluid volume excess and fluid volume deficit.
* The causes, signs and symptoms, and treatments of electrolyte imbalances.
* The complications associated with fluid and electrolyte imbalances.

LET'S GET THE NORMAL STUFF STRAIGHT FIRST

The topic of fluids and electrolytes (F & E) is the foundation for understanding many different disease processes. Virtually every client admitted to the hospital has blood drawn as the first step in the diagnostic process—to evaluate fluids and electrolytes. Nursing practice requires diligent monitoring and in-depth understanding of fluids and electrolytes. We'll study this topic the **right way,** to help you understand fluids and electrolytes inside and out.

✚ Fluids

Fluids are good! Fluids:

1. Move electrolytes and oxygen into and out of cells as needed.
2. Aid digestion.
3. Cleanse the body of waste.
4. Regulate body temperature.
5. Lubricate joints and mucous membranes.

Fluids are located in 2 places in relation to the body's cells:

1. ICF (intracellular): fluid inside the cell.
2. ECF (extracellular): any fluid outside the cell.

There are 2 types of extracellular fluid:

* Intravascular fluid: called plasma; the liquid part of blood in the extracellular compartment; total of 3 L of fluid.
* Interstitial fluid: fluid in between cells that bathes the cells; includes the lymphatic fluids; total of 9 L of fluid.[1,2]

Total body water

Total body water (TBW) is the entire amount of water in the body, usually documented as a percentage.

* Water is the numero uno body fluid and is the most critical element needed for life. Life is sustained for only a few days without water.
* In a healthy adult, TBW comprises 45% to 75% of the body's weight, with the average being 60%. TBW varies by individual.

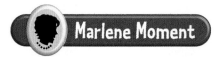

Marlene Moment

I knew that extra weight couldn't ALL be fat. It's just water, and water is good for me!

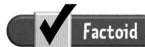

Factoid

Because women have less body fluid than men, females are more prone to dehydration than males.

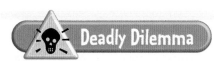

Deadly Dilemma

Elderly clients can become dehydrated very quickly if intake and output is not monitored accurately.

- When someone loses too much water, they are dehydrated. Notice I said "WATER"; this will become important later in the chapter when we study sodium imbalances.
- When more than one-third of the body's fluid is absent, life-threatening situations can occur.
- Fat has a tiny amount of water; lean tissue (muscle) has heaps of water.
- It's not fair, but babes (females) have more body fat than dudes (males); therefore, females have less body fluid.
- Elderly clients have a decreased amount of body fluid due to less body fat, which makes them a high risk for dehydration.[1,2]

Adequate fluids

A person can have adequate fluids in the body, but for some physiological reason maybe the fluids are not being pumped around to all the vital organs by the heart like they should. Because of this malfunction, the vital organs don't realize the fluids are there, and thus they don't access them. In turn, the body goes into shock because it doesn't realize that fluids are available.

CASE IN POINT A client with streptococcal toxic shock syndrome experiences severe hypotension—68/42 mm Hg. The heart is not pumping out adequate blood to the vital organs due to the hypotension. The vital organs assume there is no blood available, although the client has not lost any blood. As a result, the body goes into shock. Even though the correct volume of blood exists inside the body, it's not going where it needs to (maybe it's pooling in the venous system). The client's body responds by shouting, "Hey, I'm in shock!"

CASE IN POINT A client is stung by a bee and all of his vessels vasodilate—a response occasionally seen in allergic reactions. The same amount of fluid volume is in the body because the client hasn't lost any fluids, but the blood vessel is now larger. This enlarged vessel makes it SEEM like there are inadequate fluids circulating in the body. Once again, the body THINKS it is in shock and reacts accordingly.

Where do we get fluids?

About 90%—2500 mL—of our fluids come from ingested substances, such as food and drink. These substances break down into water. Fluids also come from IV substances, blood, blood products, and the accumulation from metabolic oxidation.[1,2]

FLUID INTAKE The usual fluid intake per day in a healthy adult looks something like this:

Ingested fluids	1300 mL
Water in foods	1000 mL
Oxidation	300 mL
	2600 mL

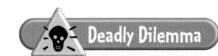

Deadly Dilemma

When major organs aren't being perfused with adequate fluids they can die. Vascular collapse—or shock—can occur when there are not enough fluids to keep the blood vessels open.

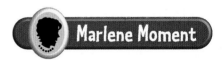

Marlene Moment

Notice I said we get 90% of our fluids through **ingestion,** not **indigestion.**[1,2]

Acceptable fluid intake and loss on a daily basis for a healthy adult is 1500 to 3000 mL.[1,2]

How do we lose fluid?

We lose fluid by 2 ways: sensible and insensible. Skin loss can be sensible or insensible.

1. Sensible fluid loss: loss that is SEEN.
   - Occurs through the skin.
   - Includes urine, sweat, and feces.
   - Approximately 500 mL/day is lost through the skin.
   - The kidneys excrete 800 to 1500 mL/day of fluid depending on the individual's intake.[1,2]

2. Insensible fluid loss: loss that is NOT SEEN.
   - Occurs through the kidneys, intestinal tract, lungs, and skin.
   - Includes water evaporation from the skin.
   - Exhalation from the lungs accounts for approximately 500 mL/day fluid loss.
   - Approximately 100 to 200 mL/day is lost through gastrointestinal output.[1,2]

Abnormal fluid loss

Abnormal fluid loss results from a physiologic imbalance. Examples include:

- Fever or an increased room temperature, which escalates fluid loss through the lungs and skin.
- Severe burns, which cause increased fluid loss (skin can't hold fluid in if it's damaged).
- Hemorrhage where the vascular volume decreases at an accelerated rate (for example, bleeding during surgery, trauma, or a ruptured aneurysm).[1,2]

Other abnormal fluid losses may be seen in Table 1-1:

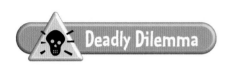

Rapid breathing causes increased fluid loss.

Table 1-1

Abnormal fluid loss	Definition
Emesis	Vomiting of fluid
Fistulas	Abnormal opening that secretes fluid
Secretions	Drainage from wounds or suction tubes
Wound exudates	Fluid from surgical drains
Paracentesis	A procedure where fluid is extracted from the abdomen (the peritoneum)
Thoracentesis	A procedure where fluid is extracted from the space between the visceral and parietal pleura (linings around the lungs)
Diaphoresis	Excessive sweating during illness

Source: Created by author from Reference #1.

DEHYDRATION   The 2 types of dehydration are:

1. Mild dehydration: 2% loss of body weight, which equals 1 to 2 L of body fluid.

2. Marked dehydration: 5% loss of body weight, which equals 3 to 5 L of body fluid.[1,2]

CASE IN POINT   A loss of 20% or more of body fluid can result in death unless drastic measures to rehydrate the client are taken.[1,2] For example, in a burn client, the damaged vessels cannot hold fluid in, so large amounts of fluid shift out of the vascular space. This is why fluid replacement is one of the most important aspects of burn treatment, especially in the first 24 hours.

Making sense of the numbers

Client input should always be close to the output. If a client takes in 3000 mL of fluid in 24 hours and puts out only 500 mL, this client is retaining too much fluid. This could lead to life-threatening problems such as fluid volume overload, congestive heart failure (CHF), or pulmonary edema. As nurses, this is why we must not just **LOOK** at the numbers, but we must make sense of them.

A quick way to estimate fluid balance is to compare the intake to the output. You should **always** make this comparison when checking the intake and output (I & O) record in order to detect or prevent any complications for your clients.

✚ Electrolytes

What are electrolytes? Electrolytes are elements that, when dissolved in water, acquire an electrical charge—positive or negative. Body fluid is mainly a mixture of water and electrolytes. If either water or electrolytes get out of whack—causing lack of homeostasis—then your clients may encounter potentially life-threatening problems.

The following are the vital electrolytes:

- Sodium (Na^+)
- Potassium (K^+)
- Calcium (Ca^{2+})
- Magnesium (Mg^{2+})
- Chloride (Cl^-)
- Phosphate (HPO_4^{2-})[1]

How do we measure electrolytes?

There are many important things we can learn about our clients by studying the "numbers" of electrolytes. Let's review how electrolytes are actually measured. There are 3 measurements used to count the number of electrolytes in the serum, sometimes referred to as plasma and vascular space the plasma and vascular space. The unit of measurement varies from laboratory to laboratory.

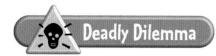

When administering insulin, especially IV insulin, watch the serum potassium level. It can drop, thus leading to life-threatening arrhythmias.

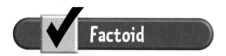

The only kind of insulin that can be given IV is regular insulin.[1]

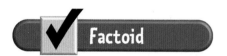

PTH makes serum calcium increase.

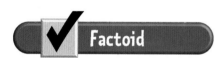

Calcitonin causes serum calcium to decrease.

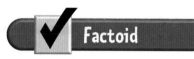

Anytime serum calcium increases, the phosphorus level decreases, and vice versa.

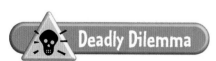

A severe excess or deficit of magnesium or potassium can lead to life-threatening complications: respiratory arrest, seizures, or life-threatening arrhythmias.

1. mg/100 mL (milligrams/100 mL): measures the weight of the particle in a certain amount of volume. This is the same as mg/dL (deciliter).
2. mEq/L: milliequivalent is one-thousandth of an equivalent—the amount of a substance that will react with a certain number of hydrogen ions. This is measured per liter of fluid. Simply put, this is atomic weight.
3. mmol/L (millimoles/liter): millimole is one-thousandth of a mole per liter of fluid. Basically, this measurement offers an in-depth analysis of the electrolyte being evaluated.[1,2]

Where do electrolytes live in the body?

Electrolytes can be found all over the body.

1. Potassium: found inside the cell; the most plentiful electrolyte in the body.
2. Magnesium: found inside the cell; second most plentiful electrolyte in the body.
3. Sodium: numero uno electrolyte in the extracellular fluid.
4. Phosphorus: found inside the cell and in the bones.
5. Calcium: found mainly in bones and teeth; some floats around in the blood as well.
6. Chloride: found inside the cell, the blood, and the fluid between cells.[1,2]

Raging hormones!

Hormones help keep electrolytes within normal range. Here's how:

1. Insulin: moves potassium from the blood (vascular space) to the inside of the cell, causing the serum K^+ to drop.
2. Parathyroid hormone (PTH): moves calcium from the bone into the blood when serum calcium levels are low. This causes the serum calcium to increase.
3. Calcitonin: moves calcium into the bones as needed. When the serum calcium is too high, calcitonin kicks in and moves calcium from the blood into the bone. This causes serum calcium to decrease. Calcitonin occurs naturally in the body, but it may be given in drug form as well.[1]

How do we get rid of excess electrolytes?

Excess electrolytes are excreted by:

• Urine, feces, and sweat.
• Aldosterone: causes sodium and water **retention** while causing potassium **excretion** through the urine.
• PTH: increases urine excretion of phosphorus and decreases urine excretion of calcium.[1,2]

What causes decreased oral electrolyte intake?

Table 1-2 explores the causes of decreased oral electrolyte intake and why this occurs.

Table 1-2

Cause	Why
Anorexia	Lack of appetite
Feeling weak	Lack of energy to take in nutrients
Shortness of breath	Some clients need all of their energy to breathe and will neglect eating in the process (shortness of breath may ↑ with eating, so client chooses not to eat)
GI upset	When you are nauseated, do you feel like eating?
Income	Not able to afford nutritious foods
Fad dieting (low in potassium)	Intentionally limiting oral intake

Source: Created by author from Reference #1.

Abnormal electrolyte losses

Fluid loss can cause an excessive deficit of electrolytes, which may leave your patient in a pickle! The relationship between fluid loss and electrolyte deficit is shown in Table 1-3.

Table 1-3

Problem	Why
Vomiting	Causes expulsion of ALL stomach contents, which contains a lot of electrolytes (especially potassium and chloride)
Nasogastric (NG) suction	Electrolytes are sucked out of the stomach
Intestinal suction	Most electrolytes are absorbed in the intestine; if the intestine is being suctioned then electrolytes can't be absorbed properly
Drainage (from wounds or fistulas)	All body fluid contains electrolytes; drainage causes a decrease of body fluid, resulting in a loss of electrolytes
Paracentesis	Removing fluid from the body causes a decrease in electrolytes
Diarrhea	Intestines are rich with magnesium. Diarrhea causes loss of magnesium and prevents magnesium from staying in the GI tract long enough to be absorbed
Diuretics	Causes excretion of potassium through the kidneys (depends on the type of diuretic)
Kidney trauma, illness, disease	Causes loss or retention of electrolytes

Source: Created by author from Reference #1.

CASE IN POINT   A common nursing order is "nothing by mouth" (NPO). When your patients are NPO, remember that the kidneys are still functioning and excreting potassium—that's just what kidneys like to do. This could lead to a potassium deficit in your clients, which can be life threatening if the electrolyte isn't replaced. Usually when a client is NPO, the physician will write an order for IV fluids with added potassium in the solution to maintain homeostasis.

What causes electrolyte excess in the blood?

Table 1-4 gives the causes and reasons of electrolyte excess in the blood.

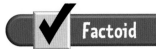

Factoid

Depleted electrolytes must be replaced.

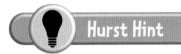

Hurst Hint

When administering medications, make it a habit to check how each particular drug can affect electrolyte balance.

Table 1-4

Cause	Why
Kidney trauma, illness, or disease	When the kidneys are sick, electrolytes can accumulate in the blood; the kidneys aren't able to excrete the excess—especially magnesium and potassium
Massive blood transfusions	Preservatives in blood can contain a lot of calcium; the longer blood sits in the blood bank, cells begin to rupture—or hemolyze. When cells rupture, potassium is released from the cell into the bag of blood. Therefore, several blood transfusions could increase the serum potassium, especially if the kidneys aren't working properly (excess potassium is excreted through the kidneys)
Tumors	Certain types can cause calcium to leach from the bone and move into the blood
Crushing injuries	Cells rupture, causing potassium and phosphorus to release into the bloodstream
Chemotherapy	Destroys and ruptures cells, which releases potassium and phosphorus into the bloodstream

Source: Created by author from Reference #1.

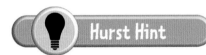

Hurst Hint

If your client has an illness that impairs kidney function, you must monitor for potassium retention—hyperkalemia—which can lead to life-threatening arrhythmias.

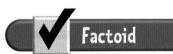

Factoid

Alcoholics may have many electrolyte imbalances due to poor nutrition and decreased absorption of electrolytes.

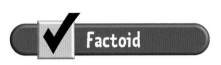

Factoid

It is standard treatment to utilize IV therapy when caring for someone with a fluid and electrolyte imbalance.

✚ Organs that support fluid and electrolyte homeostasis

Several major organs maintain fluid and electrolyte balance in the body. Patients can have a disease or an alteration in any of these organs, which may affect fluid and electrolyte balance. During your schooling, you will learn specific nursing interventions to help your clients regain and maintain homeostasis. Let's look at the major organs that maintain fluid and electrolyte homeostasis.

Kidneys

The kidneys (Fig. 1-1):

- Maintain sodium and water balance.
- Regulate fluid and electrolyte balance by controlling output.
- Filter 170 L of plasma per day.
- Regulate fluid volume and osmolality (concentration of particles in a solution).
- Activate the renin–angiotensin response as needed.
- When not taking fluid in by mouth, the urine output will drop. Why? The kidneys aren't getting enough perfusion/blood flow to produce urine OR the kidneys are trying to compensate by holding on to fluid.

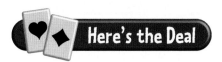

Here's the Deal

The renin–angiotensin response kicks in when blood volume is low. This causes retention of sodium and water in the vascular space to replenish lost blood volume.

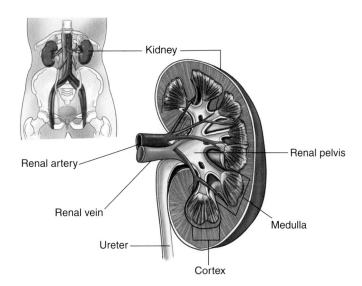

◀ Figure 1-1. Kidney.

Kidney

Renal artery

Renal vein

Ureter

Renal pelvis

Medulla

Cortex

CASE IN POINT   Anytime the kidneys are not perfusing adequately, permanent kidney damage can occur. It only takes 20 minutes of poor perfusion to promote acute tubular necrosis.[1,2] Acute tubular necrosis results in damage to the renal tubules, usually from ischemia during shock. If you don't recognize decreased kidney perfusion, renal failure and possible patient death can result.

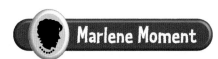

Marlene Moment

The renin–angiotensin response . . . just like Martha Stewart says, "It's a good thing."

Cardiovascular system

- Pumps and carries fluids and other good stuff throughout the body, to the vital organs, especially to the kidneys; a client must have a BP of at least 90 systolic to maintain adequate organ perfusion.
- Cardiac output is the amount of fluid the left ventricle is pumping out. Consistent and adequate cardiac output leads to adequate tissue perfusion.
- Blood vessels can constrict in response to decreased volume. When blood pressure drops below 90 systolic, blood vessel constriction may occur.
- When blood vessels constrict, BP increases. When blood vessels dilate, BP decreases. This compensatory response helps maintain tissue perfusion and fluid and electrolyte homeostasis.[1,2]

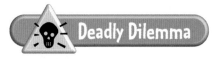

Deadly Dilemma

Clients with renal failure cannot excrete excess volume as they need to, which can result in serious conditions such as pulmonary edema or heart failure.

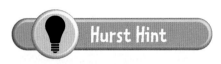

Hurst Hint

Always think left ventricle when you think about cardiac output.

CASE IN POINT   Pretend a balloon is a vein or an artery. Take your hand and squeeze the balloon. When you squeeze the balloon what happens to the pressure in the balloon? It goes up. DON'T POP THE BALLOON! This is the exact principle that occurs when the blood vessels constrict the vascular volume.

LEFT VENTRICLE WEAKNESS   Things that weaken the left ventricle and lead to decreased cardiac output are shown in Table 1-5:

Table 1-5

Cause	Why
Myocardial infarction (MI)	Damaged cardiac muscle can't pump effectively, causing cardiac output to drop
Bradycardia	When pulse is decreased the heart is unable to pump as much blood out so cardiac output decreases
Excessive tachycardia	The ventricles of the heart do not have time to completely fill with blood when the heart is beating fast, so less blood is pumped out
Low fluid volume	Not enough volume exists to fill the heart chambers, resulting in decreased cardiac output
Arrhythmias	Some arrhythmias decrease cardiac output because the heart does not pump effectively due to a glitch in the cardiac electrical system. Arrhythmias are no big deal until they affect cardiac output
High blood pressure	If the heart is having to pump blood out against a high pressure, not as much blood can set out to the body. Therefore, cardiac output decreases
Drugs	Can affect heart contractions, thus impacting heart rate and cardiac output

Source: Created by author from Reference #1.

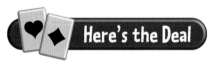

Here's the Deal

Clients who experience rapid breathing either due to a high ventilator setting or anxiety may need increased fluids to maintain homeostasis.

Lungs

Short and sweet: The lungs regulate fluid by releasing water as vapor with every exhalation. Every time you exhale, water is lost.

Adrenal glands

The adrenal glands (Fig. 1-2) secrete aldosterone. Aldosterone:

* Retains sodium and water.
* Excretes potassium at the same time.
* Builds up vascular volume, which makes the BP go up (because sodium and water are being retained in vascular space).

Remember, more vascular volume means more blood pressure.

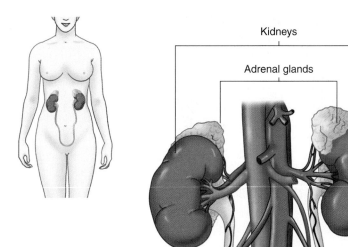

Kidneys

Adrenal glands

◀ Figure 1-2. Adrenal glands.

DEFINE TIME

Excrete: to move **out** of the body (urethra excretes urine).

Secrete: to give off **into** the body (cells secrete mucus).

Pituitary gland

The pituitary gland (Fig. 1-3) stores antidiuretic hormone (ADH), which causes retention of **water.** As water is retained in the vascular space, vascular volume and blood pressure increase.

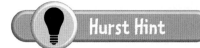

Hurst Hint

More vascular volume means more blood pressure.

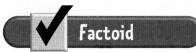

Factoid

Retention of sodium and water causes potassium excretion, because sodium and potassium have an inverse relationship.

◀ Figure 1-3. The pituitary gland.

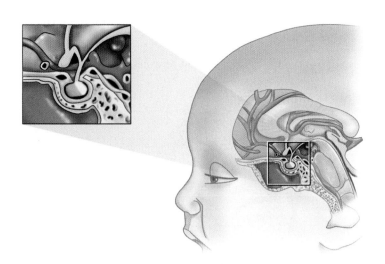

Parathyroid glands

The parathyroid glands (Fig. 1-4) secrete parathyroid hormone (PTH). This causes an increase in serum calcium by pulling it from the bones and placing the calcium in the blood.[1,2]

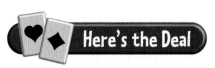

Here's the Deal

When more blood is flowing through the kidneys, if the kidneys are functioning properly; thus they produce more urine.

▶ Figure 1-4. Parathyroid glands.

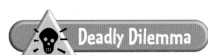

Deadly Dilemma

It is your responsibility to make sure that clients with an impaired thirst mechanism remain hydrated.

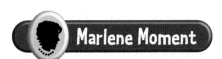

Marlene Moment

When you eat the entire industrial-size bag of salty chips all by yourself, you become thirsty because your serum sodium goes up. You are able to respond to your thirst mechanism by preparing yourself a lovely beverage to quench your thirst. (A patient may not be able to quench their thirst without your help)

▶ Figure 1-5. Thyroid gland.

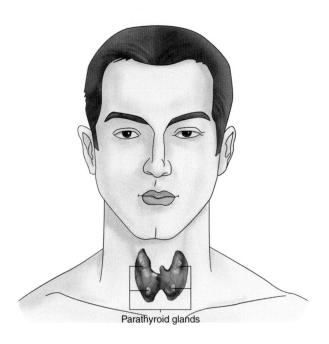

Parathyroid glands

Thyroid gland

The thyroid gland (Fig. 1-5) releases thyroid hormones. These hormones increase blood flow in the body by:

- Providing energy

- Increasing pulse rate
- Increasing cardiac output

- Increasing renal perfusion
- Increasing diuresis

- Ridding of excess fluid[1,2]

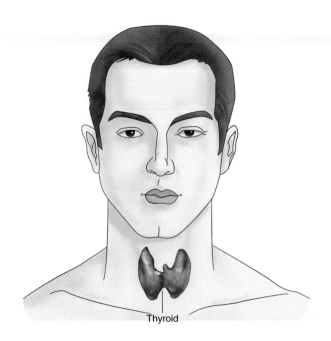

Thyroid

Hypothalamus

The amount of fluid the body desires is monitored by the thirst response, which is controlled by the hypothalamus (Fig. 1-6).

- Most adults can respond to their thirst mechanism. Clients who are elderly, confused, unconscious, or very young (infants) may not be able to respond to their thirst mechanism.[1,2]

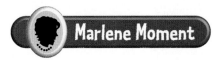

Marlene Moment

As Kramer on the television show *Seinfeld* said, "These pretzels are making me thirsty!" Remember that?

◀ Figure 1-6. Hypothalamus.

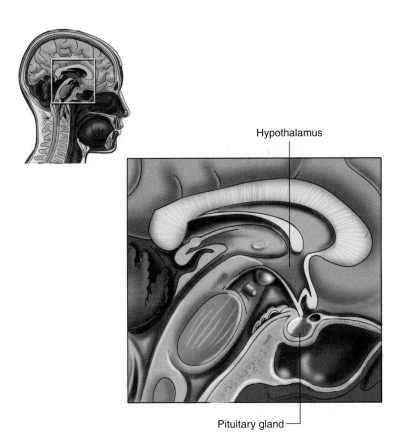

Hypothalamus

Pituitary gland

Small intestine

The small intestine absorbs 85% to 95% of fluid from ingested food and delivers it into the vascular system.[1,2]

Lymphatic system

The lymphatic system moves water and protein back into the vascular space.

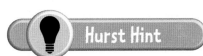

Hurst Hint

As serum sodium increases, so does thirst.

✛ Substances that can alter fluid balance

There are 2 specific goodies in our body that can alter fluid balance:

1. Plasma protein.
2. Glucose.

Plasma protein

Plasma protein holds on to fluid in the vascular space. There are several types of plasma proteins, but the most abundant is albumin.

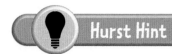

Anytime you see unexplained swelling in a client, consider asking the physician to order a serum albumin blood test.

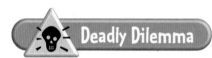

By the time you get an acutely ill diabetic client who is in diabetic ketoacidosis (DKA) into the intensive care unit, he may have zero output! This is an emergency that needs immediate attention or the kidneys could die forever!

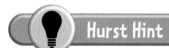

When a client goes into DKA, the urine output will go through 3 phases: polyuria, oliguria, and then anuria. IV fluids must be started prior to the anuria stage to prevent kidney failure!

CASE IN POINT If a client is badly burned, malnourished (decreased protein intake), or has a disease where the liver is not making adequate amounts of albumin, problems can occur. Adequate albumin needed to hold fluid in the vessels may not exist; therefore, the fluid may leak out of the vessels into the tissues and cause shock. These clients look as if they are in a fluid volume excess because they are so swollen from fluid accumulation in the tissues and interstitial spaces. The fluid is in the body, it just isn't in the vascular space.

Glucose

The vascular space likes the particle-to-water ratio to be equal. In this case the particle is glucose. The body doesn't like it when the balance gets out of whack.

CASE IN POINT When the blood sugar is very high, as in diabetics, the blood has too many glucose particles compared to water in the vascular space. This causes particle-induced diuresis (PID), sometimes called osmotic diuresis. The kidneys monitor the blood for fluid, electrolyte, and particle imbalances. When the kidneys sense the increased number of glucose particles, they want to help the blood rid the excess. But think about this: Have you ever excreted just a sugar particle? No! You would have remembered that! The glucose is excreted out of the body through the urine, which is made up of many substances including water and electrolytes. Polyuria occurs as the kidneys excrete the excess sugar. The kidneys continue to filter the **blood** to decrease the serum glucose, resulting in fluid loss from the vascular space. If this goes on long enough, hypovolemia and shock can result. Once shock occurs, polyuria ceases. Oliguria results, which could lead to anuria. Now the kidneys feel used and are really ticked off! The kidneys tried to help the blood get rid of the glucose particles, and as a result vascular volume dropped. The kidneys say, "Look what you've done to me! I was trying to help you, blood, and now you are trying to kill me!" Why are the kidneys so emotional? Because they are the **first** organs to die when there is inadequate fluid in the body. Remember, it only takes 20 minutes of poor kidney perfusion for acute tubular necrosis to occur.

DEFINE TIME

- Oliguria is urine output < 400 mL/day.
- Anuria is the absence of urine output.[1,2]

LET'S GET DOWN TO SPECIFICS

Almost every hospitalized client has some sort of fluid and electrolyte imbalance. These imbalances can impede patient progress and account for a longer hospital stay. Let's look at the most common fluid and electrolyte imbalances.

✚ Fluid volume deficit

Simply put, fluid volume deficit (FVD) results when fluid loss exceeds fluid intake.

What is it?

In FVD, sodium and water are lost in equal amounts from the vascular space. FVD is:

- Also called hypovolemia or isotonic dehydration.
- Not the same as dehydration.

What causes it and why?

- Decreased intake or poor appetite—Fluids must be taken in to replace what is being burned in routine metabolism.
- Drugs that affect fluids and electrolytes—Some drugs cause fluid and electrolyte losses (diuretics).
- Diuresis—Many diseases can causes the body to excrete fluid (Diabetes Insipidus, Addison's disease.)
- Forgetting to drink and eat—Patients with Alzheimer's disease or other forms of dementia may forget to eat/drink. Unconscious clients or immobile clients may be physically unable to get to water/food.
- Poor response to fluid changes—The kidneys may not respond as they once did to fluid problems (kidneys should decrease excretion of fluids if a fluid volume deficit is present).

Table 1-6 shows other causes and reasons for FVD.

Table 1-6

Cause	Why
Vomiting	Stomach loses electrolytes and fluid
Diarrhea	Loss of fluid and electrolytes from the "other end"
GI suction	Mechanical removal of fluid and electrolytes with an NG tube
Diuretics	Excessive excretion of fluid and electrolytes through the kidneys
Impaired swallowing	Decreased oral intake of fluids and electrolytes
Tube feedings	Contain nutrients needed to survive EXCEPT water
Fever	Causes fluid loss (sweating)
Laxatives	Excessive use causes fluid and electrolyte loss
Hemorrhage	Loss of blood volume at a fast rate
Third spacing	Blood volume drops when fluid leaves the vascular space

Source: Created by author from Reference #1.

Signs and symptoms and why

Table 1-7 shows the signs and symptoms associated with FVD and why these occur.

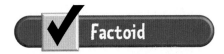
Factoid

Dehydration is when **water is lost** and **sodium is retained.**

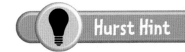
Hurst Hint

If a client loses fluids from her body long enough—it doesn't matter how the fluid is lost—the vascular volume will eventually drop. The faster the fluid loss, the quicker the client becomes symptomatic.

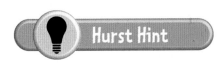
Hurst Hint

Ask your client, "How are your rings fitting?" If the rings are looser than normal, this could be a sign of fluid loss.

Table 1-7

Signs and symptoms	Why
Acute weight loss	Water weighs about 8 lbs/gallon; I liter weight is 2.2 lbs or 1 kg. Weight loss may mean water loss (not fat)
Decreased skin turgor (tenting occurs)	Decreased skin elasticity caused by decreased tissue perfusion
Postural hypotension (orthostatic hypotension)	Fluid deficit causes BP drop from supine or sitting position to upright position
Increased urine specific gravity	What little urine that is being excreted will be concentrated as not much fluid is present in the body
Weak, rapid pulse	Heart pumps faster to move fluid
Cool extremities	Peripheral vasoconstriction shunts blood to vital organs and away from extremities
Dry mucous membranes	Decreased fluids causes membrane dryness
Decreased BP	Less vascular volume leads to lower blood pressure
Decreased peripheral pulses	Blood shunted away from extremities; poor tissue perfusion
Oliguria	Body holding on to what fluid is available
Decreased vascularity in the neck and hands	Not enough fluid to keep vasculature open
Decreased central venous pressure (CVP)	Less vascular volume leads to lower central venous pressure
Increased respiratory rate	Maintain oxygen distribution throughout the body

Source: Created by author from Reference #1.

Quickie tests and treatments

Laboratory testing for FVD include serum electrolytes, BUN, and creatinine. Treatment measures include oral fluid replacement if tolerated and IV fluid (IVF) replacement. If the deficit is due to hemorrhage or blood loss, blood products are administered to increase vascular volume.

What can harm my client?

Be on the lookout for complications of FVD including:

- Shock.
- Poor organ perfusion, leading to acute tubular necrosis and renal failure.
- Multiorgan dysfunction due to poor perfusion.
- Decreased cardiac output.
- Congestive heart failure.

If I were your teacher, I would test you on . . .

There is a lot of information to know regarding FVD, including:

- Causes and reasons for FVD.
- Signs and symptoms and explanations for FVD.

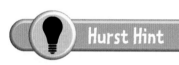

Hurst Hint

When blood is concentrated—called hemoconcentration—the hemoglobin, hematocrit, osmolarity, glucose, blood urea nitrogen (BUN), and serum sodium increase.

- Concepts related to I & O and daily weight monitoring.
- IVF replacement: types of fluids used, calculation of administration rates.
- Interventions to reverse hypovolemia: oral rehydration therapy, IVF.
- Monitoring urine output including appropriate output amounts.
- Care of the client experiencing orthostatic hypotension.
- How FVD affects laboratory values.
- Monitoring for fluid overload.
- Administration of blood products and associated complications.
- Pump function and maintenance.

✚ Fluid volume excess

In short, fluid volume excess (FVE) results when fluid intake exceeds fluid loss.

What is it?

Fluid volume excess is:

- Excessive retention of water and sodium in the extracellular fluid (ECF).
- Also called hypervolemia or isotonic overhydration.

What causes it and why

Table 1-8 demonstrates the causes of FVE and why it occurs.

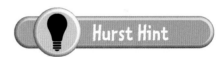

Hurst Hint

The heart moves fluid forward; otherwise, the fluid backs up into the lungs causing pulmonary edema.

Table 1-8

Causes	Why
Renal failure	Kidneys aren't able to remove fluid
CHF	Decreased kidney perfusion due to decreased cardiac output leads to excessive fluid retention
Cushing syndrome	Excess steroids associated with the disease cause fluid retention
Excessive sodium: from IV normal saline or lactated ringers or foods	Causes fluid retention in the vascular space
Blood product administration	Blood products go directly into the vascular space expanding the volume
Increased ADH	ADH tells the body to retain water in the vascular space
Medications	For example, steroids cause fluid retention
Liver disease	Excess production of aldosterone, which causes sodium and water retention
Hyperaldosteronism	Sodium and water retention in the vascular spaces
Burn treatment	After 24 hours postburn, the damaged vessels start to repair and hold fluid. Rapid hydration therapy can cause fluid overload. After 24 hours, fluid begins to shift from the interstitial space to the vascular space
Albumin infusion	Causes fluid retention (albumin/protein holds fluid into the vascular space)

Source: Created by author from Reference #1.

Signs and symptoms and why

Table 1-9 shows the signs and symptoms associated with FVE and why these occur.

Table 1-9

Signs and symptoms	Why
Jugular vein distension (JVD)	Vascular space is full, causes distension of jugular veins
Bounding pulse, tachycardia	Heart pumps hard and fast to keep the fluid moving forward
Abnormal breath sounds	Excess fluid collects in the lungs; lungs sound wet
Polyuria	Kidneys excrete the excess fluid
Decreased urine specific gravity	Kidneys are trying to get rid of excess fluid which causes urine to be diluted
Dyspnea and tachypnea	Excess fluid in the lungs impairs respiratory efforts
Increased BP	More vascular volume leads to increased blood pressure
Increased central venous pressure (CVP)	More vascular volume leads to increased central venous pressure
Edema	Vascular spaces leak fluid into the tissues
Productive cough	Fluid collects in the lungs causing a productive cough; the body is trying to rid of the excess fluid through mucous
Weight gain	Fluid retention causes weight gain

Source: Created by author from Reference #1.

Quickie tests and treatments

Tests:

- Serum Electrolytes: If the serum sodium is decreased this would mean there is too much free water in the vascular space. If the sodium is normal, this would mean sodium and water had been retained equally. All electrolytes are important to review with FVE, but the sodium in particular will help determine the cause of the FVE and the particular treatment that is needed.

- BUN and Creatinine: If these values are elevated it could mean the kidneys are not functioning properly and therefore not excreting fluid appropriately causing FVE.

- Chest x-ray: If the heart is enlarged, as can be seen with an x-ray, this could mean congestive heart failure.

Treatments:

- Loop diuretics: Furosemide (Lasix) may be used to pull fluid off the patient. Be sure and watch for Hypokalemia when administering this drug.

- Potassium-Sparing Diuretics: Spironolactone (Aldactone) will pull fluid off the patient, but not potassium as Lasix does. Be sure and watch for hyperkalemia with this drug.
- Dietary Sodium Restrictions: Sodium/salt causes fluid retention so the client must be careful to limit this in their diet.
- Treat the cause: As there are many different things that can cause FVE, the treatment must be individualized for the specific cause.

What can harm my client?

The major complications of FVE that can harm your client are CHF and pulmonary edema.

If I were your teacher, I would test you on . . .

If Aunt Marlene were giving the test, you would be asked questions about:

- The causes and their reasons for FVE.
- Signs and symptoms of FVE and explanations.
- Recognition and emergency treatment of pulmonary edema.
- Assessment and description of abnormal breath sounds.
- Medications and their side effects used to treat FVE.
- How FVE affects laboratory values.
- Concepts related to I & O and daily weights.
- IVF calculations.
- Safety, function, and maintenance of an IV pump.
- Proper, focused physical assessment specific for fluid volume excess.

✚ Sodium imbalances

The following apply to the electrolyte sodium:

- Chief electrolyte in ECF.
- Assists with generation and transmission of nerve impulses.
- An essential electrolyte of the sodium–potassium pump in the cell membrane.
- Food sources: bacon, ham, sausage, catsup, mustard, relishes, processed cheese, canned vegetables, bread, cereals, snack foods.
- Excess sodium is excreted by kidneys.
- Excretion of sodium retains potassium.
- Normal adult sodium level is 135 to 145 mEq/L.
- Helps maintain the volume of body fluids.

Renin–angiotensin system

ECF (vascular volume) decreased → Renin produced by kidneys → Angiotensin I converted to angiotensin II → Aldosterone secreted → Sodium and water retained.

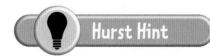

Hurst Hint

In fluid volume deficit and fluid volume excess, the osmolarity and serum sodium are not affected as the client loses fluid and sodium proportionately. To get a change in either one of these 2 things, the fluid level in the vascular space must either go up or down.

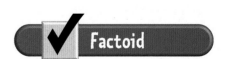

Factoid

Sodium is the only electrolyte that is affected by water. Sodium level decreases when there is too much water in the body. Conversely, sodium level increases with less water in the body.

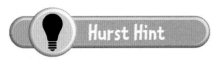

Hyponatremia: what is it?

Hyponatremia is serum sodium less than 135 mEq/L.[1]
Hyponatremia is:

* Not enough sodium in the ECF (vascular space).

* Possibly, there is too much water diluting the blood which makes serum sodium go down.

* Anytime there is a sodium problem there is a fluid problem as well.

What causes it and why

Table 1-10 shows the causes of hyponatremia and what is responsible for them.

Table 1-10

Causes	Why
Excessive administration of D5W	Water dilutes the sodium level
Diuretics	May cause excessive loss of sodium
Wound drainage	Loss of sodium
Psychogenic polydypsia	Excessive, rapid oral intake of fluids dilutes the blood
Decreased aldosterone	Sodium and water are excreted while potassium is retained
Low-sodium diet	Not enough sodium in the diet, which causes decreased blood levels of sodium
Syndrome of inappropriate antidiuretic hormone (SIADH)	Large amount of water is retained in the vascular space, causing dilution of blood; blood dilution causes decreased serum sodium because the sodium is measured in relation to the water in the blood
Vomiting and sweating	Loss of fluids and sodium (probably losing more sodium than water)
Replacing fluids with water only	Sodium is not replenished, leading to low blood levels

Source: Created by author from Reference #1.

Signs and symptoms and why

The signs and symptoms and rationales given in Table 1-11 are associated with hyponatremia.

Table 1-11

Signs and symptoms	Why
Lethargy and confusion	Decreased excitability of cell membranes; brain does not function well with low levels of sodium
Muscle weakness	Decreased excitability of cell membranes
Decreased deep tendon reflexes (DTRs)	Decreased excitability of cell membranes
Diarrhea	GI tract motility increases
Respiratory problems	Late symptom; respiratory muscles become weak and can't function properly

Source: Created by author from Reference #1.

Quickie tests and treatments

Tests:

- The main diagnostic test for hyponatremia is serum electrolytes (blood work); this is the quickest and simplest way to see what the serum sodium actually is.

Treatment: Depends on the cause

- When determining treatment you must know whether the serum sodium is low due to low intake or extreme loss of sodium alone OR is the hyponatremia due to excessive WATER in the vascular space which would dilute the serum sodium. Knowing this will effect the treatment.
- 0.9% normal saline IV (Normal Saline [0.9%] has sodium in the solution. This is a quick way to increase the serum sodium. More concentrated forms of IV sodium are available as well [3% Saline]. Be sure and watch for FVE with any of these solutions as this fluid will increase the volume of the vascular space).
- Increase Dietary Sodium (helps increase serum sodium).
- If appropriate, discontinue drugs/treatments that could be causing sodium loss.

What can harm my client?

Seizures and brain damage are the major complications associated with hyponatremia. Also, consider what *caused* the hyponatremia when determining what could harm your patient.

If I were your teacher, I would test you on . . .

Test questions would cover the following information:

- Causes of hyponatremia and their explanation.
- Hyponatremia signs and symptoms and the reasons for them.
- Seizure precautions and management.
- Neurological assessment.
- Food sources of sodium.
- Normal value of sodium.
- Assessment of deep tendon reflexes (DTRs). (Changes in DTR may indicate a neuro problem)
- Monitoring fluid balance.
- Treatment and care of the patient with hyponatremia.

Hypernatremia: what is it?

- Hypernatremia is serum sodium greater than 145 mEq/L.[1]
- Hypernatremia is similar to dehydration: there is too much sodium and not enough water in the body.

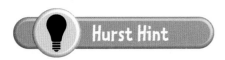
Hurst Hint

Anything that causes an increased "water" loss or excessive sodium intake can cause hypernatremia.

What causes it and why

Table 1-12 details the causes of hypernatremia.

Table 1-12

Causes	Why
Administration of IV normal saline without proper water replacement	Too much sodium, not enough water
Hyperventilation	Exhalation causes water loss, which causes sodium level to appear increased
Watery diarrhea	Fluid loss from the GI tract; water loss causes increased sodium concentration
Hyperaldosteronism	Retention of large amount of sodium
Renal failure	Kidneys not able to excrete excess sodium
Heat stroke	Water loss exceeds sodium loss causing increased sodium concentration in the blood
NPO status	Decreased intake causing hemoconcentration and increased sodium
Infection	Fever associated with infection causes loss of water and concentration of sodium
Diabetes insipidus	Excess water loss resulting in sodium concentration

Source: Created by author from Reference #1.

Signs and symptoms and why

The signs and symptoms and corresponding rationales for hypernatremia are listed in Table 1-13.

Table 1-13

Signs and symptoms	Why
Tachycardia	Heart is trying to pump what little fluid is left around the body to ensure adequate organ perfusion
Dry, sticky mucous membranes	Decreased saliva
Thirst	Brain sending signals that fluids are needed to dilute the sodium
Changes in level of consciousness (LOC)	Increased sodium interferes with brain function
Decreased heart contractility	Late hypernatremia causes decreased excitability of muscles; high serum sodium decreases the movement of calcium into the cardiac cells, causing decreased contraction and cardiac output
Seizure	Early hypernatremia causes increased muscle excitability
Muscle twitching	Early hypernatremia causes increased muscle excitability
Muscle weakness	Late hypernatremia causes decreased muscle response
Decreased DTRs	Late hypernatremia causes decreased muscle response

Source: Created by author from Reference #1.

Quickie tests and treatments

Tests:

* The quickest way to determine hypernatremia is serum electrolytes (blood work)

Treatment:

* When treatment is being determined, the cause of hypernatremia must be considered as the treatment is very individualized/specific depending on the cause.
* Diuretics may be used to pull of excess sodium. This can be tricky as the client could lose too much fluid/water as well which could make the serum sodium go even higher.
* Restrict all forms of sodium: Foods can have excess sodium as well as drugs and IV fluids.

What can harm my client?

As with hyponatremia, seizures and brain damage are the major complications associated with hypernatremia. Don't forget the complications associated with fluid problems as well.

If I were your teacher, I would test you on . . .

The key concepts of hypernatremia that are important to remember are:

* Causes and explanations for hypernatremia.
* Signs and symptoms of hypernatremia and the reasons behind them.
* Normal value of sodium.
* Food sources of sodium.
* Neurological assessment including DTRs.
* Safety precautions for patients with hypernatremia.
* Importance of recognizing signs and symptoms of cardiac output.
* Interventions and importance of reversing hypernatremia carefully and slowly.

✚ Potassium imbalances

The following are true regarding potassium:

* Makes skeletal and cardiac muscle work correctly.
* Major electrolyte in the intracellular fluid.
* Potassium and sodium are inversely related (when one is up, the other is down).
* Plays a vital role in the transmission of electrical impulses.
* Food sources: peaches, bananas, figs, dates, apricots, oranges, melons, raisins, prunes, broccoli, potatoes, meat, dairy products.
* Excreted by the kidneys.
* Stomach contains large amount of potassium.
* Normal potassium level: 3.5 mEq/L to 5.0 mEq/L.[1]

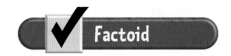

Factoid

In clients with hypo- or hypernatremia, think BRAIN first.

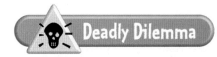

Deadly Dilemma

When the sodium level in the body increases or decreases rapidly, fatal complications can result. Rapid shifts in the serum sodium are dangerous!

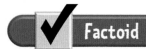

Factoid

Paralytic ileus can occur from severe hypokalemia. Abdominal distension will probably be next since there is no peristalsis.

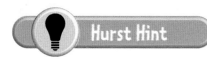

Hurst Hint

Remember, arrhythmias can lead to decreased cardiac output, resulting in hypotension.

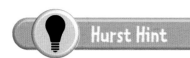

Hurst Hint

When we think about hypokalemia usually we think about muscle cramps first. However, don't forget the client can have muscle weakness too!

Hypokalemia: what is it?

Hypokalemia is a serum potassium below 3.5 mEq/L.[1]

What causes it and why

The causes of hypokalemia are shown in the Table 1-14.

Table 1-14

Causes	Why
Diuretics, thiazide diuretics	Potassium is excreted through urine
Steroids	Retains sodium and water and excretes potassium
GI suction	Removes potassium from the GI tract
Vomiting	Loss of potassium from the GI tract
Diarrhea	Loss of potassium from the GI tract
NPO status; poor oral intake	Not taking in enough potassium
Age	Kidneys lose potassium with age
Cushing syndrome	Sodium and water are retained, potassium is excreted
Kidney disease	Poor resorption of potassium
Alkalosis	Potassium moves into the cell dropping serum potassium
IV insulin	Drives potassium back into the cell dropping serum potassium

Source: Created by author from Reference #1.

Signs and symptoms and why

The signs and symptoms and corresponding rationales for hypokalemia are given in Table 1-15.

Table 1-15

Signs and symptoms	Why
Muscular weakness, cramps, flaccid paralysis	Potassium is needed for skeletal and smooth muscle contraction, nerve impulse conduction, acid–base balance, enzyme action, and cell membrane function
Hyporeflexia	Muscle cells require potassium for cell membrane excitability
Life–threatening arrhythmias	Heart cells require potassium for nerve impulse transmission and smooth muscle contraction
Slow or difficult respirations	Respiratory muscles are weakened
Weak, irregular pulse	Cardiac muscles are weakened
Decreased bowel sounds	Hypomotility of GI tract
EKG changes: ST segment depression; flat T-wave; inverted T-wave	Potassium needed for nerve impulse conduction
Decreased LOC	Potassium needed for excitability of brain cell membranes

Source: Created by author from References #1 and #3.

Quickie tests and treatments

Tests:

* The quickest way to determine hypokalemia is by looking at the serum electrolytes (blood work/blood chemistries) to determine if the serum K^+ is too low.
* EKG (shows flattened T wave, depressed ST segment, and a U-wave). The EKG will also be assessed for potentially life threatening arrhythmias such as Premature Ventricular Contractions (PVC's) and other ventricular arrhythmias such as ventricular tachycardia or ventricular fibrillation.

Treatments:

* The primary cause of hypokalemia must be determined so a specific treatment plan can be developed.
* High potassium diet (to replace K^+)
* IV or oral potassium chloride (increases serum K^+. When administering IV K^+ be sure and check for proper kidney function/good urine output. If the kidneys are not working well, then IV K^+ can cause a rapid increase in the serum K^+ which could lead to a life threatening arrhythmia). A good rule to remember when administering IV K^+ is not to exceed 20 mEq/hour. If the serum K^+ is increased too rapidly the heart could stop (cardiac arrest).

What can harm my client?

Hypokalemia can cause life-threatening arrhythmias, such as ventricular tachycardia, ventricular fibrillation, and asystole. Respiratory depression may also occur.

If I were your teacher, I would test you on . . .

Aunt Marlene would ask questions about:

* Causes of hypokalemia and the reasons behind them.
* Signs and symptoms of hypokalemia and the corresponding explanations.
* Recognition of life-threatening arrhythmias and emergency treatment.
* Food sources of potassium.
* Interventions to correct potassium imbalance.
* Special considerations when administering potassium medications.
* Focused physical assessment specific for hypokalemia.
* Recognition of a paralytic ileus.
* Monitoring the urine output associated with potassium chloride infusions.
* Care of the IV site associated with potassium chloride infusions.
* Precautions to take when administering IV-K^+

Hyperkalemia: what is it?

Hyperkalemia is serum potassium greater than 5.0 mEq/L.[1]

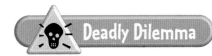

Deadly Dilemma

Clients taking a cardiac glycoside with a diuretic should be monitored closely for hypokalemia, which can potentiate the cardiac glycoside and cause toxicity.[3]

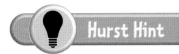

Hurst Hint

A client taking a diuretic may be switched to a potassium-sparing diuretic to prevent further urinary loss of potassium.[3]

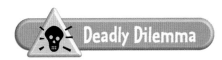

Deadly Dilemma

In severe hyperkalemia, ascending flaccid paralysis of the arms and legs may be seen; this paralysis moves distal to proximal.

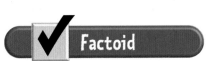

Factoid

Regarding potassium imbalances, the severity of the symptoms always depends on how fast the serum potassium is rising or falling.

What causes it and why

Table 1-16 details the causes and reasons behind them for hyperkalemia.

Table 1-16

Cause	Why
Renal failure	Kidneys aren't able to excrete potassium
IV potassium chloride overload	Too much potassium in the IV fluid
Burns or crushing injuries	Potassium is released when cells rupture
Tight tourniquets	Red blood cells rupture and release potassium when the tourniquet has been placed too tightly
Hemolysis of blood sample	Damaged cells in the sample result in a false high reading (damaged cells release potassium)
Incorrect blood draws	Drawing blood above on IV site where potassium is infusing will cause a false high reading
Salt substitutes	Usually made from potassium chloride
Potassium-sparing diuretics	Cause potassium retention
Blood transfusions	Deliver elevated levels of potassium in the transfused blood. Blood transfusions may have increased K^+ levels. As blood sits over a period of time, cells rupture and release K into blood that is going to be given to the patient
ACE inhibitors	Retain potassium
Tissue damage	Destroys cells releasing potassium into the bloodstream
Acidosis	Causes serum potassium to increase
Adrenal insufficiency (Addison's disease)	Causes sodium and water loss and potassium retention
Chemotherapy	Destroys cells releasing potassium into the bloodstream

Source: Created by author from Reference #1.

Signs and symptoms and why

Table 1-17 shows the signs and symptoms and associated rationales of hyperkalemia.

Table 1-17

Signs and symptoms	Why
Begins with muscle twitching associated with tingling and burning; progresses to numbness, especially around mouth; proceeds to weakness and flaccid paralysis	Excess potassium interferes with skeletal and smooth muscle contraction, nerve impulse conduction, acid–base balance, enzyme action, and cell membrane function
Diarrhea	Smooth muscles of the intestines hypercontract, resulting in increased motility
Cardiac arrhythmia; bradycardia; EKG changes: peaked T-wave, flat or no P-wave, wide QRS complex; ectopic beats on EKG leading to complete heart block, asystole, ventricular tachycardia, or ventricular fibrillation	Dysfunctional nerve impulse conduction and smooth muscle contraction

Source: Created by author from References #1 and #3.

Quickie tests and treatments

Tests:

- The quickest way to determine if hyperkalemia is present is to assess the serum electrolytes.
- The EKG will also be assessed to determine if any arrhythmias are present so they can be treated at once.

Treatments:

- The treatment depends on the primary cause.
- IV insulin in conjunction with 10–50% glucose IV (IV insulin will lower the serum K^+ by pushing it into the cell. However, insulin is going to lower the serum glucose the same way. This is why the glucose must be given with the insulin to prevent hypoglycemia)
- Administration of sodium polystyrene sulfonate (Kayexalate) with 70% sorbitol (Kayexalate, which can be given po or by enema) will decrease serum K^+ by causing excretion through the GI tract). When caring for a client receiving Kayexalate, be sure and watch their serum sodium as hypernatremia can occur. Kayexalate will decrease the serum K^+ and increase the serum sodium as these two electrolytes have an inverse relationship. You may have to increase the patient's water intake with this drug to offset hypernatremia/dehydration.
- Diuretics (to increase renal excretion of K^+).
- 10% calcium gluconate IV (to decrease myocardial irritability).
- Hemodialysis (if the kidneys are not working properly, which is a major cause of hyperkalemia, the serum K^+ will probably increase. Therefore, hemodialysis may be needed to perform the functions of the kidneys. Hemodialysis will wash the K^+ out of the blood until the serum K^+ is at the proper level. It will be needed as long as the kidneys are not functioning adequately).
- Peritoneal dialysis (a procedure where K^+ can be washed out of the blood).
- Limit high potassium foods.
- Limit drugs which could cause retention of K^+ (aldactone).

What can harm my client?

Be sure to monitor clients with hyperkalemia for dehydration, neurological changes, and life-threatening arrhythmias.

If I were your teacher, I would test you on . . .

Potential test items include:

- Causes of hyperkalemia and what's behind them.
- Signs and symptoms of hyperkalemia and the rationales.
- Recognition of life-threatening arrhythmias and emergency treatment.
- Cardiopulmonary resuscitation (CPR) techniques.
- Food sources of potassium.
- Medication management of hyperkalemia.
- Prevention and patient education of hyperkalemia.

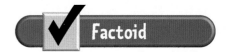

Factoid

Remember, anytime an arrhythmia occurs, cardiac output is affected, which decreases BP.

✚ Calcium imbalances

The following points pertain to calcium:

- Acts like a sedative on muscles.
- Most abundant electrolyte in the body.
- Has an inverse relationship to phosphorus.
- Necessary for nerve impulse transmission, blood clotting, muscle contraction, and relaxation.
- Needed for vitamin B_{12} absorption.
- Promotes strong bones and teeth.
- Who needs extra calcium? Children, pregnant women, lactating women.
- Food sources: milk, cheese, dried beans.
- Must have vitamin D present to utilize calcium.
- If blood levels of calcium decrease, the body takes calcium from the bones and teeth. (to build the blood level back up)
- Parathyroid hormone (PTH) increases serum calcium by pulling it from the bones and putting it in the blood.
- Calcitonin decreases serum calcium by driving the blood calcium back into the bones.
- Normal calcium: 9.0 to 10.5 mg/dL.[1]

Hypocalcemia: what is it?

Hypocalcemia occurs when the serum calcium level drops below 9.0 mg/dL.[1]

What causes it and why

Table 1-18 explores the causes and their explanations for hypocalcemia.

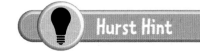

Hurst Hint

When calcium is decreased, think "not sedated."

Table 1-18

Cause	Why
Decreased calcium intake	Causes calcium levels in the blood to decrease
Kidney illness	Causes excessive calcium excretion
Decreased vitamin D	Vitamin D is needed to absorb and utilize calcium properly
Diarrhea	Increased excretion of calcium
Pancreatitis	Pancreatic cells retain calcium. Pancreatitis causes the pancreas to lose calcium
Hyperphosphatemia	Increased serum phosphorus causes decreased serum calcium
Thyroidectomy	If the parathyroids are accidentally removed during a thyroidectomy, PTH levels decrease. PTH causes an increase in serum calcium; without it, serum calcium will decrease
Medications (calcium binders)	Decrease serum calcium

Source: Created by author from Reference #1.

Signs and symptoms and why

The signs and symptoms and associated rationales for hypocalcemia are listed in Table 1-19.

Table 1-19

Signs and symptoms	Why
Muscle cramps	Inadequate calcium causes the muscles to contract
Tetany	Inadequate calcium causes the muscles to contract
Convulsions	Inadequate calcium causes impaired nerve transmissions and the muscles to contract
Arrhythmias	Impaired electrical impulses in the heart
Positive Chvostek's sign	Inadequate calcium causes hyper-excitability of the facial muscles
Positive Trousseau's sign	Inadequate calcium causes hyper-excitability of the hand muscles
Laryngeal spasm	Inadequate calcium causes contracture of the larynx
Hyperactive DTRs	Inadequate calcium causes improper nerve conduction, resulting in hyperactivity of the reflexes
Cardiac changes: decreased pulse, prolonged ST interval, prolonged QT interval, decreased myocardial contractility	Calcium regulates depolarization in the cardiac cells.If calcium is decreased, depolarization is impaired
Respiratory arrest	Respiratory muscles become rigid, decreasing airflow
LOC changes	Brain requires calcium to function
Increased gastric activity	Inadequate calcium causes hyperactivity

Source: Created by author from Reference #1.

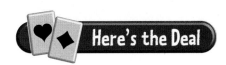

Here's the Deal

A positive Chvostek's sign occurs when the cheek over the facial nerve is tapped and the facial muscle twitches. A positive Trousseau's sign occurs when the BP cuff is pumped up and the hand begins to twitch and spasm.

Quickie tests and treatments

Tests:

* The quickest way to determine if the serum calcium is low is to assess the electrolytes.
* An EKG may be performed to determine if any arrhythmias are occurring due to calcium's effect on the heart.

Treatments:

* As usual, the specific treatment is totally dependent on the cause of the hypocalcemia.
* IV calcium (to increase serum calcium). Client MUST be on a heart monitor as this drug can cause the QRS complex to widen. You should

be SCARED if the QRS starts to widen because it can widen all the way out to a flat line (asystole)! I didn't have to go to nursing school to know a flat line is BAD!

- Vitamin D therapy (this vitamin helps the body utilize the calcium that is present).
- Increase dietary calcium (helps increase the serum calcium).

What can harm my client?

Seizures, laryngospasm, respiratory arrest, and arrhythmias are all conditions that must be closely monitored in your patients with hypocalcemia.

If I were your teacher, I would test you on . . .

Aunt Marlene would ask test questions on:

- Causes of hypocalcemia and the explanations for them.
- Signs and symptoms of hypocalcemia and their rationales.
- Seizure precautions and management.
- Laryngospasm and respiratory arrest precautions and management.
- Treatment of hypocalcemia including drug therapy.
- Proper diet for hypocalcemic clients.
- Normal values of serum calcium.
- Food sources of calcium.
- Precautions and techniques for IV administration of calcium.
- Be aware there are various forms of potential calcium salts (calcium gluconate, calcium chloride, calcium gluceptate).

Hypercalcemia: what is it?

Hypercalcemia is a serum calcium level that exceeds 10.5 mg/dL.[1]

What causes it and why

Table 1-20 explores the causes and their reasons for hypercalcemia.

Table 1-20

Cause	Why
Hyperparathyroidism	Excessive PTH that causes the serum calcium to increase
Immobilization	Calcium leaves the bones and moves into the bloodstream
Increased calcium intake	Increases serum calcium
Increased vitamin D intake	Increases serum calcium
Thiazide diuretics	Causes calcium retention
Kidney illness	Can cause retention of calcium

Source: Created by author from Reference #1.

Signs and symptoms and why

Table 1-21 looks at the signs and symptoms and corresponding rationales of hypercalcemia.

Hurst Hint

Excess calcium: think SEDATED.

Table 1-21

Signs and symptoms	Why
Decreased DTRs	Excess calcium causes a sedative effect and decreases deep tendon reflexes
Muscle weakness	Excess calcium causes a sedative effect and weakens muscles
Renal calculi	Excess calcium is trapped in the kidneys
Pathological fractures	Bones are brittle because calcium has moved from the bone into the blood
Central nervous system (CNS) depression: lethargy, coma, confusion	Excess calcium sedates the nervous system
Early cardiac changes: increased P-wave; decreased ST interval; wide T-wave; increased BP	Mild hypercalcemia increases cardiac activity
Late cardiac changes: decreased pulse moving to cardiac arrest	Severe hypercalcemia decreases cardiac activity
Respiratory arrest	Sedated respiratory muscles; decreased oxygenation
Decreased bowel sounds	Hypoperistalsis occurs because intestines are sedated
Increased urine output	Kidneys working to get rid of excess calcium, which depletes the vascular space
Increased clotting times	Excess calcium clots blood quickly
Kidney stones	Excess calcium promotes stone formation

Source: Created by author from Reference #1.

Quickie tests and treatments

Tests:

- The quickest way to determine if the serum calcium is too high is to assess the serum electrolytes.
- EKG (will be assessed to determine if the hypercalcemia is causing arrhythmias).
- X-ray (to assess for osteoporosis and other bone changes, urinary calculi (kidney stones).
- Urinalysis (to assess the level of calcium in the urine).

Treatment:

- Treatment is dependent on the initiating cause of hypercalcemia.
- Normal Saline IV (dilutes the blood which will decrease the concentration of calcium in the vascular space)

- IV phosphate (when phosphorus is given IV the serum phosphorus is going to go up. The higher the serum phosphorus goes, the lower the serum calcium will go as these two electrolytes have an inverse relationship)

What can harm my client?

The life-threatening complications of hypercalcemia are respiratory depression and arrhythmias.

If I were your teacher, I would test you on . . .

My test would include:

- Causes of hypercalcemia and their explanations.
- Signs and symptoms of hypercalcemia and the corresponding rationales.
- Interventions to reverse hypercalcemia.
- Medication therapy and related side effects.
- Teaching the client about weight-bearing exercises.
- Emergency interventions for arrhythmias and respiratory arrest.
- Focused physical assessment specific to hypercalcemia.
- Monitoring for deep vein thrombosis (DVT).
- Monitoring DTRs.
- Implications of decreased bowel sounds.
- Nursing interventions for kidney stone management.

✚ Phosphorus imbalances

Phosphorus:

- Promotes the function of muscle, red blood cells (RBCs), and the nervous system.
- Assists with carbohydrate, protein, and fat metabolism.
- Food sources: beef, pork, dried peas/beans, instant pudding.
- Has an inverse relationship with calcium.
- Regulated by the parathyroid hormone.
- Normal phosphorus is 3.0 to 4.5 mg/dL.[1]

Hypophosphatemia: what is it?

Hypophosphatemia is serum phosphate that is below 3.0 mg/dL.[1]

What causes it and why

This is easy. Just refer to the charts under hypercalcemia. **Hypophosphatemia** looks just like **hypercalcemia.**

Signs and symptoms and why

This is easy. Just refer to the charts under hypercalcemia. **Hypophosphatemia** looks just like **hypercalcemia.**

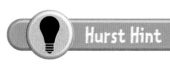

Hurst Hint

Remember that phosphorus and calcium have an inverse relationship!

Quickie tests and treatments

Tests:

- The quickest way to assess hypophosphatemia is to look at the serum electrolytes.
- X-ray (looking for skeletal changes; remember, if the phosphorus is low the serum calcium will be high; the calcium that is now in the blood came from the bone leaving the bones brittle and weak; may see osteomalacia or rickets).

Treatment:

- Supplemental Phosphorus (can be given po, or IV; may be added to tube feedings).
- IV phosphorus is given when phosphorus drips below 1 mg/dL and when the GI tract is functioning properly
- Additional treatments depend on the underlying cause.

What can harm my client?

The life-threatening complications of hypophosphatemia are respiratory depression and arrhythmias.

If I were your teacher, I would test you on . . .

- Causes of hypophosphatemia and the explanations for them.
- Signs and symptoms of hypophosphatemia and their rationale.
- Interventions to reverse hypophosphatemia.
- Medication therapy and related side effects.
- Emergency interventions for arrhythmias and respiratory arrest.
- Focused physical assessment specific to hypophosphatemia.
- Monitoring for DTRs.
- Implications of decreased bowel sounds.

Hyperphosphatemia: what is it?

Hyperphosphatemia is a serum phosphate level that is above 4.5 mg/dL.[1]

What causes it and why

The rest is easy! Just refer to the charts under hypocalcemia.
Hyperphosphatemia looks just like **hypocalcemia.**

Signs and symptoms and why

The rest is easy! Just refer to the charts under hypocalcemia.
Hyperphosphatemia looks just like **hypocalcemia.**

Quickie tests and treatments

The easiest way to determine if hyperphosatemia is present is to check their electrolyte levels.

Tests:

- X-ray (may be done to assess for any skeletal changes. May have an unusual amount of calcium being deposited into the bone. Remember, if the phosphorus level is high, the calcium level is low. The calcium is being pushed into the bone).

Treatment:

- The underlying cause of the hyperphosphatemia must be treated.
- Administration of vitamin D preparations such as calcitrol (rocaltrol): remember, the serum calcium will be low with this condition; vitamin D helps the body utilize whatever calcium is present.
- Administration of phosphate-binding gels (this drug will bind phosphorus and therefore lower the serum phosphorus level; however, this will also make the serum calcium go up).
- Restriction of dietary phosphorus (to help decrease serum phosphorus).
- Possibly dialysis (to remove the excess phosphorus).

What can harm my client?

The complications associated with hypocalcemia can harm your client. Seizures, laryngospasm, respiratory arrest, and arrhythmias are all conditions that must be closely monitored in your patients with hyperphosphatemia.

If I were your teacher, I would test you on . . .

Aunt Marlene would ask test questions on:

- Causes of hyperphosphatemia and why.
- Signs and symptoms of hyperphosphatemia and why.
- Seizure precautions and management.
- Laryngospasm and respiratory arrest precautions and management.
- Treatment of hyperphosphatemia including drug therapy.
- Proper diet for hyperphosphatemia client.
- Normal values of serum phosphorus.
- Precautions and techniques for IV administration of vitamin D preparations.

✚ Magnesium imbalances

Magnesium:

- Present in heart, bone, nerves, and muscle tissues.
- Second most important intracellular ion.
- Assists with metabolism of carbohydrates and proteins.
- Helps maintain electrical activity in nerves and muscle.
- Also acts like a sedative on muscle.
- Food sources: vegetables, nuts, fish, whole grains, peas, beans.

- Magnesium levels are controlled by the kidneys (excreted by kidneys).
- Normal magnesium: 1.3 to 2.1 mEq/L.[1]
- Can cause vasodilatation.

Hypomagnesemia: what is it?

Hypomagnesemia is a serum magnesium level below 1.3 mEq/L.[1]

What causes it and why

Table 1-22 explores the causes and background of hypomagnesemia.

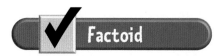

The majority of magnesium comes from our dietary intake.

Table 1-22

Cause	Why
Diarrhea	Intestines store large amounts of magnesium; diarrhea depletes these stores
Diuretics	Excretion of magnesium in urine
Decreased intake	Depletes magnesium stores and does not replenish them
Chronic alcoholism	Alcoholics are malnourished, which leads to decreased magnesium
Medications	Some drugs cause increased excretion of magnesium

Source: Created by author from Reference #1.

Signs and symptoms and why

Table 1-23 explores the signs and symptoms and related rationales of hypomagnesemia.

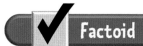

Decreased magnesium levels increase nerve impulses. Think: NOT SEDATED.

Table 1-23

Signs and symptoms	Why
Increased neuromuscular irritability	Decreased levels of magnesium can cause neuromuscular irritability
Seizure	Decreased levels of magnesium can cause neuromuscular hyperactivity
Hyperactive DTRs	Decreased levels of magnesium can cause neuromuscular hyperactivity
Laryngeal stridor	The larynx is smooth muscle; if there is not enough magnesium to sedate it, spasms will occur
Positive Chvostek's and Trousseau's signs	Decreased levels of magnesium can cause muscular spasms
Cardiac changes: arrhythmias; peaked T-waves; depressed ST segment; ventricular tachycardia; ventricular fibrillation; irregular heartbeat	The heart is a smooth muscle. If there is not enough magnesium to sedate it, impaired nerve conduction and muscle spasms can occur

(Continued)

Table 1-23. (*Continued*)

Signs and symptoms	Why
Dysphagia	The esophagus is a smooth muscle; if there is not enough magnesium to sedate it, muscle tightness will occur
Hypertension	Decreased magnesium causes vasoconstriction; constriction makes BP go up
Decreased GI motility	GI muscles contract stalling peristalsis; paralytic ileus may occur
Changes in LOC	Confusion or psychosis may be caused by central nervous system excitability due to decreased magnesium

Source: Created by author from Reference #1.

Quickie tests and treatments

The simplest way to determine if someone's magnesium level is too low is to assess the serum electrolytes.

Tests:

- Urinalysis (to assess the magnesium level in the urine; remember, magnesium is excreted through the kidneys)
- EKG (as magnesium can have an effect on the heart, the EKG will be assessed to determine if any arrhythmias are occurring).
- New diagnostic tests include nuclear magnetic resonance spectroscopy and ion-selective electrode tests which can measure ionized serum magnesium levels very accurately.

Treatment:

- As always, the underlying cause must be identified and treated.
- Increased dietary magnesium (will help increase the serum magnesium level)
- Magnesium salts (will help increase the serum magnesium levels)
- Magnesium sulfate IV (to increase the Mg levels. Make sure the kidneys are working because a lot of magnesium is excreted through the kidneys. Don't forget magnesium acts like a central nervous system depressant (sedative) so watch those respirations and the deep tendon reflexes [DTR's will depress prior to the respirations so assess these frequently])

What can harm my client?

Be sure to monitor your clients for the following life-threatening complications of hypomagnesemia:

- Laryngospasm.
- Aspiration due to dysphagia.
- Arrhythmias.

If I were your teacher, I would test you on . . .

Possible testing material includes:

- Causes of hypomagnesemia and details on them.
- Signs and symptoms and background for hypomagnesemia.
- Emergency management of arrhythmias and laryngospasm.
- Monitoring swallowing mechanism to prevent aspiration.
- Medications used to reverse hypomagnesemia.
- Importance of monitoring bowel sounds.
- Safety precautions for clients experiencing LOC changes.

Hypermagnesemia: what is it?

Hypermagnesemia is a serum magnesium level above 2.1 mEq/L.[1]

What causes it and why

Table 1-24 explores the causes of hypermagnesemia.

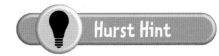

Remember magnesium acts like a sedative. "THINK SEDATED" with hypermagnesemia.

Table 1-24

Cause	Why
Renal failure	Kidneys are unable to excrete magnesium
Increased oral or IV intake	Body cannot process excessive magnesium
Antacids	Many antacids contain a large amount of magnesium, which can build up in the blood, making it difficult for the kidneys to excrete the excess in a timely manner

Source: Created by author from Reference #1.

Signs and symptoms and why

Table 1-25 explores the signs and symptoms and rationales associated with hypermagnesemia.

Table 1-25

Signs and symptoms	Why
BP decreases	Magnesium causes vasodilation, which decreases BP
Facial warmth and flushing	Excess magnesium dilates the capillary beds
Drowsiness to comatose state depending on severity of imbalance	Excess magnesium acts like a sedative
Decreased DTRs	Excess magnesium reduces electrical conduction in the muscles, making them sluggish
Generalized weakness	Excess magnesium reduces electrical conduction in the muscles, making them sluggish
Decreased respirations to respiratory arrest depending on severity of imbalance	Hypoactive respiratory muscles
Cardiac changes: decreased pulse, prolonged PR, wide QRS, cardiac arrest	Central nervous depression and smooth muscle relaxation

Source: Created by author from Reference #1.

Quickie tests and treatments

Check the serum electrolytes to determine how high the serum magnesium level is.

Tests:

- EKG: As magnesium can have a significant effect on the heart the EKG will be assessed to determine if any arrhythmias are present.

Treatments:

- Specific treatment always depends on the primary cause of the hypermagnesemia.
- Decrease magnesium salt administration especially in clients with renal failure (to prevent the magnesium level from going any higher; hopefully this will help the serum magnesium level to drop into a normal range)
- If in an emergency situation, respiratory support may be needed as excess magnesium can suppress the respirations.
- Hemodialysis with magnesium free dialysate (since a kidney problem may be present, hemodialysis may be needed to help decrease the serum magnesium).
- Loop diuretics (to help the body excrete the excess magnesium [assuming the kidneys are working properly]).
- 0.45% saline solution and/or IV calcium gluconate to help balance the magnesium levels.

What can harm my client?

The major complications associated with hypermagnesemia are respiratory arrest, cardiac arrest, and hypotension.

If I were your teacher, I would test you on . . .

My test on hypermagnesemia would cover:

- Causes of hypermagnesemia and why?
- Signs and symptoms of hypermagnesemia and why?
- Management of respiratory arrest.
- Management of cardiac arrest.
- Management of hypotension.
- Interventions to reverse hypermagnesemia.
- Importance of monitoring vital signs.

SUMMARY

A client's condition can change rapidly if she develops a fluid and electrolyte imbalance. You must be able to recognize signs and symptoms of fluid and electrolyte imbalances, prevent possible complications due to these imbalances, evaluate lab work critically, and implement appropriate nursing interventions. If you would like to hear Aunt Marlene discuss fluids and electrolytes, call her office e 601-833-1961 and order her CDs. You'll love F and E . . . believe it or not and your med-surg scores will soar! ☺

PRACTICE QUESTIONS

1. The client at the highest risk for fluid volume deficit is a:

  1. 36-year-old client with the flu.

  2. 4-month-old client with diarrhea.

  3. Healthy 80-year-old client with a fractured wrist.

  4. 26-year-old pregnant client with nausea and vomiting.

  Correct answer: 2. The adult clients in answer choices 1, 3, and 4 can communicate their needs and independently replace their fluids. A baby cannot communicate his needs, such as thirst, or independently replace his fluids. Also, the younger and older populations are always more prone to dehydration.

2. A 32-year-old client has a nursing diagnosis of fluid volume excess (FVE). A nurse examining the client would expect to find:

  1. Postural hypotension.

  2. Cool extremities.

  3. Moist mucous membranes.

  4. Weak, rapid pulse.

  Correct answer: 3. Postural hypotension, cool extremities, and a weak, rapid pulse are all signs of fluid volume deficit (FVD). Moist mucous membranes are the only sign and symptom listed consistent with fluid volume excess.

3. A client presents to the emergency department (ED) with tachycardia, elevated blood pressure, and seizures. Further assessment reveals a history of chronic alcoholism, causing the nurse to suspect:

  1. Magnesium deficit.

  2. Sodium deficit.

  3. Potassium excess.

  4. Calcium excess.

  Correct answer: 1. Alcoholics tend to have hypomagnesemia as their primary electrolyte imbalance due to a poor dietary intake. A sodium deficit can cause seizures, but the other symptoms are not consistent with hyponatremia. The symptoms in the question are not consistent with hyperkalemia. Hypercalcemia weakens muscles, and therefore would not cause seizures.

4. A client's calcium level is 8.8 mg /dL. An appropriate nursing intervention is:

  1. Notify the physician immediately.

  2. Administer oral calcium supplements as ordered.

  3. Limit intake of foods rich in calcium.

  4. No intervention required at this time.

Correct answer: 4. A normal calcium level is 8.8 mg/dL, so no intervention is needed at this time. There is no need to notify the physician, as this is not a critical value. Calcium supplements are administered in hypocalcemia. High-calcium foods are limited in hypercalcemia.

5. The nurse expects the client with hypophosphatemia to also experience:

    1. Hyperalbuminemia.

    2. Hypercalcemia.

    3. Hypernatremia.

    4. Hyperkalemia.

    Correct answer: 2. Phosphorus has an inverse relationship with calcium. If the phosphorus level is low, the calcium level is high. Sodium and potassium do not have a significant relationship with phosphorus. Hyperalbuminia is not an electrolyte state and is an inappropriate answer.

6. Why does excessive administration of D5W cause hyponatremia?

    1. The kidneys excrete the excess potassium.

    2. The lungs exhale the excess vapor.

    3. Water in the solution dilutes the serum sodium level.

    4. Dextrose is the solution concentrates the sodium level.

    Correct answer: 3. Excessive administration of D5W causes the water in the solution to dilute the sodium level, causing hyponatremia. The remaining answer selections are inappropriate.

7. When reviewing a client's laboratory results, the nurse recognizes which is a normal value for potassium?

    1. 4.3 mEq/L

    2. 2.8 mEq/L

    3. 8.7 mEq/L

    4. 6.5 mEq/L

    Correct answer: 1. The normal value for potassium is 3.5 to 5.0 mEq/L.

8. A client presents to the emergency department (ED) with chest pain after completing an hour of vigorous exercise. The nurse knows he should expect which laboratory result?

    1. Decreased hematocrit.

    2. Increased osmolality.

    3. Decreased urine specific gravity.

    4. Increased hemoglobin.

Correct answer: 2. The client is most likely dehydrated from excessive exercise. The chest pain can cause hypoxemia. Dehydration concentrates the blood. Concentration makes the lab values increase. Therefore, the hematocrit and urine specific gravity increase. The hemoglobin decreases since the client experiences chest pain causing the hypoxemia. Osmolality increases in the presence of dehydration.

9. The nurse knows that when caring for the client on a telemetry unit, an elevated U-wave seen on an EKG is specific to which electrolyte imbalance?

   1. Hypomagnesemia.

   2. Hypermagnesemia.

   3. Hyperkalemia.

   4. Hypokalemia.

   Correct answer: 4. Hypokalemia is the only electrolyte imbalance that could possibly cause a U-wave on an EKG.

10. A client is being discharged from the hospital after being treated for a decreased potassium level. In order for the client to maintain an appropriate potassium level, the nurse suggests which food when providing discharge teaching?

   1. Baked potatoes.

   2. Peas.

   3. Fowl.

   4. Nuts.

   Correct answer: 1. Of the foods listed, baked potatoes are highest in potassium.

References

1. Hurst M. *Finally Understanding Fluids and Electrolytes* [audio CD-ROM]. Ambler, PA: Lippincott Williams & Wilkins; 2004.

2. Chernecky C. *Real-World Nursing Survival Guide: Fluids and Electrolytes.* Philadelphia: Saunders; 2002.

3. Allen KD, Boucher MA, Cain JE, et al. *Manual of Nursing Practice Pocket Guides: Medical-Surgical Nursing.* Ambler, PA: Lippincott Williams & Wilkins; 2007.

Bibliography

Hurst Review Services. www.hurstreview.com.

Kee JL, Paulanka BJ. *Fluids and Electrolytes with Clinical Applications: A Programmed Approach.* 6th ed. Albany, NY: Delmar Publishers; 2000.

Springhouse Editors. *Nurse's Quick Check: Fluids and Electrolytes.* Ambler, PA: Lippincott Williams & Wilkins; 2005.

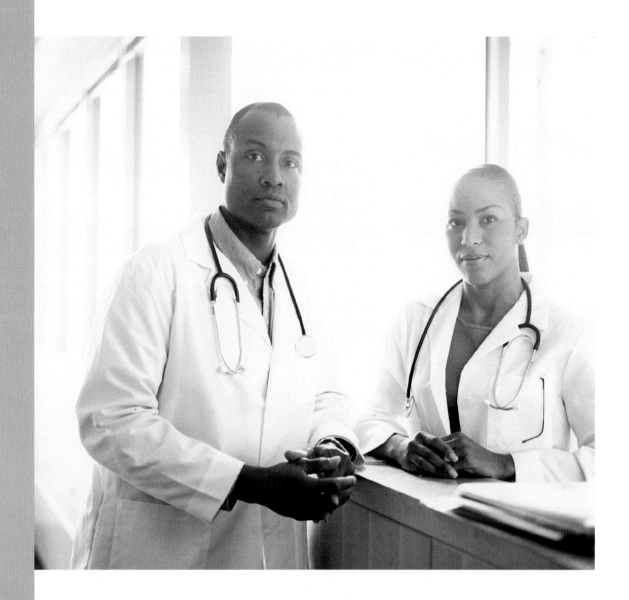

2 Acid–Base Balance

OBJECTIVES

In this chapter, you'll review:

- The key basics of acid–base imbalance.
- Specific causes, signs and symptoms, and rationales of respiratory acidosis and alkalosis and metabolic acidosis and alkalosis.
- Diagnostic tests, treatments, and possible complications of respiratory acidosis and alkalosis and metabolic acidosis and alkalosis.

LET'S GET THE NORMAL STUFF STRAIGHT FIRST

Like fluids and electrolytes, acid–base balance is very important to your nursing practice because many diseases and disorders include a malfunction of acid–base homeostasis. For example: Postop clients can easily develop respiratory acidosis; a hysterical patient may develop respiratory alkalosis; a client with diabetes can develop metabolic acidosis; and a pregnant patient may develop metabolic alkalosis from excessive vomiting. As you can see, nurses of all specialties need to understand acid–base balance. So let's get it started in here!

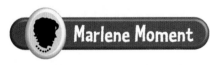

Factoid

When a "P" appears in front of CO_2 or O_2, this means the blood was drawn from an artery (see Fig. 2-1). "P" means partial pressure. Sometimes you will see it written as PaO_2 or $PaCO_2$.

▶ Figure 2-1. Blood gases test.

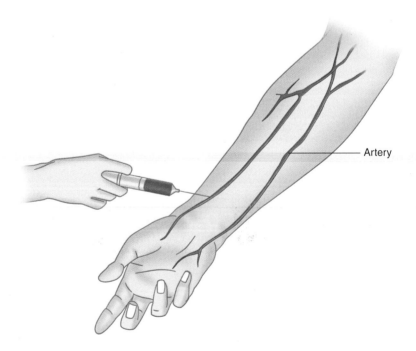

Artery

Marlene Moment

Arterial blood gases are drawn from an artery (duh!) and this hurts!

✚ Let's start with the basics

Normal arterial blood gases (ABGs) look as shown in Table 2-1:

Table 2-1

Normal ABGs		
pH	Hydrogen ion concentration	7.35–7.45
PCO_2	Partial pressure of carbon dioxide	35–45 mm Hg
PO_2	Partial pressure of oxygen	80–100 mm Hg
HCO_3^-	Bicarbonate	22–26 mEq/L

Source: Created by author from Reference #1.

Quiz time

Before we get too much into this, I am going to ask you some basic questions. Ready?

1. Q: What makes an acid an acid?

   A: The hydrogen ion (H^+).

2. Q: What makes a base a base?

   A: The bicarbonate ion (HCO_3^-).

3. Q: If many hydrogen ions (H^+) are present in a liquid, is this liquid an acid or a base?

   A: An acid.

4. Q: What happens to the pH of this liquid?

   A: The pH decreases. The more acidic a solution, the lower the pH.

5. Q: Does this liquid, if infused into a client, make the client acidic (acidotic) or basic (alkalotic)?

   A: Acidotic, because hydrogen ions are acidic.

6. Q: If a lot of base is in a liquid, is this liquid acidic or basic?

   A: You know the answer is basic!

7. Q: What happens to the pH of this liquid?

   A: The pH increases because the more basic (alkaline) a solution, the higher the pH.

8. Q: If this liquid is infused into a client, does the client become acidotic or alkalotic?

   A: Alkalotic, because the client has high levels of bicarbonate (a base) in the blood.

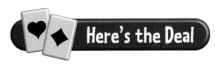 **Here's the Deal**

The major lung chemical is carbon dioxide (CO_2)—an acid. The major kidney chemicals are bicarbonate (HCO_3^-) and hydrogen (H^+).

AN OVERVIEW OF ACID–BASE IMBALANCES

We are now going to quickly review the general acid–base imbalances that can occur and their affect on homeostasis. Let's first look at carbon dioxide (CO_2). Here we go!

Ok, I have another question for you: Is carbon dioxide an acid or a base? It's an acid! Always think of carbon dioxide as an acid because the minute carbon dioxide gets inside the body it mixes with water and turns into carbonic acid. This is why you always have to think of carbon dioxide as an acid. We get rid of carbon dioxide by one way only . . . exhaling.

When there is a lot of carbon dioxide buildup in the body, the client becomes acidotic because carbon dioxide is what? Yes, an acid!

- If carbon dioxide is retained in the body, which organs are not working correctly? Remember, carbon dioxide can only be excreted by the lungs. So, if carbon dioxide is building up in the body, then the lungs are not doing their job of excreting the carbon dioxide.

- If a client is in respiratory acidosis or alkalosis, is the problem with the lungs or the kidneys? The lungs! **Think: respiratory equals lungs!**

- If the lungs are sick, which organ is going to compensate for malfunctioning lungs? The kidneys! If the lungs cannot get rid of the excess carbon dioxide, then the kidneys are going to go to work to try to correct the problem. The kidneys goal right now is to get the pH back into normal range. The kidneys use bicarbonate (base) and hydrogen (acid) in an effort to correct the pH. In this instance, when there is too much CO_2 (acid), the kidneys will kick in and secrete bicarbonate into the blood and excrete hydrogen out of the body.

- **If the lungs are getting rid of <u>too much</u> CO_2 (acid), as with hyperventilation, then the** patient will become alkalotic. Now, the pH is out of range so the kidneys will try to correct it with the same two chemicals, bicarb and hydrogen. Since the kidneys are trying to correct alkalosis, they will **excrete** bicarb from the body and **retain** hydrogen.

- If a client is in metabolic acidosis or alkalosis, is the problem with the lungs or the kidneys? The kidneys! **Think: metabolic equals kidneys!**

- Do the kidneys compensate slowly or quickly? The kidneys are very slow in their compensation, but they are much more efficient than the lungs. It can take the kidneys anywhere from 24 hours to 3 days to start their compensation duties.

- If the kidneys are sick, which organ/organs are going to compensate for the malfunctioning kidneys? The lungs! The lungs are going to compensate by either blowing off the excess carbon dioxide (by increasing respirations) or retaining carbon dioxide (by slowing respirations). How the respiration will change, depends on whether the client is experiencing metabolic acidosis or alkalosis.

- Do the lungs (Fig. 2-2) compensate slowly or quickly? Quickly.

REST AND RECAP TIME   Now's a good time to take a little rest and recap what we've covered thus far.

- Hydrogen is an acid. Bicarbonate is a base.

- The more acidic the blood, the lower the pH.

- The more basic (alkaline) the blood, the higher the pH.

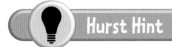

The kidneys are slow to compensate, but when they do . . . they do a good job!

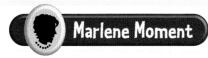

Later, I don't want to hear you say, "The kidneys are going to blow off carbon dioxide!" Hello? Kidneys cannot blow off anything . . . only the lungs can exhale. Whatever!

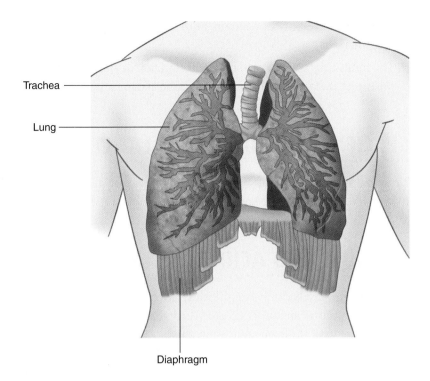

◀ Figure 2-2. Lungs.

Trachea

Lung

Diaphragm

✚ Respiratory acidosis and alkalosis overview

● The lungs have one chemical: carbon dioxide.

● In an acid–base imbalance such as respiratory acidosis or alkalosis, the lungs are sick. That is why the name "respiratory" is included in the name of the disorder.

● Anytime the lungs are sick and are causing respiratory acidosis or respiratory alkalosis, the problem is due to carbon dioxide.

● To correct a respiratory imbalance, the **compensating organs** are the kidneys, because the lungs can't compensate for themselves if they are sick.

● When the lungs are sick, the kidneys compensate by manipulating the chemicals bicarbonate and hydrogen to correct the imbalance and bring the pH back into normal range again. This is done by secreting bicarbonate and excreting hydrogen.

● The kidneys are slow but effective in compensating for respiratory acidosis or respiratory alkalosis.

✚ Metabolic acidosis and alkalosis overview

● The problem ORGANS in metabolic acidosis and metabolic alkalosis are the kidneys. Bicarbonate and hydrogen are considered the **problem chemicals** when the kidneys are sick.

● Since the kidneys are sick, they aren't able to maintain homeostasis/normal pH. A different organ must come into play here.

● In metabolic acidosis or metabolic alkalosis the **compensating organs** are the lungs.

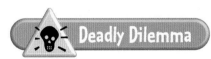

Deadly Dilemma

The brain likes to the body pH to be perfect all the time. When the pH gets out of whack, neuro and level of consciousness (LOC) changes can occur. This is why with **any** acid–base imbalance you must monitor the client's LOC.

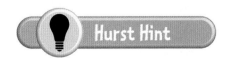

Hurst Hint

All diseases, disorders, and imbalances vary in degree from client to client.

- The lungs have only one chemical to work with: the acid, carbon dioxide (CO_2).
- The lungs can blow off or retain Carbon Dioxide **quickly** when working to correct metabolic acidosis or metabolic alkalosis.

SPECIFIC ACID–BASE IMBALANCES

Now that we understand the general principles associated with acid–base imbalance let's look at the specific disorders in detail.

CALCIUM AND ACID–BASE IMBALANCES

Blood calcium levels can be significantly affected by acid base imbalances. Let's looks at how calcium is affected during acidosis and alkalosis.

There are two kinds of calcium in the blood; Calcium that is bound to a plasma protein and calcium that is not bound to plasma protein. When calcium is **bound**, it might as well be invisible/absent/not present/doesn't count. It's the unbound calcium that can have an effect on our body.

Unbound calcium is "active". Bound calcium is "inactive".

Note: Hydrogen ions will not let calcium bind to plasma proteins. The more H^+ ions that are present, more free/unbound calcium will be present as well.

Acidosis: If the blood is acidotic there must be a lot of hydrogen (acid) too. The more acid the blood, the more unbound calcium is present. Therefore, acidosis makes serum calcium go up! Remember, calcium acts like a sedative on all muscles of the body.

Alkalosis: Alkalosis causes calcium to bind with plasma proteins. Therefore, alkalosis causes serum calcium to go down! Since, calcium (sedative) is low, the muscles will not be relaxed; instead, the muscles will be tight and begin to twitch.

✚ Respiratory acidosis

What is it?

Respiratory acidosis is an acid–base imbalance that occurs when the pH is decreased—below 7.35—and the partial pressure of carbon dioxide (PCO_2) is increased—greater than 45 mm Hg. (Note: Anytime you see the words partial pressure you are to know we are talking about arterial blood.) Carbon dioxide builds up in the blood because the client has some disorder, which causes the client to hypoventilate and retain carbon dioxide. Since the client retains this acid, this causes the pH to go down. This imbalance can be acute, as in sudden cessation of breathing, or chronic, such as in lung disease.[1–3]

DEFINE TIME   Hypercapnia is a buildup of carbon dioxide in the blood to levels greater than 45 mm Hg.[1]

Hurst Hint

The only way carbon dioxide can build up in the blood is by a significant decrease in respiration. If breathing slows down, then the acid carbon dioxide is not exhaled effectively and it builds up in the blood, causing acidosis.

Marlene Moment

You are going to work with some health care workers who believe every client should have a PRN sleeping pill at bedtime. Beware, not every client can handle these types of drugs as the respiratory rate can decrease significantly in some patients!

What causes it and why

The first thing to think of when trying to figure out causes of respiratory acidosis is "breathing." Respiratory acidosis always begins with a breathing problem. Something causes decreased alveolar ventilation, which in turn causes carbon dioxide retention (Table 2-2).

Table 2-2

Causes	Why
Respiratory arrest	Not exhaling CO_2
Some drugs (narcotics, sedatives, hypnotics, anesthesia, ecstasy)	Suppresses respirations, causing retention of CO_2
Sleep apnea	Suppresses respirations, causing retention of CO_2
Excessive alcohol	Suppresses respirations, causing retention of CO_2
Surgical incisions (especially abdominal), broken ribs	Pain with deep breathing, causing retention of CO_2
Collapsed lung (pneumothorax, hemothorax)	Unable to blow off excess CO_2, causing a buildup in the blood
Weak respiratory muscles (myasthenia gravis, Guillain–Barré syndrome)	Poor respiratory exchange, causing buildup of CO_2
Airway obstruction (poor cough mechanism, laryngeal spasm)	Poor respiratory exchange, causing buildup of CO_2
Brain trauma (specifically medulla)	Decreased respiratory rate
High-flow O_2 in chronic lung disease	Decreases client's drive to breathe; hypoxia
Severe respiratory distress syndrome	Decreased blood flow to the lungs and decreased gas exchange results in CO_2 retention

Source: Created by author from Reference #3.

Signs and symptoms and why

Remember, the signs and symptoms of respiratory acidosis will vary depending on the initial cause (Table 2-3).

Table 2-3

Signs and symptoms	Why
Neurological changes: headache, confusion, blurred vision, lethargy, coma, decreased deep tendon reflexes (DTRs)	Excess acid causes brain vessels to vasodilate, leading to brain swelling and increased intracranial pressure (ICP); CO_2 can cross the blood–brain barrier, causing changes in pH
Papilledema	Increased ICP

(Continued)

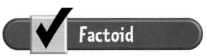

Anytime poor gas exchange exists, CO_2 builds up in the blood. Respiratory acidosis will likely occur.

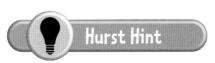

Many diseases and illnesses result in poor gas exchange: chronic obstructive pulmonary disease (COPD), emphysema, bronchitis, pneumonia, asthma, increased mucous, pulmonary edema, and pulmonary embolism. The list can go on forever.

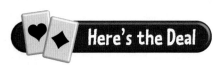

Here's the Deal

When a client has a <u>chronic</u> lung problem, her drive to breathe will no longer be hypercapnia, but will be hypoxia. As long as the client is hypoxic, she will breathe spontaneously. If a lot of oxygen is administered, the client isn't hypoxic anymore, causing her to STOP breathing.

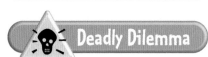

Deadly Dilemma

In respiratory acidosis the client is breathing too slowly, too shallow, or not breathing at all. In all 3 situations, the client is retaining CO_2. Think hypoventilation first!

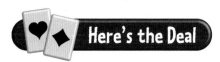

Here's the Deal

Just because compensation occurs in respiratory acidosis does not mean the primary cause is being corrected. The problem that caused respiratory acidosis must be corrected simultaneously with the acidosis.

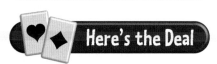

Here's the Deal

When respiratory acidosis occurs suddenly, hypertension is seen first due to hypercapnia then progressing to hypotension as it worsens.

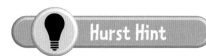

Hurst Hint

Hypoxia may be the first sign of respiratory acidosis. The early signs of hypoxia are restlessness and tachycardia. Early hypoxia: restlessness, tachycardia.

Table 2-3. (*Continued*)

Signs and symptoms	Why
Hyperkalemia	Acidosis causes K^+ to increase in the blood. To compensate for the respiratory acidosis, H^+ (acid) moves out of the blood into the cell where K^+ is now living. Now the blood is less acid. However, K^+ does not want to live with H^+ inside the cell, so K^+ moves into the bloodstream causing the serum K^+ to go up
Decreased muscle tone; decreased DTRs	Increased H^+ levels and hyperkalemia and hypercalcemia
Hypotension	Vasodilation with severe respiratory acidosis
Restlessness; tachycardia	Increased CO_2 level leads to decreased O_2 level (hypoxia)
Arrhythmias	Hyperkalemia, hypoxia
Cardiac arrest	As the acidosis worsens, the electricity in the heart slows, causing bradycardia and cardiac arrest
Acidic urine	Kidney compensation has begun (kidneys excreting hydrogen)
Warm skin	Vasodilation

Source: Created by author from Reference #3.

Quickie tests and treatments

Tests and treatments vary. They depend on the patient and/or the problem.

- Treat the cause.
- Airway clearance: possible intubation.
- Mechanical ventilation with PEEP.
- Goal is to have the client blow off the excess CO_2.
- Administer drugs to open up the airways and thin out secretions so they can be coughed up.
- Increase fluids to liquefy secretions so they can be coughed up more easily.
- Oxygen therapy.
- Respiratory therapy: breathing treatments.
- Elevate head of bed (HOB) for lung expansion.
- Monitor ABGs.
- Monitor for electrolyte imbalances.
- Monitor pulse oximetry.
- Administration of Pulmocare: a tube feeding sometimes used to decrease CO_2 retention.[3]

DEFINE TIME   PEEP stands for positive end-expiratory pressure, a setting on a mechanical ventilator. On end expiration, the mechanical ventilator exerts pressure down into the lungs to keep the alveoli from collapsing. Therefore, gas exchange is improved.

MORE ON OXYGEN THERAPY   Administer low-dose oxygen to clients with chronic lung conditions and high doses to those with acute conditions even if they have chronic lung disease. You are confused by this, aren't you? The rule is to give low-flow oxygen to clients with chronic lung disease. Why? As long as they are a little hypoxic, they will continue to breathe. We want our patients to breathe! If you give a chronic lunger too much O_2 they will no longer be hypoxic. You will have taken away their drive to breathe (hypoxia) so they stop! Give high-flow oxygen to chronic lung patients in an acute situation like respiratory arrest. Why? They have stopped breathing and need 100% oxygen STAT. If the chronic lunger has already stopped breathing then we no longer have to worry about what we just talked about until they breathe again.

What do the ABGs look like?

In respiratory acidosis, the ABGs look as shown in Table 2-4.

Table 2-4

ABGs in respiratory acidosis	
pH	Less than 7.35 (acidosis makes pH go down)
PCO_2	Greater than 45 mm Hg (CO_2 is being exhaled properly so it builds up in blood)
PO_2	Less than 80 mm Hg (when CO_2 is up, O_2 is down)
HCO_3^-	Normal until kidney compensation starts; then will start to rise above 26 mEq/L

Source: Created by author from References #1 and #3.

What can harm my client?

Respiratory acidosis is brought on by different things. What can harm your client is dependent on the initial cause of the imbalance. So don't forget to focus on the initial problem.

- Respiratory arrest.
- Arrhythmias: leading to cardiac arrest and shock.
- Severe decrease in LOC.

If I were your teacher, I would test you on . . .

- Causes of respiratory acidosis and why.
- Signs and symptoms of respiratory acidosis and why.
- Function and safety regarding mechanical ventilation.
- ABG draws and values.
- Focused cardiopulmonary assessment.
- Prevention and care of electrolyte imbalances.

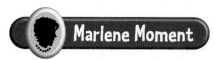

When caring for a restless client who is worrying you to death by wrapping her IV tubing around her head and climbing out of bed, don't say, "I'm gonna see what the doc has ordered to calm her down!" Think about hypoxia first!

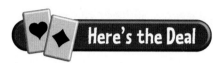

Hypoxia causes the heart rate to increase to pump what little oxygen is left to the vital organs. Bradycardia occurs because the heart is not receiving enough oxygen. Late hypoxia: cyanosis, bradycardia.

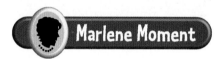

I didn't have to go to nursing school to figure out something is wrong when Paw-Paw turns purple. Identify hypoxia early before it goes too far!

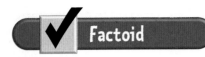
Factoid

Acute respiratory acidosis causes hyperkalemia. With chronic respiratory acidosis, the K^+ may be normal as the kidneys have time to readjust and get the K^+ back into the normal range.

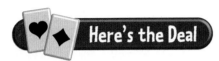
Here's the Deal

Anytime a client is on PEEP, your primary nursing assessment is to listen for bilateral breath sounds. Why? Because the pressure exerted from the mechanical ventilator can pop a lung!

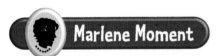
Marlene Moment

A popped lung is not a good thing!

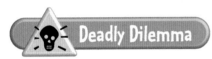
Deadly Dilemma

If the PO_2 is not brought back up to at least 60 mm Hg, cardiac arrest could occur.[3]

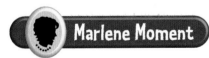
Marlene Moment

Maybe you are hysterical over a test for which you are studying. When you are hysterical you breathe rapidly and blow off CO_2. Be careful, you may throw yourself into respiratory alkalosis!

- Oxygen therapy, equipment, and safety.
- Compensation mechanisms.

Table 2-5 shows a recap of Respiratory Acidosis.

Table 2-5

Recap of respiratory acidosis
The name "respiratory" tips you off to the fact that a lung problem exists
Since it is a lung problem, the problem chemical is the acid carbon dioxide (CO_2)
Acidosis from a lung problem is due to irregular breathing. Perhaps the client is hypoventilating—breathing only 2 to 4 times a minute, causing retention of carbon dioxide (CO_2). Maybe the client has stopped breathing altogether—possibly not exhaling carbon dioxide (CO_2) at all
The client retains all of this carbon dioxide (CO_2), which causes a buildup of acid in the body
This buildup of acid causes the pH to decrease

Source: Created by author from Reference #3.

✚ Respiratory alkalosis

What is it?

Respiratory alkalosis is an acid–base imbalance where the PCO_2 is less than 35 mm Hg and the pH is greater than 7.45. Basically, the pH is increased and the CO_2 is decreased. As in respiratory acidosis, the lungs are the cause of the problem in respiratory alkalosis.

- The only way the PCO_2 can decrease in the blood is through excessive exhalation—hyperventilation.
- When the lungs are impaired, the kidneys compensate with their own chemicals—bicarbonate and H^+.
- The kidneys will retain H^+ because this is acid. We want to keep acid in order to replace the acid being lost from the hyperventilation.
- The kidneys will excrete bicarbonate because this is base. This excretion of the base will help raise acid levels and restore the body to a normal pH.
- Respiratory alkalosis means that the client has lost excessive CO_2 (acid), thus making the client alkalotic.

DEFINE TIME   Hypocapnia occurs when the CO_2 is low; hypercapnia occurs when the CO_2 is high. Hyperapnia is hyperventilation.

What causes it and why

Respiratory alkalosis is caused by excess respirations that result in excess loss of CO_2 as shown in Table 2-6.

Table 2-6

Causes	Why
Hysteria; anxiety	Rapid respirations
High mechanical ventilator setting	Rapid respirations
Aspirin overdose	Aspirin stimulates the respiratory center, causing increased respirations
Pain (having a baby)	Increased respirations
Fever	Increased respirations
Sepsis	Increased respirations
High altitudes	Less oxygen causes increased respirations
Anemia	Fewer red blood cells (RBCs) to carry oxygen, causing hypoxia. Hypoxia causes increased respirations to produce more oxygen

Source: Created by author from References #1 and #3.

Signs and symptoms and why

Table 2-7 shows the signs and symptoms of respiratory alkalosis.

Table 2-7

Signs and symptoms	Why
Hyperventilation	Increased respirations causing excess loss of CO_2
Light-headedness, dizziness, fainting	Hypocapnia causes vasoconstriction of brain vessels; blood flow to brain is decreased
Rapid pulse	Hypocapnia triggers receptors in the medulla that increase heart rate
Hypokalemia	H^+ ions move out of the cell into the bloodstream to decrease alkalinity. K^+ moves into the cells trying to get away from H^+, which decreases serum K^+
Arrhythmias	Hypokalemia

Source: Created by author from Reference #3.

CASE IN POINT   Let's pretend your client is hysterical. He is screaming, crying, and breathing quickly. The client shouts, "I'm getting dizzy! I think I'm gonna faint!" Before you know it, he hits the floor. Well, now. Are you going to wait until the kidneys kick in to compensate? Are you going to say, "Everybody stand back, the kidneys are about to kick in!" I don't think so! You know it will take a few days for kidney compensation to begin. Instead, you calm the client; have him slow down his breathing; have him breathe into a paper bag—not plastic, you don't want him to suffocate, do you? When the client exhales into the paper bag he will re-inhale his own CO_2. Yeah! It's his CO_2; let him have it back!

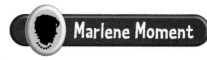

Marlene Moment

Labor and delivery nurses beware. During labor, the client may hyperventilate and exhibit signs and symptoms of a stroke (numbness of the face) and add to the drama of the situation.

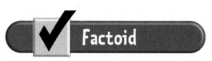

Factoid

Aspirin overdose initially causes respiratory alkalosis as ASA ↑'s respirations, but over time metabolic acidosis can occur as ASA is acidic.

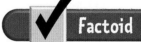

Factoid

Hypocapnia stimulates the autonomic nervous system, which cause anxiety, changes in respiration, tingling, and sweating.

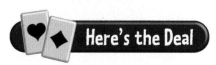

Here's the Deal

Calcium acts like a sedative. Hypocapnia decreases serum calcium so the muscles may get tight. This can lead to tetany and seizures!

Quickie tests and treatments

- Treat the cause.
- Monitor vital signs, especially respirations.
- Monitor electrolytes.
- Administer antianxiety medications as ordered.
- Place on mechanical ventilator to control respiratory rate in severe cases.
- Monitor ABGs.
- Calm the client.
- Have client breathe into paper bag or rebreather mask to encourage CO_2 retention.[3]

What do the ABGs look like?

In respiratory alkalosis, the ABGs look like shown in Table 2-8.

Table 2-8

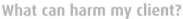

ABGs in respiratory alkalosis	
pH	Greater than 7.45 (alkalosis makes pH go up)
PCO_2	Less than 35 mm Hg (because it is being exhaled)
PO_2	Greater than 100 mm Hg
HCO_3^-	Normal until kidney compensation starts; then will be less than 22 mEq/L

Source: Created by author from References #1 and #3.

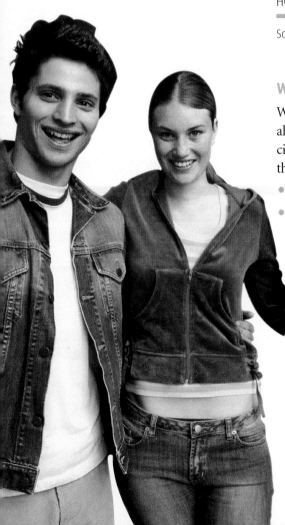

What can harm my client?

What harms your client is totally dependent on what causes the respiratory alkalosis. For example, if the cause is due to an aspirin overdose, then specific complications for this event exist. Remember to focus on the cause of the imbalance.

- Life-threatening arrhythmias.
- Seizures.

If I were your teacher, I would test you on . . .

- Be able to identify ABG values and choose appropriate acid/base imbalance according to the values given.
- Causes of respiratory alkalosis and why.
- Signs and symptoms of respiratory alkalosis and why.
- Prevention of and monitoring for electrolyte imbalances.
- Interventions to reverse respiratory alkalosis.
- Seizure precautions.
- Recognizing and treating arrhythmias.
- Compensation mechanisms. (H^+ and K^+ swap places)

Table 2-9 shows a recap of respiratory alkalosis.

Table 2-9

Recap of respiratory alkalosis
The name "respiratory" tips you off to the fact that a lung problem exists
Since it is a lung problem, the problem chemical is the acid carbon dioxide (CO_2)
Excessive exhalation causes PCO_2 to decrease in the blood. Acid is lost
When the lungs are impaired, the kidneys compensate with their own chemicals—bicarbonate and H^+. The kidneys will retain H^+ because this is acid. We want to keep acid since the body is losing acid from the excessive exhalation. The kidneys will excrete bicarbonate—a base—in order to create a more acidic environment and return the pH to normal
Respiratory alkalosis means that the client has lost excessive CO_2 (acid), thus making the client alkalotic

Source: Created by author from Reference #3.

✚ Metabolic acidosis

What is it?

Metabolic acidosis is an acid–base imbalance where the pH is less than 7.35 and the bicarbonate level is less than 22 mEq/L. Acid (H^+ ions) builds up in the body, or too much bicarbonate has been lost from the body. Basically, the pH is decreased and the bicarbonate level is decreased. The less bicarb you have in the body, the more acid you will be.

* In metabolic disorders, the problem is not with the lungs but with the kidneys.
* Which chemicals are associated with the kidneys? Bicarbonate and H^+.
* The decrease in the alkaline substances (bases) causes a build up of acids in the body, causing acidosis.
* Which organ will compensate? The lungs will compensate by increasing respirations in an effort to blow off excess CO_2 (acid) and therefore increase pH.
* The lungs will start compensating in just few minutes, but it's not enough to correct the imbalance at this point.

What causes it and why (Table 2-10)

Table 2-10

Causes	Why
Diabetic ketoacidosis, malnutrition, starvation	The body breaks down fat for energy, producing the acid ketones. Ketones are a byproduct of fat metabolism. Ketones are acids!
Lactic acidosis	Arterial disorders decrease oxygenated blood in the tissues. This causes the body to switch from aerobic metabolism (using oxygen) to anaerobic metabolism (without oxygen). The end product of anaerobic metabolism is a buildup of lactic acid, causing acidosis, ie., occlusion of lower extremity artery

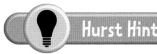

Hurst Hint

When acid builds up in the body, acidosis occurs and pH goes down. When too much bicarbonate (base) is lost from the body, this leaves the body too acidic, again causing acidosis.

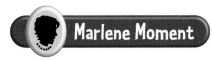

Marlene Moment

We always blame "metabolic" disorders on the kidneys, but just between you and me, it's not always the kidneys' fault.

(Continued)

Table 2-10. (*Continued*)

Causes	Why
Shock	Oxygenated blood is not delivered throughout the body, causing anaerobic metabolism and a buildup of lactic acid
Kidney illness	Decreased secretion or resorption of bicarbonate into the blood; decreased excretion of H^+ ions
Gastrointestinal (GI) illness: diarrhea	Lower GI contents are alkaline and diarrhea causes a loss of base solutions from the body, resulting in acidic blood
Drugs: Diamox, Aldactone	Diamox causes loss of bicarbonate; Aldactone causes K^+ retention and an increase of serum K^+. The blood pushes the K^+ into the cell to decrease serum K^+. This is a normal compensatory mechanism. When K^+ is pushed into the cell, H^+ is pushed out of the cell into the bloodstream, causing acidosis (remember, H^+ is acid)
Aspirin overdose	Acid is the end product of aspirin metabolism

Source: Created by author from Reference #3.

Signs and symptoms and why

The signs and symptoms of metabolic acidosis are due to the cause of the imbalance. For example, if renal failure is the initial cause, you will see signs and symptoms related to renal failure; if diabetic ketoacidosis is the initial cause. Some general signs and symptoms are found in (Table 2-11).

Table 2-11

Signs and symptoms	Why
Hyperkalemia	H^+ builds up in the blood and the body compensates by pushing the excess H^+ ions into the cells (where they can't be seen). When H^+ moves into the cell, this disturbs K^+ (whose favorite place to live is in the cell <u>alone</u>), who moves out into the bloodstream. This causes an increase in serum K^+
Arrhythmias	Bradycardia, peaked T-waves, prolonged PR interval, widened QRS
Increased respiratory rate	Medulla in the brain is stimulated by excess H^+ ions. Kussmau respirations compensate by blowing off CO_2 (acid). Eventually, PCO_2 decreases
Headache, decreased LOC, coma	The brain does not like it when the pH is out of normal range
Muscle twitching and burning, oral numbness, weakness, flaccid paralysis (severe hyperkalemia)	Hyperkalemia
Weakness, flaccid paralysis, tingling and numbness in the arms and legs	Hyperkalemia and hypercalcemia

Source: Created by author from Reference # 3.

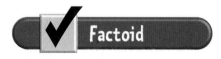

Factoid

Hyperkalemia begins with muscle twitching, then proceeds to weakness and flaccid paralysis.

DEFINE TIME   A Kussmau respiration is an increase in rate and depth of respiration. When Kussmau respirations are present, CO_2 is being blown off in increased amounts.

Quickie tests and treatments

* Monitor ABGs.
* Treat the cause.
* Monitor and manage hyperkalemia.
* Monitor and manage arrhythmias.
* Monitor and manage hypercalcemia.
* Administer sodium bicarbonate IV to decrease acidity of blood.
* Monitor LOC closely.
* Administer lactated Ringers (LR) given IV to increase base level.
* Institute seizure precautions (brain doesn't like it when the pH is messed up).

What do the ABGs look like?

In metabolic acidosis, the ABGs look as shown in Table 2-12.

Table 2-12

ABGs in metabolic acidosis	
pH	Less than 7.35
PCO_2	Will decrease to less than 35 mm Hg as it is blown off (compensation is occuring)
PO_2	Normal
HCO_3^-	Less than 22 mEq/L

Source: Created by author from References #1 and #3.

What can harm my client?

The initial problem or cause associated with metabolic acidosis will determine the complications to watch out for. A couple of universal precautions are:

* Life-threatening arrhythmias.
* Cardiac arrest.

If I were your teacher, I would test you on . . .

* Causes of metabolic acidosis and why.
* Signs and symptoms and why of metabolic acidosis.
* Changes in ABGs.
* Compensation mechanisms.
* Prevention and management of complications.
* Medication administration and possible side effects.

Table 2-13 shows the recap of metabolic acidosis.

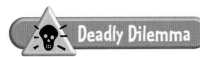 **Deadly Dilemma**

Administering sodium bicarbonate can be very dangerous, as it can actually intensify acidosis due to changes at the cellular level (changes which are way over my head!). Sodium bicarbonate should be used only as a quick, temporary fix for increased acid levels and should be given according to specific ABG values rather than generously as we used to do in the past during code situations.

Table 2-13

Recap of metabolic acidosis
The problem is with the kidneys, not the lungs.
Bicarbonate (base) and H+ (acid) are associated with the kidneys.
Metabolic acidosis can be caused by loss of bicarbonate through diarrhea, and renal insufficiency. The decrease in the alkaline substances (bases) causes a buildup of acids in the body. It can also be caused by diseases that increase acid levels (OFA)
The lungs compensate increasing respiratory rate and depth to blow off CO_2 and increase pH. This is called a Kussmau respiration.

Source: Created by author from Reference #3.

✚ Metabolic alkalosis

What is it?

Metabolic alkalosis is an acid–base imbalance where the pH is greater than 7.45 and the bicarbonate level is greater than 26 mEq/L. There is an excess of base in the body and a loss of acid. Basically, pH is increased and bicarbonate is increased.

- The lungs did not cause the problem; that is why it is a metabolic problem and not a respiratory one.
- Metabolic means the "kidneys", which involve bicarbonate and H+.
- The lungs compensate by retaining CO_2 by means of hypoventilation. This compensates for the alkalosis and helps the pH go down into normal range.

What causes it and why

Table 2-14 gives the causes of metabolic alkalosis.

Table 2-14

Causes	Why
Vomiting; bulimia; nasogastric (NG) tube suctioning	Removes stomach acid leaving the body alkaline
Excess antacid ingestion	Increases serum alkaline levels; kidneys may not be able to get rid of excess
Blood transfusions	Preservative citrate is converted to bicarbonate (when blood is administered, the client is getting bicarb too)
Sodium bicarbonate	IV administration in code situations may leave the client too alkaline
Thiazide and loop diuretics	Loss of chlorine, which impedes manufacture of hydrochloric (HCL) acid, making the body alkaline. Chlorine depletion enhances bicarbonate resorption, increasing alkalinity

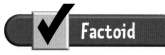

Factoid

Metabolic alkalosis is the most common acid–base imbalance. It accounts for 50% of all acid–base disturbances.[1,3]

Hurst Hint

When bicarbonate builds up in the blood, alkalosis occurs and the pH goes up. A deficit of acid in the body will also cause alkalosis.

(Continued)

Table 2-14. (*Continued*)

Causes	Why
Baking soda	Home remedy for GI upset; very alkaline
Hypokalemia	Hypokalemia causes H^+ to move into the cell, forcing K^+ into the bloodstream, increasing serum K^+. This is a normal compensatory mechanism to correct the hypokalemia. This causes a decrease in available hydrogen needed to make hydrochloric acid (HCL) which will make the client more alkalotic (less acid makes more base)
Activation of renin–angiotensin system	H^+ ions secreted into the nephron add bicarbonate to the vascular space, making the blood alkaline
Steroids	Sodium and water retention and K^+ loss. Refer to *hypokalemia* to see how this causes alkalosis
Dialysis	High bicarbonate dialysate is used to correct metabolic acidosis in end-stage renal disease (ESRD). The dialysate is alkalinic
Licorice	Sodium and water retention and K^+ loss. Refer to *hypokalemia* to see how this causes alkalosis

Source: Created by author from Reference #3.

Signs and symptoms and why

Table 2-15 gives the general signs, symptoms and the associated reasons for ABGs.

Table 2-15

Signs and symptoms	Why
Arrhythmias, flattened T-wave	Hypokalemia
Decreased respirations, hypoventilation	Respiratory compensation to retain CO_2. Receptors in medulla of brain are depressed due to excess of bicarbonate; eventually, PCO_2 will rise
Hypokalemia	Vomiting may have caused initial imbalance. As K^+ moves into the cells, serum K^+ drops. H^+ moves into the bloodstream, increasing serum acidity
Tightening of muscles, tetany, LOC changes, seizures, tingling in fingers and toes	Hypocalcemia; alkalosis causes calcium to bind with albumin, making the calcium inactive
LOC changes	The brain doesn't like it when pH is out of balance; hypocalcemia
Hepatic encephalopathy	Alkalosis causes increased ammonia production

Source: Created by author from Reference #3.

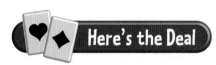

Here's the Deal

Licorice is 50 times sweeter than sugar. It is used to flavor chewing tobacco and cigars. Although rare, it could cause hypokalemia.

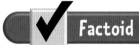

Factoid

The kidneys have the ability to make extra bicarbonate when needed and reabsorb it through the kidney tubules.

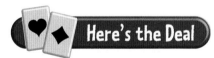

Here's the Deal

The two most common causes of metabolic alkalosis are loss of stomach acid and diuretics.

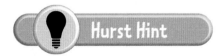

Hurst Hint

Ammonia as seen in hepatic encephalopathy acts like a sedative.

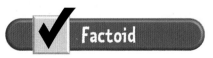

Factoid

Alkalosis inhibits the respiratory center in the medulla.[3]

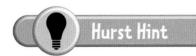

The ABGs of metabolic alkalosis will look like: pH greater than 7.45 and HCO_3^- greater than 26 mEq/L. If compensation has begun, PCO_2 will increase.

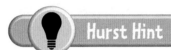

Acidosis: Think hyperkalemia and hypercalcemia.
Alkalosis: Think hypokalemia and hypocalcemia.

What do the ABGs look like?

In metabolic alkalosis, the ABGs look as shown in Table 2-16.

Table 2-16

ABGs in metabolic alkalosis	
pH	Greater than 7.45
PCO_2	Normal; increases with compensation
PO_2	Remains the same
HCO_3^-	Greater than 26 mEq/L

Source: Created by author from References #1 and #3.

Quickie tests and treatments

- Treating the cause of the acid–base imbalance (antiemetics for vomiting, etc.).
- Monitoring ABGs for further complications.
- Treating arrhythmias.
- Stopping client bicarbonate intake.
- Monitoring potassium levels and correcting hypokalemia.
- Monitoring respirations and LOC.
- Assessing for hypotension.
- Treating dehydration if present.
- Assessing DTRs.
- Administering ammonium chloride IV in severe cases to increase acidity (increases H^+).
- Administering acetazolamide (Diamox) to increase excretion of bicarbonate through the kidneys.[1,2]

What can harm my client?

Metabolic alkalosis can cause the following life-threatening illnesses:

- Arrhythmias.
- Cardiac arrest.
- Seizures.

If I were your teacher, I would test you on . . .

- Be able to identify specific imbalances of acid/base according to situations and ABG values given.
- Causes of metabolic alkalosis and why.
- Signs and symptoms of metabolic alkalosis and why.
- Signs and symptoms of hypokalemia and related treatment.
- Signs and symptoms of hypocalcemia and related treatment.
- Seizure precautions and management.
- Monitoring for changes in ABGs and management.

Table 2-17 shows the recap of metabolic alkalosis.

Table 2-17

Recap of metabolic alkalosis
The problem is with the kidneys, not the lungs
Bicarbonate (base) and H⁺ (acid) are associated with the kidneys
Metabolic alkalosis can be caused by increased bicarbonate through diuretic therapy, prolonged nasogastric suctioning, and excessive vomiting, resulting in ↑ pH levels
The lungs compensate by retaining CO_2 by means of hypoventilation. This compensates for the alkalosis

Source: Created by author from Reference #3.

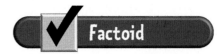

Clients may have combined acid imbalances at the same time, such as respiratory acidosis and metabolic acidosis.

SUMMARY

The respiratory and renal systems can be both the cause and "cure" for pH imbalances. Remember that the lungs control carbon dioxide levels and the kidneys control bicarbonate levels. By monitoring your client's carbon dioxide, bicarbonate, and pH levels you can successfully prevent and treat any acid–base imbalances.

PRACTICE QUESTIONS

1. Which lab values indicate metabolic acidosis?

1. pH — 7.40, PCO_2 — 38, HCO_3^- — 23.

2. pH — 7.33, PCO_2 — 30, HCO_3^- — 18.

3. pH — 7.28, PCO_2 — 48, HCO_3^- — 29.

4. pH — 7.46, PCO_2 — 30, HCO_3^- — 25.

Correct answer: 2. In metabolic acidosis, the result of a kidney illness, the pH is decreased, as is the bicarbonate level due to acidosis. Answer (1) represents normal values. Answer (3) signifies respiratory acidosis due to the low pH, high PCO_2, and high HCO_3^-. Answer (4) indicates alkalosis due to the high pH level.

2. The ability of the body's regulatory system to correct acid–base imbalances is a process called:

1. Compensation.

2. Modification.

3. Ventilation.

4. Diffusion.

Correct answer: 1. Compensation is a defense mechanism of the body to self-correct acid–base imbalances. Modification indicates change, but not necessarily a correction. Ventilation is air movement in and out of the lungs. Diffusion is the mixing of molecules or ions.

3. The process of excreting bicarbonate out of the body to correct an acid–base imbalance occurs through the:

1. Lung.

2. Kidney.

3. Liver.

4. Pancreas.

Correct answer: 2. The kidney is the only organ that deals with bicarbonate. The lung manipulates carbon dioxide. The liver metabolizes nutrients and detoxifies medications. The pancreas secretes insulin, glucagon, and somatostatin.

4. A client with diabetes mellitus is admitted to the hospital complaining of lethargy, weakness, headache, nausea, and vomiting. The physician orders arterial blood gas testing. The nurse suspects the lab results will confirm:

1. Metabolic acidosis.

2. Metabolic alkalosis.

3. Respiratory acidosis.

4. Respiratory alkalosis.

Correct answer: 1. The major acid–base imbalance associated with diabetes is metabolic acidosis.

5. A client is admitted to the emergency department (ED) with a diagnosis of respiratory alkalosis. The nurse recognizes a symptom of this condition as:

1. Nausea.

2. Kussmaul respirations.

3. Hyperventilation.

4. Bradycardia.

Correct answer: 3. The major cause of respiratory alkalosis is hyperventilation. Nausea is too nonspecific and is a symptom of many illnesses. Kussmaul respirations are seen with metabolic acidosis. The client in respiratory alkalosis is usually experiences tachycardia due to hypoxia, not bradycardia.

6. When performing an assessment of a client admitted with metabolic alkalosis, the nurse should ask about the use of?

1. Aspirin.

2. Acetaminophen.

3. Antacids.

4. Antihistamines.

Correct answer: 3. Antacids are very alkaline, and too many of them can cause metabolic alkalosis. The other medications typically do not cause metabolic alkalosis.

7. Arterial blood gas values of pH — 7.28, pCO_2 — 50, HCO_3^- — 24 indicate the presence of which acid–base imbalance?

   1. Metabolic acidosis.

   2. Metabolic alkalosis.

   3. Respiratory acidosis.

   4. Respiratory alkalosis.

   Correct answer: 3. In metabolic acidosis the pH is low, but the PCO_2 is low too because the client has Kussmaul respirations in an effort to blow off excess CO_2 (acid). In metabolic alkalosis, the pH is high. In respiratory alkalosis, the pH is high.

8. The nurse should watch for which electrolyte imbalance in a client who has chronic respiratory acidosis?

   1. Hyperkalemia.

   2. Hypomagnesemia.

   3. Hyperphosphatamia.

   4. Hypocalcemia.

   Correct answer: 1. In acidosis, H^+ is pushed into cells and K^+ comes out of the cells into the bloodstream; therefore, the client is hyperkalemic. This is a normal compensatory mechanism. Magnesium is not significantly affected in acidosis nor is phosphorus. In acidosis, calcium levels tend to go up, resulting in hypercalcemia.

9. Lactated Ringers IV is ordered by the client's physician to reverse which acid–base imbalance?

   1. Metabolic acidosis.

   2. Metabolic alkalosis.

   3. Respiratory acidosis.

   4. Respiratory alkalosis.

   Correct answer: 1. Lactated Ringers IV is given in metabolic acidosis to increase the base level. It is not given in other acid–base imbalances listed. IV push bicarbonate may be given in respiratory acidosis.

10. A client's ABG results are pH — 7.47, CO_2 — 38, HCO_3^- — 29. The nurse should further assess:

   1. Shock.

   2. Headache.

   3. Numbness and tingling of the extremities.

   4. Increased pulse and respiratory rate.

Correct answer: 3. These ABGs are consistent with metabolic alkalosis. Numbness and tingling are associated with metabolic alkalosis due to hypocalcemia. Shock is associated with metabolic acidosis. Headache is typically associated with acidosis. Increased pulse and respiratory rate are associated with respiratory alkalosis.

References

1. Pagana KD, Pagana TJ, eds. *Diagnostic and Laboratory Test Reference.* 6th ed. St Louis: Mosby; 2003.

2. Beers MH. *The Merck Manual of Medical Information.* 2nd home ed. New York: Pocket Books; 2004.

3. Hurst M. *Finally Understanding Fluids and Electrolytes* [audio CD-ROM]. Ambler, PA: Lippincott Williams & Wilkins; 2004.

4. Allen KD, Boucher MA, Cain JE, et al. *Manual of Nursing Practice Pocket Guides Medical-Surgical Nursing.* Ambler, PA: Lippincott Williams & Wilkins; 2007.

Bibliography

Hurst Review Services. www.hurstreview.com.

Kee JL, Paulanka BJ. *Fluids and Electrolytes with Clinical Applications: A Programmed Approach.* 6th ed. Albany, NY: Delmar Publishers; 2000.

Springhouse Editors. *Nurse's Quick Check: Fluids and Electrolytes.* Ambler, PA: Lippincott Williams & Wilkins; 2005.

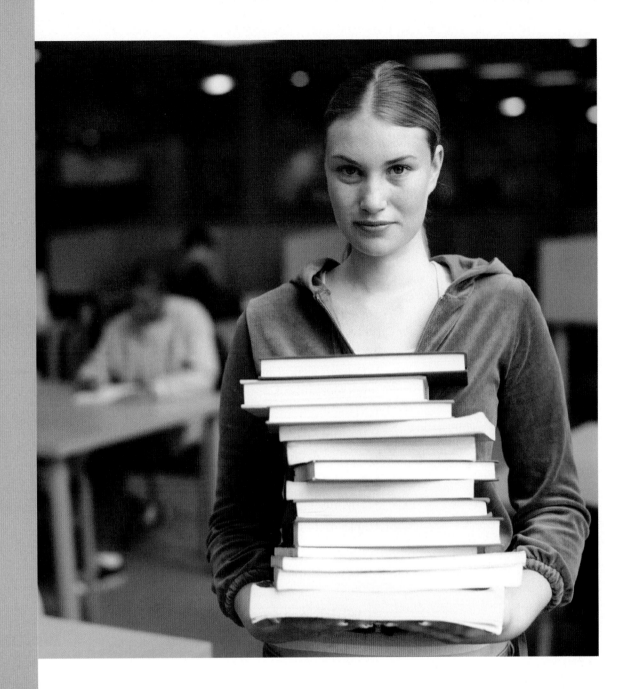

3 Immune System

OBJECTIVES

In this chapter, you'll review:

* The function, involved organs, and response categories of the immune system.

* The signs and symptoms associated with common immune illnesses.

* Need-to-know information regarding common immune illnesses including diagnostic tests, treatments, and possible complications.

LET'S GET THE NORMAL STUFF STRAIGHT FIRST

The immune system consists of specialized cells and structures that protect the body against invasion by harmful substances. Specifically, the immune system:

1. Defends against infection by protecting the body against invading microorganisms.

2. Maintains homeostasis by removing old cells, primarily by the spleen.

3. Identifies circulating cells and destroys mutant cells.

The primary immune organs are the:

* Lymph nodes.
* Thymus.
* Spleen.
* Tonsils.
* Bone marrow.

✚ Which organ does what?

The following chart (Table 3-1) displays the roles of the major immune organs (Fig. 3-1).

Table 3-1

Organ	Function
Lymph nodes	Filter bacteria and foreign cells
Thymus	Produces T-cells
Spleen	Filters blood; produces lymphocytes and monocytes; destroys bacteria
Tonsils	Produce lymphocytes to fight pathogens entering the nose and mouth
Bone marrow	Source of lymphocytes and macrophages; recognizes and removes old cells; contains stem cells that evolve into B-cells, T-cells, and phagocytes

Source: Created by author from Reference #1.

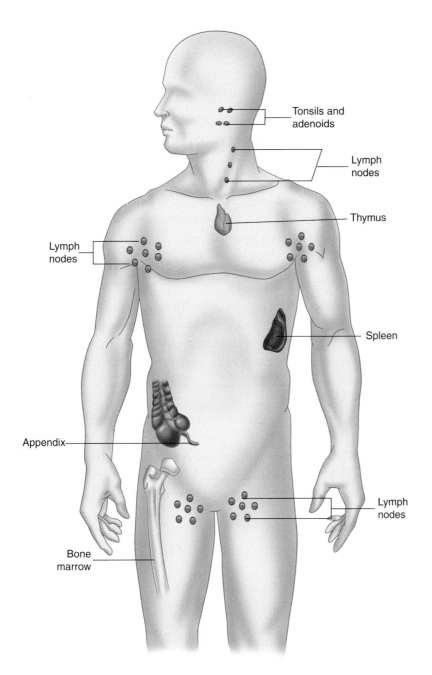

◀ Figure 3-1. Primary organs of the immune system.

Tonsils and adenoids

Lymph nodes

Thymus

Lymph nodes

Spleen

Appendix

Lymph nodes

Bone marrow

How does the immune response work?

The immune system recognizes foreign cells—called antigens—that are not a normal part of the body. The immune system responds to these antigens by producing antibodies that attack and destroy the invading antigens. The body does this according to 2 categories:

1. Antibody-mediated immunity (AMI or humoral immunity): antibodies (gammaglobulins and immunoglobulins) dissolved in the blood, lymph, and other body fluids bind to the antigen and trigger a response to it. B-cells (lymphocytes) found mostly in spleen and lymph nodes produce these antibodies.

2. Cell-mediated immunity (CMI): highly developed ability to differentiate self from nonself. Provides a surveillance system for ridding body of self cells that might harm the body. CMI helps prevent development

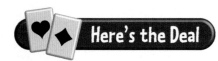

T-cells can be killer, helper, or suppressor T-cells. Killer cells destroy the invading cell; helper cells help B-cells secrete immunoglobulin; suppressor cells reduce AMI (humoral response).

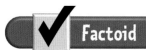

B-cells are responsible for AMI by differentiating into plasma cells, which excrete large amounts of immunoglobulin.

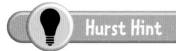

Immunoglobulins are a fancy name for antibodies. There are 5 types of immunoglobulins: IgA, IgD, IgE, IgG, and IgM.

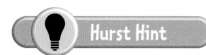

Common items used in the hospital setting that have latex are tape, ambu bags, bulb syringes, oxygen masks, electrode pads, catheters/drains, stethoscope tubing, BP tubing, gloves, injection ports, stretchers (mattresses), and tourniquets.

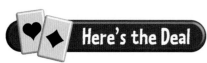

The more you come in contact with latex, the greater the chance you will develop an allergy to it one day. So if you are using a lot of latex condoms you may want to mix it up a little! And use sheep skin every now and then.

of cancer and metastasis after exposure to carcinogens. Leukocytes involved are T-cells. T-cells bind to the surface of other cells that display the antigen and trigger a response. The response may involve other lymphocytes and any other leukocytes (white blood cells).[1]

LET'S GET DOWN TO SPECIFICS

Let's get down to the specific illnesses that can occur when the immune system is not in homeostasis. This lack of immune homeostasis causes an immune response. Let's look at how various altered immune responses can present themselves in your patients.

✚ Latex allergy

Latex allergy affects 10% to 30% of health care workers and 1% to 5% of the general population in the United States. It is most prevalent in patients with spina bifida and urogenital abnormalities.[2,3] Latex allergy is only one type of hypersensitivity reaction caused by an altered immune response.

What is it?

Latex allergy is a hypersensitivity reaction to one or more proteins found in natural rubber latex. After exposure, there is an increased production of IgE that leads to histamine release. A reaction can be caused by direct contact with latex or by inhaling the latex particles that mix with cornstarch used on balloons or in gloves to keep them from sticking together.

What causes it and why

Table 3-2 displays the causes and why of latex allergy.

Table 3-2

Causes	Why
Defect in bone marrow cells	Decreased production of lymphocytes and macrophages needed to fight off antigens
Deformed bladder or urinary tract	Repeated exposure to urinary latex products increases the risk of latex allergy (frequent intermittent catheterization)
History of multiple surgeries	Repeated exposure to latex increases the risk of developing latex allergy
History of allergies	Immune response is already increased, which can cause a reaction to latex
Food allergies to banana, avocado, kiwi, passion fruit, strawberry, tomato, and chestnut	Contain some of the same allergens found in latex
Spina bifida	Early and repeated exposure to latex in the health care setting increases the risk of developing latex allergy

Source: Created by author from References #1, #2, and #3.

Signs and symptoms and why

The signs and symptoms of latex allergy can range from contact dermatitis to life-threatening anaphylactic reaction (Type I hypersensitivity reaction). The immune system triggers certain cells to produce immunoglobulin E (IgE) antibodies to fight the latex allergen. The IgE antibodies signal the immune system to release histamine and other chemicals, which cause many signs and symptoms. Table 3-3 shows the signs and symptoms and related rationales for latex allergy.

Table 3-3

Signs and symptoms	Why
Hives, welts, urticaria, pruritus	Histamine release from mast cells that exist deep within the skin; causes blood vessel dilatation and increased capillary permeability
Swelling of affected area	Histamine dilates blood vessels and increases capillary permeability causing inflammation
Runny nose	Histamine causes mucus production and decreased ciliary action
Sneezing	Histamine response to allergen
Headache	Histamine response to allergen
Red, itchy, teary eyes	Histamine response to allergen
Sore throat, hoarse voice	Drainage of nasal mucus into the throat causes multiple attempts to clear the throat by coughing resulting in a sore throat and hoarse voice
Abdominal cramps	Histamine causes constriction of smooth muscle
Chest tightness, wheezing, stridor	Bronchoconstriction caused by histamine stimulation of smooth muscle
Hypotension	Vasodilation; vessels start to leak due to mast cell invasion
Tachycardia	Vascular volume decreases causing an increase in heart rate because the heart tries to pump what little fluid is left around the body

Source: Created by author from References #2 and #3.

Quickie tests and treatments

Radioallergosorbent test shows specific IgE antibodies to latex. Patch testing results in hives with itching and redness. Treatments include:

- Airway, airway, airway!
- Preventing exposure (wrap BP cuffs and stethoscopes in cloth or use "special" equipment).
- Corticosteroids.
- Antihistamines.
- Histamine-2 receptor blockers.
- Epinephrine 1:1000.
- Oxygen therapy.

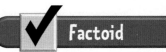

About half of all children with spina bifida are allergic to latex.[2]

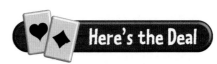

Symptoms develop within 5 to 30 minutes and go away when the latex is removed.[3]

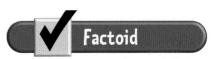

The nutritionist may want to counsel the client to avoid the following foods as they have similar allergens to latex: banana, avocado, kiwi, passion fruit, strawberry, tomato, and chestnut.

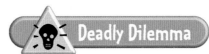

Although most hospitals have needle less systems in place, keep in mind when adding medication to the IV bag etc. When adding medication to the IV bag of a client with latex allergy, inject the drug through the spike port, not the rubber latex port.[3] You could introduce latex into the bloodstream and that's not nice!

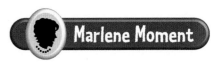

It's not nice to send regular balloons to people with latex allergies. You should send Mylar balloons instead . . . if you're a nice person, that is.

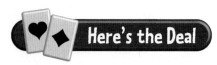

The client with latex allergy should wear a medical alert bracelet at all times!

Be sure to put clients with a latex allergy either in a private room or in a room with another client with latex allergy.

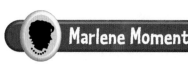

If your client has a latex allergy, get ready to wear those fancy purple latex-free gloves!

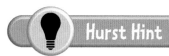

Always ask your clients about allergies and encourage them to wear a medi-alert bracelet listing known allergies.

- Volume expanders.
- IV vasopressors.
- Aminophylline (Truphylline) and albuterol (Proventil).[3]

What can harm my client?

The life-threatening complication of latex allergy is anaphylaxis. Make sure you are familiar with the signs and symptoms, nursing interventions, medical treatments, and client teaching related to anaphylaxis.

If I were your teacher, I would test you on . . .

- Teaching the client to wear medical identification jewelry.
- Signs and symptoms of latex allergy and why.
- The causes and why of latex allergy.
- Medication administration and possible side effects.
- Techniques to keep the client's environment latex free.
- Signs, symptoms, and interventions of anaphylaxis.
- Skin care of rash and hives.
- Focused assessment addressing respiratory and hemodynamic status.

✚ Anaphylaxis at a glance

What is it?

- Severe type 1 rapid hypersensitivity reaction.
- Dramatic, acute reaction to an allergen.

What causes it?

- Systemic exposure to sensitizing agents: chemicals, foods, drugs, enzymes, hormones, insect venom, vaccinations.

Signs and symptoms and why (Table 3-4)

Table 3-4

Signs and symptoms	Why
Urticaria, sweating, sneezing, rhinorrhea	Histamine release
Sudden feelings of doom, fright, anxiety	Hypoxia; IgE activation
Cyanosis	Hypoxia
Cool, clammy skin	Blood being shunted to vital organs
Tachypnea, wheezing, stridor	Hypoxia related to laryngeal edema; smooth muscle constriction
Hypotension, shock	Vasodilation; capillaries leaking fluid due to weakness from mast cell invasion
Chest tightness	Bronchial constriction
Dizziness, drowsiness, headache	Hypoxia
Seizures	Hypoxia
Severe abdominal cramps, nausea, diarrhea; urinary incontinence	Constriction of smooth muscles

Source: Created by author from Reference #3.

Quickie tests and treatments

- Determine the cause and maintain the airway!
- Patient's history and signs and symptoms establish the diagnosis.
- Skin testing may help identify a specific antigen, but can cause severe allergic reaction.
- Maintain a patent airway.
- Cardiopulmonary resuscitation (CPR).
- Oxygen therapy.
- Endotracheal tube, if needed.
- Epinephrine 1:1000 aqueous solution, subQ, or IV.
- Corticosteroids to reduce inflammatory reaction.
- Diphenhydramine (Benadryl) IV.
- Vasopressors to support blood pressure.
- Norepinephrine (Levophed) to restore blood pressure.
- Volume expander infusions.
- Dopamine (Dobutrex) to support blood pressure.
- Aminophylline (Truphylline) IV to dilate bronchi.
- Antihistamines to counteract histamine reaction. [3]

What can harm my client?

- Respiratory arrest, cardiac arrest, or both.
- Vascular collapse.
- Immediate threat of death.

If I were your teacher, I would test you on . . .

- Patient safety during emergency treatment.
- Causes of anaphylaxis.
- Signs and symptoms of anaphylaxis.
- Monitoring for adverse reactions to medications and treatments.
- Peripheral IV insertion and care.
- Complications associated with skin or scratch testing.
- Client and family education.

✚ Osteoarthritis

There are more than 100 types of arthritis and the cause of most types is unknown. Osteoarthritis (OA), also called osteoarthroses or degenerative joint disease (DJD), affects nearly 21 million Americans.[4]

What is it?

OA (see Fig. 3-2) is the progressive deterioration and/or loss of cartilage in the joints, particulary the hips, knees, vertebral column, and hands. This breakdown of cartilage—which cushions the joints—causes the bones to rub together resulting in pain, stiffness, and loss of movement in the joint. The cartilage becomes soft, opaque, yellow, and thin resulting in fissures, pitting, ulcerations, bone spurs, and bone cysts.[1]

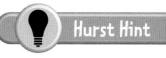

Hurst Hint

When the client begins to improve, fluid may shift from the tissue back into the vascular space. This is when you should watch for fluid volume overload.

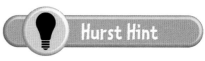

Hurst Hint

Some muscles contract and constrict and some muscles vasodilate. Airways usually constrict in anaphylaxis and blood vessels usually dilate causing BP to drop.

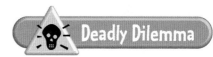

Deadly Dilemma

Treat any sign of an allergic reaction as if it is an emergency. It could be a mild reaction or could turn into a fatal reaction within minutes.

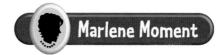

Marlene Moment

Never be afraid to call for help or call a code if you feel your patient is having an allergic reaction. It's better to overreact and save a life than to underreact and let someone die.

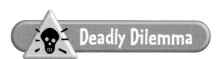

Deadly Dilemma

If you ever give an injection, especially if it is an antibiotic, make sure the client stays in the office or ED for at least 30 minutes afterward so you can monitor for signs of a reaction.

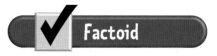

Factoid

Osteoarthritis is the most common form of arthritis.

▶ Figure 3-2. **A.** A joint with severe osteoarthritis. **B.** The areas affected by osteoarthritis.

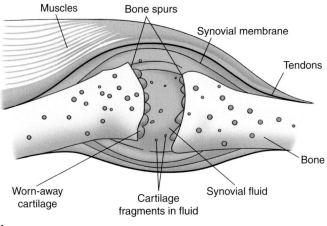

Muscles

Bone spurs

Synovial membrane

Tendons

Bone

Worn-away cartilage

Cartilage fragments in fluid

Synovial fluid

A

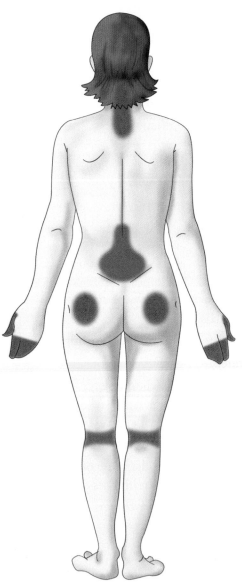

B

What causes it and why

Table 3-5 gives the causes and associated reasons for osteoarthritis.

Table 3-5

Causes	Why
Aging	Water content of the cartilage increases and the protein makeup of cartilage degenerates; this causes joint degeneration
Metabolic disorders	Hormones and chemicals associated with diabetes and blood disorders can cause early cartilage wear and joint degeneration
Joint trauma	Joint structure is compromised, causing deterioration
Obesity	Added weight to the joints causes mechanical stress on the cartilage
Congenital abnormalities	Joints are vulnerable to mechanical wear, causing early degeneration and loss of joint cartilage
Genetics	Found in multiple members of same family implying genetic predisposition

Source: Created by author from References #1 and #4.

Signs and symptoms and why

Table 3-6 gives the signs and symptoms of osteoarthritis.

Table 3-6

Signs and symptoms	Why
Pain and stiffness of the joint; most common symptom	Inflamed synovium, irritation of nerve endings, friction between bones, decreased cartilage
Immobility of the joint	Pain and stiffness
Joint swelling, warmth	Immune reaction that sends increased leukocytes to the area
Muscle atrophy	Decreased movement of the body area due to pain
Crepitus	Decreased cartilage causes bone to rub together
Heberdon's nodes	Bony enlargement of distal finger joints due to repeated inflammation
Bouchard's nodes	Bony enlargement of proximal finger joints due to repeated inflammation
Numbness and tingling in the affected areas, especially at night	Nerve involvement, progression of the disease

Source: Created by author from References #1 and #4.

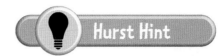

Osteoarthritis: think weight-bearing joints first.

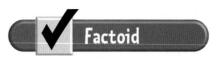

Women tend to have more hand involvement while men tend to have more hip involvement.[1]

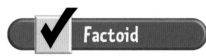

African Americans have more knee but less hand involvement than other groups.[1]

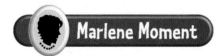

Roughly 70% of folks over the age of 70 have OA in their hands.[1] Isn't it bad enough that we start to sag everywhere and can't remember where we put our dentures as we age?

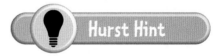

The pain and stiffness associated with osteoarthritis is increased after periods of extended rest or after exercise (especially weight bearing and standing). If the pain is worse with exercise, it improves with rest; if the pain is worse after sleep, it gets better with movement.

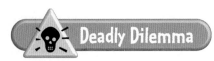

Deadly Dilemma

Most total joint repair patients are expected to bear weight within the first 24 to 48 hours postsurgery. Make sure that hazards such as catheter tubing, IV pumps, linens, and shoes are cleared out of the client's way as they take those first steps.

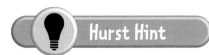

Hurst Hint

Osteoarthritis can affect joints unilaterally (one bad knee) whereas rheumatoid arthritis almost always affects bilateral joints.

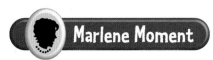

Marlene Moment

Hyaluronic acid, a fairly new OA drug, is made from rooster combs. For you city folks, that's the Mohawk-like crown on a rooster's head!

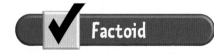

Factoid

RA affects mostly women.[1]

Quickie tests and treatments

OA is diagnosed by physical exam: swollen, painful joints; limited range of motion (ROM); and joint nodules. X-ray may show narrowing of the joint space. Bone scan, MRI, and CT may be used to diagnose vertebral OA. Blood tests are not useful in diagnosing OA. Treatments include:

- Weight reduction.
- Exercise.
- Heat.
- Assistive orthotic devices.
- NSAIDs.
- Acetaminophen.
- COX-2 inhibitors (if not contraindicated).
- Opioids.
- Intra-articular corticosteroids.
- Topical analgesics.
- Glucosamine and chondroitin.
- Hyaluronic acid.
- Invasive: arthroscopy, osteotomy, total joint repair.[1,4]

What can harm my client?

- Surgical complications such as deep vein thrombosis (DVT) and pulmonary embolism (PE).
- Falls and other safety concerns.
- Surgical infection.
- Displacement of the prosthetic implant.

If I were your teacher, I would test you on . . .

- Medication administration and possible side effects.
- The causes of OA and why.
- The signs and symptoms of OA and why.
- Postsurgical complications and management.
- Client teaching regarding weight control and exercise.
- Home care of osteoarthritis.
- Postop positioning and weight-bearing exercises.
- Postop discharge teaching.[1]

✚ Rheumatoid arthritis

Rheumatoid arthritis (RA) affects 1% of the U.S. population or 2.1 million Americans.[5] There is no cure for RA, but researchers are making tremendous progress in the management of the disease through the development of new drugs, exercise, joint protection techniques, and self-care regimens.[5]

What is it?

Rheumatoid arthritis (see Fig. 3-3) is an autoimmune disease characterized by systemic inflammation that affects the synovial lining of the joints. The client with RA experiences periods of exacerbation and remission.

WHAT IS AN AUTOIMMUNE DISEASE?   Autoimmune diseases are caused when the body does not turn off the immune system to fight foreign invaders. Because of this, the body produces antibodies against its own healthy cells because it has run out of foreign enemies to fight. The body continues the fight against itself, which results in debilitating and life-threatening illnesses.

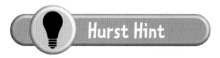

Hurst Hint

Think bilateral and symmetrical joint pain especially after awakening; this discomfort last for 30 minutes or longer with rheumatoid arthritis.

◄ Figure 3-3. **A.** Normal joint. **B.** Joint affected by rheumatoid arthritis.

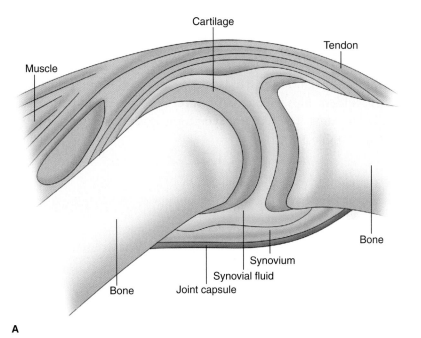

A

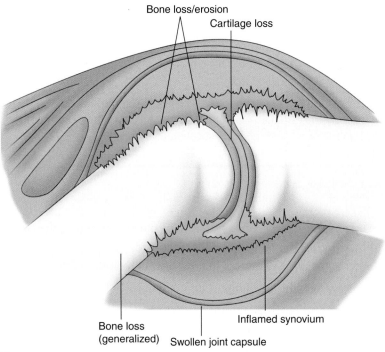

B

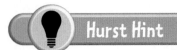

Hurst Hint

Pain associated with rheumatoid arthritis is mainly seen with movement in the early stages; as the disease progresses, the pain is constant due to increased prostaglandin release and joint destruction.

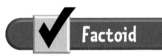

Factoid

Many clients with rheumatoid arthritis report increased fatigue and weakness in the early afternoon.

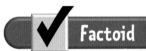

Factoid

Many of the symptoms that do not include the joint are due to the initial inflammatory response kicking in prior to any joint involvement.

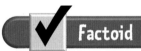

Factoid

Sjögren's syndrome—dry eyes and mouth— is the most common syndrome associated with rheumatoid arthritis.

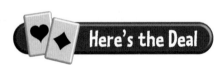

Here's the Deal

Nodules appear over bony prominences like the elbow and occur only in those patients who have rheumatoid factor. Nodules are associated with progressive and destructive disease.[1]

What causes it and why (Table 3-7)

Table 3-7

Causes	Why
Autoimmune disease	Antibodies attack the synovium of the joint affecting the cartilage, tendons, and ligaments. The illness progresses as cartilage, bone, and ligaments are destroyed. The joints become fused
Genetic transmission	Genetic marker HLA-DR4 increases the likelihood of RA being passed down in families

Source: Created by author from Reference #1 and #5.

Signs and symptoms and why

RA symptoms begin in the hands, wrists, and feet. It progresses to the knees, shoulders, hips, elbows, ankles, cervical spine, and temporomandibular joints. The onset of symptoms is acute, bilateral, and symmetric (Table 3-8).

Table 3-8

Signs and symptoms	Why
Swelling in small joints	Increased T- and B-cells to the area; blood vessels form in the synovial lining; inflammation
Pain, stiffness, and fatigue, especially upon awakening	Increased T- and B-cells to the area; blood vessels form in the synovial lining; inflammation
Warm, swollen, effusions; rheumatoid nodules	Neutrophils accumulate in the synovial fluid; inflammation can cause warmth as well
Increase in severity of physical signs and symptoms	Chemicals begin to break down the cartilage
Joint instability, contractures, decreased range of motion (ROM), joint deformities	Cartilage breaks down; bones erode; ligaments become lax
Deformities of the hands and feet; examples ulnar drift, swan-neck or boutonniere deformity	Misalignment resulting from swelling, progressive joint destruction, and partial dislocation of bones

Source: Created by author from References #1 and #5.

The symptoms can become systemic in nature, affecting the organs and blood vessels, resulting in organ failure.[1]

Other signs and symptoms that do not include the joints are:

- Anorexia, weight loss, fatigue, and malaise.
- Dry eyes and mucous membranes.
- Leukopenia and anemia.
- Paresthesia of the hands and feet.

- Low-grade fever.
- Lymphadenopathy.
- Raynaud's phenomenon.[1,5]

Quickie tests and treatments

Diagnostics include:

- History and physical.
- Antinuclear antibody (ANA) test, positive.
- Increased erythrocyte sedimentation rate (ESR), white blood cells (WBC), platelets, and anemia.
- Positive rheumatoid factor; presence alone does not confirm RA.
- Red blood cell (RBC) count, decreased.
- C4 complement component, decreased.
- C-reactive protein, positive.
- Arthrocentesis: cloudy, milky, dark yellow synovial fluid with increased leukocytes.
- Bone scan, MRI, CT scan, joint scan.
- X-ray: bony erosions, narrowed joint spaces.[1]

Treatment includes:

- Cold therapy during acute episodes.
- Heat therapy to relax muscles.
- Physical therapy.
- Weight control.
- Aspirin.
- NSAIDs.
- Antimetabolite: methotrexate (Rheumatrex).
- Antirheumatic: hydroxychloroquine (Plaquenil).
- Corticosteroids: prednisone (Deltasone).
- Gold therapy: gold sodium thiomalate (Myochrysine).[1]

What can harm my client?

- Infection.
- Malnutrition.
- Immobility.
- Systemic involvement resulting in organ failure.

If I were your teacher, I would test you on . . .

- Psychosocial care of the RA client.
- Medication administration and monitoring for side effects.
- Management of sleep disturbance, anorexia, pain, and fatigue.
- Safety precautions and measures for this population.
- Signs and symptoms and why of RA.

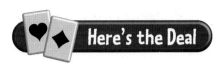

Here's the Deal

Corticosteroids are the most effective RA medication for unremitting inflammation and pain. Antirheumatic agents like methotrexate are effective, but they need time in the body before they become effective.

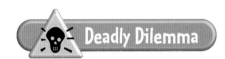

Deadly Dilemma

Remember that those clients with progressive RA need to be careful regarding temperature changes and should wear proper foot and hand attire because of paresthesias in the hands and feet.

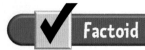

Factoid

When a client has SLE, every organ of the body can become affected at some point.

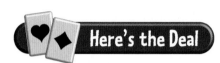

Here's the Deal

Many women have flare-ups during their menstrual cycle due to the added stress on the body. Therefore, flare-ups decrease with menopause.

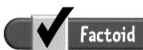

Factoid

SLE mainly affects women between 15 and 40 years; it affects African Americans more than Caucasians.[1]

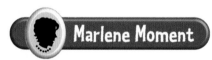

Marlene Moment

One of my favorite clients was a young lady with lupus. I cared for her for many weeks in the ICU: braided her hair, polished her fingernails, and made sure she was as comfortable as possible. Later, she was moved to the floor where she coded and passed away. I will never forget her dimples. Some patients never leave us. . . .

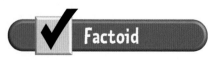

Factoid

With SLE, think "autoimmunity."

- What causes RA and why.
- Diagnostic testing for RA.

✚ Systemic lupus erythematosus (SLE) at a glance

What is it?

- Autoimmune disorder that involves most organ systems.
- Characterized by periods of exacerbation and remission.

What causes it?

- Dysfunctional immune system that causes overproduction of autoantibodies.
- Results in inflammation of the veins and arteries.
- Source is a combination of genetics, hormones, environmental factors, viruses, and medications.

Signs and symptoms

(The "why" is not always identifiable with autoimmune disorders. As you can see many different systems can be affected.) Think inflammation:

- Arthritis: joint swelling, tenderness, pain.
- Skin rash.
- Butterfly rash across the bridge of the nose and cheeks.
- Skin lesions that worsen during flares and exposure to sunlight.
- Alopecia, especially during flare-ups.
- Oral and nasal ulcers.
- Pleuritic pain with deep inspiration.
- Pericarditis, which causes chest pain.
- Atherosclerosis.
- Fatigue.
- Glomerulonephritis, renal illness.
- Hypertension.
- Impaired cognitive function, depression, psychosis.
- Lymphadenopathy, splenomegaly, hepatomegaly.
- Anemia, leukopenia, thrombocytopenia.[1]

Quickie tests and treatments

Tests include:

- ANA, positive.
- Decreased complement fixation.
- Decreased hemoglobin, hematocrit, white blood cells, platelets.
- Increased erythrocyte sedimentation rate (ESR).
- Lupus erythematosus cell preparation, positive.
- Rheumatoid factor, positive.
- Proteinuria and hematuria on urinalysis.[1]

Treatments include:

- Aspirin.
- NSAIDs.
- Antianemics: ferrous sulfate (Feosol).
- Antirheumatic: hydroxychloroquine (Plaquenil).
- Cytotoxic drugs: methotrexate (Folex).
- Steroids: prednisone (Deltasone).
- Immunosuppressants: azathioprine (Imuran).
- Scheduled rest periods.
- If renal failure, hemodialysis or kidney transplant.
- Dietary iron, protein, vitamins.
- Plasmapheresis.[1]

What can harm my client?

- Infection.
- Malnutrition.
- Renal failure.
- Seizures.
- Heart disease.
- Severe depression or psychosis that may lead to suicide.

If I were your teacher, I would test you on . . .

- Signs and symptoms and causes of SLE.
- Patient teaching: exposure to sunlight, smoking cessation, stress reduction, skin care.
- Medication administration and monitoring of side effects (especially steroids!).
- Signs and symptoms of renal failure, depression, psychosis.
- Teaching patient to avoid hair spray, hair coloring, blow dryers, oral contraceptives, facial powders.
- Monitoring for infection and change in vital signs.

✚ Gout

Gout is an immune disorder with metabolic origins. Gout affects more males that females and the incidence increases with age and body mass index.[1]

What is it?

Primary gout is due to severe dieting or starvation, excessive intake of foods high in purines (shellfish, organ meats), or heredity. Secondary gout is caused by drug therapy (diuretics), an increase in cell turnover (leukemia), and an increase in cell breakdown. Uric acid deposits build up in the joints, mainly in the feet and legs, causing painful arthritic joints.

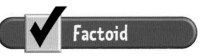

Factoid

When all of the blood elements are depressed, the term "pancytopenia" is used. "Pan" meaning everything. Lupus clients may have blood problems due to increased numbers of circulating antibodies.

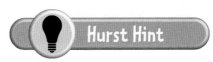

Hurst Hint

A flare-up may be close at hand if the client starts to complain of GI symptoms like nausea or diarrhea.

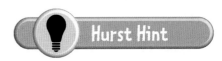

Hurst Hint

Encourage your client to relax, relax, relax! Yoga, meditation, and exercise are great ways to relax. Remember this too when scheduling your client for procedures while in hospital.

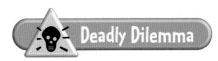

Deadly Dilemma

Since the client's immune system is depressed, she should always check with her physician prior to receiving any immunization or flu shot.

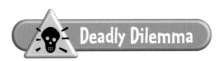

Deadly Dilemma

SLE: When clients are on steroids, they should never stop taking them suddenly. This can lead to an Addisonian crisis, shock, and death!

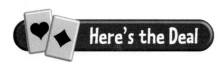

SLE: Since long-term steroid therapy is a major treatment, the bones may become affected as steroids cause osteoporosis and decrease blood supply to joints. The hip is the major area of complaint.

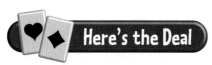

SLE: Fatigue exacerbates lupus.

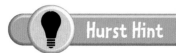

SLE: Don't forget to teach your client to wear sunscreen, long sleeves, and big hats!

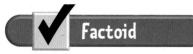

SLE: Watch for proteinuria, as this is the most common kidney problem the lupus client experiences.

Gout occurs intermittently, but can lead to chronic disability, severe hypertension, and renal disease. Compliance with a treatment regimen leads to a good prognosis.[1]

What causes it and why

Table 3-9 shows the causes and reasons for gout.

Table 3-9

Causes	Why
Increased uric acid	Over-secretion of uric acid or a renal defect that decreases secretion of uric acid
Genetic predisposition	Can be passed down in families

Source: Created by author from Reference #1.

Signs and symptoms and why

Table 3-10 shows the signs and symptoms for gout.

Table 3-10

Signs and symptoms	Why
Pain, inflammation of joints, especially great toe	Urate crystals form in the joints, especially in the toe due to gravity
Tophi of the great toe, hands (Fig. 3-4), ear	Repeated attacks and continued buildup of urate crystals deposit in peripheral areas of the body
Kidney stones	Kidneys not able to excrete excess uric acid
Joint enlargement	Loss of joint motion
Back pain	Kidneys tender due to excess buildup of uric acid

Source: Created by author from Reference #1.

▶ Figure 3-4. Tophi of the hands.

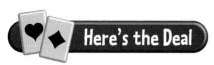

SLE: The leading cause of death in SLE clients is kidney disease.

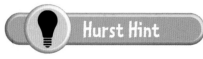

SLE: The good news is lupus is usually controllable with close supervision.

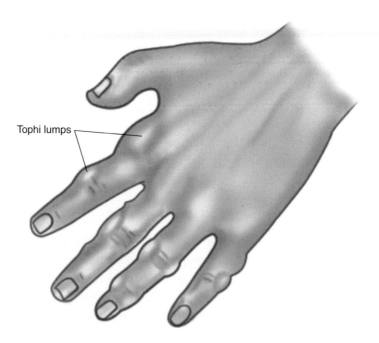

Tophi lumps

Quickie tests and treatments

- Arthrocentesis of inflamed joint or tophus: urate crystals present.
- Serum concentration of uric acid greater than 7 mg/dL.
- X-ray shows cartilage and bone damage.
- Alkaline ash diet to increase urine pH.
- Antigout drugs: allopurinol (Zyloprim).
- Uricosuric drugs: probenecid (Benemid).
- Corticosteroids: betamethasone (Celestone).
- Alkalinizing drugs: sodium bicarbonate.
- NSAIDs.[1]

What can harm my client?

The most prevalent complication with gout is renal illness, which although rare, can lead to kidney failure.

If I were your teacher, I would test you on . . .

- Patient teaching regarding avoiding alcohol and high-purine foods.
- Patient teaching regarding weight reduction.
- Causes and signs and symptoms of gout.
- Positioning of involved extremities (especially during acute episodes).
- Nonpharmacological measures to relieve pain.
- Administration and monitoring of pain medications.
- Interventions to prevent renal calculi, kidney illness.
- Monitoring for side effects of antigout drugs.

✚ Fibromyalgia

Fibromyalgia is seen in 3% to 6% of the general population—mostly women, and is most commonly diagnosed in individuals between the ages of 20 and 50.[1]

What is it?

Fibromyalgia is a syndrome of multiple etiologies that affects the immune and central nervous systems and many organs. It is a syndrome of chronic pain and not a disease of inflammation.[1]

What causes it and why

Patients with fibromyalgia have abnormal levels of substance P, which amplifies pain signals to and from the brain. For these patients, it is as if the pain volume is turned way up, causing persistent and chronic pain. Serotonin, which normally reduces the intensity of pain signals, is found in low levels in fibromyalgia patients. Serotonin also plays an important role in sleep regulation. Fibromyalgia patients have sleep disturbances, which also contribute to the increased pain. A history of viral or immune illnesses and physical trauma are believed to contribute to fibromyalgia as well.

Signs and symptoms and why

Table 3-11 shows the signs and symptoms of fibromyalgia.

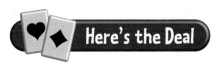

SLE: Clients with SLE should avoid birth control pills, sulfa drugs, and penicillin, as all of these can cause flare-ups! We don't like flare-ups!

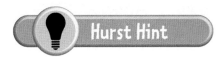

Gout: Some people call gout "gouty arthritis."

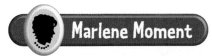

Gout: Patients with gout need to steer clear of beer, wine, anchovies, liver, sardines, kidneys, sweetbreads, lentils, shellfish, and all other organ meats. No more liver and onions at the local cafeteria!

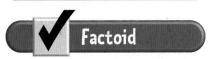

Gout: Do you know what sweetbreads really are? No, not a muffin . . . intestines! Yum! In the country we call them chitterlings. The proper pronunciation is "chitlins." Avoid all organ meats if you are "gouty."

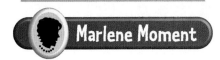

Gout: Jeffrey Dahmer wouldn't have been compliant on this diet due to his love of organ meats!

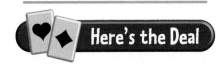

Gout: A gouty attack can be precipitated by anything that promotes dehydration: diuretics, extreme diets, or happy hour!

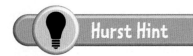

Hurst Hint

Gout: The first thing to think of with gout is this: Big, hot, red toe!

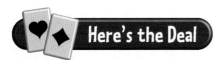

Here's the Deal

Gout: Even the sheets touching the toe or affected joint can increase pain.

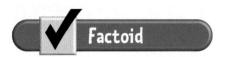

Factoid

Gout: When taking probenecid, the client should avoid aspirin, because when taken together they increase uric acid retention. Not good!

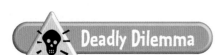

Deadly Dilemma

Gout: If a gout client is on steroids and NSAIDs, watch for GI bleeding as these drugs are very irritating to GI system.

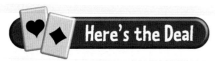

Here's the Deal

Gout: Clients with gout better drink a lot of water to flush out the excess uric acid . . . about 2-3 L/day is groovy!

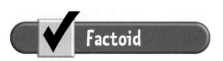

Factoid

Gout: Choose acetaminophen rather than aspirin as a test answer, as aspirin can bring on gouty attacks.

Table 3-11

Signs and symptoms	Why
Chronic pain	Abnormal levels of substance P
Chronic fatigue	Abnormal levels of serotonin, sleep disturbances, pain
Cognitive changes: short-term memory deficit, brain fog, word mix-ups, lack of concentration	Sleep deprivation
Paresthesias	Disturbances in the function of neurons in the sensory pathway
Restless leg syndrome	Neurological dysfunction; exact cause unknown
Lack of coordination	Neurological dysfunction, sleep deprivation

Source: Created by author from Reference #6.

Other signs and symptoms of fibromyalgia may include:

- Migraine headaches.
- Abdominal pain.
- Irritable bowel syndrome.
- Skin color changes.
- Temporomandibular joint (TMJ) disorder.[6]

Quickie tests and treatments

There is no clear diagnostic test to determine fibromyalgia. Laboratory tests and x-rays are used to rule out other conditions. Fibromyalgia is diagnosed by the presence of widespread pain in combination with tenderness at specific locations and chronic fatigue.

Treatments include:

- Regular, moderate exercise program.
- Scheduled periods of rest.
- Relaxation techniques, stretching, keeping warm, high-quality sleep.
- Tricyclic agents: amitriptyline (Elavil).
- Selective serotonin reuptake inhibitors (SSRIs): fluoxetine (Prozac).
- Anxiolytic agents: clonazepam (Klonopin).
- Muscle relaxants: cyclobenzaprine (Flexeril).
- Antiseizure agents: pregabalin (Lyrica).
- NSAIDs.[6]

What can harm my client?

Fibromyalgia is not life-threatening, although the physical symptoms can be very uncomfortable. Patients may have difficulty dealing with the psychosocial aspects of the syndrome such as:

- Depression.
- Anxiety.
- Grief: not able to participate in life activities as once able.
- Frustration: no clear treatment, lack of understanding from family, friends, health care providers.
- Anger.

If I were your teacher, I would test you on . . .

- Teaching the patient about scheduling rest periods, decreasing stress, and techniques to help induce sleep.
- Medication administration and possible side effects.
- Causes and signs and symptoms of fibromyalgia.
- Psychosocial care of clients with fibromyalgia.

✚ Chronic fatigue syndrome at a glance

What is it?

- Chronic fatigue syndrome (CFS) is a syndrome of multiple etiologies that affect the immune and central nervous systems and many organs.
- Debilitating, severe chronic fatigue that affects most body systems with periods of exacerbation and remission.

What causes it?

When dealing with immune disorders, the "why's" are not always identifiable.

- Immune dysfunction.
- Infectious agents.
- Hormonal abnormalities.
- Nutritional deficiencies.[7]

Signs and symptoms

- Severe, incapacitating fatigue not improved by bed rest and worsened by physical or mental activity.
- Decreased physical activity and stamina.
- Difficulties with memory and concentration.
- Impaired sleep.
- Persistent muscle pain.
- Joint pain (without redness or swelling).
- Headaches.
- Tender lymph nodes.
- Increased malaise following exertion.
- Sore throat.
- Irritable bowel.

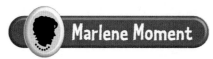

Marlene Moment

Gout: "I'll have the beef consommé, meat with intestines and mushroom gravy, asparagus, and a double Crown and Coke, please (I need some fluid to wash down my Lasix)." I've been longing for a good gout attack!

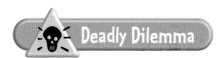

Deadly Dilemma

Gout: Colchicine, an antigout drug, can cause GI upset. Be sure to monitor your patients for this side effect.

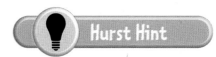

Hurst Hint

Gout: Think fluids when caring for these patients! They must keep their kidneys flushed to prevent stone formation.

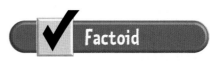

Factoid

Gout: Clients with gout need to be on a low-fat diet because fat decreases excretion of uric acid. We want to get rid of uric acid!

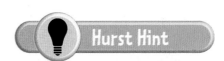

Hurst Hint

Gout: Heat may be used to increase blood flow and remove waste products from the affected area; whereas cold packs may be used to decrease pain and inflammation.

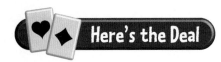

Here's the Deal

Gout: You must remind your patients to have their serum uric acid levels checked periodically to ensure the effectiveness of the treatment plan and patient compliance.

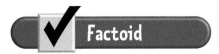

Factoid

Fibromyalgia: Fibromyalgia is not a psychological or muscular illness as once believed.

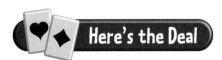

Here's the Deal

Fibromyalgia: Fibromyalgia is most common in young to middle-aged women.

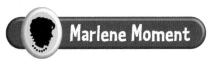

Marlene Moment

Fibromyalgia: It is known that patients with fibromyalgia do not hit deep, restorative sleep. I'm getting sleepy, sleepy, sleepy . . . just thinking about it!

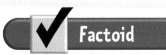

Factoid

Fibromyalgia: To be diagnosed with fibromyalgia, a client must have discomfort at 11 or more designated tender points called "trigger points."

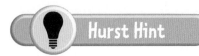

Hurst Hint

Fibromyalgia: Fibromyalgia clients should not chew gum and should avoid foods that are difficult to chew, as this stresses the TM joint.

- Depression or psychological problems (irritability, mood swings, anxiety, panic attacks).
- Chills and night sweats.
- Visual disturbances (blurring, sensitivity to light, eye pain).
- Allergies or sensitivities to foods, odors, chemicals, medications, or noise.
- Brain fog.
- Difficulty maintaining upright position, dizziness, balance problems, or fainting.[7]

Quickie tests and treatments

- No diagnostic tests available.
- Clinical diagnosis using patient history and physical.
- Treat the symptoms (massage helps).
- Moderate activity and exercise.
- Scheduled rest periods.
- Stress management.
- Tai chi, acupuncture, herbs.
- Dietary supplements like evening primrose oil, fish oil, and vitamins may help, but not proven scientifically.
- Tricyclic agents: amitriptyline (Elavil).
- Antiviral drugs: acyclovir (Zovirax).
- Selective serotonin reuptake inhibitors (SSRIs): fluoxetine (Prozac).
- Anxiolytic agents: clonazepam (Klonopin).
- NSAIDs.
- Antihistamines.
- Antihypertensive beta-blockers: atenolol (Tenormin).[7]

What can harm my client?

- Lack of medical management or treatment.
- Severe depression that leads to suicide.
- Severe hypotension.

If I were your teacher, I would test you on . . .

- Patient education regarding diet, exercise, stress reduction, relaxation techniques.
- Medication administration and possible side effects.
- The causes and signs and symptoms of CFS.
- Nonpharmacological and pharmacological pain management.

SUMMARY

The immune system protects us from illness and is effective most of the time. When the immune system is compromised, the body falls prey to illness and disease that can challenge homeostasis. Nurses play a key role in maintaining client health by monitoring immune function and preventing immune dysfunction. Understanding the key concepts of immune function and related illnesses can help you provide optimum outcomes for your patients.

PRACTICE QUESTIONS

1. The following choices are risk factors for osteoarthritis (OA) except:

1. Obesity.

2. Genetic susceptibility.

3. Heart disease.

4. Increased age.

Correct answer: 3. Obesity, genetic susceptibility, and increased age are all risk factors for osteoarthritis. Heart disease is not.

2. When taking care of the client diagnosed with gout, the nurse monitors for an increased level in:

1. Uric acid.

2. Calcium.

3. Sodium.

4. Creatinine.

Correct answer: 1. Increased uric acid is specific to gout. Increased levels of calcium, sodium, and creatinine are not specific to gout.

3. The most effective medication therapy used for treating systemic lupus erythematosus (SLE) is:

1. NSAIDs.

2. Corticosteroids.

3. Immunosuppressive agents.

4. Antimalarials.

Correct answer: 2. Corticosteroids are the most effective treatment for SLE. While antimalarials, immunosuppressive agents, and NSAIDs may be a part of treatment, they are not as effective as corticosteroids in combating inflammation and pain.

4. A 26-year-old female client presents to the emergency department (ED) with complaints of joint swelling, fatigue, and weight loss. While interviewing the client, the nurse notes a rash extending from the client's bridge of the nose to both cheeks. The nurse recognizes this symptom as unique to:

1. Rheumatoid arthritis.

2. Gout.

3. Scleroderma.

4. Systemic lupus erythematosus.

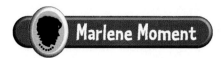

Marlene Moment

Fibromyalgia: Some fibromyalgia patients equate their pain to running a marathon every single day! Others equate their daily fatigue as being similar to that experienced with the flu! Can you imagine?

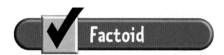

Factoid

Fibromyalgia: Stress and exertion can make fibromyalgia worse.

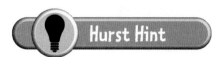

Hurst Hint

Fibromyalgia: Fibromyalgia patients typically look healthy and have no outward signs of pain or discomfort.[6]

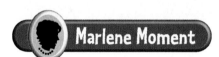

Marlene Moment

CFS: Many people want to call CFS a psychiatric disorder, which it is not. If a client has swollen lymph nodes, inflamed oropharynx, and fever . . . this pretty much rules out the pure psychiatric diagnosis. Duh!

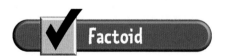

Factoid

CFS: CFS is mainly seen in women, especially Hispanics.

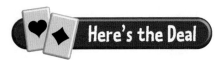

CFS: To be diagnosed with CFS, the client must report extreme fatigue for 6 months or longer, which usually follows flu-like symptoms. In addition, the client must report at least 4 other symptoms such as sore throat, muscle or joint pain, headaches, and fatigue after waking from sleep.

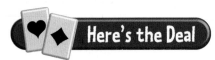

CFS: It was once believed that CFS was caused by the Epstein–Barr virus. However, new studies show this doesn't necessarily cause CFS, but the virus could quicken the onset of CFS symptoms.[7]

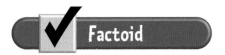

CFS: Too much rest may make CFS worse.

Correct answer: 4. A butterfly rash extending from the bridge of the nose to both cheeks is unique to systemic lupus erythematosus (SLE). The butterfly rash is not present in rheumatoid arthritis, gout, or scleroderma.

5. A 24-year-old female client is found to have a latex allergy. Which item poses the least risk for this client?

1. Condom.

2. Feminine hygiene pad.

3. Balloon.

4. Brazil nut.

Correct answer: 4. Condoms, feminine hygiene pads, and balloons may all contain latex. Foods such as banana, avocado, kiwi, passion fruit, strawberry, and chestnut contain some of the same allergens found in latex. Brazil nuts are not linked to latex allergy.

6. A laboratory result of positive C-reactive protein is indicative of which immune disorder?

1. Rheumatoid arthritis.

2. Osteoarthritis.

3. Gout.

4. Systemic lupus erythematosus.

Correct answer: 1. A positive C-reactive protein may be present in rheumatoid arthritis. C-reactive protein is not present in osteoarthritis, gout, or systemic lupus erythematosus.

7. An 8-year-old client is admitted to the emergency department (ED) with symptoms of an allergic response as a result of ingesting jelly beans. The initial action by the nurse should be:

1. Obtain a complete medical history from the parents.

2. Assess for dyspnea or laryngeal edema.

3. Place the client on a cardiac monitor.

4. Administer an antihistamine.

Correct answer: 2. The initial intervention by the nurse is to assess for dyspnea or laryngeal edema associated with an allergic reaction and anaphylaxis. The other answer options are appropriate nursing measures to take after assessing and managing for an open airway.

8. The nurse is teaching a client about the management of fibromyalgia. Which is the most appropriate statement made by the nurse?

    1. "You will feel awful every day for the rest of your life."

    2. "You can beat this illness by exercising vigorously 2 hours every day."

    3. "You will have days when you feel OK and others when you don't feel well."

    4. "You must adhere to the low-sodium, low-fat diet to keep symptoms at bay."

Correct answer: 3. Fibromyalgia is characterized by periods of exacerbation and remission. The client will have days where she feels good and others when she feels poorly. Moderate exercise alternated with rest periods is recommended for fibromyalgia patients. Clients with fibromyalgia may find that certain foods trigger their symptoms, such as chocolate and alcohol, but they do not need to adhere to a low-sodium, low-fat diet.

9. Clients with chronic fatigue syndrome often have difficulty sleeping. Which factor is not associated with the sleeping aspect of chronic fatigue syndrome?

    1. Frequent awakening.

    2. Restless legs.

    3. Nocturia.

    4. Vivid dreaming.

Correct answer: 3. Nocturia, waking in the night with the urge to urinate, is not associated with the sleep disturbances of chronic fatigue syndrome. Clients with chronic fatigue syndrome have difficulty falling asleep, hypersomnia, frequent awakening, intense and vivid dreaming, restless legs, and nocturnal myoclonus. Most CFS patients experience nonrestorative sleep as compared to their pre-illness experience.

10. Fibromyalgia is caused by abnormal levels of:

    1. Melatonin.

    2. Substance P.

    3. Norepinephrine.

    4. Lutropin.

Correct answer: 2. Patients with fibromyalgia have abnormal levels of substance P and serotonin, which contribute to the chronic pain and sleep disturbances.

References

1. Smeltzer SC, Bare BG, eds. *Brunner & Suddarth's Textbook of Medical-Surgical Nursing*. 10th ed. Philadelphia: Lippincott Williams & Wilkins; 2004.

2. American Latex Allergy Association. *Latex Allergy Statistics*. Available at: http://www.latexallergyresources.org/topics/LatexAllergyStatistics.cfm. Accessed January 2, 2007.

3. Allen KD, Boucher MA, Cain JE, et al. *Manual of Nursing Practice Pocket Guides: Medical-Surgical Nursing*. Ambler, PA: Lippincott Williams & Wilkins; 2007.

4. Arthritis Foundation. *Osteoarthritis Fact Sheet*. Available at: http://www.arthritis.org/conditions/Fact_Sheets/OA_Fact_Sheet.asp. Accessed January 3, 2007.

5. Arthritis Foundation. *Rheumatoid Arthritis Overview*. Available at http://www.arthritis.org/conditions/DiseaseCenter/RA/ra_overview.asp. Accessed January 3, 2007.

6. Arthritis Foundation. *Fibromyalgia*. Available at: http://www.arthritis.org/conditions/DiseaseCenter/Fibromyalgia/fibromyalgia_symptoms.asp. Accessed January 3, 2006.

7. Centers for Disease Control and Prevention. *Chronic Fatigue Syndrome*. Available at http://www.cdc.gov/cfs/. Accessed January 3, 2007.

Bibliography

Hurst Review Services. www.hurstreview.com.

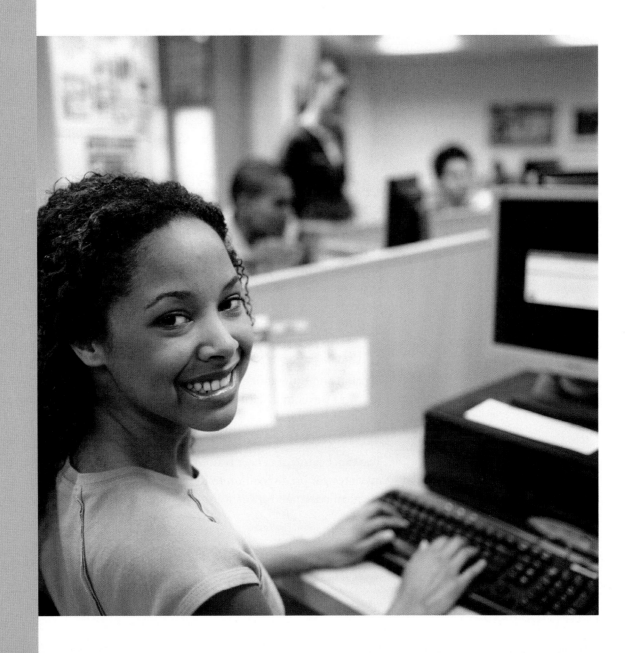

CHAPTER

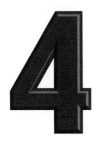

Oncology

OBJECTIVES

In this chapter, you'll review:

- The causes and risk factors of common cancers.
- The signs and symptoms associated with common cancers.
- Need-to-know information regarding common cancers including diagnostic tests, treatments, and possible complications.

LET'S GET THE NORMAL STUFF STRAIGHT FIRST

Oncology may look like an enormous topic that you'll never be able to tackle, right? Wrong! We will work together to master the need-to-know oncology information! Let's begin with what you do know: Oncology is the branch of medicine that deals with tumors, including their development, diagnosis, treatment, and prevention.[1] Cancer is any disease characterized by abnormal cell growth and development caused by damaged DNA. In cancer, the malignant cells can no longer perform division and differentiation normally. They can invade surrounding tissues and travel to distant sites in the body, wreaking all kinds of havoc.

✚ What causes cancer and why

The exact cause of cancer is not known, but there are several factors that may create a predisposition to developing cancer. Table 4-1 demonstrates the most common factors for developing cancer.

Table 4-1

Lifestyle	Genetics	Environment	Personal
Tobacco use	Family history	Radiation	Age
Alcohol		Viruses	Fitness
Diet		Infections	Occupation
Sexual behavior		Environmental carcinogens	Immune function
Obesity			Race
Stress			Reproductive history
			Hormones

Source: Created by author using Reference #2.

Nonmalignant versus malignant

Cancer is the result of wild and unchecked growth of abnormal cells. When these cells begin their growth, they may become nonmalignant cancer cells or malignant cancer cells. The nonmalignant cancer cells can create problems by displacing normal tissue or creating lumps and bumps where there shouldn't be any. These problems are generally self-limiting and can easily be treated by removing the growth, so long as the growth is in a place where it can be removed. Nonmalignant cancers become a problem when they are difficult to remove or they are poorly differentiated—not neatly enclosed. If a nonmalignant cancer spreads in a tentacle-like manner, winding around healthy tissue and organs, it can become just as deadly as a malignant tumor by cutting off the blood supply to the healthy tissues or organs.

Malignant cancers grow wildly and like to spread to other tissues or organs throughout the body. These malignant cells take over the normal cells and damage that tissue or organ, and then spread (generally through the lymph system) to other tissues and organs. Left untreated, malignant cancers may kill your patient.

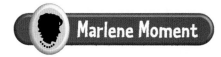

Just because cancer cells are non-malignant doesn't mean that they aren't trouble!

✚ Signs and symptoms and why

The signs and symptoms of cancer are very well known and are advertised regularly by the American Cancer Society. The seven warning signs of cancer create the acronym CAUTION:

Change in bowel or bladder habits.

A sore that does not heal.

Unusual bleeding or discharge.

Thickening or lump in the breast or elsewhere.

Indigestion or difficulty swallowing.

Obvious changes in a wart or mole.

Nagging cough or hoarseness.[3,4]

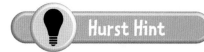

It is extremely important that you use the CAUTION acronym when taking a patient history.

Cancer cells grow like crazy and travel to all parts of the body to set up housekeeping where they are not wanted or needed. The result is metastasis of the malignant cells. New sites are invaded by the cells, the cells multiply, and metastatic tumors appear. These tumors can affect body tissues and organs by causing the signs and symptoms listed above.

LET'S GET DOWN TO THE SPECIFICS

For the remainder of this chapter, we will focus on the most commonly diagnosed cancers in the United States according to the North American Association of Central Cancer Registries (NAACCR) and the American Cancer Society (ACS).[5,6] I will provide you with the need-to-know core content to help you understand the pathology, signs and symptoms, and patient care of common cancers. This understanding will help you excel in the classroom and in the clinical setting.

✚ Let's begin with breast

According to the American Cancer Society, breast cancer is the leading site for cancer among women.[7] Although breast cancer mainly affects women, men are at a low risk for developing the disease and should be aware of the risk factors including family history. Both men and women should report any change in their breasts to a physician immediately.

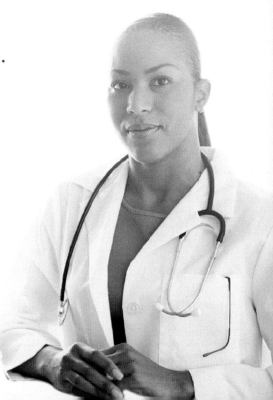

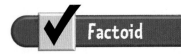

Factoid

Sixty percent of breast cancers occur after age 60. The risk is at its greatest after age 75.[2]

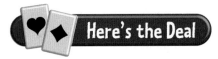

Here's the Deal

Hormones that increase breast maturation may increase the chance for cell mutations.

What is it?

Breast cancer is the growth of malignant cells lining the ducts or lobules of the breast that spread by way of the lymphatic system and the bloodstream. The malignant cells travel through the right side of the heart to the lungs and to the other breast, chest wall, liver, bone, and brain.[4]

Breast cancer is classified as:

- Adenocarcinoma: the most common form that arises from the epithelial tissues.
- Intraductal: develops within the ducts.
- Infiltrating: occurs in the parenchymal tissue.
- Inflammatory (rare): grows rapidly, causing the overlying skin to become edematous, inflamed, and indurated.
- Lobular: involves the lobes of the glandular tissue.
- Medullary or circumscribed: enlarging tumor that grows rapidly.[4]

What causes it and why

The exact cause of breast cancer is unknown. However, several risk factors that may increase the chances of developing breast cancer are listed in Table 4-2.

Table 4-2

Risk factors	Why
Family history of breast cancer	Breast cancer in the client's mother, sister, or daughter (first-degree relatives) increases the risk of developing breast cancer 2 to 3 times
Age	Longer exposure to estrogens that can cause cell mutations
Breast cancer gene	There are 2 separate genes for breast cancer. These genes are seen in less than 1% of women; however, if a female has one of these genes it increases her chances of getting breast cancer by 50% to 85%
Early onset of menses	The earlier a client starts menses, the greater the chance of developing breast cancer due to longer exposure of estrogen that may cause cell mutations
Late menopause	Longer exposure to estrogens that may cause cell mutations
Estrogen therapy	Most studies do not show a relationship between estrogen use and breast cancer, but use of estrogens is still listed as a risk factor as the jury is still out on this topic
Endometrial or ovarian cancer	Immunosuppression and hormonal changes that cause cell mutations
First pregnancy after age 35	Longer exposure to estrogen that causes cell mutations
Nulligravida (never pregnant)	Doubles the risk for breast cancer; longer exposure to estrogens that causes cell mutations
Radiation exposure, especially before age 30	Causes cell mutations and immunosuppression
Alcohol or tobacco use	Make it easier for cancer-causing substances to enter and damage individual cells. Alcohol may temporarily increase the concentration of estrogens that circulate in the blood, causing cell mutations
Obesity	Risk is higher for postmenopausal, obese women due to estrogen changes and high-fat diet
High-fat diet	Fat triggers estrogen, fueling tumor growth

Source: Created by author from References #2 and #4.

Signs and symptoms and why

The signs and symptoms of breast cancer are caused by the travel of the malignant cells to body tissues and organs where they clump to form tumors. Half of all breast cancers develop in the upper outer quadrant of the breast, while the nipple is the second most common site, followed by the upper inner quadrant, the lower outer quadrant, and finally, the lower inner quadrant.[4]

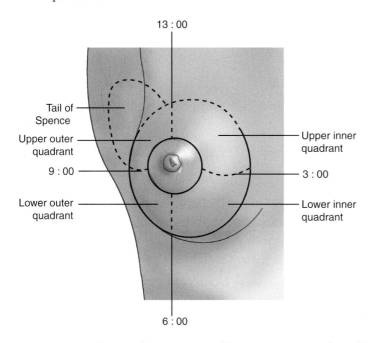

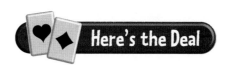

Early menstruation, late menopause, pregnancy in later age, and never becoming pregnant increase the risk for breast cancer due to longer exposure to estrogens, which may increase cancer growth.

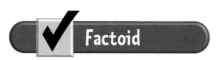

Most clients with breast cancer have no identifiable risk factors. In many cases, it is still a guessing game.

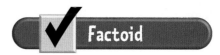

Specific genes have been linked to breast cancer, confirming the possibility of inheritance of the disease.

The most common signs and symptoms of breast cancer are found in Table 4-3.

Table 4-3

Signs and symptoms	Why
Painless lump or mass on palpation	Cells clump to form tumors but don't carry pain nerve impulses
Clear, milky, or bloody discharge	Cells of breast tissue do not function properly
Asymmetry of breasts	Tumor growth in one breast
Change in skin tissue—dimpling, inflammation	Tumor pulls and retracts skin tissue
Change in breast tissue—thickening	Tumor growth displaces breast tissue
Nipple retraction or scaly skin around nipple	Tumor growth displaces breast tissue
Arm edema	Lymph nodes responsible for tissue drainage may be affected causing the edema; arm edema may indicate metastasis
Enlargement of the cervical, supraclavicular, or axillary lymph nodes	Lymph node involvement; not able to function effectively

Source: Created by the author from Reference #4.

Quickie tests and treatments

I'm not going to cover all of the diagnostic tests, medications, and treatments for breast cancer, but I'll highlight the main ones you should know. Breast cancer is best detected by monthly self-breast examination (SBE).

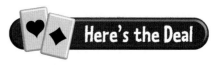

In more than 80% of the cases, the client discovers the lump herself.

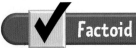

Factoid

In the early stages, the tumor may be movable; in later stages, the tumor fixes itself and becomes nonmovable.

Hurst Hint

The most common tumor location is the upper outer quadrant of the breast. This area includes the tail of Spence that reaches up under the arm.

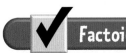

Factoid

Peau d'orange is a change in breast skin that resembles the pitted skin of an orange.

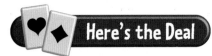

Here's the Deal

A rare type of breast cancer is called Paget's disease, which involves the nipple epithelium.

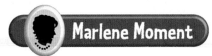

Marlene Moment

It is critical that all women know how to perform SBE. This is one of the earliest and easiest ways to detect a lump or mass. Don't be shy! Spread the word!

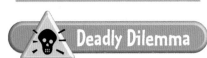

Deadly Dilemma

When caring for a postoperative mastectomy patient, post a sign in **BIG, BOLD** print above the patient's bed that warns not to perform venipunctures or blood pressure monitoring on the affected arm.

Screening mammography is recommended for all women over age 40 every 1 to 2 years and every year for women over age 50. Calcification on mammography is indicative of breast cancer. Once the tumor is located via mammography, a tissue sample is taken by fine-needle aspiration for biopsy to identify the type and stage of the tumor.

Treatments include:

- Surgery.
- Chemotherapy.
- Radiation.
- Analgesics.
- Antiemetics.
- Chemotherapy agents: cyclophosphamide (Cytoxan), methotrexate (Folex).
- Hormonal therapy: tamoxifen (Nolvadex).[7]

What can harm my client?

You should be aware of certain actions that may cause harm to your patients with breast cancer. As the nurse, it is your professional duty and responsibility to keep your patients free from harm. The following can potentially harm your patient with breast cancer:

- Performing venipuncture or blood pressure monitoring on the affected arm. (The arm associated with the side where mastectomy was performed)
- Malnutrition.
- Infection.
- Severe immunosuppression.
- Abduction or external rotation to the affected arm.[4]

If I were your teacher, I would test you on . . .

Items that may appear on your test are:

- Importance of providing emotional support to breast cancer patients and their families.
- Self-breast exam (SBE) techniques.
- Teaching clients to prepare for a mammogram. (No lotions, powder, deodorant)
- Postoperative positioning.
- Preventing postoperative complications.
- Treatment-related complications, such as leukopenia, thrombocytopenia, bleeding, nausea, vomiting, and anorexia.
- Importance of protecting arm on side where mastectomy occurred (there are many things the client should avoid such as taking BP using this arm to avoiding sunburn).

✚ Prostate, not prostrate

Prostate cancer is the most common cancer, other than skin cancers, in American men. The American Cancer Society (ACS) estimates that during 2006 about 234,460 new cases of prostate cancer were diagnosed in the

United States. About 1 man in 6 will be diagnosed with prostate cancer during his lifetime, but only 1 man in 34 will die of it. Prostate cancer accounts for about 10% of cancer-related deaths in men. A little over 1.8 million men in the United States are survivors of prostate cancer.[8]

What is it?

Prostate cancer (Fig. 4-1) is the slow growth of cancer cells in the form of tumors that originate in the posterior prostate gland, which may progress to widespread bone metastasis and death. Primary prostatic lesions can invade the ejaculatory ducts and seminal vesicle. Androgens have been shown to speed tumor growth.[4,9]

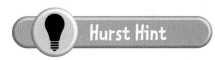

Hurst Hint

I can promise you that you will be asked questions about the positioning, recovery exercises, and care of the affected arm in a mastectomy patient. Better review it!

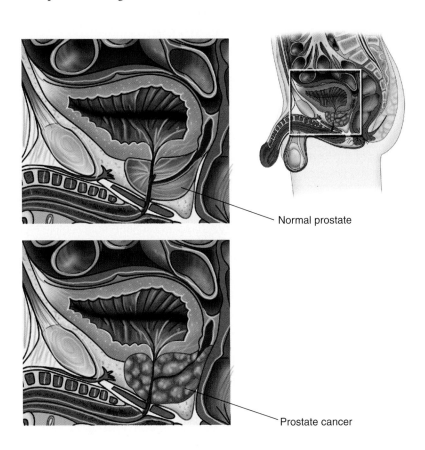

Normal prostate

Prostate cancer

◀ Figure 4-1. Prostate cancer.

What causes it and why

The exact causes of prostate cancer are unknown, but risk factors are shown in Table 4-4.

Table 4-4

Risk factors	Why
Age over 50 years	The aging process produces biochemical reactions that contribute to abnormal cell growth
Family history	There are a few specific genes that may be responsible for prostate cancer that are passed down in families
High-fat diet	Fat can trigger hormone growth that can feed tumors
Testosterone	Does not cause prostate cancer, but feeds its growth

Source: Created by author from Reference #10.

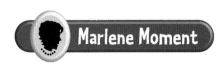

Marlene Moment

Some people pronounce prostate "prostrate." The prostate is a male reproductive organ. Prostrate means to be reduced to helplessness—a common feeling for nursing students!

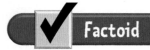

Signs and symptoms and why

Prostate cancer usually has no symptoms, especially in the early stages. Symptoms can occur when the cancer grows into the prostate gland and narrows the urethra. Common signs and symptoms are shown in Table 4-5.

Table 4-5

Signs and symptoms	Why
Difficulty initiating a urinary stream	Tumor pressure on the prostate gland, narrowed urethra
Dribbling	Infection, narrowed urethra
Painless hematuria	Infection
Urine retention	Nerve damage due to tumor pressure; bladder cannot empty completely as enlarged prostate is closing off urethra
Pain with sexual orgasm	Tumor pressure
Firm nodular mass with sharp edge	Tumor growth
Edema of the scrotum or leg (advanced disease)	Tumor growth, impaired lymphatics
Hard lump in the prostate region (advanced disease) change in voiding patterns (nocturia, frequency, urgency) decreased force of stream	Tumor growth as prostate is enlarged causing constriction on urethra, the bladder cannot empty completely
Bone pain	Bone metastasis

Source: Created by author from Reference #4.

Quickie tests and treatments

The American Cancer Society recommends that men older than age 40 receive a digital rectal exam and prostate-specific antigen (PSA) test yearly.
   Diagnostic tests:

- Transrectal prostatic ultrasonography.
- Bone scan.
- Excretory urography.
- Magnetic resonance imaging (MRI).
- Computed tomography (CT).[4]

Treatment varies with the stage of cancer, but can include:

- Chemotherapy.
- Radiation.
- Hormonal therapy.
- Radical prostatectomy.
- Transurethral resection of the prostate.
- Chemotherapy agents: mitoxantrone (Novantrone), vinblastine (Velban), paclitaxel (Taxol).
- Prednisone.

- Opioids.
- Bisphosphonates.
- Corticosteroids.[11]

What can harm my client?

Your care of the patient with prostate cancer should focus on therapies to reduce incontinence and pain. Keep in mind the following that can potentially jeopardize your patient's progress to recovery:

- Malnutrition.
- Infection.
- Severe immunosuppression.
- Dehydration.
- Weakness.
- Osteoporosis (side effect of treatments).
- Excessive bleeding or bruising.[12]

If I were your teacher, I would test you on . . .

- Signs and symptoms of prostate cancer and why they occur.
- Who is at risk of prostate cancer.
- Importance of providing emotional support to patients and their families.
- Monitoring pain and providing comfort measures.
- Proper wound assessment and care.
- Preventing postoperative complications.
- Teaching perineal exercises, such as Kegel exercises, to strengthen the pelvic muscles and decrease incontinence.
- Providing options for impotence.
- Importance of follow-up care and regular screening.
- Detailed care and teaching postop prostatectomy.
- What is a PSA test?

✚ Lung cancer

Lung cancer (Fig. 4-2) accounts for about 13% of all new cancers, with 70% of the people diagnosed with lung cancer being older than age 65. For men, 1 in 13 will develop lung cancer, and for women, it is 1 in 17.[13] Lung cancer is associated with a poor prognosis, with only 13% of patients surviving 5 years after diagnosis.[4]

What is it?

Lung cancer results from malignant tumors arising from the respiratory epithelium. The most common types of lung cancer are:

1. Epidermoid: squamous cell, which may cause bronchial obstruction.

2. Adenocarcinoma: metastasizes through the blood stream to other organs.

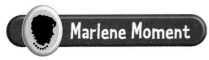

Marlene Moment

Now let's face it . . . a digital rectal exam is no fun for anyone. However, it can save lives when it comes to cancer detection!

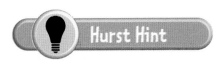

Hurst Hint

The majority of cancer patients are at risk for malnutrition. It is important to offer small meals and snacks, which include the patient's favorite foods. Maintaining metabolic demands is crucial in the fight against any cancer.

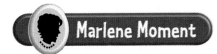

Marlene Moment

Kegel exercises aren't just for women!

► Figure 4-2. **A.** Healthy lung.
B. Smoker's lung with carcinoma.

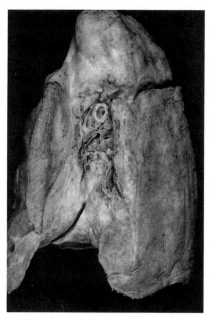
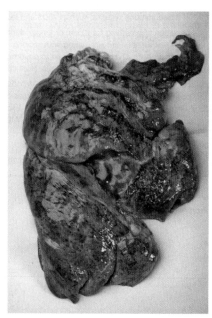

A   B

3. Oat cell: small cell, which metastasizes very early through the lymph vessels and bloodstream to other organs.

4. Anaplastic: large cell, which metastasizes extensively throughout the body.[4]

What causes it and why

The exact cause of lung cancer is unknown, but common risk factors are included in Table 4-6.

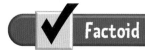
Factoid

In some cases, lung cancer is due to metastasis from other organs, such as the adrenal glands, brain, bone, kidneys, and liver.

Table 4-6

Risk factors	Why
Genetic predisposition	First-degree relatives of lung cancer patients have a 2 to 3.5 times greater risk of developing lung cancer
Tobacco smoking	Cellular damage
Exposure to environmental pollutants	Cellular damage
Exposure to occupational pollutants	Cellular damage

Source: Created by author from Reference #4.

♥ ♦ Here's the Deal

The symptoms of lung cancer may be caused by airway obstruction due to tumor growth, bronchial cell changes, and tumors that are thought to cause mucus production.[4]

Signs and symptoms and why

The most common signs and symptoms of lung cancer are found in Table 4-7.

Table 4-7

Signs and symptoms	Why
Cough	Usually first and most common symptom; irritants in the lungs
Finger clubbing	Chronic hypoxia
Enlarged liver	Immunosuppression; metastasis
Chest pain	Tumor growing into chest wall
Hemoptysis	Cancer growing into underlying vessels
Edema of the face, neck, upper torso	Tumor compressing the vena cava
Decreased breath sounds	Bronchial constriction
Chills and fever	Infection
Hoarseness	Cancer invading vocal cords
Superior vena cava syndrome	Tumor compressing vena cava causing upper body/facial swelling
Wheezing	Bronchial constriction; tumor narrowing the airway
Pleural friction rub	Tumor spreads into pleural space
Dyspnea	Tumor in lungs
Enlarged lymph nodes	Advanced disease and metastasis
Recurrent bronchitis, pneumonia	Immunosuppression; infection
Fatigue, weakness	Late sign
Anorexia, weight loss	Late sign

Source: Table created by author from Reference #4.

Quickie tests and treatments

Diagnostics:

- Bronchoscopy.
- Chest x-ray.
- Lung scan.
- Lung biopsy (Fig. 4-3).
- Sputum study.

Treatments:

- Oxygen therapy.
- Radiation.
- Chemotherapy.
- Immunotherapy.
- Surgery.
- Analgesics.
- Antiemetics.

▶ Figure 4-3. Lung biopsy.

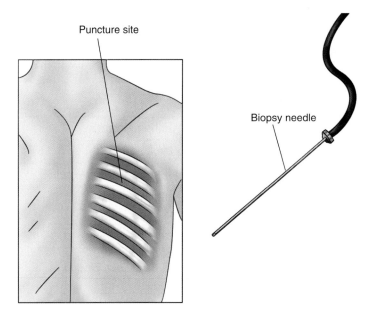

Puncture site

Biopsy needle

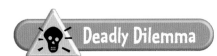

Deadly Dilemma

It is crucial that you always monitor the functioning of respiratory equipment, such as oxygen tubing and accessories, oxygen concentrator, mechanical ventilator, and suctioning machine.

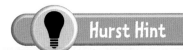

Hurst Hint

One sure fire way to test patency of a nasal cannula is to immerse the cannula in a cup of water. If bubbles appear, the oxygen is flowing through the cannula.

- Antineoplastics: cyclophosphamide (Cytoxan), cisplatin (Platinol).
- Diuretics.[4]

What can harm my client?

Patients with lung cancer are extremely ill. This is why it is imperative that you perform a proper assessment of these patients including the related equipment used in their treatment. Frequent monitoring of oxygen status, tissue perfusion, airway clearance, and vitals signs is crucial. Other factors to monitor include the risk for:

- Infection.
- Recurrent cancer.
- Malnutrition.
- Dehydration.
- Respiratory failure.
- Electrolyte abnormalities.
- Risk of bleeding.
- Pooling of secretions.
- Immobility.
- Poor mouth and skin care.
- Malfunctioning equipment (oxygen concentrator, mechanical ventilator, suctioning machine).[4]

If I were your teacher, I would test you on . . .

If I were giving you a test on lung cancer, I would ask questions about:

- Palliative care measures.
- Postoperative care of the patient receiving wedge resection, segmental resection, lobectomy, or pneumonectomy. (Which ones require chest tubes postop, definitions)

- Postoperative complications and wound care.
- Collaboration with the social worker, dietician, and physical therapist.
- Chest tube function.
- Hydration and nutrition status.
- Sputum and oxygen monitoring.
- Referral of smokers to cessation programs and psychological therapy.
- Proper patient positioning according to which part of lung was removed or if the entire lung was removed.

✚ Colorectal cancer

Colorectal cancer refers to cancer that develops in the colon or the rectum. Colorectal cancer is the third most common cancer diagnosed in both American men and women. Colorectal cancer is the cause of death in approximately 56,000 Americans a year. However, the death rate from colorectal cancer has been decreasing for the past 15 years. This decrease may be because there are fewer cases, more of the cases are diagnosed early, and treatments have improved.[14]

What is it?

In many patients, colorectal cancer starts as a noncancerous polyp, which develops on the lining of the colon or rectum. Adenomas are the types of polyps that have the potential to become cancerous. Colorectal cancers develop slowly over a period of several years.[14]

What causes it and why

While the cause of colorectal cancer is unknown, there are several associated risk factors, as seen in Table 4-8.

Table 4-8

Risk factors	Why
Intake of excessive saturated animal fat	Red meats increase certain bacteria that are carcinogenic to the bowel
Low-fiber, high-carbohydrate diet	Decreases intestinal peristalsis; carcinogens stay in contact with the intestinal wall for extended periods
Diseases of the digestive tract	Decreased absorption of nutrients; decreased peristalsis which increases time carcinogens stay in contact with intestinal wall
Age older than 50 years	More than 90% of people diagnosed with colorectal cancer are older than 50[14]
History of ulcerative colitis	Chronic inflammation of colon can lead to many types of cancer
Chronic constipation	Prolonged exposure to carcinogens
Diverticulosis	Prolonged exposure to bacteria and carcinogens
Family polyposis	Environmental or genetic susceptibility

Source: Created by author from Reference #4 and #14.

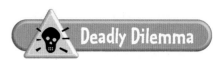

All cancer patients are weak, thus making them a safety risk. Remember, patient safety always comes first!

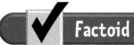

The bigger the polyp, the greater the risk for colorectal cancer.

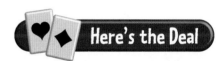

High-risk clients must be taught the importance of a high-fiber, low-fat diet—reducing red meats. Also, teach importance of rectal exams yearly after age 40 and yearly colonoscopies after age 50.[4]

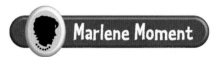

Although there's nothing like a good steak dinner, encourage your patients to include chicken, fish, lean pork, and high-fiber foods into their diets to reduce the risk of colorectal cancer!

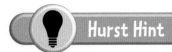

Hurst Hint

An early sign of colorectal cancer is rectal bleeding; a late sign is pain.

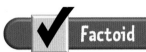

Factoid

Tumors in the left (descending) colon will cause an obstruction earlier because of its smaller diameter. Obstruction in the right (ascending) colon does not occur until later in the disease because this area has a larger diameter.

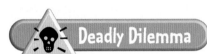

Deadly Dilemma

Clients may have ribbon-shaped or pencil-shaped stools due to colorectal obstruction.

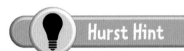

Hurst Hint

Early diagnosis is the key to possibly curing colorectal cancer.

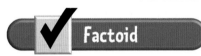

Factoid

Aspirin (and other NSAIDs) may decrease the risk for colorectal cancer due to antiinflammatory effects.

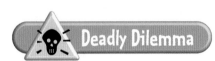

Deadly Dilemma

Barium examination should not come before a colonoscopy because barium sulfate interferes with this test.[4]

Signs and symptoms and why

The growth of tumors in the colon constricts the intestine, which contribute to the signs and symptoms of colorectal cancer. Common signs and symptoms associated with colorectal cancer are found in Table 4-9.

Table 4-9

Signs and symptoms	Why
Black, tarry stools	Bleeding from the colon
Nausea and vomiting	May be sign of obstruction
Abdominal cramping, distension, aching, and pressure	Bowel contents may be trapped due to tumor blockage irritating the bowel; obstruction could be forming
Diarrhea and constipation	Tumor encircling the intestine; blockage occurs causing constipation then bowel content works its way through causing diarrhea
Anorexia and weight loss	Tumor consuming calories
Rectal pressure	Tumor growth
Melena	Blood in stool from tumor invading intestine
Abdominal visible masses	Tumor growth
Abdominal fullness	Tumor causing pressure and distension
Enlarged inguinal and supraclavicular lymph nodes	Metastasis
Pallor	Bleeding causing anemia
Weakness	Anemia from bleeding
Abnormal bowel sounds	Obstruction

Source: Table created by author from Reference #4.

Quickie tests and treatments

Diagnostic tests:

- Fecal occult blood test, positive.
- Barium enema.
- Biopsy.
- Colonoscopy.
- Digital rectal exam.
- Lower gastrointestinal (GI) series.
- Hematology: decreased hemoglobin and hematocrit.
- Sigmoidoscopy.

Treatments:

- Radiation.
- Chemotherapy.
- Surgery.
- Antiemetics.
- Antineoplastics.
- Folic acid derivative: leucovorin (Citrovorum factor).[4]

What can harm my client?

Your nursing care should include monitoring pain, bowel and bladder function, and vital signs. Provide good nursing care to prevent these possible complications:

* Rectal hemorrhage.
* Infection.
* Electrolyte imbalance.
* Blockage of the GI tract.
* Fatigue.
* Malnutrition.
* Dehydration.[4]

If I were your teacher, I would test you on . . .

Guaranteed, on your nursing school test you will be asked information about:

* GI assessment.
* Daily weight to assess electrolyte status.
* Emergency nursing interventions associated with intestinal obstruction.
* Signs/symptoms of intestinal obstruction.
* Monitoring patient stools; collecting a stool sample.
* Postoperative care and prevention of postoperative complications.
* Postoperative patient positioning.
* Total parenteral nutrition (TPN).
* Patient teaching and management of a colostomy.
* Referral to support services, such as the Colon Cancer Alliance or the American Cancer Society.
* Patient preparation and teaching associated with barium enema, colonoscopy.
* Bowel sound changes associated with intestinal obstruction.

✛ Bladder cancer

Approximately $2.9 billion is spent each year in the United States on the treatment of bladder cancer. Bladder cancer affects more men than women in all ethnic groups. The incidence of bladder cancer is higher in Caucasians than African Americans, but the mortality rates are almost the same due to the later stage at diagnosis among African Americans. Bladder cancer is mostly seen in men.[15]

What is it?

Bladder cancer is a malignant tumor that develops on the bladder wall or grows into the wall, invading the underlying muscles. It may metastasize to the periaortic lymph nodes, prostate gland, rectum, ureters, and vagina.[4]

What causes it and why

The exact cause of bladder cancer in unknown. However, the disease is associated with certain risk factors (Table 4-10).

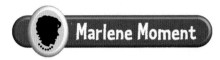

Marlene Moment

No rushing for a pass, WWF wrestling, or bench presses allowed after colorectal surgery!

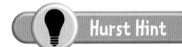

Hurst Hint

Postop colorectal surgical patients should be kept in semi-Fowler's position to promote emptying of the GI tract. This could be a test question!

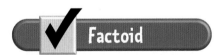

Factoid

Bladder cancer is the most common cancer of the urinary tract.[15]

Table 4-10

Risk factors	Why
Chronic bladder irritation and infection in patients with renal calculi	Irritation and infection causes cell mutations
Indwelling urinary catheters	Irritates mucosa, causing cell mutations
Use of cyclophosphamide (Cytoxan)	Carcinogen that infiltrates the urine
Exposure to industrial chemicals and radiation	Carcinogens that cause cell mutations
Excessive intake of coffee, phenacetin, sodium, saccharin, sodium cyclamate	Carcinogens that infiltrate the urine
Cigarette smoking	Contributes to almost 50% of the cases, and smoking cigars or pipes also increases the risk

Source: Created by author from References #4 and #15.

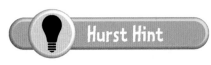

Hurst Hint

Since hematuria is painless and sometimes intermittent, this causes some clients to delay treatment.

Signs and symptoms and why

Carcinogens in the urine can lead to bladder cancer, resulting in the signs and symptoms shown in Table 4-11.

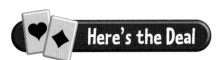

Here's the Deal

Bladder cancer likes to metastasize to the bones.

Table 4-11

Signs and symptoms	Why
Suprapubic pain after voiding	Caused by invasive lesions; pressure exerted on the tumor; obstruction
Flank pain and tenderness	Obstructed ureter
Painless hematuria with or without clots	Major sign of bladder cancer; due to tumor invasion
Urinary frequency, urgency, dribbling, irritability, nocturia	Infection or obstruction which decreases urine outflow
Dysuria, anuria	Infection or obstruction
Fever, chills	Infection

Source: Created by author from Reference #4.

Quickie tests and treatments

Diagnostic tests:

- Urinalysis: detection of blood and malignant cells.
- Hematology: decreased red blood cell count, hemoglobin, and hematocrit.
- Cystoscopy.
- Cytologic examination.
- Excretory urography.

- Ultrasonography.
- Bone scan: detects metastasis.

Treatments:
- Chemotherapy.
- Surgery.
- Transfusion therapy with packed red blood cells.
- Analgesics.
- Antispasmodics: phenazopyridine (Pyridium).
- Sedatives: oxazepam (Serax).
- Chemotherapy agents: thiotepa (Thioplex), doxorubicin (Adriamycin), mitomycin (Mutamycin).[4]

What can harm my client?

It is important that your nursing assessment and interventions focus on the patient's renal status, pain, and maintaining adequate fluid balance. Factors that may harm your patient are:
- Infection.
- Malnutrition.
- Ineffective coping mechanisms.
- Dehydration.
- Inactivity.
- Myleosuppression.
- Chemical cystitis.
- Skin rash.[4]

If I were your teacher, I would test you on . . .

The following are good testable items:
- Postoperative care and complications.
- Monitoring for hematuria or infection in the urine.
- Maintaining continuous bladder irrigation.
- Fluid and nutritional needs.
- Side effects of medications.
- Postradiation patient teaching.
- Providing supportive care to the patient and family.
- Postchemotherapeutic care.
- Teaching regarding potential client changes in sexual activity.
- Stoma assessment and care (ileal conduit).
- Teaching patient not to engage in heavy lifting or contact sports.
- Urinary diversions (ileal conduit, urostomy)
- Care of patient with bladder spasms.
- Importance of monitoring urine output.
- Risk factors for bladder cancer.

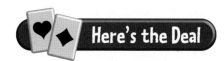

Mouth sores and oral pain are common problems for patients undergoing chemotherapy. These can lead to anorexia and malnutrition. Follow your facility's protocol for caring for mouth sores and oral pain.

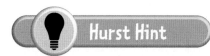

As for all postoperative patients or patients with limited activity tolerance, it is important to teach and assist with turning, coughing, and deep breathing techniques to prevent the pooling of lung secretions that may result in infection.

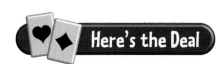

Cold packs applied to skin that has recently undergone radiation can cause skin damage. Warn your patients against this practice!

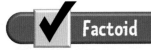

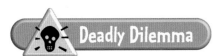

Non-Hodgkin lymphoma is increasingly seen in the geriatric population (due to decreased immune system) and those with impaired immune systems.

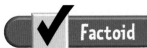

Patients with immune deficiencies due to inherited conditions, drug treatment, organ transplantation, or HIV infection have more of a chance of developing lymphoma than people without an immune deficiency.[18]

✚ Non-Hodgkin lymphoma

Non-Hodgkin lymphoma (NHL) is the fifth most common cancer in this country, not counting nonmelanoma skin cancers. A person's risk of developing non-Hodgkin lymphoma during his or her lifetime is about 1 in 50. The prognosis for these patients is poor, but with today's treatments about 30% to 50% of people can live at least 5 years. The rate of non-Hodgkin lymphoma has doubled since the 1970s. However, incidence rates are stabilizing due to the decline in AIDS-related NHL.[16]

What is it?

Non-Hodgkin lymphoma is a cancer of the lymphoid tissue and is three times more common than Hodgkin's disease.[4] There are approximately 30 types of non-Hodgkin lymphomas, which make classification difficult.[17]

What causes it and why

The exact cause of non-Hodgkin lymphoma is unknown. However, immunologic or viral contributing factors may play a role.[17] In non-Hodgkin lymphoma, tumors grow throughout the lymph nodes and lymphatic organs—spleen or bone marrow—and spread from there. *B-lymphocytes* (B-cells) and *T-lymphocytes* (T-cells) are the two main types of lymphocytes. In the United States, 85% of all cases of non-Hodgkin lymphoma come from B-lymphocytes (B-cells) and 15% from T-lymphocytes (T-cells).[17]

Signs and symptoms and why

Signs and symptoms (Table 4-12) depend on what area of the body is attacked, and include:

Table 4-12

Signs and symptoms	Why
Anorexia; weight loss	Malnutrition, immunosuppression
Painless, swollen lymph glands	Cellular growth
Malaise	Spreading of disease, body trying to fight disease
Fatigue	Spreading of disease, body trying to fight disease
Fever	Spreading of disease, body trying to fight disease
Night sweats	Spreading of disease, body trying to fight disease
Difficulty breathing, cough	Spreading of disease, body trying to fight disease
Enlarged tonsils, adenoids	Spreading of disease, body trying to fight disease, immune response
Rubbery cervical and supraclavicular nodes	Spreading of disease, immune response
Anemia, thrombocytopenia, leukopenia	All blood elements are decreased

Source: Created by author from References #4, #17, and #18.

Quickie tests and treatments

Diagnostics:

- Biopsy.
- Bone marrow aspiration (Fig. 4-4).

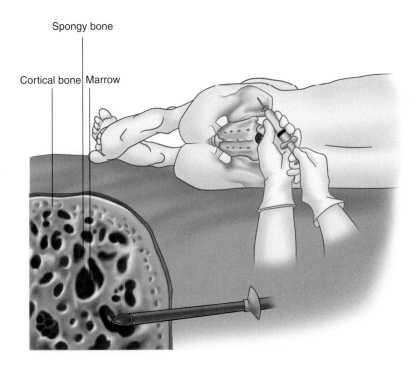

Spongy bone

Cortical bone | Marrow

◀ Figure 4-4. Bone marrow aspiration.

- Chest x-ray.
- Blood chemistries: anemia, elevated calcium.

Treatments:

- Radiation.
- Chemotherapy agents: vincristine (Oncovin), doxorubicin (Adriamycin).
- Small, frequent meals.
- Increased fluid intake.
- Limited activity.
- Frequent rest periods. [4]

What can harm my client?

Your patient assessment should focus on detecting complications associated with lymphoma. Factors that may harm your patient include:

- Infection.
- Bleeding.
- Electrolyte imbalance.
- Jaundice.
- Malnutrition.
- Dehydration.
- Poor mouth and skin care.
- Adverse reactions to blood transfusions.[4]

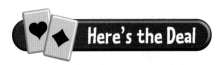

Here's the Deal

Lymphoma patients fatigue easily due to anemia. Showing patients how to schedule rest periods to improve immune function and decrease weakness is an important nursing intervention.

If I were your teacher, I would test you on . . .

Aunt Marlene would test you on:

* Medications and their side effects.
* Nonpharmacological measures to relieve pain, such as relaxation techniques.
* Appropriate diet for these patients.
* Patient teaching regarding scheduled rest periods.

✚ Melanoma of the skin

Cancer of the skin is the most common of all cancers. Melanoma accounts for about 4% of skin cancer cases, but it causes most skin cancer deaths. The American Cancer Society estimates that in 2006 there were 62,190 new cases of melanoma in this country. About 7910 people will die of this disease.[19]

What is it?

Skin cancer is caused by a malignant primary tumor of the skin. The most common sites are the head and neck in men, legs in women, and back in people exposed to excessive sunlight.[4] There are four common types:

1. Superficial spreading melanoma: develops between ages 40 and 50 and is the most common type.
2. Nodular melanoma: develops between ages 40 and 50, invades the dermis, and metastasizes early.
3. Acral-lentiginous melanoma: most common among Hispanics, Asians, and blacks; occurs on the palms of the hands, soles of the feet, and under the tongue.
4. Lentigo maligna melanoma: most benign, rare, and slow growing. Occurs between ages 60 and 70 due to a lentigo maligna on an exposed skin surface.[4]

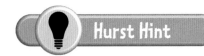

The number of new cases of melanoma in the United States is on the rise.[19] Therefore, you should include questions regarding sun exposure in your patient history.

What causes it and why?

Skin cancer is caused from ultraviolet rays from the sun that damage the skin. Other causes include:

* Radiation.
* Chemical irritants.
* Heredity.
* Immunosuppressive drugs.
* Infrared heat or light.

The majority of skin cancers arise from a pre-existing nevus. Malignant melanoma spreads through the lymph system and bloodstream, metastasizing to the regional lymph nodes, skin, liver, lungs, and central nervous system.[4]

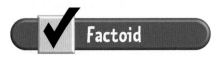

Skin cancer can also be caused by chronic irritation or friction to an area of skin.

Signs and symptoms and why

Malignant melanoma follows an unpredictable course, resulting in many possible signs and symptoms, as seen in Table 4-13.

Table 4-13

Signs and symptoms	Why
Sore that doesn't heal	Cancer cells affect normal cell membranes, inhibiting repair
Changes in moles, birthmarks, freckles, scars, or warts	Cancer cells change the skin layers, resulting in skin changes
Persistent lump or swelling	Tumor growth
Nevus that increases in size, changes color, becomes inflamed or sore, itches, ulcerates, bleeds, changes texture, or pigment regresses	Cancer cells change the skin layers, resulting in skin changes
Lesions appearing on the ankles or inside surfaces of the knees	Cancer cells change the skin layers, resulting in skin changes
Pigmented lesions on the palms, soles, or under the nails	Cancer cells change the skin layers, resulting in skin changes
Elevated tumor nodules that may bleed	Tumor growth, infection
Flat nodule with smaller nodules scattered over the surface	Cancer cells change the skin layers, resulting in skin changes
Waxy nodule with telangiectasis	Cancer cells change the skin layers resulting in skin changes
Irregular bordered lesion with tan, black, or blue colors	Cancer cells change the skin layers, resulting in skin changes

Source: Table created by author from Reference #4.

Quickie tests and treatments

Diagnostics:

- Skin biopsy.
- Chest x-ray: assists in staging.
- Hematology: anemia, elevated erythrocyte sedimentation rate (ESR), abnormal platelet count, abnormal liver function studies.

Treatments:

- Radiation.
- Chemotherapy.
- Biotherapy.
- Immunotherapy.
- Immunostimulants.
- Cryosurgery.
- Curettage.
- Antiemetics.
- Antineoplastics.

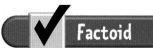

Factoid

The signs and symptoms of melanoma of the skin result from changes to the skin layers and the spread of the cancer cells to other body areas via the lymph system and bloodstream.

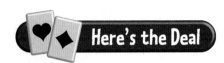

Skin cancer is very serious! It can quickly metastasize to the lymph nodes, skin, liver, lungs, and central nervous system.

- Alkylating agents: carmustine (BiCNU).
- Antimetabolites: fluorouracil (Adrucil).[4]

What can harm my client?

Patients with malignant melanoma require close, long-term follow-up care to detect metastasis and recurrences.[4] Possible harmful factors to these patients include:

- Malnutrition.
- Sun exposure.
- Infection.
- Medication side effects.[4]

If I were your teacher, I would test you on . . .

Patients should be encouraged to express their feelings about changes in body image and fear of dying (if applicable). I can promise you that your teacher will test you on therapeutic communication techniques, to use to help these patients cope with their illness. Other testable material may include:

- Teaching patients about skin care and sun avoidance.
- Importance of a well-balanced diet.
- Postoperative care and prevention of complications.
- Postchemotherapy and postradiation nursing care.
- Effective skin assessment.

✚ Uterine cancer

In 2006, approximately 41,200 new cases of uterine cancer, which encompasses the body of the uterus, were diagnosed in the United States, with 95% of these being endometrial cancers. An estimated 7350 women in the United States died from cancer of the uterine corpus during 2006. According to estimates from various studies, uterine sarcomas (including carcinosarcomas, leiomyosarcomas, and endometrial stromal sarcomas) account for around 4% of cancers of the uterus, equaling approximately 1600 cases in 2006.[20]

What is it?

Uterine sarcoma is a cancer that starts from tissues such as muscle, fat, bone, and fibrous tissue of the uterus. A malignant tumor grows in the connective tissue, bone, cartilage, or striated muscle that spreads into neighboring tissue or by way of the bloodstream.[21] More than 95% of cancers of the uterus are carcinomas—cancers that develop from epithelial cells of the lining layers of that organ.[20] Cervical cancers develop in the lower part of the uterus above the vagina. Endometrial cancers develop in the upper part of the uterus. This section will only focus on uterine sarcoma.

What causes it and why

The direct cause of uterine cancer in unknown. Related risk factors are shown in Table 4-14.

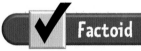

Female patients who have received high-energy radiation as a therapy to treat some cancers are at an increased risk for developing a second type of cancer, such as uterine sarcomas. These cancers are typically diagnosed 5 to 25 years after exposure to radiation.[22]

Table 4-14

Risk factors	Why
Age over 50 years	Longer exposure to estrogens that can cause cell mutations
History of endometrial hyperplasia	Cellular mutations
Estrogen replacement therapy (ERT)	Exposure to estrogens that can cause cell mutations
Overweight	Fat triggers estrogen, fueling tumor growth
Hypertension	Unclear if risk is due to hypertension alone or obesity that coincides with hypertension
Diabetes	Many diabetics are obese and hypertensive
History of other cancers	Immunosuppression, presence of cancer cells
History of taking tamoxifen for breast cancer treatment or prevention	Tamoxifen interferes with the activity of estrogen
Radiation, especially before age 30	Causes cellular mutations

Source: Created by author from References #21, #22, and #23.

Signs and symptoms and why

The signs and symptoms that may point to uterine cancer are seen in Table 4-15.

Table 4-15

Signs and symptoms	Why
Bleeding and spotting	The most common early sign due to cellular changes
Vaginal discharge	Cellular changes
Pelvic pain	Tumor growth and pressure
Pelvic mass	Tumor growth
Feeling of "fullness" in the pelvis	Tumor pressure

Source: Created by author from References #21, #22, and #23.

Quickie tests and treatments

Diagnostic tests:

- Biopsy.
- Hysteroscopy.
- Dilation and curettage (D & C).
- Cystoscopy.
- Proctoscopy.
- Transvaginal ultrasound.
- Computed tomography (CT).
- Positron emission tomography (PET) scan.
- Magnetic resonance imaging (MRI).
- Chest x-ray.[23]

Deadly Dilemma

About 85% of patients diagnosed with uterine sarcoma have symptoms of postmenopausal bleeding or spotting (bleeding between periods). This is why post-menopausal women should be taught to immediately report any bleeding or spotting to their health care provider.[23]

Treatments:

- Chemotherapy.
- Radiation.
- Surgery.
- Chemotherapy agents: cisplatin (Platinol), gemcitabine (Gemzar).
- Hormone therapy: megestrol acetate (Megace), medroxyprogesterone acetate (Provera).

Treatments depend on the type and stage of cancer and the patient's overall medical condition.[24]

What can harm my client?

Your nursing assessment and interventions should focus on pain, emotional support, and complications related to therapy, such as:

- Infection.
- Bleeding.
- Bruising.
- Shortness of breath.
- Malnutrition.[24]

If I were your teacher, I would test you on . . .

On the day of the big test, you may be questioned about:

- Patient comfort interventions.
- Biopsy techniques and postcare.
- Medication administration.
- Postoperative care and prevention of postoperative complications.
- Communication with the health care team (dietician, physical therapist, and social worker) to assist in optimal care of the cancer patient.

Marlene Moment

If I hear that you are not attending to the psychosocial needs of your cancer patients, I'll come and get you!

SUMMARY

Cancer is an ever-changing field of nursing care. The nursing elements that are most important are ensuring comfort and addressing the psychosocial needs of the client and the family. Cancer may be disfiguring, debilitating, and expensive, thus creating opportunities for the health care team to work together to ensure positive outcomes for cancer patients.

PRACTICE QUESTIONS

1. While administering a chemotherapeutic agent, the nurse suspects extravasation at the client's IV site. The first nursing action is:

   1. Place ice over the infiltration site.

   2. Stop the medication administration.

   3. Administer antidote.

   4. Apply warm compresses to the IV site.

Correct answer: 2. The primary nursing action is to stop the medication administration to prevent further damage to the vessels. Placing ice over the infiltration site and administering an antidote are not appropriate first actions. Applying a warm compress over the IV site is incorrect, as this would cause vasodilation, furthering tissue damage.

2. The most common cancer in males is:

   1. Prostate.

   2. Lung.

   3. Colorectal.

   4. Testicular.

   Correct answer: 1. Prostate cancer accounts for 29.4% of males; lung cancer 15.8%; colorectal cancer 11.2%; and testicular cancer less than 2%.

3. A 28-year-old female client is undergoing brachytherapy for uterine cancer. A primary nursing action is to:

   1. Encourage the client's small children to visit.

   2. Provide adequate skin care to the site.

   3. Tell the client that any body fluids emitted may be radioactive.

   4. Place a lead apron over the client.

   Correct answer: 3. Those who come in contact with the client or her body fluids are at risk for radiation exposure. Therefore, small children and pregnant women should not come in contact with these clients. Brachytherapy includes an internal site, so skin care management is inappropriate. The nurse should wear the lead apron, not the client.

4. A client presents with mild stomatitis while undergoing chemotherapy. An appropriate nursing intervention is to:

   1. Rinse with mouthwash three times a day (TID).

   2. Use a soft toothbrush.

   3. Provide cold foods.

   4. Floss twice a day.

   Correct answer: 2. Using a soft toothbrush minimizes trauma to the oral mucosa. Using a mouth wash TID can dry out the oral membranes due to the alcohol content. Foods of extreme temperature should be avoided. Flossing may cause trauma to the gums.

5. It is recommended by the American Cancer Society for women age 50 and over, who have no family history of breast cancer, to have a mammogram:

   1. Every year.

   2. Every 2 years.

   3. Every 3 years.

   4. Every 5 years.

Correct answer: 1. The ACS recommends screening mammography for all women over age 40 every 1 to 2 years and every year for women over age 50.

6. Which is recommended by the American Cancer Society to decrease cancer risk?

   1. Physical exam once a year.

   2. Drink 8 to 10 glasses of water daily.

   3. Increase dietary fiber.

   4. Exercise at least three times a week.

   Correct answer: 3. ACS recommends increasing dietary fiber to decrease breast, colon, and prostate cancer. Drinking 8 to 10 glasses of water daily and exercises three times a week are not specific to cancer prevention. An annual physical exam will not decrease cancer risk.

7. When caring for the client undergoing chemotherapy, the nurse teaches the client and family:

   1. Not to receive any immunizations.

   2. Discontinue any birth control pills.

   3. Blood in the urine is normal.

   4. Ibuprofen may be taken for temperature greater than 101 degrees Fahrenheit.

   Correct answer: 1. Immunizations can cause an adverse reaction in chemotherapy patients due to their decreased antibody response. Clients should continue birth control, since most antineoplastics are teratogenic. Blood in the urine is a sign of thrombocytopenia and should be reported to the physician. NSAIDs should not be administered because they can prolong bleeding time and the client's platelets are already compromised by the chemotherapy agent.

8. Cruciferous vegetables appear to decrease cancer risk. The following are considered cruciferous vegetables except:

   1. Broccoli.

   2. Cabbage.

   3. Spinach.

   4. Brussels sprouts.

   Correct answer: 3. Spinach is a carotenoid vegetable, not a cruciferous one. Broccoli, cabbage, and brussels sprouts are all cruciferous vegetables.

9. Which surgery involves removing organs or tissues that are likely to develop cancer?

　1. Palliative.

　2. Prophylactic.

　3. Diagnostic.

　4. Reconstructive.

Correct answer: 2. Prophylactic surgery is performed to prevent cancer of certain organs or tissues. Palliative surgery promotes client comfort when a cure is not available. Diagnostic surgery retrieves tissue samples for definitive cancer diagnosis. Reconstructive surgery maintains optimal function or a cosmetic effect after curative or radical surgeries.

10. The antineoplastic agents that act by altering the DNA structure are:

　1. Mitotic spindle poisons.

　2. Hormonal agents.

　3. Antimetabolites.

　4. Alkylating agents.

Correct answer: 4. Alkylating agents alter DNA structure. Mitotic spindle poisons stop metaphase. Hormonal agents alter cellular growth. Antimetabolites interefere with biosynthesis or metabolites.

References

1. Anderson K, ed. *Mosby's Medical, Nursing, & Allied Health Dictionary*. 4th ed. St. Louis: Mosby; 1994.

2. American Cancer Society. *What Are the Risk Factors for Cancer?* Available at: www.cancer.org/docroot/CRI/content/CRI_2_4_2x_ What_are_the_risk_factors_for_cancer_72.asp?sitearea= Accessed December 14, 2006.

3. American Cancer Society. *ACS History*. Available at: www.cancer.org/ docroot/AA/content/AA_1_4_ACS_History.asp. Accessed December 14, 2006.

4. Allen KD, Boucher MA, Cain JE, et al. *Manual of Nursing Practice Pocket Guides: Medical-Surgical Nursing*. Ambler, PA: Lippincott Williams & Wilkins; 2007:295,222,183,177,82,54.

5. The North American Association of Central Cancer Registries. *Five Most Commonly Diagnosed Cancers in the U.S.* Available at: www.naaccr.org/ index.asp?Col_SectionKey=11&Col_ContentID=48 Accessed December 16, 2006.

6. American Cancer Society. *2006 Estimated U.S. Cancer Cases*. Available at: http://www.cancer.org/docroot/PRO/content/PRO_1_1_Cancer_ Statistics_2006_Presentation.asp. Accessed December 16, 2006.

7. American Cancer Society. *Breast Cancer Facts and Figures 2005–2006*. Available at: www.cancer.org/downloads/STT/CAFF2005BrF.pdf. Accessed December 14, 2006.

8. American Cancer Society. *What Are the Key Statistics about Prostate Cancer?* Available at: www.cancer.org/docroot/CRI/content/CRI_2_4_ 1X_ What_are_the_key_statistics_for_prostate_cancer_36.asp?rnav=cri. Accessed December 16, 2006.

9. American Cancer Society. *What Is Prostate Cancer?* Available at: www.cancer.org/docroot/CRI/content/CRI_2_4_1X_What_is_ prostate_cancer_36.asp?rnav=cri. Accessed December 16, 2006.

10. American Cancer Society. *What Are the Risk Factors for Prostate Cancer?* Available at: www.cancer.org/docroot/CRI/content/CRI_2_4_ 2X_What_are_the_risk_factors_for_prostate_cancer_36.asp?sitearea= Accessed December 16, 2006.

11. American Cancer Society. *Prostate Guide: Chemotherapy.* Available at: www.cancer.org/docroot/CRI/content/CRI_2_4_4X_Chemotherapy_ 36.asp?rnav=cri. Accessed December 16, 2006.

12. National Comprehensive Cancer Network. *Side Effects of Prostate Cancer Treatments.* Available at: www.nccn.org/patients/patient_gls/ _english/_prostate/5_side-effects.asp. Accessed December 16, 2006.

13. American Cancer Society. *What Are the Key Statistics about Lung Cancer?* Available at: www.cancer.org/docroot/CRI/content/CRI_2_ 4_1x_What_Are_the_Key_Statistics_About_Lung_Cancer_15.asp?site area=. Accessed December 16, 2006.

14. American Cancer Society. *What Is Colorectal Cancer?* Available at: www.cancer.org/docroot/CRI/content/CRI_2_6X_Colorectal_Cancer _Early_Detection_10.asp?sitearea=&level= Accessed December 16, 2006.

15. National Cancer Institute. *Snapshot of Bladder Cancer.* Available at: http://planning.cancer.gov/disease/Bladder-Snapshot.pdf. Accessed December 17, 2006.

16. American Cancer Society. *What Are the Key Statistics about Non-Hodgkin Lymphoma?* Available at: www.cancer.org/docroot/CRI/ content/CRI_2_4_1X_What_are_the_key_statistics_for_non-Hodgkins_lymphoma_32.asp?rnav=cri. Accessed December 17, 2006.

17. American Cancer Society. *What Is Non-Hodgkin Lymphoma?* Available at: www.cancer.org/docroot/CRI/content/CRI_2_4_1X_ What_Is_Non_Hodgkins_Lymphoma_32.asp. Accessed December 17, 2006.

18. American Cancer Society. *Do We Know What Causes Non-Hodgkin Lymphoma?* Available at: www.cancer.org/docroot/CRI/content/ CRI_2_4_2X_Do_we_know_what_causes_non-Hodgkins_ lymphoma_32.asp?rnav=cri. Accessed December 17, 2006.

19. American Cancer Society. *How Many People Get Melanoma Skin Cancer?* Available at: www.cancer.org/docroot/CRI/content/CRI_ 2_2_1X_How_many_people_get_melanoma_skin_cancer_50.asp? rnav=cri. Accessed December 17, 2006.

20. American Cancer Society. *What Are the Key Statistics about Uterine Sarcoma?* Available at: www.cancer.org/docroot/CRI/content/CRI_2_4_ 1X_What_are_the_key_statistics_for_uterine_sarcoma_63.asp?rnav= cri. Accessed December 18, 2006.

21. American Cancer Society. *What Is Uterine Sarcoma?* Available at: www.cancer.org/docroot/CRI/content/CRI_2_4_1X_What_is_ uterine_sarcoma_63.asp?rnav=cri. Accessed December 18, 2006.

22. American Cancer Society. *What Are the Risk Factors for Uterine Sarcoma?* Available at: www.cancer.org/docroot/CRI/content/CRI_2_4_ 2X_What_are_the_risk_factors_for_uterine_sarcoma_63.asp?rnav= cri. Accessed December 18, 2006.

23. American Cancer Society. *How Is Uterine Sarcoma Diagnosed?* Available at: www.cancer.org/docroot/CRI/content/CRI_2_4_3X_ How_is_uterine_sarcoma_diagnosed_63.asp?rnav=cri. Accessed December 18, 2006.

24. American Cancer Society. *How Is Uterine Sarcoma Treated?* Available at: www.cancer.org/docroot/CRI/content/CRI_2_4_4X_How_is_ uterine_sarcoma_treated_63.asp?rnav=cri. Accessed December 18, 2006.

Bibliography

Hurst Review Services. www.hurstreview.com.

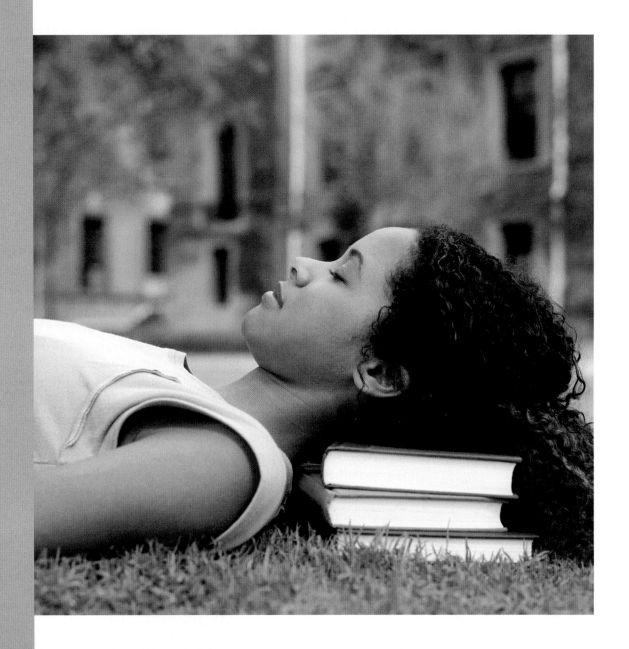

CHAPTER

5

Respiratory System

OBJECTIVES

In this chapter, you'll review:

- Normal respiratory anatomy and function.
- Illnesses and diseases of the respiratory system.
- Essential information regarding respiratory diagnostic tests, treatments, and client care.

LET'S GET THE NORMAL STUFF STRAIGHT FIRST

Occasionally you find bodily physical systems, terminology, and functions that just make sense. That is true of the respiratory system (Fig. 5-1)! The respiratory system sustains oxygen (O_2) and carbon dioxide (CO_2) levels in the blood while maintaining acid–base balance in the body. Ok, so here's the scoop. You breathe air in through your nose and mouth, where it is warmed and filtered. It travels down through a series of tubes such as the pharynx, larynx, and trachea. It moves through the mainstem bronchus to either the left or right bronchi (Fig. 5-2), which end in even smaller tubes called bronchioles. (Think tributaries of a river!) The bronchioles are surrounded by small groups of bubbles or air sacs—alveoli. The alveoli are infiltrated with small blood vessels where the exchange of O_2 and CO_2 takes place. The oxygen from the inspired air passes through to the blood, and the carbon dioxide takes the place of the oxygen and travels the same path back out as exhaled gas (expiration). Hence, the name "gas exchange." See how it all just **sounds** right?

▶ Figure 5-1. Respiratory system.

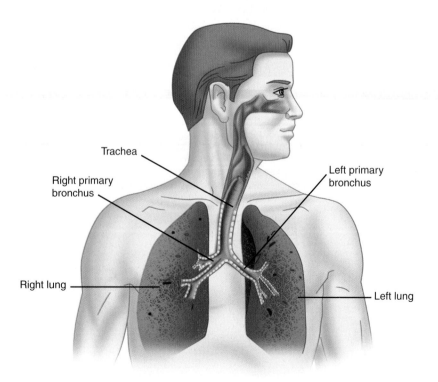

Trachea

Left primary bronchus

Right primary bronchus

Right lung

Left lung

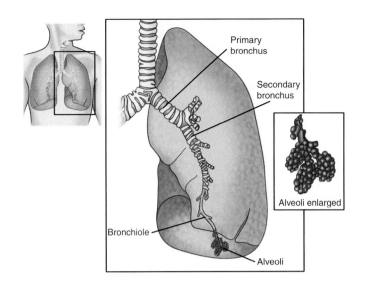

◀ Figure 5-2. Bronchus, bronchiole, and alveoli.

✚ ABGs

Remember in Chapter 2 (Acid–Base Balance) we discussed arterial blood gases (ABGs)? Good! Then a quickie review of the respiratory function in acid–base balance is all that is going to be needed here!

Here's a quick question: Is CO_2 considered an acid or a base? An acid! When it mixes with water in the body, it becomes carbonic acid. The only way to get rid of CO_2 is exhalation. CO_2 buildup due to hypoventilation in the body causes an acidotic state. Conversely, blowing off too much CO_2 due to hyperventilation causes an alkalotic state. Just remember that at the initial onset of a respiratory illness acidosis or alkalosis may be present in an attempt to compensate for the disease or injury. No problems, right?

✚ Hypoxia versus hypoxemia

These terms seem to be very confusing and need to be formally defined before we travel any further down the respiratory pathway.

- Hypoxemia is a decrease in the oxygen concentration of the blood.
- Hypoxia is a general oxygen deficiency or reduced oxygen content in the inspired air.

Therefore, hypoxia can lead to hypoxemia.[1]

✚ Breath sounds

Table 5-1 simplifies breath sounds.

Table 5-1

Type of breath sound	What it sounds like	Why
Crackles	Crackling paper or slight popping sound	Air moving through a very moist area as with pulmonary edema
Rhonchi	Bubbles	Air moving through fluid-filled airway
Stridor	High-pitched crow, usually heard during inspiration	Air being forced through a swollen upper airway
Wheezing	Whistling	Airway constricted by fluid or secretions; bronchospasm; tumor

Source: Created by author from Reference #1.

LET'S GET DOWN TO THE SPECIFICS

The respiratory system plays a very important role in the overall health of all the other bodily systems. Now that we have explored an overview of the respiratory system anatomy, let's discuss a few of the most common respiratory diseases and illnesses.

✛ Acute respiratory distress syndrome

Acute respiratory distress syndrome (ARDS) is the sudden inability of the body to sufficiently oxygenate the blood, and usually occurs in critically ill patients.[2] ARDS clients have a high mortality rate and should be treated as quickly as possible.

What is it?

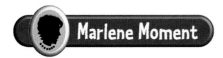

Marlene Moment

Another name for ARDS is Da-nang lung . . . not "the dang lung." This name originated from trauma doctors treating war victims with ARDS.

ARDS is a medical emergency in which the lungs—due to direct or indirect injury—fill with fluid.[2,3] This results in low arterial oxygen levels. ARDS is known for its rapid onset after the first sign of respiratory distress, usually within 24 to 48 hours of the original disease.

Other names for ARDS are shock lung, stiff lung, wet lung, or white lung. If not treated quickly, death can result in less than 48 hours. Half to 70% of the people who develop ARDS die.[1] For those clients who recover, they have little or no lung damage; some have persistent cough, shortness of breath, and increased sputum.

What causes it and why

Causes of ARDS include:

- Anaphylaxis.
- Aspiration.
- Burns.
- Drug overdose.
- Embolus.
- Heart surgery.
- Injury to the chest.
- Near drowning.
- Inhalation of toxic gases.
- Massive blood transfusions.
- Pneumonia.
- Sepsis.
- Shock.

Everything listed above can cause direct or indirect lung injury. Table 5-2 outlines some of the lung changes that occur as a result of this injury.

Table 5-2

Why
1. Injury reduces blood flow to the lungs. Hormones are released; platelets aggregate
2. Hormones damage the alveolar capillaries, increasing permeability, causing fluids to shift into interstitial space
3. Proteins and fluids leak out of capillaries, causing pulmonary edema
4. Decreased blood flow to the alveoli decreases surfactant; alveoli collapse; gas exchange is impaired
5. CO_2 crosses alveoli and is expired; blood O_2 and CO_2 levels decrease
6. Pulmonary edema increases; inflammation leads to fibrosis. Lungs become tight and cannot effectively exchange gases

Source: Created by author from References #1 to #3.

Signs and symptoms and why

The signs and symptoms of ARDS are very subtle and change as the condition of the patient worsens. Initially, clients may have hyperventilation due to the attempt to compensate for the decrease in oxygenation. The accessory muscles may be used as the client attempts to move more air through the stiff lungs. The client feels short of breath and anxiety and restlessness may occur. The heart rate will increase due to the heart's effort to deliver more blood to be oxygenated. Chest auscultation reveals crackles resulting from the fluid buildup in the lungs. As the pulmonary edema progresses, the client will change to hypoventilation as the CO_2 is retained. Cyanosis may develop due to the inability of the lungs to exchange gases. Table 5-3 shows the signs, symptoms and associated reasons for ARDS.

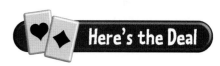 **Here's the Deal**

Hypoxemia in spite of supplemental oxygen is the hallmark sign of ARDS.[2]

Table 5-3

Signs and symptoms	Why
Shortness of breath	Hypoxia
Tachycardia	Hypoxia
Confusion	Hypoxia
Lethargy	Hypoxia
Mottled skin or cyanosis	Hypoxia
Restlessness, apprehension	Hypoxia
Crackles, wheezing	Fluid buildup in the lungs
Low O_2 level in blood	Poor gas exchange
Retractions	Increased work of breathing in an effort to expand the stiffened lung
Metabolic acidosis	Compensatory mechanisms are failing
Respiratory acidosis	Poor gas exchange causes buildup of CO_2 in the blood
Multiple organ system failure	Bodily chemicals released during ARDS affect all organs
Pneumonia	Decreased immune response; can't fight infection
Cyanosis	Decreased gas exchange

Source: Created by author from References #1 to #3.

Quickie tests and treatments

Tests:

- ABG analysis. If the client is on room air, the PaO_2 is usually less than 60 mm Hg and the $PaCO_2$ is usually less than 35 mm Hg. This is due to the increasing inability of the lungs to exchange gases due to the presence of fluid buildup.
- Chest x-ray. Shows fluid where air normally appears; early bilateral infiltrates; ground glass appearance; white-outs. Caused by lungs filling with fluid; white-outs of both lungs apparent when hypoxemia is irreversible.[3]

Treatments:

- Monitor respiratory status.
- Assess lung sounds: initially you will not hear adventitious breath sounds as the airways fill with fluid last.
- Keep condensation out of ventilator tubing; this ensures oxygen is getting to client.
- Monitor ABGs.
- Monitor the ventilator when positive-pressure mechanical ventilation (PPMV) is used; worry about pneumothorax anytime positive pressure is being used.
- Use an in-line suction system to prevent disconnecting the ventilator from the ET tube.
- Administer sedatives or neuromuscular blocking agents to paralyze the respiratory muscles and improve ventilation.
- Treat blood gas imbalances.
- Administer vasopressors to maintain BP, diuretics to reduce pulmonary edema, steroids to stabilize the cell membrane.
- Administer tube feedings to maintain/improve nutritional status.[3]

What can harm my client?

- Pulmonary edema.
- Respiratory failure.
- Pneumothorax.
- Multiple organ system failure.
- Pulmonary fibrosis.
- Ventilator associated pneumonia.
- Cardiac arrest due to ventricular arrhythmia.

If I were your teacher I would test you on . . .

- Causes of ARDS and why it occurs.
- Signs and symptoms and why of ARDS.
- Monitoring ABGs.

- Respiratory assessment.
- Mechanical ventilation.
- How PEEP affects the body.
- Importance of monitoring a pneumothorax when on PEEP.
- Care of the client receiving a neuromuscular blocking agent.
- Care of the client on a vasopressor.
- Other drugs used in the treatment of ARDS.
- Acid base imbalance with ARDS.

✚ Sleep apnea

Sleep apnea is a condition where airflow to the lungs decreases during sleep. There are three types of sleep apnea: (1) obstructive—the most common, (2) central, and (3) mixed. As the name implies, obstructive sleep apnea is due to an actual occlusion in the airway. In central sleep apnea, the drive to breathe is reduced by the nervous system, usually due to heart failure. In central sleep apnea there is no respiratory effort. In general, when clients refer to sleep apnea they are referring to obstructive sleep apnea (OSA), which we will discuss further in this section.

What is it?

OSA occurs when airflow is blocked in the throat or upper airway and can't enter the lungs. OSA is seen mainly in obese male clients who sleep on their backs. Breathing stops for a period of time, which allows CO_2 to increase and O_2 to decrease in the blood and the brain.

Apnea lasts at least 10 seconds and occurs a minimum of 5 times per hour.[1]

What causes it and why

Table 5-4 gives the causes for sleep apnea.

Table 5-4

Causes	Why
Upper airway obstruction; can be congenital	Narrowed airway decreases gas exchange
Obesity	Fat accumulates around the neck, putting pressure on the airway and making it susceptible to collapse
Alcohol consumption	Impairs respiratory center in the brain
Brainstem medulla failure	Medulla regulates breathing
Emphysema	Decreases available oxygen supply

Source: Created by author from Reference #1.

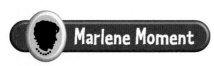

Signs and symptoms and why

Table 5-5 gives the signs and symptoms of sleep apnea.

Table 5-5

Signs and symptoms	Why
Cognitive impairment	Lack of sleep
Increased daytime sleepiness; lethargy	Lack of nighttime sleep
Loud snoring—most common symptom	Obstruction causes air to be forced through a small opening, creating the snoring sound
Apnea	CO_2 increases and O_2 decreases in the blood and the brain
Gasping, choking	Hypoxia
Sudden awakenings	Body signals client to sit up and clear the obstruction
Involuntary day napping	Poor nighttime sleep
Angina at night	Hypoxia
Decreased libido	Fatigue
Morning headache	Hypercapnia

Source: Created by author from Reference #1.

Quickie tests and treatments

Tests:

- Sleep studies with oximetry monitoring.
- EEG.
- Evaluation of the neck and upper airway for structural changes.

Treatments:

- Weight management.
- Continuous positive-airway pressure (CPAP). (Helps keep airway open)
- Smoking cessation.
- Alcohol consumption reduction.
- Discontinue drugs that cause drowsiness.
- Sleep on side and elevate head to decrease snoring.
- Oral devices made by a dentist that keep the airway open.

What can harm my client?

- Accidents due to daytime sleepiness.
- Prolonged OSA may lead to complications such as hypertension, stroke, and sleep deprivation.
- Arrhythmias due to hypoxia.
- Myocardial infarction (MI).
- Congestive heart failure (CHF): chronic hypoxia works the heart too hard and causes pulmonary hypertension. (Hypoxia is a major cause of pulmonary hypertension)

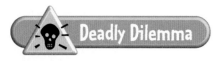

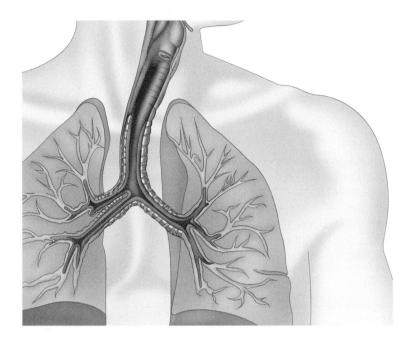

◀ Figure 5-3. Asthma.

✛ Asthma

The American Lung Association reports that 20.5 million Americans have asthma, an irritated or inflammatory disorder of the airways.[4]

What is it?

Asthma is a disease that is caused by an overreaction of the airways to irritants or other stimuli (Fig. 5-3). In normal lungs, irritants may have no effect. Asthma is considered both chronic and inflammatory and a type of chronic obstructive pulmonary disease (COPD). As a result, the client with asthma experiences bronchoconstriction, increased mucus secretions, mucosal edema, and air hunger. The episodes of asthma are usually recurrent and attacks may be due to exposure to irritants, fatigue, and/or emotional situations. Asthma is classified as either intrinsic or extrinsic (see Table 5-6). Most clients have a combination of extrinsic and intrinsic asthma.

Table 5-6

Intrinsic (nonatopic) asthma	Extrinsic (atopic) asthma
Caused by anything except an allergy	Associated with allergens like pollen, pet dander, dust mites
Can be caused by chemicals such as cigarette smoke or cleaning agents, taking aspirin, a chest infection, stress, laughter, exercise, cold air, or food preservatives	Starts in childhood/teenage years
May be due to irritation of nerves or muscles of the airway	Familial predisposition: one-third of clients have at least one family member with a diagnosis of asthma
Most episodes occur after an infection of the respiratory tract	Usually have other allergy problems like hay fever, hives, allergic rhinitis, or eczema

Source: Created by author from References #4 and #5.

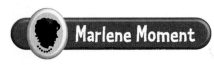

I knew it was legitimate when I said I was allergic to exercise!

What causes it and why

Airway inflammation occurs due to cells that cause inflammation— mainly lymphocytes, eosinophils, and mast cells. The inflamed airway becomes damaged and narrowed, which increases the work of breathing (see Table 5-7).

Table 5-7

Causes	Why
Environmental irritants: pet dander, dust and dust mites, cockroaches, fungi, mold, pollen, feathers, smoke, foods, cold air, food additives	Allergens cause histamine release, smooth muscles swell, airway narrows, poor gas exhange results
Stress	Hormones released during stressful times can influence gas exchange
Exercise	Increases work of breathing, making air exchange more difficult

Source: Created by author from References #4 and #5.

WHY IS THERE MORE ASTHMA NOW THAN BEFORE?   Vaccines and antibodies may have changed the way lymphocytes act in the body. Lymphocytes are supposed to fight infection, but now may actually encourage the body to release chemicals that cause the development of allergies. Additionally, children stay inside more than they used to, exposing them to insulation and artificial heat and cooling, which seems to increase exposure to allergens.[5]

Signs and Symptoms and why

The asthmatic response usually maxes out in a few hours, but can last for days and weeks, whereas the symptoms of asthma (see Table 5-8) usually occur suddenly after exposure to triggers. Most attacks occur in the morning after medications have worn off.

Status asthmaticus is a life-threatening emergency where the client is having repeated and prolonged asthma attacks unrelieved by medications.

Table 5-8

Signs and symptoms	Why
Itching on the neck	Early sign of impending attack in children; etiology unknown
Dry cough at night or with exercise	Etiology unknown
Wheezing (most noted on expiration) and bronchospasm	Leukotrienes, histamine, and other chemicals from the lung's mast cells cause bronchospasm and smooth muscle swelling, which narrows the airway
Wheezing during coughing	The higher the pitch of the wheeze, the narrower the airway
Breathlessness	Poor gas exchange
Cough (productive or nonproductive): worse at night and early morning	Excess mucus production
Mucosal edema	Histamine causes swelling of airway in the smooth muscle of the larger bronchi

(Continued)

Table 5-8. (*Continued*)

Signs and symptoms	Why
Mucus production	Histamine and leukotrienes increase mucus production; excess secretions narrow the airway further
Thick secretions	Goblet cells produce thick mucus; very hard to cough up
Sudden shortness of breath	Hypoxia
Increased respiratory rate with use of accessory muscles	Hypoxia due to worsening asthma or drug toxicity
Prolonged expiratory phase	Lungs trying to push air out
Increased pulse	Triggered by hypoxia; heart pumps harder and faster to move the limited oxygen to the vital organs
Increased blood pressure	Stress; hypoxemia can increase blood pressure
Chest tightness	Airways constricting
Diaphoresis	Anxiety; stress
Nasal flaring	Attempt to increase oxygen intake
Lung hyperinflation	Air travels into slightly opened airway lumen; on exhalation the bronchi collapse due to increased intrathoracic pressure. This causes air to become trapped
Hyperresonance to percussion	As above (air trapping in lungs)
Barrel chest	As above (air trapping in lungs)
Decreased breath sounds	Major airway obstruction
Lethargy	Hypoxia
Cyanosis	Hypoxia
Silent chest: life threatening	No air movement; PCO_2 will increase drastically
Adventitious breath sounds in lung bases	Bases of lungs fill with mucus due to increased histamine; decreases gas exchange
Respiratory alkalosis	Hyperventilation causing excessive loss of CO_2 (acid)
Decreased ability to speak	Not able to catch breath
Status asthmaticus: severe attack	Lack of response to medications; fatal if not corrected at once

Source: Created by author from References #4 and #5.

OTHER THINGS YOU NEED TO KNOW . . .

- If the asthma process continues, carbon dioxide retention will soon develop due to problems of alveolar ventilation and perfusion, therefore causing respiratory acidosis.

- Over time, chronic inflammation can cause airway remodeling, which leads to problems with airway resistance. This is one of the reasons why asthma can be a cause of COPD.

- Always consider clients admitted to a medical facility with asthma as being unstable even if they appear stable at the time of admission.

- The symptoms that accompany an emergent asthma attack include cyanosis, increasing anxiety, increasing shortness of breath, and increasing heart rate.[4]

Quickie tests and treatments

Tests:

- Skin testing for allergens.

- Pulmonary function tests (PFTs): PFTs measure how well the client is able to inhale and exhale air and how well the lungs are able to provide gas exchange. PFTs are usually diagnostic only during the attack itself. PFTs may show decreased peak flows, decreased vital capacity, and increased total lung capacity.

- Spirometry to assess amount of airway obstruction.

- Chest x-rays: helpful in determining lung hyperinflation (due to restrictive airflow), accumulation of secretions, and atelectasis.

Treatments for asthma are usually determined by the extent of the disease process:

- Desensitization if due to allergies.

- Prevention: If the environmental trigger is identified, avoidance of the precipitating irritant is the best course of action.

- Medications used to manage asthma on a daily basis are not used for treatment during an attack (see Table 5-9).

Table 5-9

Class	Medication	Comment
Bronchodilators	Theophylline (Aquaphyllin), aminophylline (Phyllocontin)	Stimulate beta-adrenergic receptors, which causes dilation of the airways; monitor blood levels with these drugs to prevent toxicity
Beta-adrenergic agonists	Albuterol (Proventil), epinephrine (AsthmaHaler Mist)	Acts on beta$_2$-adrenergic receptors in the lungs. As a result, other organs are not affected by these drugs; fewer side effects
Corticosteroids	Prednisone (Apoprednisone), hydrocortisone (Cortef), methylprednisolone (Solu-Medrol), beclomethasone (Beclodisk)	First-line drugs to reduce inflammation and swelling; inhaled form used for **prevention** (goes directly into the airway); this method limits systemic effects of steroids. Oral form used for severe cases of asthma
Mast cell stabilizers	Cromolyn (Nasalcrom), nedocromil (Tilade)	Decrease histamine, leukotrienes, bradykinins, and prostaglandins, which inflame the airway; used prophylactically
Leukotriene modifiers	Zileuton (Zyflo), montelukast sodium (Singulair), zafirlukast (Accolate)	Decrease bronchoconstriction and inflammation caused by leukotrienes; asthma preventative
Leukotriene receptor antagonists (LTRAs)	Montelukast sodium (Singulair)	Decrease bronchoconstriction and inflammation; prevent client from having to take as many high-dose inhaled steroids
Anticholinergics		Usually only given in the ED; blocks acetylcholine to prevent muscle contraction; dilates airway

Source: Created by author from References #4 and #5.

- Low-flow humidified oxygen O_2 adjusted according to ABGs, vital signs, and SaO_2.
- Teach relaxation exercises.
- Monitor ABGs.
- Monitor serum IgE: increases in allergic reactions.
- Monitor CBC: increased eosinophils.
- Keep intubation and ventilator equipment on hand.
- Chest physiotherapy to remove secretions.
- Administration of sedatives and narcotics cautiously.
- Asthma medications.

What can harm my client?

- Status asthmaticus.
- Pneumonia.
- Respiratory failure.
- Failure to get medical help during an attack that lasts 15 minutes or longer.

If I were your teacher I would test you on . . .

- Causes of asthma and related pathophysiology.
- Signs and symptoms of asthma and why they occur.
- Use of a metered dose inhaler.
- Complications associated with corticosteroid therapy.
- Asthma medications, appropriate dosages, and possible side effects.
- Respiratory assessment including evaluation of breath sounds.
- ABG interpretation.
- Management of status asthmaticus.
- Signs and symptoms of respiratory failure.
- Cardiopulmonary resuscitation (CPR).
- Prevention and patient education.
- Hydration therapy.
- Medications asthma patients should avoid and why.

✚ Chronic obstructive pulmonary disease

Chronic obstructive pulmonary disease (COPD) is the name given to a condition in which two pulmonary diseases exist at the same time, primarily chronic bronchitis and emphysema. Also, chronic asthma with either emphysema or chronic bronchitis may cause COPD.

What is it?

COPD is a condition in which obstruction to airflow impedes breathing. This is why the disease is sometimes called chronic airflow limitation (CAL). Since COPD is primarily chronic bronchitis and emphysema, we will review these two lung diseases. Chronic bronchitis occurs when the bronchi stay inflamed due to infection or irritation causing obstruction of the small and large airways. Emphysema is a condition in which the lungs have lost their elasticity, thus impeding gas exchange.

What causes it and why

Chronic bronchitis and emphysema (Fig. 5-4) are both primarily caused by cigarette smoking, making this disorder very preventable. Clients who are current smokers or have a history of smoking are at risk to develop lung infections and/or chronic inflammation. Recurrent pulmonary infections cause structural damage to the alveoli.[6] Clients with chronic bronchitis are called blue bloaters. Why? Because their excess respiratory secretions and obstruction cause hypoxia, hypercapnia, and cyanosis. Clients with chronic pulmonary emphysema are called pink puffers. Why? Because they are able to overventilate themselves and keep their ABGs somewhat normal until late in the disease.

Bronchitis signs and symptoms and why

Table 5-10 gives the signs, symptoms and associated reasons for bronchitis.

Table 5-10

Bronchitis signs and symptoms	Why
Excessive mucous production—gray, white, or yellow; early sign	Inflammation of bronchi from smoking, dust, or gas exposure; goblet cells hypersecrete mucus
Chronic cough	Body trying to rid itself of mucus
Airflow obstruction	Inflammation of bronchi causes narrowing
Dyspnea with increased intolerance to exercise; labored breathing at rest—early sign	Obstruction of airflow
Tachypnea	Hypoxia
Cyanosis	Hypoxia
Accessory muscle use	Hypoxia
Wheezes/rhonchi/crackles of expiration	Excess mucus
Prolonged expiration	Attempt to keep airway open
Polycythemia	Hypoxia causes increased RBC production as a compensatory mechanism; when hypoxic kidneys release erythropoietin it causes more RBCs to mature
Pulmonary hypertension resulting in right sided heart failure	Hypoxia increases blood pressure in the lungs increasing the workload on the right side of the heart
Edema; ascites	Right-sided heart failure; blood and fluid don't move forward but back-up causing the buildup of fluid

Source: Created by the author from Reference #6.

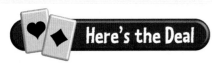

Anytime somebody has poly-cythemia, their blood is thicker, so they have an increased chance of developing a blood clot.

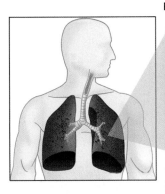

Enlarged alveoli

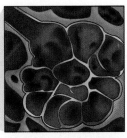

Emphysema; weakened and collapsed alveoli with excess mucus

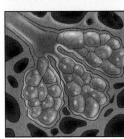

Normal healthy alveoli

◀ Figure 5-4. Chronic obstructive pulmonary disease: emphysema.

Emphysema signs and symptoms and why

Table 5-11 shows the signs, symptoms and reasons for emphysema.

Table 5-11

Emphysema signs and symptoms	Why
Dyspnea; tachypnea; air hunger	Hypoxia
Barrel-shaped chest	Hyperinflated lungs; trapped air increases AP diameter
Accessory muscle use	Increased work of breathing; increases alveolar ventilation
Prolonged expiration	Attempt to keep airway open
Grunting	Attempt to keep airway open
Clubbing of fingers and toes	Chronic hypoxia causing tissue changes
Inspiratory crackles, wheezes	Collapsed bronchioles
Decreased chest expansion	Collapsed bronchioles; not enough air to keep the lungs inflated
Decreased breath sounds	Air trapped in the alveoli
Hyperresonance on percussion	Air trapped in the alveoli
Increased total lung capacity (TLC)	Alveoli enlarge due to trapped air
Dyspnea on exertion	Hypoxia
Tachypnea	Decreased oxygenation
Pursed lip breathing; puffer breathing	Exerts back pressure into the lungs, helping to keep the alveoli open and decrease work of breathing; helps prevent alveolar collapse
Client prefers "seated" position	Improves chest expansion and oxygen flow
Weight loss	Eating interferes with breathing
Respiratory acidosis	Seen late in the disease process; poor gas exchange usually results in respiratory acidosis
Productive morning cough	Secretions pool overnight while client reclines

Source: Created by author from Reference #7.

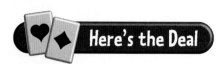

Here's the Deal

To be diagnosed with chronic bronchitis, the client must have had excessive mucus and chronic cough for at least 3 months of the past 2 years.

Quickie tests and treatments

Tests:

- Pulmonary function test.
- Pulse oximetry.
- ABGs.

Treatments:

- Smoking cessation.
- Medications: bronchodilators, steroids, mucolytics, anticholinergics, leukotriene antagonists, anxiolytics, diuretics (for right-sided heart failure).
- Immunization for influenza and pneumococcal pneumonia (Pneumovax).
- Prevent and manage respiratory infections.
- Postural drainage.
- Oxygen therapy.
- Hydration therapy.
- Monitoring ABGs.
- Small frequent meals to improve nutritional status.
- Pulmonary rehabilitation.

What can harm my client?

Clients with COPD usually only need low-flow oxygen because their drive to breathe is primarily based on their usual state of hypoxia. The chemoreceptors become insensitive to increased CO_2 levels with long-term lung disease. Increased O_2 (administering too much) may stop the hypoxic respiratory drive and cause CO_2 narcosis. Low oxygen levels are what keeps the client breathing. As long as the client is hypoxic, he will breathe. If your client receives more than 2 to 3 L/min of oxygen with an increase in PaO_2, he is no longer hypoxic and could stop breathing. Clients with COPD are very debilitated and at risk for further infections, severe respiratory failure, and safety issues such as falls.

If I were your teacher, I would test you on . . .

- Signs and symptoms of COPD and why.
- Causes of bronchitis and emphysema and why.
- Drug therapy.
- Proper positioning for clients experiencing dyspnea.
- Teaching the client pursed lip and diaphragmatic breathing.
- Infection precautions and control.
- Signs and symptoms of immunosuppression and related treatment.
- Teaching the client how to conserve energy.
- Teaching and implementing referrals for smoking cessation.
- Proper nutrition.
- Safety associated with home oxygen use.
- What ABGs look like in client with COPD (high PCO_2, low PO_2).

✚ Pulmonary edema

What is it?

Pulmonary edema occurs when capillary fluid leaks into the alveoli. Since the alveoli are filled with fluid, they don't oxygenate the blood very well and the patient will be in respiratory distress. This results in cardiac problems for the client. Pulmonary edema can be chronic or acute and can become fatal rapidly (Tables 5-12 and 5-13).

What causes it and why

Remember, anytime cardiac output drops (depending on how much) blood will back-up to lungs causing pulmonary edema.

Table 5-12

Causes	Why
Left-sided heart failure	Decreased cardiac pumping causes output to drop so blood backs-up to lungs
Left-sided myocardial infarction (MI)	Dead cardiac tissues can't pump blood causing cardiac output to drop
Valvular heart disease	Diseased valve causes backflow of blood into the heart, causing a drop in cardiac output
Arrhythmias	Decreased cardiac output
High blood pressure	Systemic high blood pressure causes an increase in aortic blood pressure; left ventricle has difficulty opening against this pressure (afterload); cardiac output drops because blood cannot escape the left ventricle

Source: Created by author from Reference #8.

Signs and symptoms and why

Table 5-13

Signs and symptoms	Why
Scared expression on client's face	Fear of not being able to breathe
Shortness of breath	Fluid in lungs; deoxygenated blood; hypoxia
Orthopnea	When client lies supine, blood moves from the legs to the heart and lungs increasing preload
Rapid, labored breathing	Fluid in the lungs; hypoxia
Tachycardia	Hypoxia
Dependent crackles developing into diffuse crackles	Fluid in lungs
Signs and symptoms of shock: cold, clammy skin; low blood pressure	Cardiac output drops making the body think it is in shock (blood is not making it to systemic circulation)
Frothy, blood stained sputum with cough; looks like beaten egg-whites	Fluid in lungs; air mixes with the fluid that contains RBCs
Cyanosis	Hypoxia
Jugular vein distension	Decreased cardiac output causes blood backup and veins to distend
FIL Respiratory acidosis	Poor gas exchange causes CO_2 retention
Restlessness	Hypoxia
S3 gallop	S1 and S2 aren't enough to pump the blood; the heart adds extra beats in an attempt to increase cardiac output
Cardiomegaly	Heart enlarges in presence of CHF (heart is overworked)

Source: Created by author from Reference #8.

Quickie tests and treatments

Tests:

- ABGs: hypoxemia, hypercapnia, or acidosis.
- Chest x-ray: diffuse haziness in lung fields, pleural effusion, cardiomegaly.
- Pulse oximetry: decreased O_2 saturation.
- Pulmonary artery catheterization: increased pulmonary artery wedge pressures. (increased wedge means pressures in left heart are increasing due to decreased ability to pump.)
- Electrocardiography: valvular disease.

Treatments:

- Supplemental oxygen (to correct hypoxia).
- Elevate the head of the bed (to help with breathing and to improve cardiac output); lower foot of bed so fluid will pool in lower extremities (this diverts some fluid away from the lungs).
- Weigh daily to monitor for fluid retention.
- Strict I & O (you want to make sure the client is putting out as much as she is taking in, or she is going to go into fluid volume excess and pulmonary edema again).
- Monitor vital signs, PA pressures, and wedge pressures as ordered.
- Treatment of underlying cause of cardiac condition.
- Consider mechanical ventilation.
- Diuretics: decrease the amount of blood returning to the right side of the heart; decrease preload.
- Positive inotropic drugs (improves heart's pumping ability).
- Nitroprusside (Nipride) IV to vasodilate arterial system; this will decrease the pressure that the LV has to pump against in the aorta (afterload). Therefore cardiac output increases.
- Nitroglycerin IV promotes vasodilation, decreases afterload.
- Naterocor (Nesiritide) IV promotes vasodilation, and as a diuretic effect also decreases wedge pressure.
- Milrinone (Primacor) IV promotes vasodilation.
- Dobutamine (Dobutrex) IV increases cardiac output.
- Morphine IV decreases anxiety and promotes vasodilation.
- If in severe CHF, consider intra-aortic balloon pump to decrease workload on the heart and to rest the weakened heart muscle.

What can harm my client?

- Increased fluid in the interstitial space leads to hypoxia, which can lead to acute respiratory failure.
- Respiratory depression from morphine.
- Arrhythmias.
- Cardiac arrest.
- Respiratory acidosis.

If I were your teacher, I would test you on . . .

- Causes of pulmonary edema and why.
- Signs and symptoms of pulmonary edema and why.
- The importance of monitoring clients receiving rapid IV fluid replacement.
- Respiratory assessment including breath sounds.
- Signs and symptoms of right-sided heart failure.
- Care of the client receiving postural drainage.
- Client education.
- Drug therapy for pulmonary edema.
- Prevention of pulmonary edema.
- Importance of reporting early signs of fluid volume excess.

✚ Pulmonary embolism

What is it?

- A thrombus that moves from a site in the body to the lungs.
- Once a thrombus moves, it is called an embolus.
- The majority of pulmonary embolisms (PEs) stem from deep vein thrombosis (DVT) in the legs.
- Some pulmonary emboli are mild and cause no symptoms, whereas others can kill a client rapidly. This depends on how much of the pulmonary arterial circulation is obstructed.
- A thrombus is not a problem as long as it stays in its place. However, if the client walks or bears weight or even has a muscle spasm, the thrombus could loosen or a piece of it could break off, forming an embolus (Tables 5-14 and 5-15).

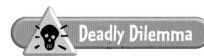

Deadly Dilemma

If you ever see air going into a central line, position the patient in left Trendelenburg. This will help move the air bubble backward instead of forward into the lungs and into the peripheral venous circulation.

What causes it and why

Table 5-14

Causes	Why
Thrombus dislodges from the legs or pelvis	Moves into the lungs
Thrombus dislodges from heart valve	Clot forms on heart valve and breaks loose; smaller growths break off and form embolus
Atrial fibrillation	Atrial quiver causing turbulent blood flow; could cause clot that travels to lungs
Central venous catheters	Clot could form on foreign body (catheter tip) and dislodge
Fractures	Especially in long bones, fat emboli could travel to the lungs
Immobility	Increases risk of DVTs
Dehydration; polycythemia vera	Blood is thick, which leads to clot formation

(Continued)

Table 5-14. (*Continued*)

Causes	Why
Pregnancy	Blood pools in lower extremities; increases risk of DVT
Vein disorders: varicose veins	Blood pools in the venous system, increasing risk of clots
Sickle cell disease	Cells lyse forming a "C" shape; they tangle and form a clot
Long car or plane trip	Blood pools in venous system of lower extremities, increasing risk of clots
Thrombophlebitis	Vein inflammation can lead to clot formation
Large air bubble in IV	Air bubble travels to right heart and then the lungs
Birth control pills/hormone replacement	Causes blood to thicken, which can lead to clot formation
Smoking while taking oral contraceptives	Blood thickens by resisting naturally occurring anticoagulants
Cancer	Some cancer cells produce clotting factors that lead to thrombus formation
Amniotic fluid	Ruptured membranes can cause an amniotic fluid bubble to enter the maternal circulation

Source: Created by author from Reference #9.

Signs and symptoms and why

Table 5-15

Signs and symptoms	Why
Shortness of breath—first sign	Clot impairs oxygenation causing hypoxia
Chest pain: sharp, substernal	Called pleuritic pain: pain increases on inspiration and decreases on expiration
Cough (hemoptysis)	Inflammation of the lungs
Restlessness; anxiety	Hypoxia
Tachycardia	Hypoxia
Low-grade fever	Inflammation
Cyanosis	Hypoxia
Crackles; pleural rub	Heard at embolism site due to inflammation
Pulmonary hypertension	Hypoxia is main cause of pulmonary hypertension; vasoconstriction in the lungs occurs in the presence of large embolus which increases pressures

Source: Created by author from Reference #9.

Quickie tests and treatments

Tests:

- ABGs: hypoxemia.
- D-dimer test positive: increases with PE; increases if clot is present in the body.
- Chest x-ray: small infiltrate or effusion.
- Lung perfusion scan: ventilation–perfusion mismatch.
- Pulmonary angiography: pulmonary filling defect; abrupt vessel ending; reveals location and extent of pulmonary embolism.
- EKG: rule out MI; detect signs of right-sided heart failure (anytime there are lung problems, the right side of the heart is stressed).
- Spiral chest computed tomography scan: positive for pulmonary emboli.
- Test for DVTs: venous studies, lower limb compression ultrasonography, impedance plethysmography, and contrast venography.

Treatments:

- Mechanical ventilation.
- Oxygen therapy.
- Anticoagulants, fibrolytics, vasopressors (for hypotension).
- Pneumatic sequential compression devices or graded compression elastic stockings to increase venous return.
- DVT medications: aspirin, clopidogrel (Plavix), dipyridamole (Persantine), enoxaparin (Lovenox).
- Vena caval ligation or placement of an umbrella filter (especially in clients who can't take anticoagulants). Prevents clots from going to lungs.
- Pulmonary embolectomy.
- Monitor the pulse oximetry (SaO_2).
- Turn client as ordered by MD, no chest physiotherapy, no back rubs (prevents emboli movement).
- Narcotics for pain: monitor respiratory rate.
- Bed rest during acute phase.
- Monitor for right sided heart failure: hypoxia in the lungs causes the blood pressure to increase in the lungs. This leads to an increased workload on the right side of the heart, resulting in heart failure.
- Incentive spirometry to expand the lungs

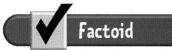

Factoid

When giving Lovenox you will see an air bubble. Do not expel it. This bubble helps prevent the loss of medicine.

What can harm my client?

- Total occlusion may be fatal.
- Pulmonary infarction.
- Respiratory failure.
- Acute right-sided heart failure (cor pulmonale).

If I were your teacher, I would test you on . . .

- Causes of pulmonary embolism and why.
- Signs and symptoms of pulmonary embolism and why.

- Medications and their contraindications.
- Most appropriate IV site for a fibrinolytic.
- How to monitor a prothrombin (PT) and partial thromboplastin time (PTT).
- Teaching for clients going home on medications.
- Hydration therapy and overhydration precautions.
- Patient education regarding dental procedures, leg positioning, bleeding precautions (especially when an coumadin and other anticlot drugs).
- Recognition of high risk patients for DVT.
- Methods to prevent venous stasis.

✚ Pneumonia

What is it?

Pneumonia is an acute infection of the lungs—bacterial or viral—that impairs gas exchange (see Tables 5-16 and 5-17). Inflammation occurs, mucus is secreted, and alveoli can fill with blood and fluid, causing atelectasis. Inflammation makes the lung stiff, making it more difficult to breathe. Hypoxia occurs from the fluid-filled alveoli, which impedes the oxygenation of the blood. Pneumonia can be localized to just a lobe of the lung or can cover an entire lung.

- Lobar pneumonia is consolidation of part or an entire lobe.
- Bronchopneumonia is consolidation of more than one lobe.

Classification of pneumonia

COMMUNITY-ACQUIRED PNEUMONIA (CAP)   Acquired outside the hospital; usually diagnosed within 48 hours of being admitted to the hospital; mainly affects the lower respiratory tract. The two presentations are:

1. Typical.

- Most common bacterial cause is *Streptococcus pneumoniae*.
- Second most common bacterial cause is *Haemophilus influenzae*.
- *Staphylococcus aureus* is another common organism.
- Common communicable viruses that cause CAP mostly affect young males: influenza, RSV, adenovirus, and parainfluenza virus.

2. Atypical.

- Most common causes are *Legionella*, *Mycoplasma*, and *Chlamydia*.

HOSPITAL-ACQUIRED PNEUMONIA (HAP)   Previously named nosocomial infection; lower respiratory tract infection not present when the client is admitted to the hospital; usually occurs within 48 hours of hospital admission.

- High-risk clients are on a ventilator; have decreased immune systems, any type of chronic lung disease, or a tracheotomy.
- The organisms causing HAPs are different from those that cause CAPs: many times these organisms are resistant to antibiotics and are very difficult to treat.

- HAPs are caused by *Pseudomonas*, *Enterobacter*, and *Staphylococcus aureus*.

OPPORTUNISTIC PNEUMONIAS

- Seen in clients with very poor immune systems: malnutrition, HIV/AIDS, transplant clients receiving steroids, cancer clients.
- Opportunistic pneumonias are caused by *Pneumocystis carinii*, cytomegalovirus, and fungi.

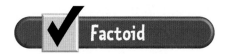

Factoid

As a rule, if you have a healthy immune system things such as *Pneumocystis carinii*, cytomegalovirus, and fungi are nothing to worry about.

Causes and why

Table 5-16

Causes	Why
Decreased cough	Decreased cough impedes lungs from expelling mucus, bacteria, and viruses
Aspiration	Bacteria that cause pneumonia reside in the oropharynx and nasopharynx and migrate to the lungs by aspiration; cause lung inflammation
Antibiotic use	Alters normal flora of lungs, allowing bacteria to grow rapidly
Smoking	Tobacco smoke decreases cilia, which impedes lungs from expelling mucus
Client illness: diabetes, AIDS, chronic lung disease	Alters normal flora of lungs, allowing bacteria to grow rapidly
Near-drowning	Aspiration of bacteria-laden water; clean water may also cause severe lung inflammation
Inhaling noxious gases	Lung inflammation; impaired gas exhange
Steroid therapy	Suppresses immune system
Malnutrition	Poor immune system
Alcoholism	Poor immune system
Clients who are NPO	If proper mouth care is not provided, bacteria will migrate from the mouth to the lungs
Clients who've undergone abdominal or thorax surgery	Postop pain impedes deep breathing, which allows fluid to accumulate in the lungs

Source: Created by author from Reference #10.

WHO IS AT RISK FOR ASPIRATION PNEUMONIA?

- Geriatric clients.
- Clients with decreased level of consciousness (LOC).
- Postop clients.
- Clients with a poor gag reflex.
- Weak clients.
- Clients receiving tube feedings.

Signs and symptoms and why

Table 5-17

Signs and symptoms	Why
Fever	Infection
Pleuritic pain	Infection and inflammation; pleural inflammation
Chills	Infection
Increased respiratory rate	Hypoxia due to decreased alveoli ventilation
Lethargy	Infection
Productive cough	Congested lungs
Shortness of breath	Hypoxia
Crackles	Congested lungs
Decreased breath sounds	Congested lungs
Dullness noted on percussion over the lungs	Consolidation of fluid and mucus in that area

Source: Created by author from Reference #10.

SPUTUM RAINBOW   The colors of sputum and their corresponding bacteria follow:

- Rust = *Streptococcus pneumoniae*.
- Pink = *Staphylococcus aureus*.
- Green with odor = *Pseudomonas aeruginosa*.

Quickie tests and treatments

Tests:

- Chest x-ray: patchy or lobular infiltrates.
- CBC: leukocytosis.
- Blood culture: positive for causative organism.
- ABGs: hypoxemia.
- Fungal/acid-fast bacilli cultures: identify etiologic agent.
- Sputum culture: positive for infecting organism.
- Assay for *Legionella*-soluble antigen in urine: positive.
- Bronchoscopy: identify etiologic agent.
- Transtracheal aspiration specimen: identify etiologic agent.

Treatments:

- Antibiotics for bacterial infection.
- Push fluids: 3 liters per day unless contraindicated to thin out secretions (the thinner the secretion the easier it will be for the patient to cough them out) rehydrate from fever.
- Humidified oxygen to reverse hypoxia and decrease work of breathing.

- Bronchodilators help to get more oxygen into the body:
    1. Sympathomimetics: albuterol (Proventil), metaproterenol (Alupent).
    2. Methylxanthines: theophylline (Theolair), aminophylline (Truphylline).
- Encourage client to cough and deep-breathe.
- Increase calories and protein in the diet. The client is burning more calories to breathe; needs protein to help fight infection.
- Consider the need for mechanical ventilation.
- Antipyretics for fever.
- Turn every two hours: prevents stasis of lung secretions.
- Elevate the head of the bed 45 degrees: easier to breathe sitting up and helps with lung expansion.
- Suction if needed.
- Monitor the ABGs, vital signs, and the pulse oximetry.
- Monitor the chest x-ray.
- Encourage frequent rest periods.
- Small frequent meals: work of breathing increases with large meal.
- Smoking cessation.
- Monitor CBC, especially WBC count.
- Drugs to liquefy secretions: guaifenesin (Anti-Tuss) or acetylcysteine (Mucomyst).
- Elderly clients and high-risk clients should have a pneumonia vaccine every 5 years.

What will harm my client?

- Respiratory failure.
- Septic shock.
- Septic shock that can lead to carditis, meningitis, and sepsis.
- Age: elderly are at greatest risk of death with any form of pneumonia.

If I were your teacher, I would test you on . . .

- Causes for pneumonia and why.
- Signs and symptoms of pneumonia and why.
- Proper handling of secretions.
- Infection precautions.
- Importance of annual flu shot.
- Medication administration and side effects.
- Chest physiotherapy.
- Respiratory assessment including abnormal findings.
- Sputum specimen and culture protocols.
- Aspiration prevention and management.

DISORDERS THAT AFFECT THE PLEURAL SPACE

The lungs have two linings surrounding them—visceral and parietal pleurae. When these linings rub together during respiration, they do so smoothly due to the presence of a little bit of lubricating fluid. If a client becomes dehydrated, the fluid becomes diminished. Due to this, you may hear a pleural friction rub during your routine respiratory assessment. In addition, blood, air, or excess fluid can accumulate between these two linings, putting pressure on the lungs, and causing a collapse of either the whole lung or one area of the lung.

✛ Pneumothorax

What is it?

Pneumothorax is when the lung collapses due to air accumulating in the pleural space (Fig. 5-5).

▶ Figure 5-5. Pneumothorax. The black area indicates air, blood, or fluid that has accumulated and collapsed the lung.

Pleural space

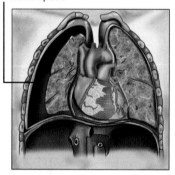

Pneumothorax

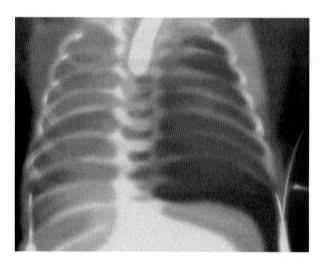

What causes it and why

There are three types of pneumothorax: open, closed, and tension. Tables 5-18 to 5-20 give their signs and symptoms.

Table 5-18

Type of pneumothorax	Cause	Why
Open	• Penetrating chest injury • Central venous catheter insertion • Chest surgery • Transbronchial biopsy • Thoracentesis • Percutaneous lung biopsy	Atmospheric air flows directly into the pleural cavity, collapsing the lung on the affected side. Also called a "sucking chest wound" or "communicating pneumothorax"
Closed	• Blunt chest trauma • Rib fracture • Clavicle fracture • Congenital bleb rupture • Emphysematous bullae rupture • Barotrauma • Erosive tubercular or cancerous lesions • Interstitial lung disease	Air enters the pleural space from within the lung, increasing pleural pressure and preventing lung expansion
Tension	• Mechanical ventilation	High levels of PEEP cause increased pressure in the lungs, which can cause the lungs to rupture
Tension	• Chest tube occlusion	If the chest tube leaving the pleural space is compressed in any way, air cannot escape from the pleural space, causing increased air pressure and collapse of the lung. The same thing can occur if the air vent on the chest tube system is covered or occluded
Tension	• Penetrating chest wound	Air in the pleural space is under higher pressure than air in the adjacent lung. Air enters the pleural space from a pleural rupture only on inspiration. This air pressure exceeds barometric pressure, causing compression atelectasis. Increased pressure may displace the heart and great vessels and cause mediastinal shift[11]

Source: Created by author from Reference #11.

Signs and symptoms of closed and open pneumothorax and why

Table 5-19

Signs and symptoms of closed and open pneumothorax	Why
Sudden sharp pleuritic pain	Inflammation at site of injury is increased with any chest wall movement
Chest does not rise or fall symmetrically	One lung is deflated
Cyanosis	Severe hypoxia
Shortness of breath	Breathing with only one lung instead of two; hypoxia
Absent breath sounds	Deflated lung
Tachycardia	Hypoxia increases heart rate
Subcutaneous emphysema	Air leaks out of lung into tissue
Distension of chest wall on affected side	Excessive air accumulates on affected side

Source: Created by author from Reference #11.

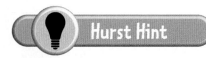

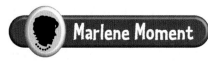

Signs and symptoms of tension pneumothorax and why

Table 5-20

Signs and symptoms of tension pneumothorax	Why
Hypotension	Pressure builds up and presses on vena cava, which decreases the amount of blood returning to the heart; decreases cardiac output
Increased pulse	Hypoxia
Increased respiratory rate	Hypoxia
Mediastinal shift	Pressure builds up on affected side and pushes everything to opposite side
Deviated trachea	As above
Distended jugular veins	Pressure builds inside thorax causing back pressure
Signs and symptoms of shock	Cardiac output decreases, not enough blood reaches the organs, the body thinks it's in shock
Hyperresonance with percussion	Affected lung side (pleural space) is full of air
Respiratory distress	One functioning lung decreases gas exchange; hypoxia

Source: Created by author from Reference #11.

What can harm my client?

- Malfunctioning chest tube, oxygen equipment, or ventilator
- Infection
- Malnutrition
- Moving a trauma patient resulting in further injury

Quickie tests and treatment

Tests:

- Chest x-ray: air in the pleural space; possible mediastinal shift.
- ABGs: low PO_2 and high PCO_2.
- Pulse oximetry: decreased initially but usually goes back to normal in 24 hours due to treatment.

Treatments:

- Bed rest to decrease need for oxygen.
- Monitor vital signs.
- Oxygen therapy.
- Chest tube placement: removes air from the pleural space so the lung can re-expand.
- Possible surgery: thoracotomy, pleurectomy.

- Pain medications: monitor respirations.
- Elevate the head of the bed: promotes maximum lung expansion, decreases work of breathing.
- If chest trauma, the doctor may place an epidural catheter to manage pain.
- If pneumothorax is due to trauma, protect the cervical spine and keep the body perfectly aligned until the doctor says the cervical spine is clear.
- Administer anxiolytics and teach relaxation techniques: client is scared because he can't breathe.
- If client has a tension pneumothorax, the initial treatment of choice is to insert a large-bore needle into the second intercostal space mid-clavicular line to relieve pressure. Next, a chest tube system is placed into the fourth intercostal space.

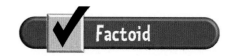

A small pneumothorax may heal itself.

If I were your teacher, I would test you on . . .

- Causes of pneumothorax and why.
- Signs and symptoms of pneumothorax and why.
- Management of chest tube system and related complications.
- Medications and potential side effects.
- Patient safety precautions.
- Measures to increase lung expansion and decrease work of breathing.
- Surgical outcomes and possible complications.

✚ Hemothorax

What is it?

A hemothorax (Fig. 5-6 and Table 5-21) is blood in the pleural cavity that can result in lung collapse.

- If client has had a hemothorax, watch for signs of hemorrhage. May need an autotransfusion (this is when blood from the pleural cavity is given back to the client IV).

What causes it and why

Damaged blood vessels in the lungs cause blood to enter the pleural cavity. The causes of blood vessel damage are:

- Blunt or penetrating chest trauma.
- Thoracic surgery.
- Pulmonary infarction.
- Neoplasm.
- Dissecting thoracic aneurysm.
- Anticoagulant therapy.
- Thoracic endometriosis.
- Central venous catheter insertion.[12]

▶ Figure 5-6. **A.** Normal anatomy of lung. **B.** Hemothorax.

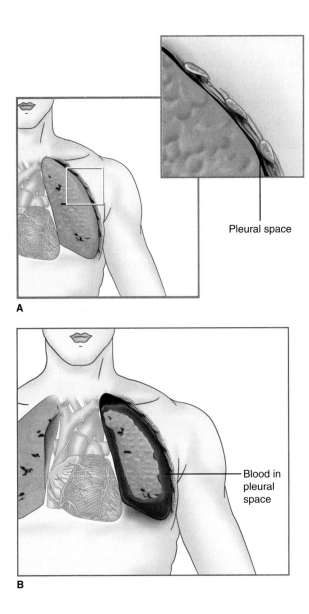

Pleural space

Blood in pleural space

A

B

Signs and symptoms and why

Table 5-21

Signs and symptoms	Why
Tachypnea	Hypoxia
Dusky skin color, cyanosis	Severe hypoxia
Diaphoresis	Pain
Hemoptysis	Blood in the lungs
Anxiety, restlessness	Hypoxia; pain
Affected side may expand and stiffen	Accumulation of excessive air (as with a stab wound)
Stupor	Decreased oxygen flow to the brain
Dullness on percussion over affected side	Filled with blood and fluid creating dull sound; collapsed lung
Decreased or absent breath sounds over affected side	Collapsed lung

Source: Created by author from Reference #12.

Quickie tests and treatments

Tests:

* Pleural fluid analysis: hematocrit greater than 50% of serum hematocrit.
* ABGs: increased PCO_2 and decreased PO_2.
* CBC: decreased hemoglobin depending on blood loss.
* Chest x-ray: positive for hemothorax.
* CT: positive for hemothorax.
* Thoracentesis: positive for blood and serosanguineous fluid.

Treatments:

* Stop hemorrhage.
* Remove blood from pleural cavity.
* Re-expansion of affected lung.
* Oxygen therapy.
* Administer analgesics.
* Chest tube (Fig. 5-7).
* Suctioning.
* Blood transfusion.
* Thoracotomy: if chest tube doesn't improve condition.

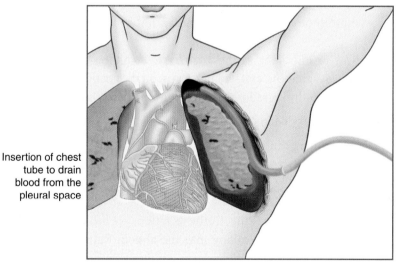

◀ Figure 5-7. Insertion of chest tube for hemothorax.

Insertion of chest tube to drain blood from the pleural space

What can harm my client?

* Adverse reaction to blood transfusion.
* Massive hemorrhage.
* Infection.
* Chest tube and oxygen equipment malfunction.

If I were your teacher, I would test you on . . .

* Pre- and postoperative care.
* Possible postoperative complications.
* Chest tube function.

- Laboratory and diagnostic tests.
- Safety protocols for administering blood products.
- Pathophysiology of hemothorax.

SUMMARY

This is a quick recap of the respiratory system. You can see how rapidly respiratory illness can progress in some clients. The respiratory system is tightly aligned with the cardiovascular system. This is why it is imperative that you always remember to perform a thorough respiratory and cardiovascular assessment on these clients to home in on any potential complications. Proper nursing assessment can save clients' lives!

PRACTICE QUESTIONS

1. Which are risk factors for obstructive sleep apnea? Select all that apply.

    1. Obesity.

    2. Smoking.

    3. Alcohol consumption.

    4. Snoring.

    Correct answers: 1, 2, & 3. Obesity, smoking, and alcohol consumption are all risk factors for obstructive sleep apnea. Snoring is a symptom of obstructive sleep apnea, not a risk factor.

2. A 52-year-old client is brought to the ED with the following symptoms: dyspnea, agitation, crackles upon auscultation, and a productive cough of pink, frothy secretion. The nurse immediately suspects:

    1. Pulmonary edema.

    2. Pulmonary embolism.

    3. Pneumonia.

    4. Pleural effusion.

    Correct answer: 1. Pink, frothy secretions are indicative of pulmonary edema due to fluid leaking into the alveoli. Pulmonary embolism is caused by an embolus obstructing a pulmonary artery, thus decreasing blood flow to the alveoli. Pneumonia does not cause pink, frothy secretions. Pleural effusion is caused by fluid entering the pleural space, not alveoli, and thus no frothy secretions are created.

3. A client with COPD is admitted to the hospital with respiratory distress where O_2 therapy is ordered. The nurse would be concerned most with which test result?

    1. Increased confusion.

    2. Increased CO_2 levels.

    3. Increased pH.

    4. Increased O_2 level.

Correct answer: 2. Increased blood O_2 levels can decrease the respiratory stimulus in the client with COPD, causing CO_2 levels to go up. O_2 therapy would decrease confusion. A decrease in pH indicates increased CO_2 levels. An increased O_2 level is expected; the CO_2 level is the biggest concern.

4. Which drug class is a quick-relief medication used to treat asthma?

   1. Corticosteroids.

   2. Diuretics.

   3. Leukotriene modifiers.

   4. Anticholinergics.

   Correct answer: 4. Anticholinergics are a quick-relief medication typically only used in the ED for management of asthma. Corticosteroids and leukotriene modifiers are long-acting. Diuretics are not used to treat asthma.

5. In taking care of a client with acute respiratory distress syndrome (ARDS), the nurse knows that a characteristic specific to ARDS is:

   1. Arterial hypoxemia unresponsive to supplemental O_2.

   2. Increased lung compliance.

   3. Pink, frothy sputum.

   4. Barrel chest.

   Correct answer: 1. Impaired gas exchange due to decreased lung compliance can cause arterial hypoxemia unresponsive to supplemental O_2, as seen in ARDS. Lung compliance is decreased in ARDS. Pink, frothy sputum is characteristic of pulmonary edema. Barrel chest is associated with emphysema.

6. Which respiratory disorder is associated with right ventricular hypertrophy?

   1. Pleural effusion.

   2. Pulmonary hypertension.

   3. Tuberculosis.

   4. Tension pneumothorax.

   Correct answer: 2. Ventricular hypertrophy occurs when the pulmonary vascular bed can no longer sustain the blood volume delivered to the right ventricle as seen in pulmonary hypertension. Pleural effusion is associated with fluid in the pleural space. Tuberculosis does not primarily affect the heart. Circulatory function is compromised with tension pneumothorax but not by right ventricular hypertrophy.

7. A client returns from a bronchoscopy procedure. Which would the nurse recognize as a complication of this procedure?

1. Aspiration.

2. Infection at incision site.

3. Gastric perforation.

4. Reaction to dye.

Correct answer: 1. The local anesthetic used impairs swallowing, which could lead to aspiration. A bronchoscopy passes a scope orally through the bronchial tubes; there is no incision site or risk of gastric perforation. Dye is not used in bronchoscopies, but it is used in lung scans.

8. A nurse is caring for a client experiencing acute atelectasis. The nurse would perform which of the following nursing interventions? Select all that apply.

1. Discourage use of pain medication.

2. Turn frequently.

3. Encourage deep breathing and coughing.

4. Encourage early ambulation.

Correct answers: 2, 3, & 4. Turning the client frequently, encouraging deep breathing and coughing, and encouraging early ambulation, move secretions. The client may require pain medication in order to turn, cough, and deep-breathe.

9. When auscultating a client's lungs, the nurse hears soft, high-pitched popping sounds upon inspiration. This is documented as:

1. Wheezes.

2. Crackles.

3. Friction rubs.

4. Rhonchi.

Correct answer: 2. Crackles are soft, high-pitched popping sounds that may be coarse or fine and are heard upon inspiration. Wheezes are a musical, high-pitched whistling sound. Friction rubs are harsh, crackling sounds made by 2 surfaces rubbing together. Ronchi sound like bubbles.

10. Surgical management of emphysema includes: Select all that apply.

1. Bullectomy.

2. Lung volume reduction surgery.

3. Lung transplant.

4. Lung biopsy.

Correct answers: 1, 2, & 3. Bullectomy is an option for clients with bullous emphysema. Lung volume reduction surgery is for clients with localized emphysema. Lung transplant is used in end-stage emphysema. Lung biopsy is done for diagnostic purposes, not treatment.

References

1. Thomas CL, ed. *Taber's Cyclopedic Medical Dictionary*. 18th ed. Philadelphia: Davis; 1997.

2. American Lung Association. *Adult (Acute) Respiratory Distress Syndrome (ARDS) Fact Sheet*. Available at: www.lungusa.org/site/pp.asp?c=dvLUK9O0E&b=35012. Accessed December 20, 2006.

3. National Library of Medicine. *Medical Encyclopedia: ARDS (Acute Respiratory Distress Syndrome)*. Available at: www.nlm.nih.gov/medlineplus/ency/article/000103.htm. Accessed December 20, 2006.

4. American Lung Association. *Facts about Asthma*. Available at: www.lungusa.org/site/pp.asp?c=dvLUK9O0E&b=22582. Accessed December 27, 2006.

5. National Library of Medicine. *Medical Encyclopedia: Asthma*. Available at: www.nlm.nih.gov/medlineplus/ency/article/000141.htm. Accessed December 27, 2006.

6. National Emphysema Foundation. *Pulmonary Disease: COPD*. Available at: http://emphysemafoundation.org/copdcbro.jsp. Accessed December 20, 2006.

7. American Lung Association. *What Is Emphysema?* Available at: www.lungusa.org/site/pp.asp?c=dvLUK9O0E&b=34706. Accessed December 20, 2006.

8. Pulmonary edema. *Nurse's 3 Minute Clinical Reference*. Springhouse, PA: Lippincott Williams & Wilkins; 2003:455–457.

9. Pulmonary embolism. *Nurse's 3 Minute Clinical Reference*. Springhouse, PA: Lippincott Williams & Wilkins; 2003:458–459.

10. *Pneumonia. Just the Facts: Pathophysiology*. Ambler, PA: Lippincott Williams & Wilkins; 2005:65–68.

11. Pneumothorax. *Nurse's 3 Minute Clinical Reference*. Springhouse, PA: Lippincott Williams & Wilkins; 2003:430–431.

12. Hemothorax. *Nurse's 3 Minute Clinical Reference*. Springhouse, PA: Lippincott Williams & Wilkins; 2003:252–253.

Bibliography

Hurst Review Services. www.hurstreview.com.

Springhouse editors. *Handbook of Pathophysiology*. 2nd ed. Philadelphia: Lippincott Williams & Wilkins; 2005.

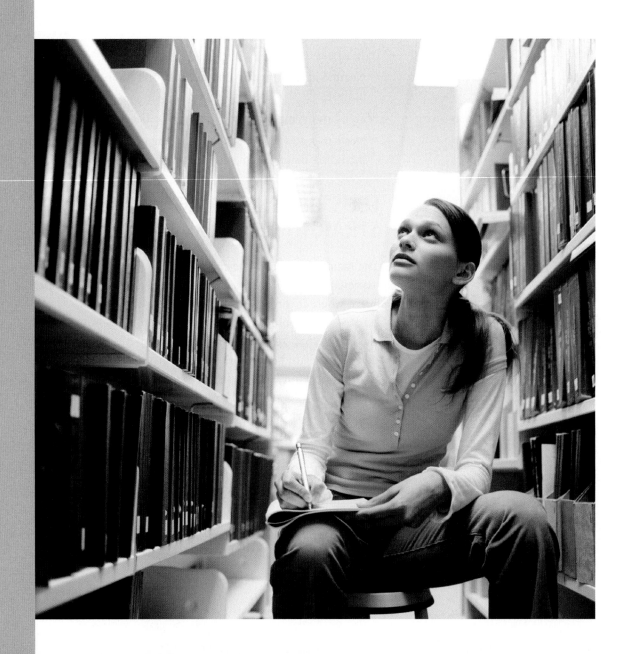

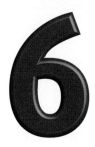

Cardiovascular System

OBJECTIVES

In this chapter, you'll review:

- Normal heart function and the pathophysiology of common cardiac illnesses.
- Signs and symptoms associated with these common cardiac problems.
- Need-to-know information regarding common cardiac problems including diagnostic tests, treatments, and possible complications.

LET'S GET THE NORMAL STUFF STRAIGHT FIRST

The major purpose of the cardiovascular system (Fig. 6-1) is to provide oxygenated blood to our cells and return deoxygenated blood to the heart, where it travels to the lungs to be reoxygenated. First of all, deoxygenated blood comes from the body, from the venous system, and travels via the inferior (from lower body) and superior (from upper body) vena cava to the right atrium. Blood flows from the right atrium to the right ventricle and out to the lungs through the pulmonary artery. The blood then picks up oxygen in the lungs and travels via the pulmonary vein to the left atrium and down to the left ventricle. From the left ventricle, oxygenated blood is pumped out through the aorta to the body.

✚ Pump you up

The entire heart acts as a pump and likes to move blood in one direction: forward. If blood is not moving forward, it backs up into the venous or arterial system. If the right side of the pump begins to fail, blood backs up into the venous system. When the left side of the heart fails, blood

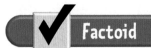

Factoid

The pulmonary artery is the only deoxygenated artery in the body. The pulmonary vein is the only oxygenated vein in the body.

▶ Figure 6-1. The heart.

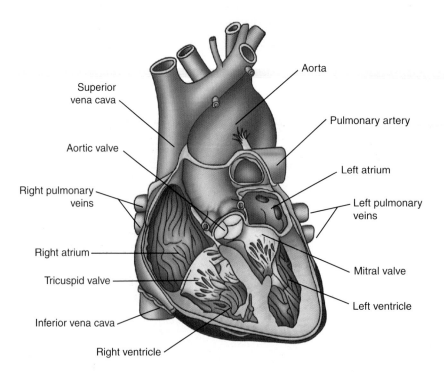

Superior
vena cava

Aorta

Aortic valve

Pulmonary artery

Right pulmonary
veins

Left atrium

Left pulmonary
veins

Right atrium

Mitral valve

Tricuspid valve

Left ventricle

Inferior vena cava

Right ventricle

backs up into the lungs, preventing blood from being pumped out to the rest of the body.

Forward blood flow out of the left ventricle can be measured using a special catheter—a thermodilution catheter. Thermodilution catheters—also called PA or Swan-Ganz catheters—are used to measure cardiac output or forward flow of blood (in the form of tissue perfusion) out of the left side of the heart. If cardiac output drops, for whatever reason, this means the left ventricle has decreased forward flow. If this decrease in forward flow is significant, the client may show signs and symptoms of decreased cardiac output. The most important skill a nurse can possess is to be competent in the assessment of the client's cardiac output. A quickie cardiac output assessment includes level of consciousness (LOC), BP, skin temp, lung sounds, urine output, and peripheral pulses.

Cardiac output

Cardiac output (CO) is defined as the amount of blood ejected from the left ventricle over one minute. The CO must remain fairly constant to achieve adequate perfusion to the body. Normal cardiac output is from 4 to 8 liters/minute.

CO is calculated using the equation:

Heart rate (HR) × stroke volume (SV) = cardiac output (CO).

Stroke volume is influenced by three factors:

1. Preload: the amount of blood returning to the right side of the heart. To remember preload, think volume—you can have too much or not enough. Ways to increase preload: increase fluid volume in the vascular space, elevate the legs, and place the client in the Trendelenberg position. Ways to decrease preload are to sit the client up with the legs down and decrease vascular volume.

2. Afterload: the pressure in the aorta and peripheral arteries that the left ventricle has to work against to get blood out. This pressure is referred to as resistance—how much resistance the ventricle has to overcome to pump blood out to the body. The aorta is naturally a high-pressure vessel, but we don't want it to go too high. Ways to increase afterload include making the client's BP go up. Now the client's left ventricle will have even more pressure to pump against. As a result, less blood will be pumped out of the heart, and cardiac output will go down. This is not nice! Ways to decrease afterload are to give your client a vasodilator or an antihypertensive. This will decrease the pressure in the aorta and therefore the heart will not have as much pressure to pump against. Then the left ventricle will say, "Thank you! Now I don't have to work as hard against that high pressure to get the blood out." Then the cardiac output will go up.

3. Contractility: the heart's ability to "squeeze" volume out of the ventricle.

✚ Whose on first?

The body has an intricate neurohormonal system that contributes to the function of the heart. Table 6-1 describes the function of the different organs or body systems in maintaining homeostasis of the cardiac system.

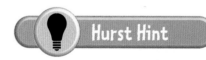

Hurst Hint

Anytime you see the words "cardiac output" (CO), you need to be thinking left ventricle.

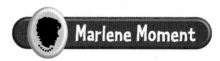

Marlene Moment

As Martha Stewart would say, "Increasing cardiac output . . . it's a good thing."

Table 6-1

Organ or body system	Function
Central nervous system	Baroreceptors and pressure-sensitive nerve endings located in the atria in the heart, carotid sinuses, and aorta sense drops in CO. A decrease in CO causes activation of the sympathetic nervous system (fight or flight response). Epinephrine (adrenaline) and norepinephrine are secreted into the blood. Epinephrine increases heart contractility, thereby increasing cardiac output. Epinephrine and norepinephrine also act as potent vasoconstrictors, so BP goes up. The parasympathetic system, when activated, basically does the opposite of the sympathetic nervous system. Activation of the parasympathetic nervous system leads to slowed heart rates and causes vasodilation
Endocrine Renin–angiotensin–aldosterone	Normally, if you have a decrease in cardiac output, the kidneys sense this decrease in perfusion and renin is secreted into the blood. Secretion of renin converts angiotensinogen (produced by the liver) into angiotensin I. In the lungs, angiotensin I is converted into angiotensin II by angiotensin-converting enzyme (ACE). Angiotensin II is a very potent vasoconstrictor. In response to circulating angiotensin, aldosterone is released from the adrenal cortex. Aldosterone causes the retention of sodium and water. Activation of this system makes blood pressure go up. Whenever you see aldosterone, think sodium AND water. Whenever you have more volume, blood pressure goes up. ACE inhibitors STOP the conversion of angiotensin I to angiotensin II, thereby decreasing blood pressure (afterload). Also, lesser amounts of circulating angiotensin II decrease aldosterone levels, resulting in less retention of sodium and water
Endocrine ADH	Antidiuretic hormone (ADH) is a hormone of the endocrine system and is "housed" in the pituitary gland in the brain. The brain, through osmoreceptors located in the hypothalamus, can sense when the blood is concentrated or dilute. In response to increases in the concentration of blood, ADH is released, and leads to water retention. Increases in water retention increase BP. (Remember, more volume, more pressure)
Endocrine B-type natriuretic peptide (BNP)	BNP was first discovered, in lesser amounts, in the brain, and is a hormone secreted primarily by cardiac cells in the ventricles in response to wall distention (volume overload). Secretion of BNP causes diuresis and vasodilation. Diuresis decreases preload (volume) in the heart, decreasing workload on the heart because there is less volume to pump. Vasodilation decreases afterload (resistance), lessening the workload on the heart. When BNP is secreted, BP goes down BNP is measured as a laboratory value and is used to classify the degree of heart failure. The higher the number, the worse the heart failure

Source: Created by author from Reference #1.

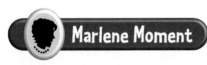

Marlene Moment

Epinephrine and norepinephrine are what you get a surge of when you come home late at night in the dark and a large man that you do not know with a mask on is waiting for you!

LET'S GET DOWN TO SPECIFICS

Cardiac illness and disease can greatly limit a client's quality of life. Some of these illnesses and diseases are life threatening, furthering the importance of the nurse's basic understanding of these illnesses and diseases.

✚ Left-sided heart failure

Congestive heart failure is classified as left-sided heart failure or right-sided heart failure.

What is it?

Left-sided heart failure occurs when the left ventricle fails and cardiac output falls. The blood backs up into the left atrium and lungs, causing pulmonary congestion (Tables 6-2 and 6-3).

What causes it and why

Table 6-2

Causes	Why
Coronary artery disease	Reduces oxygen-rich blood flow to the cardiac muscle resulting in ischemia. This decreases cardiac output. As the damaged cells begin to heal, they go through neurohormonal changes called remodeling. Remodeling is a bad thing. The "scarred" or remodeled tissue is not the same as healthy heart tissue. The remodeled cells do not contract as well as healthy heart tissue, and the client is at risk for developing congestive heart failure
Myocardial infarction	Blockage of coronary artery impedes forward blood flow, resulting in cardiac tissue ischemia. This reduces cardiac contraction and cardiac output
Myocarditis or endocarditis	Inflammation of heart muscle caused by bacterial, viral, or other infection. Damages heart muscle and impairs pumping ability
Heart valve disorders	Narrowing of heart valves causes backward flow of blood. The heart enlarges and cannot pump effectively. This decreases CO
Arrhythmias	The heart beats abnormally, leading to decreased pumping ability
Pulmonary hypertension	Damages blood vessels in the lungs, making the heart work harder to pump blood into the arteries that supply the lungs
Pulmonary embolism	Makes pumping blood into the pulmonary arteries difficult (due to blockage)
Hyperthyroidism	Overstimulates the heart, making it pump too rapidly and not empty completely with each heartbeat (if heart beats too fast, the ventricles do not have time to fill)
Hypothyroidism	Low thyroid hormones make the cardiac muscle weak, decreasing its pumping ability
Anemia	Reduction of oxygen the blood carries, so the heart must work harder to supply the same amount of oxygen to the tissues. The heart is now working harder to pump more oxygen around the body
Kidney failure	Strains the heart because the kidneys cannot remove the excess fluid from the bloodstream. This leads to decreased CO

Source: Created by author from References #1 to #8.

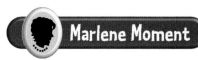

If you gotta have an MI, be sure and have a teeny, tiny one. That way when you get out of the hospital your heart will still pump pretty well.

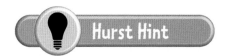

Remember, decreased forward flow is backward flow. Whenever you see backward flow, think heart failure.

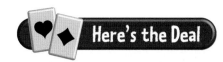

The worst-case scenario of left-side heart failure is pulmonary edema.

Signs and symptoms and why

Left-side heart failure can occur for all of the reasons cited above. When the left side of the heart fails, cardiac output decreases. Blood is not effectively pumped out to the body, thus causing poor tissue diffusion.

Table 6-3

Signs and symptoms	Why
Crackles	Indicates pulmonary congestion. If the left side of the heart is weak and cardiac output drops, there is a decrease in forward flow. A decrease in forward flow causes backward flow right into the lungs
Dyspnea	Excess fluid interferes with the lungs' ability to pick up oxygen
Nonproductive cough	Natural response to get the fluid out of the lungs to improve gas exchange
Blood tinged, frothy sputum	Blood and fluid are accumulating in lungs. Sputum will be frothy pink due to the presence of blood
Restlessness	Hypoxia
Tachycardia	The heart rate increases as a compensatory mechanism (sympathetic stimulation) in an effort to pick up and transport more oxygen to the cells
S3	Normally there are two heart sounds. S1 indicates the closing of the mitral and tricuspid valves. S2 indicates closure of the aortic and pulmonic valves. Well, when the heart fails there is an extra heart sound, called an S3 gallop. It is described as a "floppy" sort of sound caused by extra fluid in the ventricles S3 sounds like "Ken-tuc-ky"
S4	Atrial contraction against the noncompliant ventricle causes an extra heart sound S4 sounds like "Tenn-ess-ee"
Orthopnea	The client will probably have to sit up to breathe. Sitting up allows for better chest expansion and may decrease the hypoxia
Nocturnal dyspnea	The client experiences shortness of breath at night while lying flat. Lying flat causes all the blood that pools in the extremities to return to the heart (preload increases). This causes CHF or pulmonary edema
Cool, pale skin	Peripheral vasoconstriction; the heart can't work hard enough to pump the blood to the extremities to perfuse the tissues

Source: Created by author from References #4 to #8.

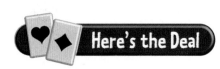

Here's the Deal

Coughing increases positive end-expiratory pressure (PEEP), which allows more time for gas exchange as the alveoli are staying open longer.

Quickie tests and treatments

Tests:

- Electrocardiography (EKG): shows heart strain, enlargement, ischemia.
- Chest x-ray: reveals pulmonary infiltrates and an enlarged heart.
- BNP level: increased.
- Echocardiogram: evaluates pumping ability of the heart and function of the valves.

- Pulmonary artery (PA) pressure monitoring: shows elevated pulmonary artery wedge pressures and left ventricular end-diastolic pressure in left-sided heart failure.

Treatments:

- Goal is to decrease workload on the heart.
- Diuretics: decrease fluid volume throughout the body.
- ACE inhibitors: dilate blood vessels decreasing workload of heart.
- Angiotensin II receptor blockers: can be used in place of ACE inhibitors.
- Beta-blockers: slow the heart rate; prevent remodeling.
- Vasodilators: cause blood vessels to dilate.
- Positive inotropic drugs: makes the heart muscle contract more forcefully.
- Anticoagulants: prevent clot formation.
- Opioids: relieve anxiety and decrease the workload on the heart especially in pulmonary hypertension.
- Oxygen therapy: improves oxygenation.
- Lifestyle modification: exercise; weight loss; reduced sodium, alcohol, and fat intake; smoking cessation; stress reduction to reduce symptoms of heart failure.
- Coronary artery bypass surgery (CABS) or angioplasty: for heart failure due to coronary artery disease (CAD).
- Heart transplant: when aggressive medical treatments are not effective.

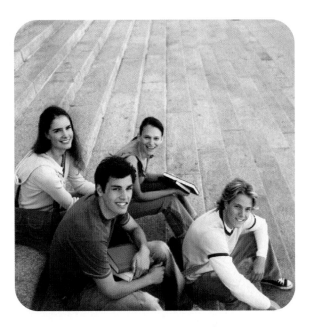

What can harm my client?

- Pulmonary edema.
- Organ failure (heart, brain, and kidney).
- Myocardial infarction.

If I were your teacher, I would test you on . . .

- Causes, signs and symptoms, and why of left-sided heart failure.
- Administration, patient monitoring, and possible side effects of medications.
- Proper nursing assessment to determine cardiac output.
- Signs and symptoms of respiratory distress.
- Patient teaching regarding lifestyle modification.
- If indicated, end-of-life care.
- Anatomy and physiology of the heart.

✚ Right-sided heart failure

What is it?

Right-sided heart failure—also known as cor pulmonale—occurs when the right ventricle doesn't contract effectively. This causes blood to back up into the right atrium and the peripheral circulation, which causes peripheral edema and engorgement of the kidneys and other organs (Tables 6-4 and 6-5).

What causes it and why

Table 6-4

Cause	Why
Left-sided heart failure	Left-sided heart failure over time will lead to right-sided heart failure. In left-sided heart failure, fluid backs up into lungs. This fluid creates increased pressures in the lungs, which is abnormal. The right side of the heart eventually becomes tired from pumping against these high pulmonary pressures. Over time the patient will experience right-sided heart failure, known as cor pulmonale
Hypertension	Heart has to pump harder to force blood into the arteries against higher pressure. The heart's walls thicken (hypertrophy) and stiffen. This causes the heart to pump less blood
Age, infiltration, infections that cause cardiac wall stiffness	Heart walls can stiffen naturally with age. Infiltration of amyloid (unusual protein not normally found in the body) can infiltrate heart walls, causing them to stiffen. Infection caused by parasites in tropical countries can cause cardiac wall stiffness
Heart valve disorders	Hinder blood flow out of the heart; heart works harder; cardiac walls thicken; diastolic dysfunction develops that leads to systolic dysfunction
Lung disorders: chronic obstructive pulmonary disease (COPD), pulmonary embolism (PE)	Cause high pressure in the lungs and can lead to right-sided heart failure. Any disease that causes hypoxia will cause the blood pressure in the lungs to go up . . . pulmonary hypertension

Source: Created by author from References #1 to #8.

Signs and symptoms and why

Table 6-5

Signs and symptoms	Why
Enlarged liver (hepatomegaly) and spleen (splenomegaly)	Blood backs up into the venous system and into the liver and spleen, causing engorgement
Epigastric tenderness	Liver and spleen have a capsule around them. This capsule does not like to stretch because it is filled with nerves and it hurts when the nerves are stretched out. When the organs become swollen, epigastric discomfort and right upper quadrant (RUQ) tenderness result
Ascites	Increased pressure in the venous system causes fluid to leak out of the vascular space into the abdominal cavity. A second reason for ascites is that the liver can no longer make albumin like it used to. Normally, albumin holds fluid in the vascular space. When albumin is low, fluid leaks out of the vascular space into the peritoneal cavity
Edema	Pressure in the venous system causes fluid to leak from the vascular space into the tissues
Anorexia, fullness, nausea	Congestion of liver and intestines
Jugular venous distension (JVD)	Blood backs up from right side of the heart into the venous system. Or, blood cannot empty into the right atrium, so it backs up into the jugular veins
Weight	Fluid retention causes an increase in weight
Nocturia	Nocturnal fluid redistribution and resorption causes urge to void at night

Source: Created by author from References #4 to #8.

Quickie tests and treatments

Tests:

- EKG: shows heart strain, enlargement, ischemia.
- Chest x-ray: reveals pulmonary infiltrates and an enlarged heart.
- BNP level: increased.
- Echocardiogram: evaluates pumping ability of the heart and function of the valves.
- Pulmonary artery (PA) pressure monitoring: shows elevated pulmonary artery wedge pressures and increased left ventricular end-diastolic pressure in left-sided heart failure.

Treatments:

- Goal is to decrease workload on the heart.
- Diuretics: decrease fluid volume throughout the body (heart isn't able to pump as much volume, so we need to get rid of excess volume).
- ACE inhibitors: dilate blood vessels, decreasing workload of heart.
- Angiotensin II receptor blockers: can be used in place of ACE inhibitors.
- Beta-blockers: slow the heart rate; prevent remodeling.
- Vasodilators: cause blood vessels to dilate (this decreases workload on the left ventricle as vasodilators drop the pressure in the aorta; cardiac output will improve as well).
- Positive inotropic drugs: make the heart muscle contract more forcefully, which hopefully will increase cardiac output.
- Anticoagulants: prevent clot formation.
- Opioids: relieve anxiety and workload on the heart especially with pulmonary hypertension.
- Oxygen therapy: treat oxygen deficiency.
- Lifestyle modification: exercise; weight loss; reduced sodium, alcohol, and fat intake; smoking cessation; stress reduction to reduce symptoms of heart failure.
- Heart transplant: when aggressive medical treatments are not effective.

What can harm my client?

- Pulmonary edema.
- Organ failure (heart, brain, and kidney).
- Myocardial infarction.

If I were your teacher, I would test you on . . .

- Causes, signs and symptoms, and why of right-sided heart failure.
- Monitoring peripheral edema and ascites.
- Measurement of jugular venous distension (JVD) and central venous pressure (CVP).
- Differentiation of right-sided and left-sided heart failure.
- Proper procedure for obtaining and documenting client weight.

✚ High-output heart failure

What is it?

High-output heart failure occurs when the cardiac output is increased but cannot meet the metabolic needs of the body (Tables 6-6 and 6-7).

What causes it and why

Table 6-6

Causes	Why
Hyperthyroidism	In hyperthyroidism, the metabolic demand is increased dramatically. Cardiac output goes up, but the demand is greater than the supply of oxygen and nutrients. The heart fails due to the lack of oxygen and nutrients
Anemia	The body compensates for decreased oxygen delivery by increasing heart rate and stroke volume. In high-output failure, the body's demand for oxygen exceeds supply. Eventually the tired heart can fail due to lack of oxygen to the actual heart muscle
Septicemia	Fevers increase metabolic demands on the body. Fighting infection also increases the metabolic demands on the body. In sepsis, the client increases CO (delivery) but the cells are unable to extract the oxygen. (In septicemia, the oxygen has a higher affinity for hemoglobin, so the hemoglobin won't "let go" of the oxygen at the cellular level)
	CO is increased, but does not meet the demands of the body
	As with all high-output failure problems, eventually the heart can fail due to lack of oxygen to the actual heart muscle
Arteriovenous fistula	An abnormal connection between an artery and a vein; short-circuits the circulation and forces the heart to pump more blood overall to deliver the usual amount of blood to the vital organs
Beriberi	Deficiency of thiamine (vitamin B_1); leads to increased metabolic demand and increased need for blood flow
Paget's disease	Abnormal breakdown and regrowth of bones, which develop an excessive amount of blood vessels; increased number of blood vessels require increased cardiac output

Source: Created by author from References #1 to #8.

Signs and symptoms and why

Table 6-7

Signs and symptoms	Why
Restlessness (early sign)	Hypoxia due to lack of oxygen at the cellular level
Tachycardia (early sign)	Hypoxia; the cells lack oxygen; heart rate (HR) increases in an effort to meet the demands of the body
Bradycardia	Heart needs oxygen and nutrients to function; if the heart is not getting adequate oxygen, it will eventually wear out, too; late sign of hypoxemia is bradycardia
Cyanosis	Late sign of hypoxemia

Source: Created by author from References #4 to #8.

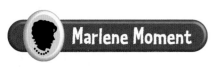

Marlene Moment

Let's not wait until someone's purple to realize something is wrong. Okay?

Quickie tests and treatment

Tests:

- T3 or T4 level: rules out hyperthyroidism.
- Hemoglobin and hematocrit level: rules out anemia.
- Echocardiogram: evaluates pumping ability of the heart and function of the valves.
- Angiogram: views blood vessels.

Treatments:

- Treat the underlying disorder.
- Red blood cell (RBC) transfusions: improves oxygenation.
- Hyperthyroidism requires medications or surgery.
- Septicemia requires antibiotics and supportive treatment.
- Arteriovenous fistula may require surgical ligation.
- Paget's disease requires medications and possible surgery.

What can harm my client?

- Heart failure.
- Infection.
- Malnutrition.
- Potential stroke.
- Falls; safety concerns.

If I were your teacher, I would test you on . . .

- Early signs of hypoxia.
- Late signs of hypoxia.
- Signs and symptoms and treatment of septicemia.
- Causes and why.
- Safety measures and prevention of client accidents.

✛ Cardiomyopathy

What is it?

There are three types of cardiomyopathy:

- Restrictive: ventricles are stiff and cannot fill properly.
- Hypertrophic: walls of the ventricles thicken and become stiff.
- Dilated: ventricles enlarge but are not able to pump enough blood for the body's needs.

In all three types of cardiomyopathy, your client may experience heart failure. If the etiology is unknown, as is often the case in hypertrophic and dilated cardiomyopathy, it is called "idiopathic" cardiomyopathy (Tables 6-8 and 6-9).

Restrictive cardiomopathy: what causes it and why

Table 6-8

Causes	Why
Diseases that change the composition of the heart muscle, making it stiff and noncompliant. Amyloidosis is one example	Often seen with multiple myeloma (bone cancer). Amyloidosis is a condition where glycoproteins are deposited within the myocardium. Accumulation of these glycoproteins in the heart alters heart function. The heart becomes stiff and rigid, resulting in a decreased volume in the ventricles and ultimately a decrease in CO. Signs and symptoms of congestive heart failure are present

Source: Created by author from References #4, #5, #6, #9, and #10.

Restrictive cardiomyopathy: signs and symptoms and why

Table 6-9

Signs and symptoms	Why
• Signs and symptoms of heart failure: bradycardia, neck vein distension, peripheral edema, liver congestion, abdominal ascites • Fatigue; weakness • Late signs include nocturnal dyspnea, S3, pink frothy sputum, cough, crackles, orthopnea, tachycardia, restlessness	The heart becomes stiff and rigid. The ventricles do not relax properly during diastole, resulting in a decreased volume in the ventricles and ultimately a decrease in CO. Your client will exhibit signs and symptoms of congestive heart failure due to decrease in forward flow of blood

Source: Created by author from References #4, #5, #6, #9, and #10.

Quickie tests and treatments

Tests:

- EKG: detects abnormalities in heart's electrical activity.
- Echocardiography (ECHO): shows enlarged atria.
- Magnetic resonance imaging (MRI): detects abnormal texture in heart muscle.
- Cardiac catheterization: measures pressures in heart chambers.
- Biopsy: identifies infiltrating substance.

Treatments:

- 70% of patients die within 5 years of symptom development.

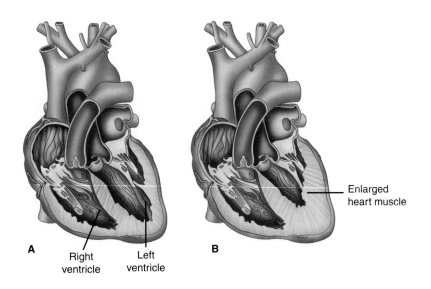

◀ Figure 6-2. **A.** Normal heart.
B. Hypertrophic cardiomyopathy.

Enlarged
heart muscle

A Right
ventricle Left
ventricle **B**

- Medications not helpful.
- Removal of blood at regular intervals: reduces amount of stored iron in clients with iron overload.
- Heart transplant.

What can harm my client?

- Infection.
- Malnutrition.
- Fall/injury.
- Depression.

If I were your teacher, I would test you on . . .

- Causes and why.
- Signs and symptoms and why.
- Cardiac physical assessment.
- Diagnostic tests.
- Nursing actions to increase oxygenation.
- End-of-life care.

Hypertrophic cardiomyopathy: what causes it and why

See Figure 6-2 and Tables 6-10 and 6-11.

Table 6-10

Causes	Why
Uncontrolled hypertension	Uncontrolled hypertension causes the ventricles and septum muscle to become hypertrophic. This causes the actual chambers of the heart to become very small and little volume ejects out of the heart, decreasing cardiac output. Less forward flow leads to backward flow
Inherited gene	The inherited gene affects the cells of the myocardium (sarcomeres) so that there is hypertrophy and asymmetry of the left ventricle
Acromegaly	Excessive growth of the heart muscle due to overproduction of growth hormone

Source: Created by author from References #3, #4, #5, #6, #9, and #10.

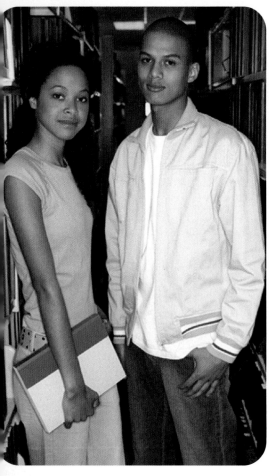

Hypertrophic cardiomyopathy: signs and symptoms and why

Table 6-11

Signs and symptoms	Why
• Fatigue; weakness • Late signs include signs and symptoms of left-sided heart failure such as nocturnal dyspnea, S3, pink frothy sputum, cough, crackles, orthopnea, tachycardia, restlessness, shortness of breath	The left ventricle becomes a large stiff muscle mass. This leaves very little room to fill the left ventricle with volume. As a result, cardiac output drops. Less ventricular filling and less forward flow results in fluid backing up into lungs. As cardiac output drops, oxygen delivery is decreased
Arrhythmias; chest pain	Especially seen with inherited HCM. As the heart hypertrophies, there is increased oxygen demand. When demand exceeds supply, myocardial ischemia occurs, leading to arrhythmias A second contributing factor is that the size of the ventricle itself impedes coronary perfusion. The stiff large muscle mass creates resistance to coronary perfusion during diastole
Palpitations	The client can sense the arrhythmias as palpitations
Faintness; dizziness	Decrease in cardiac output; decreased perfusion to the brain
Sudden cardiac death (SCD)	Lethal arrhythmias leading to death

Source: Created by author from References #4, #5, #6, #9, and #10.

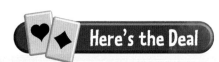

Coronary artery circulation occurs during diastole when the ventricles relax. This slows heart rate and increases diastolic time, giving the heart muscle more time for oxygen delivery.

Quickie tests and treatments

Tests:

- Chest x-ray: shows mild to moderate increase in heart size.
- Thallium scan: reveals myocardial perfusion defects.
- ECHO: shows left ventricular hypertrophy and thick intraventricular septum.
- Cardiac catheterization: measures pressures in the heart chambers if surgery is being considered.
- EKG: shows left ventricular hypertrophy; ventricular and atrial arrhythmias.

Treatments:

- Beta-adrenergic blockers: slow heart rate, reduce myocardial oxygen demands, increase ventricular filling by relaxing obstructing muscle.
- Calcium-channel blockers: increase ventricular filling by relaxing obstructing muscle.
- Antiarrhythmic drugs: reduce arrhythmias.

- Cardioversion: treats atrial fibrillation.
- Anticoagulants: reduce risk of systemic embolism with atrial fibrillation.
- Implantable cardioverter-defibrillator (ICD): treats ventricular arrhythmias.
- Ventricular myotomy or myectomy (resection of hypertrophied septum): eases outflow obstruction and relieves symptoms.
- Heart transplant: replaces malfunctioning heart.

What will harm my client?

- Not taking antibiotics prior to dental or surgical procedures to reduce risk of infective endocarditis.
- Pulmonary edema.
- Lethal arrhythmias: ventricular tachycardia and ventricular fibrillation.

If I were your teacher, I would test you on . . .

- Factors that cause hypertension to lead to heart failure.
- Medications that decrease workload on heart.
- Signs and symptoms of fluid volume excess.
- Effective client coping strategies.
- Medications that are contraindicated.
- Pre- and postop care.
- Causes and why.
- Signs and symptoms and why.
- Safety precautions.

Dilated cardiomyopathy: what causes it and why

See Figure 6-3, Tables 6-12 and 6-13.

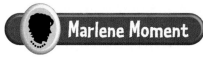

Marlene Moment

If you are on a beta-blocker, you will stay cool as a cucumber (or your vegetable of choice) if you come home one night and there is a man in a mask waiting for you in your bedroom. Why? Because beta-blockers won't let you release epinephrine and norepinephrine, so you will just kindly say, "Do I know you?"

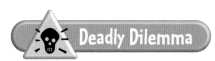

Deadly Dilemma

Many medications commonly used to treat heart failure may not help because they may decrease cardiac output even further.

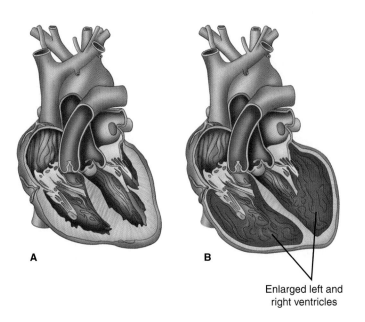

A   B

Enlarged left and right ventricles

◀ Figure 6-3. **A.** Normal heart. **B.** Dilated cardiomyopathy.

Table 6-12

Causes	Why
Chemotherapy	Toxic effects of the drugs on the myocardial cells dilate the ventricles and they cannot contract properly. Cardiac output decreases. Signs and symptoms of heart failure are observed
Alcohol and drugs	Direct toxic effects of alcohol on the myocytes (heart cells)
Coronary heart disease	Decreased oxygen delivery to the heart muscle leads to pump failure. The heart muscle dies and is replaced by scar tissue. The uninjured heart muscle stretches and thickens to compensate for the lost pumping action
Valvular heart disease	Increased volume or increased resistance to outflow in the chamber of the heart over time distends the chambers and the muscle becomes stretched, thinned, and weakened
Viral or bacterial infections	Inflammation of the heart muscle; heart muscle weakens; the heart stretches to compensate, resulting in heart failure
Hypertension	Ventricles and septum muscle hypertrophy, causing the actual chambers of the heart to become very small and little volume ejects out of the heart, decreasing cardiac output. Less forward flow leads to backward flow

Source: Created by author from References #3, #4, #5, #6, #9, and #10.

Dilated cardiomyopathy: signs and symptoms and why

Table 6-13

Signs and symptoms	Why
Shortness of breath, orthopnea, dyspnea on exertion, paroxysmal nocturnal dyspnea, fatigue, generalized weakness, dry cough at night	Left-sided heart failure: ineffective left ventricular contractility; reduced pumping ability; decreased cardiac output to body; blood backs up into the left atrium and lungs
Peripheral edema, hepatomegaly, jugular vein distension, weight gain	Right-sided heart failure: ineffective right ventricular contractility; reduced pumping ability; decreased cardiac output to lungs; blood backs up into right atrium and peripheral circulation

(Continued)

Table 6-13. (*Continued*)

Signs and symptoms	Why
Peripheral cyanosis, tachycardia	Low cardiac output
Murmur	Leaking heart valves
Arrhythmia	Stretching of the heart muscle leads to abnormal heart rhythms
Chest pain; palpitations	Arrhythmias may be felt as pain or palpitations
Syncope	Decreased cardiac output

Source: Created by author from References #4, #5, #6, #9, and #10.

Quickie tests and treatments

Tests:

- Angiography: rules out ischemic heart disease.
- Chest X-ray: shows moderate to marked cardiomegaly and pulmonary edema.
- Echocardiography: may reveal ventricular thrombi; degree of left ventricular dilation and dysfunction.
- Gallium scan: identifies clients with dilated cardiomyopathy and myocarditis.
- Cardiac catheterization: shows left ventricular dilation and dysfunction, ventricular filling pressures, and diminished cardiac output.
- Endomyocardial biopsy: determines underlying disorder.
- Electrocardiography: rules out ischemic heart disease.

Treatments:

- Oxygen therapy.
- ACE inhibitors: reduce afterload through vasodilation.
- Diuretics: reduce fluid retention.
- Beta-adrenergic blockers: treat heart failure.
- Antiarrhythmics: control arrhythmias.
- Pacemaker: corrects arrhythmias.
- Coronary artery bypass graft (CABG) surgery: manages dilated cardiomyopathy from ischemia.
- Valvular repair or replacement: manages dilated cardiomyopathy from valve dysfunction.
- Heart transplant: replaces damaged heart.
- Lifestyle modifications (smoking cessation; low-fat, low-sodium diet; physical activity; abstinence from alcohol/illicit drugs): reduces symptoms and improves quality of life.

What can harm my client?

- Pulmonary edema.
- Lethal arrhythmias.
- Malnutrition.
- Infection.

If I were your teacher, I would test you on . . .

- Causes and why.
- Signs and symptoms and why.
- Diagnostic tests.
- Medications, proper administration, and possible side effects.
- Client teaching of lifestyle modifications.
- Client care of a pacemaker.
- Complete cardiorespiratory assessment.
- Oxygen safety.

✚ Valvular heart disease

Valvular heart disease can affect any of the valves in the heart. Diseased valves may have an altered structure, which changes the blood flow. Disorders of the endocardium, the innermost lining of the heart and valves, damage heart valves. Valvular heart diseases include:

- Mitral stenosis.
- Mitral regurgitation.
- Mitral valve prolapse.
- Aortic stenosis.
- Aortic regurgitation.

See Table 6-14 for valvular heart disease at a glance.

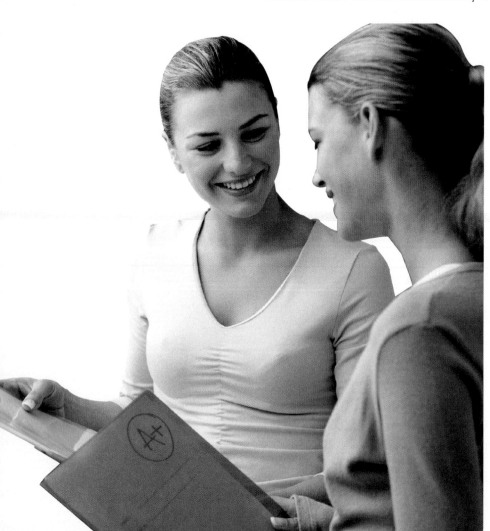

Table 6-14. Valvular Heart Disease at a Glance

Type	What is it?	Causes and why	Signs and symptoms and why	Quickie tests and treatments	What can harm my client?	If I were your teacher, I would test you on . . .
Mitral Stenosis	Mitral stenosis is narrowing of the mitral valve. The left atrium meets resistance as it attempts to move blood forward into left ventricle. Eventually the left atrium dilates and contractility decreases. Forward flow is decreased and fluid backs up into lungs. Increased volume in the lungs increases pressure in lungs. Remember: more volume, more pressure. Pulmonary hypertension in turn can lead to right-sided heart failure	• Acute rheumatic fever or infective endocarditis causes inflamed tissues. When they heal, there is scarring and thickening. This narrows the valves • Congenital abnormality causes the valve to thicken by fibrosis and calcification, obstructing blood flow • Myxoma (non-cancerous tumor in left atrium) obstructs the blood flow through the mitral valve • Blood clot reduces blood flow through the mitral valve • Adverse effect of fenfluramine and phentermine diet drug combination causes the valve to thicken by fibrosis and calcification	• Exertional dyspnea: the narrowed mitral valve decreases filling into the ventricles. Decreased volume in ventricle decreases SV and CO. Supply does not meet demand, causing exertional dyspnea. The mitral valve is narrowed, causing backward flow of volume from the left atrium into the lungs, resulting in exertional dyspnea • Orthopnea: fluid accumulates in the lungs and the client sits up to breathe better • Nocturnal dyspnea: when lying down, all the blood that pools in the extremities during the day returns to the heart. This causes more fluid in the lungs • Atrial fibrillation: the enlarged left atrium interferes	**Tests** • Echocardiography: shows blood passing through narrowed valve opening • Electrocardiography (EKG): reveals left atrial enlargement, right ventricular hypertrophy, atrial fibrillation • Chest x-ray: shows left atrial and ventricular enlargement, mitral valve calcification • Cardiac catheterization: to determine location and extent of blockage **Treatments** • Prevention of rheumatic fever • Digoxin, low-sodium diet, diuretics, vasodilators, ACE inhibitors: treat left-sided heart failure • Oxygen: increases oxygenation	• Embolitic stroke • Heart failure • Infection, especially with valve replacement surgery • Pulmonary embolism	• Causes and why • Signs and symptoms and why • Medication administration, monitoring, and possible side effects • Diagnostic tests • Proper cardiorespiratory assessment • Patient comfort techniques • Pre- and postop nursing care • Patient teaching regarding infection, prophylactic antibiotics, and lifestyle modifications

(Continued)

Table 6-14. Valvular Heart Disease at a Glance (*Continued*)

Type	What is it?	Causes and why	Signs and symptoms and why	Quickie tests and treatments	What can harm my client?	If I were your teacher, I would test you on . . .
			with normal conduction pathways. The atrium no longer contracts or contributes to left ventricular volume as before. Loss of atrial contraction decreases CO even more • Diastolic murmur: turbulent flow occurs at the narrowed valve. Murmur is heard after S2. You will hear lub (S1) dub (S2), whoosh . . . lub dub, whoosh • JVD, hepatomegaly, peripheral edema, weight gain, ascites, epigastric discomfort, tachycardia, crackles, pulmonary edema: fluid in the lungs causes increased pressures in the lungs—pulmonary hypertension. Pulmonary hypertension leads to right sided heart failure. These signs	• Anticoagulants: prevent thrombus formation around diseased or replaced valves • Prophylactic antibiotics before and after surgery and dental care: prevent endocarditis • Nitrates: relieve angina • Beta-adrenergic blockers or digoxin: slow ventricular rate in atrial fibrillation/flutter • Cardioversion: converts atrial fibrillation to sinus rhythm • Balloon valvuloplasty: enlarges orifice of stenotic mitral valve • Prosthetic valve: replaces damaged valve that can't be repaired		

Mitral Insufficiency/Regurgitation				

Mitral Insufficiency/Regurgitation

The mitral valve does not close properly during ventricular systole, causing backward flow of blood during systole. This backward flow can cause heart failure

- Infective endocarditis or rheumatic heart disease causes inflammation and damages the valve
- Coronary artery disease: ischemia and/or necrosis of the heart muscle can cause damage to the supporting structures of the mitral valve, impeding proper closure of the valve
- Aging: over time, degenerative changes can weaken the valve

- Fatigue; weakness: during ventricular systole, blood backs up into left atrium. The left side of the heart, both the atrium and ventricles, hypertrophy and dilate. Cardiac output decreases. There is an imbalance between supply and demand, causing fatigue in the client
- Pansystolic murmur: murmur heard through all of systole as blood backs up into left atrium. If S1 and S2 are audible, the murmur will be heard between these two sounds: lub, "whoosh," dub
- Angina: decreased coronary artery circulation

and symptoms are related to right-sided heart failure
- Peripheral and facial cyanosis: hypoxemia
- Hemoptysis: high pressure causes a vein or capillaries in the lungs to burst

Tests
- Auscultation: presence of heart murmur
- Electrocardiography (EKG): shows left ventricle enlargement
- Chest x-ray: shows left ventricle enlargement; fluid accumulation in the lungs
- Echocardiography: shows the faulty valve and amount of blood leaking

- Severe pulmonary edema
- Embolitic stroke
- Heart failure
- Infection, especially with valve replacement surgery
- Pulmonary embolism

Treatment
- Anticoagulants: prevent clots
- ACE inhibitors: treat mild heart failure
- Valvuloplasty: repairs the faulty valve
- Valve replacement: with a prosthetic valve

- Causes and why
- Signs and symptoms and why
- Pre- and postop care
- Proper cardiorespiratory assessment
- Diagnostic tests
- Patient teaching regarding infection and valve replacement surgery
- Medication administration, monitoring, and side effects
- Signs, symptoms, and management of thrombosis and pulmonary embolism

(continued)

Table 6-14. Valvular Heart Disease at a Glance (*Continued*)

Type	What is it?	Causes and why	Signs and symptoms and why	Quickie tests and treatments	What can harm my client?	If I were your teacher, I would test you on . . .
			• Palpitations: heartbeats are more forceful because the left ventricle has to pump more blood to compensate for the leakage back into the left atrium • Late signs include signs and symptoms of left-sided heart failure: nocturnal dyspnea; S3; pink, frothy sputum; cough; crackles; orthopnea; tachycardia; restlessness	• Prophylactic antibiotics before and after surgery and dental care: prevent endocarditis • Nitrates: relieve angina		
Mitral Valve Prolapse	The valve cusps bulge into the left atrium when the left ventricle contracts, allowing leakage of small amount of blood into the atrium	• Connective tissue disorders (systemic lupus erythematosus, Marfan's syndrome): the chordae tendineae can become elongated, which allows the mitral valve leaflets to open backward into the atrium during systole. Remember: backflow equals heart failure • Congenital heart disease: autosomal dominant	• Fatigue; weakness: during ventricular systole, blood backs up into left atrium. The left side of heart, both the atrium and ventricles, hypertrophy and dilate. Cardiac output decreases. There is an imbalance between supply and demand, causing fatigue in the client • Angina: decreased coronary artery circulation	**Tests** • Auscultation: reveals clicking sound; murmur when left ventricle contracts • Echocardiography: shows the prolapse and determines the severity of regurgitation if present • Electrocardiography (EKG): may reveal atrial or ventricular arrhythmia • Holter monitor for 24 hours: may show arrhythmia	• Arrhythmias • Infective endocarditis • Mitral insufficiency from chordal rupture	• Causes and why • Signs and symptoms and why • Medication administration, monitoring, and side effects • Proper cardiorespiratory assessment • Assessment and treatment of infection • Patient education regarding rest periods, signs of possible depression, safety measures • Antibiotics before surgical, dental, medical procedures and why? To prevent infection of the heart valve

			Treatments		Tests	
	inheritance seen in young women • Acquired heart disease (coronary artery disease [CAD], rheumatic heart disease): causes valve bulge due to inflammation	• Palpitations: heartbeats are more forceful because the left ventricle has to pump more blood to compensate for the leakage back into the left atrium • Migraine headaches: decreased cardiac output; not enough blood to the brain • Dizziness: decreased cardiac output; not enough blood to the brain • Orthostatic hypotension: decreased cardiac output; blood flow not able to rapidly adjust to client position changes • Mid-to-late systolic click; late systolic murmur: blood backing up into left atrium	• Decreased caffeine, alcohol, tobacco, stimulant intake: decreases palpitations • Fluid intake: maintains hydration • Beta-blocker: slows heart rate; reduces palpitations • Antibiotics before surgical, dental, medical procedures: prevention against bacterial infection of heart valve • Anticoagulants: prevent thrombus formation • Antiarrhythmics: prevent arrhythmias			
Aortic Stenosis	Narrowing of the aortic valve opening that increases resistance to blood flow from the left ventricle to the aorta. The left ventricle hypertrophies and weakens, leading to left-sided heart failure	• Age: degenerative changes causing scarring and calcium accumulation in the valve cusps • Rheumatic fever: causes inflammation of the cusps that leads to	• Exertional dyspnea: decreased blood supply to the enlarged heart leads to decreased CO • Angina: decreased blood supply to the enlarged heart is inadequate	• Chest x-ray: shows valvular calcification, left ventricle enlargement, pulmonary vein congestion • Echocardiography: shows decreased	• Left-sided heart failure • Right-sided heart failure • Infective endocarditis • Cardiac arrhythmias, especially atrial fibrillation	• Causes and why • Signs and symptoms and why • Medication administration, monitoring, and side effects • Proper cardiorespiratory assessment

(Continued)

Table 6-14. Valvular Heart Disease at a Glance (*Continued*)

Type	What is it?	Causes and why	Signs and symptoms and why	Quickie tests and treatments	What can harm my client?	If I were your teacher, I would test you on . . .
		scarring; usually accompanied by mitral stenosis and leakage • Birth defect: valve with two cusps instead of usual three; valve with abnormal funnel shape; calcium accumulates, causing the valve to become stiff and narrow • Atherosclerosis: lipids can increase calcium accumulation of the valves	• Syncope: sudden drop in blood pressure because the arteries in the skeletal muscles dilate during exercise to receive more oxygen-rich blood, but the narrowed valve opening prevents the left ventricle from pumping enough blood to compensate • Pulmonary congestion: left-sided heart failure • Harsh, rasping, crescendo-decrescendo systolic murmur: forced blood flow across stenotic valve	valve area, increased left ventricular wall thickness • Cardiac catheterization: increased pressure across aortic valve; increased left ventricular pressures; presence of coronary artery disease **Treatments** • Low-sodium, low-fat, low-cholesterol diet: treats left-sided heart failure • Diuretics: treat left-sided heart failure • Periodic noninvasive evaluation: monitors severity of valve narrowing • Cardiac glycosides: control atrial fibrillation • Antibiotics before medical, dental, surgical procedures: prevent endocarditis • Percutaneous balloon aortic valvuloplasty: reduces degree of stenosis • Aortic valve replacement: replaces diseased valve		• Assessment and treatment of infection • Patient education regarding diet modifications • Recognition of heart murmurs and arrhythmias • Antibiotics before surgical, dental, medical procedures and why?

Aortic Insufficiency/Regurgitation

Leakage of the aortic valve. Each time the left ventricle relaxes, blood leaks back into it. (Atria are contracting while ventricles are relaxing)

- Bacterial endocarditis, rheumatic fever: inflammatory process damages the endocardial cells, making the valves dysfunctional
- Connective tissue diseases (Marfan's syndrome): direct damage of the heart valves can occur, causing valvular regurgitation or valvular stenosis

- Left-sided heart failure such as nocturnal dyspnea, S3, pink frothy sputum, cough, crackles, orthopnea, tachycardia, restlessness: In aortic regurgitation volume is backing up through the aortic valve during diastole. In an attempt to maintain cardiac output and manage the extra volume, the left ventricle hypertrophies. Over time, though, the left ventricle fails, resulting in left-sided heart failure
- Diastolic murmur: blood is backing up into left ventricle from aorta during diastole. You will hear S1, S2, then the murmur, e.g., lub, dub, whoosh

Tests
- Chest x-ray: may show left ventricular enlargement and pulmonary vein congestion
- Echocardiography: shows left ventricular enlargement, thickening of the valve cusps, prolapse of the valve, and vegetations (accumulation of debris blood, etc.)
- Electrocardiography: shows sinus tachycardia, left ventricular hypertrophy
- Cardiac catheterization: shows coronary artery disease

Treatments
- Oxygen: increases oxygenation
- Vasodilators: reduce systolic load and regurgitant volume Valve replacement with prosthetic valve: removes diseased aortic valve
- Low-sodium diet: treats left-sided heart failure
- Diuretics: treat left-sided heart failure
- Prophylactic antibiotics before and after surgery, medical, dental care: prevent endocarditis
- Nitroglycerin: relieves angina

- Left-sided heart failure
- Pulmonary edema
- Myocardial ischemia

- Pre- and postop care
- Proper cardio-respiratory assessment
- Diagnostic tests
- Patient teaching regarding infection and valve replacement surgery
- Medication administration, monitoring, and side effects
- Signs, symptoms, and management of left-sided heart failure, pulmonary edema, MI
- Antibiotics before surgical, dental, medical procedures and why?

Source: Created by author from References #4, #5, #6, #11, and #12.

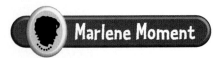

Marlene Moment

Before you run off and get that tongue ring, be sure to check for the infections that can occur (like mediastinitis) from all that bacteria draining down around your heart. Okay?

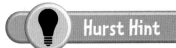

Hurst Hint

Anytime a client has a foreign (nonself) device in his body, a greater risk exists for developing an infection.

✚ Infectious cardiac disease

Infectious cardiac disease is a general term used to describe an infectious disease process of the endocardium or lining of the heart. The mitral valve is often the site affected by the infection. Microorganisms, such as bacteria or fungi, enter the blood and colonize on heart valves. This colonization makes the site extremely resistant to antibiotic treatment. An older term—bacterial endocarditis—is no longer used, as it is now known there is also a thrombotic component to the problem. The presence of the thrombus on the valve, though, increases the likelihood of infection developing. Infectious cardiac diseases include:

- Infective endocarditis.
- Pericarditis.

Infective endocarditis: what is it?

Infective endocarditis is an infection of the endocardium, heart valves, or cardiac prosthesis (Tables 6-15 and 6-16).

Infective endocarditis: what causes it and why

Table 6-15

Causes	Why
Bacteria: streptococci, staphylococci, fungi	Bacteria like to attack two organs: the kidneys and heart. When they attack the heart, they attack the valves. Once the microorganisms begin to proliferate on the valve, they can form what's called "vegetation" or purulent stuff attached to the heart valve. Fungi can proliferate on heart valves just like bacteria
Prosthetic valves	Bacteria easily stick to the foreign device
Long-term indwelling catheters	Clients with catheters—central lines, Foleys—that remain in place for extended time periods are at risk for developing an infection. This can lead to an infection in the heart valve
Recent cardiac surgery	Contamination of the area during surgery
Rheumatic heart disease; Systemic lupus erythematosus	Deposit of immune complex on the heart valve; calcification of the heart valve, making it stiff
Congenital heart defects	Malformed heart valves are more susceptible to colonization
Valvular dysfunction	Turbulent flow causes damage to the endothelial lining and can lead to a thrombus formation
IV drug abuse	IV drug abusers who do not follow aseptic technique can "inject" bacteria into the blood. Injection of bacteria into a vein follows the normal blood flow and returns to the right side of the heart. The first valve for the bacteria to attack is the tricuspid valve. This is why IV drug abusers develop tricuspid valve problems

Source: Created by author from References #4 to #6.

Infective endocarditis: signs and symptoms and why

Table 6-16

Signs and symptoms	Why
Fever	Normal response to infection. Some bacteria and fungi cannot survive in an environment with an elevated temperature
Splenomegaly: the spleen is an important immune system organ	The spleen is working overtime to protect immunity; this causes hypertrophy
Petechia	Tiny spots caused by hemorrhaging under the skin. The microemboli and septic emboli can shower any organ, including the skin, leading to clotting followed by bleeding
Hematuriae	Microemboli and septic emboli can shower any organ, especially the glomeruli, leading to clotting followed by bleeding
Cardiac murmurs	Vegetation on the valve prevents the valve from closing properly, resulting in a murmur
Pleuritic pain	Microemboli and septic emboli can shower any organ including the lungs. The inflammatory response kicks in. Tissue edema occurs and places pressure on nerve endings. This pleuritic pain may be present during inspiration or expiration
Fatigue; weakness	Vegetation on the mitral valve prevents proper closure of the valve, causing backward flow during systole, which eventually leads to heart failure. This causes fatigue and weakness
Late signs include signs and symptoms of left-sided heart failure: nocturnal dyspnea; S3; pink, frothy sputum; cough; crackles; orthopnea; tachycardia; restlessness; JVD; hepatomegaly; ascites; peripheral edema; pulmonary edema	Infection and/or clot formation on the mitral or aortic valves can lead to left-sided heart failure

Source: Created by author from References #4 to #6.

Quickie tests and treatments

Tests:

- Blood cultures: determine causative organism.
- White blood cell with differential count: elevated.
- Complete blood count and anemia panel: positive for anemia in infective endocarditis.
- Erythrocyte sedimentation rate: elevated.
- Creatinine level: elevated.
- Urinalysis: proteinuria, hematuria.
- Echocardiography: shows valvular damage.
- Electrocardiogram: atrial fibrillation.

Treatments:

- Antibiotics: given for 2 to 6 weeks IV in high doses.
- Surgery: repair or replace damaged valve and remove vegetations.

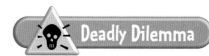

Deadly Dilemma

Chronic mitral regurgitation is not life threatening; however, it is a medical emergency when a myocardial infarction causes abrupt rupture of the supporting structures of the valve. Your client will suddenly develop severe pulmonary edema, which is life threatening.

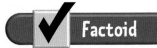

Factoid

Clients who have mechanical valves are at risk for developing clots on their valves, because like bacteria, platelets like to "stick" to foreign bodies and form clots. These clients will be placed on anticoagulants. Clients with biological valves do not require anticoagulation therapy because the natural valve does not increase platelet aggregation.

What can harm my client?

- Microemboli or septic emboli traveling to other organs.
- Stroke.
- Heart failure.
- Infection.
- Valve stenosis or regurgitation.
- Myocardial erosion.

If I were your teacher, I would test you on . . .

- Causes and why.
- Signs and symptoms and why.
- Monitoring for IV complications.
- Laboratory values.
- Pre- and postop care.
- Cardiovascular assessment.
- Monitoring renal status.
- Patient education regarding when to notify the doctor.
- Identify the location to listen for tricuspid, mitral, and aortic murmurs.

Acute pericarditis: what is it?

Acute pericarditis is an inflammation of the sac surrounding the heart (Fig. 6-4, Tables 6-17 and 6-18). The area becomes roughened and scarred. Exudates develop and pericardial effusions are possible.

▶ Figure 6-4. Pericarditis.

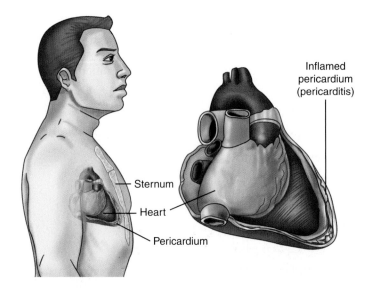

Inflamed pericardium (pericarditis)

Sternum

Heart

Pericardium

Acute pericarditis: what causes it and why

Table 6-17

Causes	Why
Myocardial infarction	The normal response to injury is to activate the inflammatory response. Once activated, inflammatory mediators migrate to the injured area. Chemical mediators such as histamine, prostaglandins, bradykinins, and serotonin cause vasodilation and increased capillary permeability. Increases in capillary permeability allow fluid and protein to leak into the surrounding tissue. Exudates of dead tissue, proteins, RBCs, and fluid may be purulent if infective and collect in the area. The inner and outermost linings become roughened and scarred
Radiation	Damage from radiation causes activation of the inflammatory response (see above)
Bacterial, fungal, or viral infections	The body attempts to "mount" an attack on the invading organisms. Immune response kicks in by activating B- and T-cell lymphocytes. The inflammatory response occurs, causing leakage of fluid into the pericardial sac
Autoimmune disorders: rheumatoid arthritis, systemic lupus erythematosus (SLE)	Activation of the inflammatory response causes increased capillary permeability. Fluid accumulates in the pericardial sac
Previous trauma or cardiac surgery	Trauma and surgery activate the inflammatory response. This can result in the accumulation of fluid in the pericardial sac

Source: Created by author from References #4 to #6.

Acute pericarditis: signs and symptoms and why

Table 6-18

Signs and symptoms	Why
Pericardial friction rub (scratchy, grating-like sound heard in systole and diastole)	Inflammation of the inner- and outermost lining of the pericardial sac causes scarring and roughening. The scraping together of the inner- and outermost layers produces a sound called a friction rub. It can best be heard at the apex of the heart
Dysphagia (difficulty swallowing)	The fluid around the heart can place pressure on the nerve endings supplying the esophagus
Chest pain: worsens with inspiration and decreases when the client leans forward; can radiate to neck, shoulders, chest, and arms	Inflammatory process stimulates the pain receptors in the heart. Leaning forward takes some of the pressure off the pleural tissue

Source: Created by author from References #4 to #6.

Chronic pericarditis: what is it?

Chronic pericarditis (Tables 6-19 and 6-20) is the result of continued irritation to the pericardial lining. The lining becomes thickened and stiff and the client may develop restrictive pericarditis.

Chronic pericarditis: what causes it and why

Table 6-19

Causes	Why
Uremia	Chronic presence of high urea levels in the blood causes irritation and inflammation to the pericardial lining. Chronic inflammation leads to thickening of the pericardial lining, causing stiffness
Autoimmune diseases: SLE, rheumatoid arthritis	Chronic irritation sets the inflammatory response into motion (see above)

Source: Created by author from References #4 to #6.

Chronic pericarditis: signs and symptoms and why

Table 6-20

Signs and symptoms	Why
Weakness	The heart chambers can no longer fill or contract effectively because they are being "squeezed" by the pericardial sac. This leads to a decrease in cardiac output, with less oxygen and nutrient delivery to the cells
Signs and symptoms of right-sided heart failure: edema, hepatomegaly, ascites, JVD	The heart is being "squeezed" and the right side of the heart cannot fill well. This results in signs and symptoms of right-sided heart failure

Source: Created by author from References #4 to #6.

Quickie tests and treatments

Tests:

- White blood cell count: elevated.
- Erythrocyte sedimentation rate: elevated.
- Serum creatinine: elevated.
- Pericardial fluid culture: identifies causative organism in bacterial or fungal pericarditis.
- Blood urea nitrogen: elevated.
- Echocardiography: shows pericardial effusion.
- Electrocardiography: shows elevated ST segment.

Treatments:

- Bed rest as long as fever and pain persist: reduces metabolic needs.
- NSAIDs: relieves pain and reduces inflammation.

- Corticosteroids: if NSAIDs are ineffective and no infection exists.
- Antibacterial, antifungal, antiviral therapy: if infectious cause.
- Pericardiocentesis: removes excess fluid from pericardial space.
- Partial pericardiectomy: creates window that allows fluid to drain into pleural space (chronic pericarditis).
- Total pericardiectomy: permits adequate filling and contraction of heart.

What can harm my client?

- Cardiac tamponade.
- Pericardial effusion.
- Infection.

If I were your teacher, I would test you on . . .

- Monitoring for drop in cardiac output.
- Causes and why.
- Signs and symptoms and why.
- Pre- and postop care.
- Infection control.
- Patient education regarding deep breathing and coughing exercises; scheduled rest periods.
- Identification of heart rhythm and sounds.
- Monitoring hemodynamic status.

✛ Cardiac tamponade

What is it?

Cardiac tamponade (Fig. 6-5, Tables 6-21 and 6-22) is caused by accumulation of fluid or blood between the two layers of the pericardium. It is the most serious complication of pericarditis.

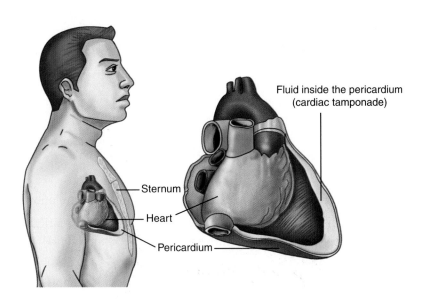

◀ Figure 6-5. Cardiac tamponade.

Fluid inside the pericardium (cardiac tamponade)

Sternum

Heart

Pericardium

What causes it and why

Table 6-21

Causes	Why
Trauma to the chest	Cardiac contusion may occur. (Bruising of the heart muscle.) Blood and fluid leak into the pericardial sac
Myocardial infarction	Inflammation at the site of the infarction leads to increased capillary permeability. Fluid can leak into the pericardial sac resulting in a tamponade
Cardiac bypass surgery	Normally blood and fluid accumulate around the heart after heart surgery. Sometimes, though, one of the sutures to a graft may burst. This may cause sudden accumulation of blood in the mediastinum, resulting in a cardiac tamponade

Source: Created by author from References #4 to #6.

Signs and symptoms and why

Table 6-22

Signs and symptoms	Why
Jugular vein distension (JVD)	Heart is "squeezed" so blood cannot fill heart. Instead blood backs up into venous system, causing distension of jugular vein
Drop in blood pressure	The heart squeezes → CO drops → decreased forward flow of volume. Remember: less volume, less pressure
Muffled heart sounds	Fluid accumulates around the heart muffling heart sounds
Pulsus paradoxus	Blood pressure drops more than 10 mm Hg with inspiration. This is because with inspiration there is even more pressure "squeezing" down on heart
Change in level of consciousness (LOC)	Decreased head perfusion due to drop in CO
Increased HR	Compensation for drop in CO
Edema	Blood backing up into the venous system

Source: Created by author from References #4 to #6.

Quickie tests and treatments

Tests:

- Chest x-ray: widened mediastinum due to blood accumulation.
- Echocardiography: detects compression of the heart, variation in blood flow in heart that occurs with breathing; shows fluid accumulation.
- Electrocardiography: fast, slow, or normal HR with no pulse.

Treatments:

- Echocardiography: monitors fluid removal.

- Pericardiocentesis: removes fluid from the pericardium.

- Percutaneous balloon pericardiotomy: drains fluid using a balloon-tipped catheter inserted through the skin.

- Subxiphoid limited pericardiotomy: drains fluid using a balloon-tipped catheter inserted through a small incision in the chest.

- Pericardiectomy: removal of the pericardium.

- Sclerotheraphy: obliterates the pericardium by causing scar tissue to form.

- Oxygen therapy: increases oxygenation and tissue perfusion.

- Intravascular volume expansion: increases blood volume and oxygenation.

- Inotropic agents: controls heart rate and decreases atrial fibrillation.

Here's the Deal

EKG may have fast, slow, or normal HR with NO pulse! That's bad! The heart is being squeezed so it cannot pump normally. The conduction system, however, remains intact. This is known as pulseless electrical activity.

What can harm my client?

- A sudden accumulation of fluid in the pericardial sac or mediastinum is a medical emergency.

- Cardiogenic shock.

- Death.

If I were your teacher, I would test you on . . .

- Assessment for cardiac output.

- Clients at risk for cardiac tamponade.

- Causes and why.

- Signs and symptoms and why.

- Pre- and postop care.

- IV administration and complications.

- Patient teaching regarding bed rest, when to notify the doctor, and postop infection prevention.

✛ Arteriosclerosis

Arteriosclerosis—hardening of the arteries—is a term for several diseases in which the wall of an artery becomes thicker and less elastic. We'll look at atherolsclerosis in detail and then quickly look at arteriolosclerosis.

Atherosclerosis: what is it?

Atherosclerosis (Fig. 6-6, Tables 6-23 and 6-24) is a condition where patchy deposits of fatty material develop in the walls of arteries, leading to reduced or blocked blood flow.

▶ Figure 6-6. Atherosclerosis.

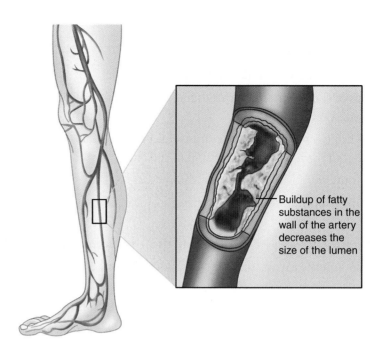

Buildup of fatty substances in the wall of the artery decreases the size of the lumen

What causes it and why

Table 6-23

Causes	Why
Repeated injury to the artery wall	Immune system involvement or direct toxicity allows materials to deposit on the artery's inner lining
High cholesterol	High levels of cholesterol in the blood injure the artery's lining, causing an inflammatory response, allowing cholesterol and other fatty materials to deposit
Infection due to bacteria or virus	Damages the lining of the artery's wall, encouraging deposits to form
Atheromas (patchy deposits of fatty material)	Form where the arteries branch because the artery's wall is injured from constant turbulent blood flow

Source: Created by author from Reference #13.

RISK FACTORS   There are many risk factors associated with atherosclerosis including:

• Smoking: decreases high-density lipoprotein (HDL), the good stuff, and increases the bad stuff, low-density lipoprotein (LDL).

• High cholesterol: risk of heart attack increases when the HDL and LDL are out of whack.

• High blood pressure: uncontrolled high blood pressure can lead to heart attack or stroke.

• Diabetes mellitus: the risk for developing atherosclerosis is 2 to 6 times higher in diabetics because sugar deposits just like fat.

- Obesity: abdominal (truncal) obesity increases the risk for diabetes, hypertension, and coronary artery disease (CAD).
- Physical inactivity: leads to obesity, high blood pressure, and CAD.
- High blood levels of homocysteine: homocysteine (an amino acid) may directly injure the lining of the arteries, making the formation of atheromas more likely.

Signs and symptoms and why

Table 6-24

Signs and symptoms	Why
High blood pressure	Atheromas grow, causing narrowing of the arteries and calcium accumulation in the arteries
Decreased peripheral pulses	Decreased elasticity of the arteries and the narrowed lumen contribute to decreased peripheral circulation
Angina	Arteries that supply the heart are narrowed
Leg cramps (intermittent claudication)	Narrowing of arteries in the legs
Stroke	Blockage of the arteries supplying the brain
Heart attack	Arteries supplying the heart are blocked
Kidney failure	Arteries supplying one or both kidneys become narrowed or blocked
Malignant hypertension	Dangerously high blood pressure caused by narrowing of the arteries

Source: Created by author from Reference #13.

Quickie tests and treatments

Tests:

- Blood pressure: monitors hypertension.
- Lipid profile: cholesterol below 200 mg/dL is desired.
- Coronary angiography: shows location and degree of coronary artery stenosis or obstruction, circulation, and condition of the artery beyond the narrowing.
- Electrocardiography: evaluates damaged heart muscle and if there is adequate blood supply.
- Cardiac catheterization: confirms presence of hardening of arteries.
- Intravascular ultrasound: views the inside walls of the arteries.
- Nuclear imaging: dye shows area of blockage.
- Exercise stress test: determines if angiography or coronary artery bypass surgery (CABS) is needed.
- Holter monitor: detects silent ischemia and angina.

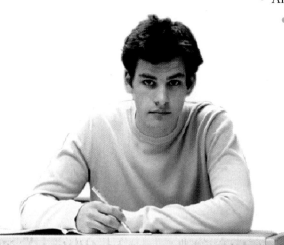

Treatments:

- Lifestyle modifications: low-fat, low-sodium, high-fiber diet; decreased alcohol intake; smoking cessation; weight loss program; exercise program.
- Nitrates: decrease cardiac pain caused by angina by vasodilating the coronary arteries, therefore supplying more blood to actual heart muscle.
- Antihypertensives: lower blood pressure.
  - Anticoagulants: prevent blood clots.
  - Percutaneous transluminal coronary angioplasty (PTCA): balloon compresses fatty plaque or blockage against vessel wall to widen diameter of blood vessel and increase blood flow.
  - Balloon angioplasty with stenting: stent expands to the size of the artery and holds it open.
  - Calcium-channel blockers: lower blood pressure.
  - Angiotensin-converting enzyme (ACE) inhibitors: widen bloods vessels, lower blood pressure.
  - Beta-blockers: reduce blood pressure and improve circulation.
  - Antiplatelets: prevent platelets from sticking together and blocking vessels.

What can harm my client?

- Stroke.
- Heart attack.
- Kidney failure.
- Malignant hypertension.
- Peripheral artery disease.

If I were your teacher, I would test you on . . .

- Causes and why.
- Signs and symptoms and why.
- Medication administration, monitoring, and side effects.
- Care of the patient during diagnostic procedures.
- Patient safety measures.
- Signs and symptoms and management of stroke, hypertension, heart attack, and kidney failure.
- Patient teaching regarding lifestyle modification, stress reduction, recognition of dangerous signs and symptoms of illness.

ARTERIOLOSCLEROSIS AT A GLANCE

- Hardening of the arterioles—small arteries.
- The walls thicken, narrowing the arterioles.
- Organs supplied by the affected arterioles do not receive enough blood. This affects the kidneys.
- Disorders occur mainly in people with high blood pressure or diabetes.
- High blood pressure and diabetes stress the walls of the arterioles, resulting in thickening.

✚ Hypertension

What is it?

Hypertension is abnormally high pressure in the arteries. Whatever the etiology, the results are the same: hypertension is the result of peripheral vasoconstriction. Vasoconstriction decreases blood flow to end organs (Table 6-25).

What causes it and why

Table 6-25

Causes	Why
Primary hypertension	Etiology unknown. It is thought, though, that there is a genetic predisposition. Gender plays a role, and men are at greater risk than women. Black males are at highest risk for the illness. Diets high in sodium, glucose, and heavy alcohol consumption are linked to hypertension. Diabetes and obesity also play a role. More recently, research indicates diets low in potassium, magnesium, and calcium are associated with hypertension
Secondary hypertension	Related to underlying disease: pheochromocytoma, hyperthyroidism, hyperaldosteronism, Cushing's syndrome, and renal disease
Pheochromocytoma	Benign tumors in the adrenal medulla secrete epinephrine and norepinephrine, leading to hypertension
Hyperthyroidism	Increase in thyroid hormone leads to increases in heart rate and cardiac output, which increases blood pressure
Hyperaldosteronism	Too much aldosterone leads to increased sodium and water. Remember, more volume, more pressure
Cushing's syndrome	Too many of all the steroids including aldosterone, which leads to increased sodium and water
Renal disease	The high pressures eventually damage the glomeruli (intrarenal failure). Now there is less blood flow (perfusion) through the kidneys. The kidneys try to fix the problem by activating renin–angiotensin–aldosterone system. This makes your client even more hypertensive and causes more damage to the glomeruli. Left untreated, this can progress to renal failure
Lifestyle: obesity, sedentary lifestyle, stress, smoking, excessive alcohol consumption, increased salt intake	Can lead to hypertension in people who have an inherited tendency to develop the illness
Arteriosclerosis	Fatty plaques collect on the artery walls, narrowing them, and leading to increased blood pressure

Source: Created by author from References #4 to #6.

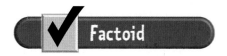

Hypertension is the number one cause of congestive heart failure.

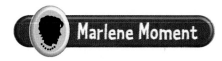

A recommendation of attending Happy Hour at least 3 to 4 times a week is not good for treating atherosclerosis or arteriosclerosis. Sorry.

CLASSIFICATION OF BLOOD PRESSURE FOR ADULTS

See Tables 6-26 and 6-27.

Table 6-26

	Systolic (mm Hg)	Diastolic (mm Hg)
Normal	<120	<80
Prehypertension	120–139	80–89
Stage I hypertension	140–159	90–99
Stage II	≥160	≥100

Source: Created by author from References #2 and #3.

Signs and symptoms and why

Table 6-27

Signs and symptoms	Why
Decreased urine output	Vasoconstriction increases pressures in the glomeruli, causing damage. This results in decreased blood supply (perfusion). Decreased kidney perfusion results in decreased urine output
Change in LOC; one-sided weakness related to a cerebral vascular accident (CVA)	Chronic hypertension damages the carotid endothelium, eventually leading to atherosclerosis. Plaques can break off from the shearing forces created by high pressures. When plaques break off in the carotid arteries, they can cause a stroke
Neurological changes related to cerebral hemorrhage	High pressures in the arterioles in the brain may cause them to rupture
Chest pain from a myocardial infarction	Hypertension causes increased rate of atherosclerosis and leads to CAD. The large "hypertrophied" left ventricle requires more blood flow for proper oxygenation. Demand exceeds supply, leading to a heart attack
Pulsatile back pain from an aortic aneurysm	Shearing hypertensive forces tearing the layers of the aorta
Heart failure signs and symptoms: Nocturnal dyspnea, S3, pink frothy sputum, cough, crackles, orthopnea, tachycardia, restlessness	Chronic hypertension causes increased workload on the left side of the heart. The left ventricle hypertrophies. The hypertrophied muscle is so large the chamber size of the left ventricle decreases. Less volume fills the ventricle, so cardiac output drops. Remember, decreased forward flow equals backward flow. In this case, flow moves backward into the lungs. As the heart pumps against this high peripheral vascular resistance (PVR) or systemic vascular resistance (SVR), it must overcome high pressures to move blood out of the heart. Eventually, the heart gets tired and begins to fail

Source: Created by author from References #2 and #3.

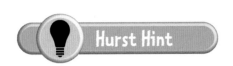

Hurst Hint

Decreased kidney perfusion always results in decreased urine output.

Quickie tests and treatments

Tests:

- Test for suspected underlying cause.
- Blood pressure monitoring.
- 24-hour blood pressure monitor: confirms consistent hypertension.
- Serum BUN: elevated.
- Serum creatinine: elevated.
- Urinalysis: positive for blood cells and albumin.
- Auscultation: check for abdominal bruit, irregular heart sounds.
- Eye examination with ophthalmoscope: views arterioles of retina is an indication that other blood vessels in the body are damaged.
- Electrocardiography (EKG): detects enlargement of the heart.

Treatments:

- Lifestyle modification: weight management; exercise regimen; smoking cessation; low-sodium, low-fat, low-cholesterol, high-fiber diet; decreased alcohol consumption; decreased stress; maintain intake of calcium, magnesium, potassium; home monitoring of blood pressure.
- Diuretics: dilate blood vessels; help kidneys eliminate sodium and water.
- Beta-blockers: decrease blood pressure; decrease chest pain.
- ACE inhibitors: dilate arterioles and lower blood pressure.
- Angiotension II blockers: lower blood pressure.
- Calcium-channel blockers: dilate arterioles and lower blood pressure.
- Direct vasodilators: dilate blood vessels and lower blood pressure.

Marlene Moment

Rule: No fat = No fun. I guess I will have to give up my fried chicken, rice and gravy, and macaroni and cheese.

What can harm my client?

- Stroke.
- Heart failure.
- Renal failure.
- Blindness.

If I were your teacher, I would test you on . . .

- Causes and why.
- Signs and symptoms and why.
- Normal versus abnormal blood pressure reading.
- Medication administration, monitoring, and side effects.
- Patient education regarding lifestyle modifications; how to monitor blood pressure at home.
- Proper blood pressure techniques.
- Signs and symptoms of end-organ damage.

+ Coronary artery disease

What is it?

Coronary artery disease is a condition in which the blood supply to the heart muscles is completely or partially blocked. CAD is due to athero-sclerosis that develops in the arteries that encircle the heart and supply it with blood. Atheromas grow, bulge into the arteries, narrowing the arteries, and partially blocking blood flow. Calcium accumulates in the atheromas. Atheromas may rupture. Blood may enter a ruptured atheroma, making it larger, and thus narrowing the artery even more. The ruptured atheroma triggers a thrombus, which may further narrow or block the artery. The thrombus can detach (becoming an embolus) and block another artery farther downstream. As the coronary artery becomes blocked, the supply of oxygen-rich blood to the heart muscle decreases, causing ischemia. This can lead to angina and MI (see Tables 6-28, 6-29 and 6-30).

What causes it and why

Table 6-28

Causes	Why
Atherosclerosis	Fatty plaques deposit and narrow the arteries over time
Congenital defects	Irregular vessel shapes can cause plaques and other debris to become trapped narrowing the vessels
Coronary artery spasm	Creates a temporary vessel blockage
Dissecting aneurysm	An aneurysm creates a bulging out of the vessel wall due to pressure. This can cause atherosclerotic plaque formation at the site of the aneurysm, which causes further weakening of the artery wall. A blood clot may form at the site and dislodge, increasing the chance of stroke
Infectious vasculitis	Inflammation of the vessels contributes to growth of plaque in the arteries
Syphilis	If left untreated, syphilis can cause inflammation of the vessels, which leads to growth of plaque in the arteries
High blood levels of C-reactive protein (CRP)	CRP levels rise when there is inflammation. The inflammation process contributes to the growth of plaque in arteries

Source: Created by author from References #4 to #6.

RISK FACTORS AND WHY

Table 6-29

Risk factors	Why
Age	The longer we live, the more time we have to develop plaques
Men are at increased risk but women approach same risk after menopause	It was thought estrogen had a cardioprotective property. Current research does not support this theory. At this time it is not clear "why" postmenopausal women are at increased risk for having an MI
Positive family history	Some families are just really good at making plaque in their coronary arteries
Diets high in cholesterol and fat	Diets high in fat lead to increased levels of LDL. This speeds up hardening of the arteries
Hypertension	Anything that damages the endothelial lining speeds up hardening of the arteries. Hypertension damages the endothelial lining of vessels
Smoking	Increases oxidation of LDL, thereby increasing fatty streaks in the vessels
Diabetes mellitus	High glucose levels damage vessels
Chronic kidney disease	There is a link between increased creatinine levels and risk for CAD
Abdominal obesity	Increased adipose tissue around the midsection of the body has been linked to increased risk for developing CAD
Sedentary lifestyle	Inactivity increases LDL levels and decreases HDL (the good kind)
Autoimmune disorders such as rheumatoid arthritis	Damages the endothelial lining of vessels

Source: Created by author from References #4 to #6.

Signs and symptoms and why

Table 6-30

Signs and symptoms	Why
MI	The arteries become narrowed due to fatty plaque buildup (atherosclerosis) and not enough oxygen reaches the heart, causing ischemia
Angina	The arteries become narrowed due to fatty plaque buildup (atherosclerosis) and not enough oxygen reaches the heart, causing ischemia. The ischemia causes chest pain
High blood pressure	Atheromas grow, causing narrowing of the arteries and calcium accumulation in the arteries
Decreased peripheral pulses	Decreased elasticity of the arteries and the narrowed lumen contribute to decreased peripheral circulation
Nausea and vomiting	Angina
Fainting	Decreased blood flow prevents oxygenation of the brain
Sweating	Angina
Cool extremities	Decreased peripheral circulation
Shortness of breath	Decreased cardiac output leads to decreased lung perfusion

Source: Created by author from References #4 to #6.

Quickie tests and treatments

Tests:

- Chest x-ray: reveals whether the heart is misshapen or enlarged due to disease and if abnormal calcification (hardened blockage due to cholesterol build up) in the main blood vessels exists.
- Electrocardiography (EKG): reveals MI, ischemic changes.
- Holter monitoring for 24 hours: reveals MI.
- Echocardiography: views heart's pumping activity. Parts that move weakly may have been damaged during a heart attack or may be receiving too little oxygen. This may indicate CAD.
- Stress test: determines safe exercise prescription and presence of ischemia.
- Angiogram: dye used in conjunction with x-ray outlines blockages.
- Electron beam computerized tomography (EBCT): also called an ultrafast CT scan, detects calcium within fatty deposits that narrow coronary arteries. If a substantial amount of calcium is discovered, CAD is likely.
- Magnetic resonance angiography (MRA): checks arteries for areas of narrowing or blockages—although the details may not be as clear as those provided by an angiogram.
- Myocardial perfusion imaging with thallium 201 during treadmill exercise: shows ischemia as "cold spots."

Treatments:

- Beta-blockers: interfere with epinephrine and norepinephrine, thus reducing heart rate and blood pressure.
- Nitrates: dilate blood vessels; decrease pain.
- Antiplatelets: thin blood and decrease chances of clot.
- Calcium-channel blockers: prevent blood vessels from narrowing and counter coronary artery spasm.
- ACE inhibitors: reduce risk of heart attack.
- Angioplasty and stent placement (percutaneous coronary revascularization): opens artery wall; some stents slowly release medication to help keep the artery open.
- Coronary artery bypass surgery: graft created to bypass blocked coronary arteries using a vessel from another body part. This allows blood to flow around the blocked or narrowed coronary artery. Because this requires open heart surgery, it's most often reserved for cases of multiple narrowed coronary arteries.
- Coronary brachytherapy: if the coronary arteries narrow again after stent placement, radiation may be used to help open the artery again.
- Laser revascularization: laser beam makes tiny new channels in the wall of the heart muscle. New vessels may grow through these channels and into the heart to provide additional paths for blood flow.

What can harm my client?

- MI.
- Myocardial ischemia.
- Angina.
- Complete coronary artery blockage can cause ventricular fibrillation and sudden cardiac death (SCD).
- Arrhythmias.
- Heart failure.
- Stroke.

If I were your teacher, I would test you on . . .

- Causes and why.
- Signs and symptoms and why.
- Risk factors and why.
- Client preparation for diagnostic tests.
- Medication administration, monitoring, and side effects.
- Patient education regarding lifestyle modification.
- Signs and symptoms, and nursing interventions for MI, heart failure, angina, arrhythmia, and stroke.
- Patient and family support.

✚ Abdominal aortic aneurysm

Note: Cerebral aneurysms are not discussed in this section. See Tables 6-31 and 6-32. (Refer to Chapter 9 for more information on cerebral aneurysms.)

What is it?

An aortic abdominal aneurysm (bulge in the wall of the aorta) is located in the part of the aorta that passes through the abdomen.

What causes it and why

Table 6-31

Causes	Why
Atherosclerosis	Atherosclerotic changes lead to weakening of the aorta
Hypertension	Every ventricular contraction causes a shearing or pulsatile force exerted on the walls of the aorta. Continued exposure of the weakened area to the shearing force causes a sac-like area to form
Hereditary connective-tissue disorders (Marfan's syndrome)	Genetic connective-tissue diseases cause weakening of the aortic wall
Blunt trauma	Weakening of the aortic wall. Most common etiology for saccular aneurysms
Infections (syphilis)	Causes inflammation which weakens the aortic wall
Thrombus formation	Blood flow inside the aneurysm is slow; calcium can deposit in the wall of an aneurysm

Source: Created by author from References #4 to #6.

Signs and symptoms and why

Table 6-32

Signs and symptoms	Why
Change in LOC	Widening of the artery occurs at the site where the aneurysm occurs. Blood slows within the widened area of the aorta. The area distal, in this case the brain, receives less flow. Less perfusion to the head results in decreased LOC
Pulsatile mass in periumbilical area	Enlargement of the aorta
Systolic bruit over aorta	Turbulent blood flow
Lumbar pain that radiates to the flank and groin; severe, persistent abdominal and back pain	Pressure on lumbar nerves; ruptured aneurysm
Weakness, sweating, tachycardia, hypotension	Hemorrhage

Source: Created by author from References #4 to #6.

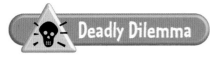

Deadly Dilemma

A ruptured abdominal aneurysm is often fatal.

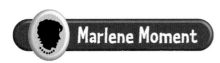

Marlene Moment

It's not good to wait until your client is complaining of severe, burning back pain to think, "Oh, maybe it's an aneurysm."

Quickie test and treatments

Tests:

- Pain is usually a late clue. Most patients have no symptoms and are diagnosed by chance during a routine physical.
- Palpitation: pulsating mass in midline of abdomen; tenderness, pain.
- Auscultation: bruit.
- Abdominal x-ray: detects aneurysm with calcium deposits in its wall.
- Ultrasonography: shows size of aneurysm.
- Computed tomography (CT) of abdomen: determines size and shape of aneurysm.
- Magnetic resonance imaging (MRI) of abdomen: determines size and shape of aneurysm.

Treatments:

- Risk factor modification: decrease cholesterol and blood pressure to prevent expansion and rupture of aneurysm.
- Beta-blockers: reduce risk of aneurysm expansion and rupture; decrease blood pressure.
- Resection of aneurysm and replacement of damaged aortic section with Dacron graft: repairs aneurysm.
- Monitor for signs of acute blood loss (decreasing blood pressure; increasing pulse and respiratory rate; cool, clammy skin; restlessness; decreased sensorium): detects signs of rupture.
- Emergency surgery: for rupture or threatened rupture.

What can harm my client?

- Shock from hemorrhage.
- Kidney failure.
- Organ failure.
- Permanent lumbar nerve damage.
- Infection.
- Death.

If I were your teacher, I would test you on . . .

- Causes and why.
- Signs and symptoms and why.
- Risk factors.
- Signs and symptoms, and nursing management of shock and hemorrhage.
- Medication administration, monitoring, and side effects.
- Patient education regarding lifestyle modification.

✚ Thoracic aortic aneurysm

What is it?

Thoracic aortic aneurysm occurs in the part of the aorta that passes through the chest (thorax). It is an abnormal widening of the ascending, transverse, or descending part of the aorta (Tables 6-33 and 6-34).

What causes it and why

Table 6-33

Causes	Why
High blood pressure	Every ventricular contraction causes a shearing or pulsatile force exerted on the walls of the aorta. Continued exposure of the weakened area to the shearing force causes a sac-like area to form
Syphilis	Causes an aneurysm to form in the part of the aorta nearest the heart
Blunt injury to the chest	Weakens the aortic wall
Atherosclerosis	Atherosclerotic changes lead to weakening of the aorta
Bacterial infections, usually at an atherosclerotic plaque	Causes inflammation and weakens the aortic wall
Rheumatic vasculitis	Causes inflammation and weakens the aortic wall
Coarctation of the aorta	A narrowing of the aorta between the upper-body artery branches and the branches to the lower body. This blockage can increase blood pressure in the arms and head, reduce pressure in the legs, and strain the heart. Aortic valve abnormalities often accompany coarctation

Source: Created by author from References #4 to #6.

Signs and symptoms and why

Table 6-34

Signs and symptoms	Why
Dysphagia	Aneurysm exerts pressure on the esophagus
Shortness of breath	Thoracic aneurysm exerts pressure in the chest
Chest pain	Ascending aortic aneurysms can interfere with coronary artery perfusion
Decreased pulses	Decreased blood flow to extremities
Cool hands; numbness, tingling	Decreased blood flow to extremities
May have large variation in blood pressure between upper and lower extremities	Location of the aneurysm interferes with blood flow to the lower extremities. When blood is pumped into the widened area, the aneurysm, it slows down. Blood flow distal to the aneurysm is decreased
Hoarseness	Pressure on nerve to voice box (larynx)
Horner's syndrome: constricted pupil, drooping eyelid, sweating on one side of face	Pressure on nerves in the chest
Pain high in the back, radiates to chest and arms	Ruptured thoracic aortic aneurysm
Shock	Internal bleeding

Source: Created by author from References #4 to #6.

Quickie tests and treatment

Tests:

- Pain is usually a late clue. Most patients have no symptoms and are diagnosed by chance during a routine physical.
- Chest x-ray: displaced windpipe; widening of aorta and mediastinum.
- CT: detects size and location of aneurysm.
- MRI: detects size and location of aneurysm.
- Transesophageal ultrasonography: determines size of aneurysm.
- Aortography: lumen of aneurysm, size, and location.
- Electrocardiography: rules out MI.
- Echocardiography: identify location of aneurysm root.

Treatments:

- Risk factor modification: decrease cholesterol and blood pressure to prevent expansion and rupture of aneurysm.
- Beta-blockers: reduce risk of aneurysm expansion and rupture; decrease blood pressure.
- Resection of aneurysm and replacement of damaged aortic section with Dacron graft: repairs aneurysm.
- Monitor for signs of acute blood loss (decreasing blood pressure; increasing pulse and respiratory rate; cool, clammy skin; restlessness; decreased sensorium): detects signs of rupture.

- Emergency surgery: for rupture or threatened rupture.
- Whole blood transfusions: if needed in presence of hemorrhage.
- Analgesics: relieve pain.
- Antibiotics: fight infection.
- Calcium-channel blockers: lower blood pressure.

What can harm my client?

- Shock from hemorrhage.
- Kidney failure.
- Organ failure.
- Permanent lumbar nerve damage.
- Infection.
- Death.

If I were your teacher, I would test you on . . .

- Causes and why.
- Signs and symptoms and why.
- Risk factors.
- Administration of blood products; client monitoring while receiving blood products.
- Signs, symptoms, and nursing management of shock and hemorrhage.
- Medication administration, monitoring, and side effects.
- Patient education regarding lifestyle modification.

✚ Aortic dissection

What is it?

An aortic dissection is a fatal disorder in which the inner lining of the aortic wall tears. When the aorta tears, blood surges through, separating (dissecting) the middle layer of the wall from the still-intact outer layer. This forms a new false channel in the wall of the aorta (Tables 6-35 and 6-36).

What causes it and why

Table 6-35

Causes	Why
High blood pressure	Pressure of the blood flow deteriorates the artery's wall
Hereditary connective-tissue disorders: Marfan's syndrome, Ehlers–Danlos syndrome	Artery wall becomes less elastic and prone to tearing
Birth defects of heart and blood vessels: coarctation of the aorta, patent ductus arteriosus, defects of the aortic valve	Artery wall becomes less elastic and weak making it more prone to tearing
Arteriosclerosis	Artery wall becomes less elastic and more prone to tearing
Injury	Weakens the artery wall making it prone to tearing

Source: Created by author from References #4 to #6.

Signs and symptoms and why

Table 6-36

Signs and symptoms	Why
Severe pulsating chest and back pain	As the aneurysm increases in size with each shearing force, the layers of the aorta rip apart
Cyanosis to lower extremities	With every ventricular contraction, blood is being pumped out of the aorta and into the dissected area. This results in little or no perfusion distal to the dissection
Decrease pulses to lower extremities	With every ventricular contraction, blood is being pumped out of the aorta and into the dissected area. This results in little or no perfusion distal to the dissection
Pallor, cold, tingling or numbness to extremities	With every ventricular contraction, blood is being pumped out of the aorta and into the dissected area. This results in little or no perfusion distal to the dissection
Sudden drop in blood pressure	With every ventricular contraction, blood is being pumped out of the aorta and into the dissected area. This results in little or no perfusion distal to the dissection
Abdominal aortic dissections: extreme difference in upper and lower extremity blood pressures.	Perfusion may occur above the dissection for a period of time (upper extremities). For the reasons cited above, distal to the aneurysm there will be little or no perfusion
Abdominal pain	Mesentery arteries are blocked
Tingling; inability to move a limb	Nerve damage caused by blockage of spinal arteries

Source: Created by author from References #4 to #6.

Quickie tests and treatments

Tests:

* Palpation of pulses: diminished.
* Auscultation: murmur.
* Chest x-ray: shows widened aorta.
* CT with radiopaque dye: detects aortic dissection.
* Transesophageal echocardiography: detects even very small aortic dissections.

Treatments:

* Admission to ICU.
* Beta-blockers: given IV to reduce heart rate and blood pressure.
* Surgery: rebuilds aorta with graft; valve repair if indicated.
* Lifetime therapy of beta-blockers or calcium-channel blockers with ACE inhibitor: reduces stress on the aorta by lowering blood pressure.

What can harm my client?

- Hypovolemic shock.
- Death.
- Stroke.
- MI.
- Kidney failure.
- Cardiac tamponade.

If I were your teacher, I would test you on . . .

- Causes and why.
- Signs and symptoms and why.
- Client care during diagnostic procedures.
- Pre- and postop care.
- Medication administration, monitoring, and side effects.
- Signs and symptoms, and management of cardiac tamponade.
- Signs and symptoms, and management of complications like MI.
- Patient education regarding lifetime medication regimen.

CASE IN POINT   Two clients present to the ED. One client has a history of kidney stones, is doubled over in pain, and has hematuria. The other client's upper extremity blood pressures are far greater than the lower extremity blood pressures, and the client is complaining of severe back pain. Which client do you see first? Hey ya'll, pain never killed anybody! And, even though hematuria indicates possible kidney stones in this situation, kidney stones never killed anybody! You've never picked up the morning newspaper to read "Man Dies of Kidney Stone"? No!

You better go see that other client first, who is exhibiting signs and symptoms of aortic dissection.

✚ Peripheral vascular disease

Peripheral vascular diseases (PVDs) are diseases of the blood vessels (arteries and veins) located outside the heart and brain. The term peripheral arterial disease (PAD) or peripheral artery occlusive disease (PAOD) is used for a condition that develops when the arteries that supply blood to the internal organs, arms, and legs become completely or partially blocked as a result of atherosclerosis.

Peripheral artery disease: what is it?

Peripheral artery disease results in reduced blood flow in the arteries of the trunk, arms, and legs. Arteries carry oxygenated blood to the body. If, for whatever reason, your client has an arterial problem distal to the damaged artery, that area is not getting enough oxygen. When tissues do not get enough oxygen, the body moves from aerobic to anaerobic metabolism. Anaerobic metabolism causes a buildup of lactic acid. Lactic acid irritates nerve endings, causing pain. This section explores some of the illnesses that cause damage to the peripheral arteries (Tables 6-37–6-50).

Peripheral artery disease: what causes it and why

Table 6-37

Causes	Why
Atherosclerosis in the peripheral arteries, usually occurs in the lower extremities	Atherosclerosis occurs in the peripheral arteries just as it does in the coronary arteries, leading to narrowing of the arteries. This impairs circulation to the extremity. Vessels can become completely obstructed by clot formation in the affected area
Fibromuscular dysplasia	Abnormal growth of muscle in the artery wall that causes narrowing
Tumor; cyst	Causes pressure outside the artery
Thrombus	Causes sudden, complete blockage in an already narrowed artery
Embolus	Travels in the bloodstream and lodges someplace other than place of origin
Thoracic outlet syndrome	Blood vessels and nerves in the passageway between the neck and chest become compressed

Source: Created by author from References #4 to #6.

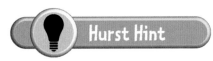

Hurst Hint

When assessing circulation remember the 5 P's:

Pulselessness
Paresthesia
Pallor
Pain
Paralysis

Peripheral artery disease: signs and symptoms and why

Table 6-38

Signs and symptoms	Why
Pain	Narrowing of the vessel impedes circulation, so that arterial blood isn't getting to the tissue. Oxygen demand exceeds supply
Leg cramps (intermittent claudication)	Usually present during walking or exercise because not enough oxygen is getting to the leg muscles
Coldness	Decreased blood supply to the extremity results in decreased temperature
Numbness, tingling (paresthesia)	Decreased circulation to the neurovascular system
Muscle atrophy	Impaired circulation. Any muscle with decreased blood supply will atrophy
Hair loss on the affected extremity	Impaired tissue perfusion
Thickening of nails and dry skin	Impaired tissue perfusion
Decreased peripheral pulses	Decreased circulation
Ulcerations to toes and fingers	Impaired tissue perfusion leads to ischemic ulcers
Gangrene	Black, crunchy toes due to loss of tissue perfusion and presence of tissue necrosis
Pallor	Impaired tissue perfusion
Decreased pulses	Impaired perfusion
Paralysis	No perfusion for a long period of time can result in paralysis

Source: Created by author from References #4 to #6.

Quickie tests and treatments

Tests:

- Arteriography: shows type, location, and degree of obstruction; establishment of collateral circulation.
- Ultrasonography and plethysmography: show decreased blood flow distal to the occlusion.
- Electrocardiogram: may show presence of cardiovascular disease.

Treatments:

- Antiplatclcts: thin the blood, prevent clot formation.
- Lipid-lowering agents: lower cholesterol.
- Antihypertensives: lower blood pressure.
- Thrombolytics: dissolve blood clots.
- Anticoagulants: thin the blood; prevent clot formation.
- Exercise: to improve circulation and help with weight control (determined by physician).
- Foot care: to prevent injury.
- Modify lifestyle risk factors for atherosclerosis (diet, weight control, alcohol, tobacco, inactivity, stress level): to improve quality of life.
- Angioplasty: used to avoid surgery and relieve symptoms.
- Surgery: depends on severity of symptoms.

What can harm my client?

- Limb loss.
- Severe ischemia.
- Skin ulceration.
- Gangrene.

If I were your teacher, I would test you on . . .

- Causes and why.
- Signs and symptoms and why.
- Proper assessment of circulation, tissue perfusion, and extremity sensitivity.
- Wound care and related client teaching.
- Psychological support for limb loss.
- Medical management of phantom pain. If amputation has been performed.
- Patient education regarding injury prevention.

✚ Buerger's disease

What is it?

Buerger's disease is inflammation and blockage of small and medium-sized arteries of the extremities. It is most common in males who are heavy smokers.

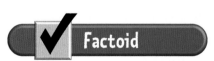

Factoid

What is phantom pain? Pain sensed by the brain as coming from a limb that has been amputated. Often, the pain will be sensed as coming from the ankle, foot, and/or toes. The pain is real and often has to be treated.

What causes it and why

Table 6-39

Causes	Why
Heavy smoking; chewing tobacco	Triggers inflammation and constriction of the arteries. Autoimmune vasculitis

Source: Created by author from References #4 to #6.

Signs and symptoms and why

Table 6-40

Signs and symptoms	Why
Claudication in the feet and hands	Pain due to insufficient blood flow during exercise or at rest
Numbness; tingling in the limbs	Emotional disturbances, nicotine, chilling
Raynaud's phenomenon	Distal extremities—fingers, toes, hands, feet—turn white upon exposure to cold
Skin ulcerations, redness/cyanosis, and gangrene of fingers and toes	Insufficient blood flow

Source: Created by author from References #4 to #6.

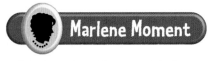

Marlene Moment

There's nothing like some black, crunchy toes in a pair of Birkenstock sandals.

Quickie tests and treatments

Tests:

* Segmental limb blood pressures: demonstrate distal location of lesions or occlusions.
* Doppler ultrasound: visualizes vessels to detect patency/occlusion.
* Contrast angiography: detects occlusion.

Treatments:

* Immediate smoking and tobacco-chewing cessation.
* Regional sympathethic block or ganglionectomy: produce vasodilation and increase blood flow.
* Amputation of affected area: restores blood flow.
* Antiplatelets: thin the blood, prevent clot formation.
* Lipid-lowering agents: lower cholesterol.
* Antihypertensives: lower blood pressure.
* Thrombolytics: dissolve blood clots.

What can harm my client?

* Continued smoking and tobacco chewing.
* Inability to cope with stress.

- Side effects of medications.
- Postop infection.
- Limb loss.
- Severe ischemia.
- Skin ulceration.
- Gangrene.

If I were your teacher, I would test you on . . .

- Causes and why.
- Signs and symptoms and why.
- Pre- and postop surgical care.
- Coping strategies of amputation.
- Management of phantom pain.
- Patient education regarding injury prevention.
- Proper assessment of circulation, tissue perfusion, and extremity sensitivity.
- Wound care and related client teaching.

✚ Raynaud's disease and Raynaud's phenomenon

What is it?

Raynaud's disease occurs when the small arteries (arterioles) in the fingers or toes constrict tightly in response to cold.

What causes it and why

Table 6-41

Causes	Why
Exposure to cold	Arterial constriction associated with Raynaud's disease
Strong emotion	Arterial constriction associated with Raynaud's disease
Injury	Arterial constriction associated with disease or phenomenon
Drugs: beta-blockers, clonidine, antimigraine drugs	Arterial constriction can worsen Raynaud's phenomenon
Nicotine	Arterial constriction can worsen Raynaud's phenomenon

Source: Created by author from References #4 to #6.

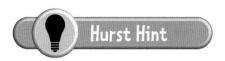
✔ Factoid

Raynaud's phenomenon is less common than Raynaud's disease. It may be associated with scleroderma, rheumatoid arthritis, atherosclerosis and other connective tissue diseases. We use the term Raynaud's disease when the cause is unknown and phenomenon when the cause is associated with connective tissue diseases and autoimmune diseases.

💡 Hurst Hint

Raynaud's disease is usually benign. Raynaud's phenomenon can be associated with a poorer prognosis.

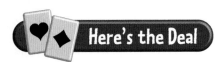

When you think of Raynaud's disease, picture this: the fingers turn white (ischemia), then blue (continued ischemia), then red (vasospasm resolved and sudden return of blood flow).

Signs and symptoms and why

Table 6-42

Signs and symptoms	Why
Numbness; tingling relieved by warmth	Cold triggers constriction of small arteries in fingers and toes
Blanching on skin of the fingers	Decreased peripheral vascularization
Blanching that progresses to cyanosis and redness	Warming improves circulation and restores normal color and sensations
Smooth, shiny, tight skin	Scleroderma, lupus; recurrent and prolonged episodes
Small, painful sores on tips of fingers or toes	Decreased sensation leads to injury

Source: Created by author from References #4 to #6.

Quickie tests and treatments

Tests:

- Arteriography: reveals vasospasm.
- Blood laboratory tests: detect underlying disorders.

Treatments:

- Avoidance of cold exposure and mechanical or chemical injury.
- Smoking cessation.
- Sympathectomy (nerves cut or blocked): if conservative treatment fails to prevent ischemic ulcers.
- Sedatives, biofeedback: control anxiety.
- Calcium-channel blockers: lower blood pressure.

What can harm my client?

- Further exposure to cold.
- Inability to cope with stress.
- Side effects of medications.
- Ischemia.
- Gangrene.
- Amputation.

If I were your teacher, I would test you on . . .

- Causes and why.
- Signs and symptoms and why.
- Medication administration, monitoring, and side effects.
- Coping strategies.
- Patient education regarding smoking cessation, avoiding exposure to exacerbating elements, and underlying disorder(s) if relative.
- Monitoring for effective circulation, ischemia, gangrene.

✚ Peripheral venous disease

Peripheral venous disease is a general term for damage, defects, or blockage in the peripheral veins. These veins carry blood from the hands and feet to the heart to receive oxygen. Peripheral venous disease can occur almost anywhere in the body but is most common in the arms and legs.

Veins are thin-walled distensible vessels that when working properly, collect blood and return blood to right side of the heart. Two mechanisms, muscle contractions and venous valves, help blood return to right side of the heart. When muscles are tense, they "squeeze" down on the vein, pushing blood back toward the right side of the heart. Valves help prevent backward blood flow.

We only want blood to flow in one direction, forward. If blood isn't going forward, it stagnates causing irritation, inflammation, and damage. A clot can even form in the damaged area. Venous congestion occurs and venous ulcers can form. These ulcerations are found on the insides or outsides of the ankles, where blood tends to stagnate.

Varicose veins: what are they?

Varicose veins are abnormally enlarged superficial veins of the lower extremities. They occur most often in the saphenous veins located on the insides of the lower extremities.

Varicose veins: what causes them and why

Table 6-43

Causes	Why
Familial predisposition	Unknown
Congenital weakness of the vein	Weakened area becomes dilated, distended, and tortuous
Obesity, pregnancy, abdominal tumors, prolonged standing, major surgeries, prolonged bed rest.	Increase venous congestion in the lower extremities. Venous congestion can lead to dilation and distention of the weakened vein. Eventually the valves in the lower extremities become incompetent and the vein further dilates
Trauma	Weakens vein integrity

Source: Created by author from References #4 to #6.

Varicose veins: signs and symptoms and why

Table 6-44

Signs and symptoms	Why
Edema	Increased hydrostatic pressure eventually causes leaking out of the vascular space into the tissue
Cramping or pain in affected extremity	Increased pressure from venous engorgement and edema
Heaviness in affected extremity	Edema and venous engorgement
Itching, redness, rash	Warmth created while wearing socks or stockings
Phlebitis	Spontaneously, or from injury

Source: Created by author from References #4 to #6.

Quickie tests and treatments:

Tests:

- Palpation: May feel the veins when they are not visible.
- X-ray: assesses functioning of deep veins.
- Ultrasonography: assesses functioning of deep veins.

Treatments:

- Elevating the legs: relieves symptoms but does not prevent new varicose veins from forming.
- Elastic stockings (support hose): compress the veins and prevent them from stretching and hurting.
- Surgical stripping: removes varicose veins.
- Sclerotherapy (injection therapy): seals the veins, so blood no longer flows through them.
- Laser therapy: cuts or destroys tissue.

What could harm my client?

- Infection.
- Venous stasis ulcers.
- Clots.

If I were your teacher, I would test you on . . .

- Causes and why.
- Signs and symptoms and why.
- Client education regarding prevention of varicose veins and relief of symptoms.
- Pre- and postop surgical care.
- Signs and symptoms, and management of infection.
- Signs and symptoms, and management of clots.
- Proper circulatory assessment.

✛ Thrombophlebitis

What is it?

Thrombophlebitis is an acute condition characterized by inflammation of vessels with thrombus formation. It may occur in the superficial or deep veins (deep vein thrombosis).

What causes it and why

Table 6-45

Causes	Why
Estrogen therapy, oral contraceptives	Increased activity of clotting factors; smoking + oral contraceptives = blood clot
Hypercoagulability states: sepsis; thrombophilias (lack of antithrombin III or protein C deficiency)	Body's coagulation cascade is working overtime

(Continued)

Table 6-45. (*Continued*)

Causes	Why
Right-sided heart failure	Right side of the heart does not pump blood forward as it should. Blood moves backward into the venous system. Pooling of blood in lower extremities causes irritation and inflammation. The clotting cascade is triggered by inflammation causing red blood cells (RBCs), white blood cells (WBCs), and platelets (PLTs) to form a clot (thrombus)
Pregnancy and childbirth	Enlarged uterus places pressure on the vena cava, decreasing venous return. This leads to pooling of blood in the lower extremities. Stagnation of blood irritates and inflames the vessels. The clotting cascade is triggered by the inflammatory process
Orthopedic surgery	Prolonged immobility leads to venous pooling and stagnation of blood. Stagnation of blood irritates and inflames the vessels. The clotting cascade is triggered by inflammation. RBCs, WBCs, and PLTs adhere to form a thrombus
Obesity	Increased intra-abdominal pressure decreases venous return. Stagnation of blood irritates the vessels, causing inflammation. The clotting cascade is triggered by inflammation
Dehydration	Blood is thickened. All of the blood cells—RBCs, WBCs, and PLTs—are too close together. Clotting can occur
Smoking	Vasoconstricting effects of nicotine are associated with hypercoagulability
Prolonged immobility: postoperative clients, bed-ridden clients, persons who experience prolonged travel, and spinal cord injury clients	Pumping action of muscles is needed to make blood return to the right side of the heart. Stagnation of blood irritates the vessels, causing inflammation. The clotting cascade is triggered by inflammation

Source: Created by author from References #4 to #6.

Signs and symptoms and why

Table 6-46

Signs and symptoms	Why
Heat; erythema	Heat and redness occur as a result of vasodilation in the area. Mobilization of histamine and bradykinin in response to endothelial injury causes vasodilation
Swelling	Mobilization of the biochemical mediators (histamine and bradykinin) in response to endothelial injury causes increased capillary permeability and accumulation of fluid in the tissue
Pain	Swelling exerts pressure on nerve endings in the area

Source: Created by author from References #4 to #6.

Quickie tests and treatments

Tests:

● Doppler ultrasonography: confirms diagnosis by checking leg for clots.

Treatments:

● Prevention of pulmonary embolism.

● Elevate the affected leg: prevents thrombus enlargement.

● Anticoagulants: thin the blood.

- Thrombolytics: dissolve the thrombus.
- Filter (umbrella) placement: traps emboli before they can reach the lungs.
- PCD (pneumatic compression devices) or sequential compression devices (SCDs): prevent clot from moving to lungs.
- Hydration: prevents dehydration.
- Thromboembolic disease (TED) hose (elastic stockings): decrease swelling.
- Surgery: to repair the valves of the veins.

What can harm my client?

- Homan's sign assessment.
- Pulmonary embolism.
- Chronic venous insufficiency.

If I were your teacher, I would test you on . . .

- Causes and why.
- Signs and symptoms and why.
- Pre- and postop client care.
- Medication administration, monitoring, and side effects.
- Proper vascular assessment techniques.
- Signs, symptoms, and management of pulmonary embolism.
- Patient education regarding prevention.

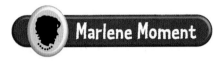

Marlene Moment

Homan's sign assessment has been deemed unsafe as part of the vascular assessment because you can actually dislodge a clot!

✚ Chronic venous insufficiency

What is it?

Chronic venous insufficiency means your client has problems with venous stasis (blood slowing down or pooling) in the lower extremities. This occurs in the late stages of DVT and causes destruction to the valves in the deep veins and connecting veins of the legs.

What causes it and why

Table 6-47

Causes	Why
Clients who are obese, sedentary, pregnant	These conditions increase intra-abdominal pressure. Increased intra-abdominal pressure causes decreased venous return. Blood begins to pool in the legs
Traveling for long periods of time without exercise	When legs are placed in the dependent position, blood has to work against gravity to return to the right side of the heart. Blood begins to pool in the lower extremities
Clients who require bed rest; spinal cord injuries	Blood returns to the heart by the pumping action of muscle contractions. Without adequate muscle contractions, blood pools in the lower extremities
Congestive heart failure (bi-ventricular failure)	Right side of the heart does not pump blood forward like it used to. When blood is not moving forward, it goes backward into the venous system. Pooling of blood in the lower extremities occurs. Pressures inside the vascular space (hydrostatic) exceed tissue pressures. Fluid leaks out of the vascular space and into the tissue

Source: Created by author from References #4 to #6.

Signs and symptoms and why

Table 6-48

Signs and symptoms	Why
Edema	Pooling of blood in the lower extremities. Eventually the pressure in the vascular space exceeds the pressure in the tissue. Fluid leaks out of vascular space and into the tissue. Pitting edema may be evident
Pain	Edema places pressure on nerve endings
Leg heaviness	Increased weight of extremity from edema
Scaly, itchy, reddish brown skin on the inside of the ankle	Red blood cells escape from swollen veins into the skin
Calf permanently enlarges and feels hard	Scar tissue develops and traps fluid in the tissues. Ulcers are more likely to develop

Source: Created by author from References #4 to #6.

Quickie tests and treatments

Tests:

- Doppler ultrasonography: confirms diagnosis by checking leg for clots.

Treatments:

- Prevention of pulmonary embolism.
- Elevate the affected leg: prevents thrombus enlargement.
- Anticoagulants: thin the blood.
- Thrombolytics: dissolve the thrombus.
- Filter (umbrella) placement: traps emboli before they can reach the lungs.
- PCDs (pneumatic compression devices) or sequential compression devices (SCDs): prevent clot from moving to lungs.
- Hydration: prevents dehydration.
- TED hose (elastic stockings): decrease swelling.
- Surgery: to repair the valves of the veins.

What can harm my client?

- Pulmonary embolism.

If I were your teacher, I would test you on . . .

- Causes and why.
- Signs and symptoms and why.
- Pre- and postop client care.
- Medication administration, monitoring, and side effects.
- Proper vascular assessment techniques.
- Signs, symptoms, and management of pulmonary embolism.
- Patient education regarding prevention.

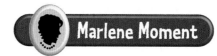

Marlene Moment

When you have symptoms associated with chronic venous insufficiency, you may want to reconsider wearing that Guess mini skirt. Why? Because the public has rights too!

✚ Acute coronary syndrome (ACS)

What is it?

Acute coronary syndrome (ACS) is an umbrella term used to describe any symptoms of acute myocardial infarction (heart attack).

What causes it and why

Table 6-49

Causes	Why
Atherosclerosis	Plaques occlude the vessels, causing a decrease in blood flow to the heart. Myocardial ischemia results in angina
Embolism	Lipid laden plaques that are "spongy" or soft tend to break off. A clot then forms over that area. This clot can partially or totally occlude the vessels

Source: Created by author from References #4 to #6.

RISK FACTORS

- Family history of heart disease.
- Obesity, sedentary lifestyle.
- Smoking.
- High-fat, high-cholesterol diet.
- Menopause.
- Stress.
- Diabetes.
- Hypertension.
- Hyperlipoproteinemia. (↑ lipids in the blood)

Signs and symptoms and why

Table 6-50

Angina/MI	Signs and symptoms	Why
Angina	• Chest pain: burning, squeezing, crushing; may radiate to left arm, neck, jaw, shoulder blade; relieved by nitroglycerin	• Myocardial ischemia
MI	• Chest pain: severe, persistent, crushing, squeezing; may radiate to left arm, jaw, neck, or shoulder blade; unrelieved by rest or nitroglycerin	• Coronary artery occlusion
	• Perspiration; anxiety; hypertension; feeling of impending doom	• Pain; sympathetic nervous system stimulation
	• Fatigue; shortness of breath; cool extremities; hypotension	• Heart is not able to pump enough blood to maintain adequate tissue and organ perfusion
	• Nausea and vomiting	• Pain; vagal stimulation

Source: Created by author from References #4 to #6.

Quickie tests and treatments

Tests:

- Troponin levels: elevated; troponin is released into the bloodstream when cardiac cells die.
- Creatine phosphokinase (CPK), MB isoenzyme of CPK (CPK-MB): elevated; enzymes that are released from the cells when there is myocardial cell death.
- Serial electrocardiograms (EKGs): necrotic tissue is electrically silent.
- WBCs: elevated (leukocytosis).

Treatments for angina:

- Oxygen therapy: delivers oxygen to the heart muscle.
- Nitrates: dilate arteries and veins to reduce myocardial oxygen consumption.
- Beta-adrenergic blockers: reduce heart's workload and oxygen demands.
- Calcium-channel blockers: treat angina caused by coronary artery spasm.
- Antiplatelets: minimize platelet aggregation and danger of coronary occlusion.
- Antilipemics: reduce elevated serum cholesterol or triglyceride levels.
- Coronary artery bypass surgery or percutaneous transluminal coronary angioplasty: for obstructive lesions.

Treatments for MI:

- Thrombolytic therapy (unless contraindicated) within 3 hours of onset of symptoms: restores vessel patency and minimizes necrosis. If a thrombolytic is about to be administered, be extra careful in site selection. You would not choose the jugular vein. Why? Since the major complication of a thrombolytic is hemorrhage, you wouldn't want to get caught holding excessive pressure on someone's neck even if it is to stop bleeding, or you are going to get fired and go to jail!
- Percutaneous transluminal coronary angioplasty (PTCA): to open blocked or narrowed arteries.
- Oxygen: increase oxygenation of blood.
- Nitroglycerin sublingually: to relieve chest pain (unless systolic blood pressure <90 mm Hg or heart rate <50 or >100 beats/minute).
- Morphine: to relieve pain.
- Aspirin: to inhibit platelet aggregation.
- IV heparin (for patients who have received tissue plasminogen activator): to promote patency in affected coronary artery.
- Lidocaine, transcutaneous pacing patches (or transvenous pacemaker), defibrillation, or epinephrine: to combat arrhythmias.
- IV nitroglycerin for 24 to 48 hours (in patients without hypotension, bradycardia, or excessive tachycardia): to reduce afterload and preload and relieve chest pain.

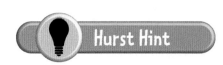

Hurst Hint

In caring for your clients with acute coronary syndrome, remember MONA greets every client. **M**orphine, **O**xygen, **N**itroglycerin, **A**spirin.

What can harm my client?

- Lethal arrhythmias.
- Cardiogenic shock.
- Heart failure causing pulmonary edema.
- Pericarditis.
- Cerebral or pulmonary emboli.

If I were your teacher, I would test you on . . .

- Causes of angina and MI and why.
- The differences between angina and MI signs and symptoms and why.
- CPR techniques.
- Proper cardiopulmonary and vascular assessment.
- Significance of diagnostic tests.
- Medication administration, monitoring, and side effects.
- Oxygen safety.
- IV monitoring and complications.
- Patient education regarding lifestyle modification.

SUMMARY

In this chapter you have reviewed the key cardiac diseases, their causes, signs and symptoms, and treatments. Always remember to assess your clients thoroughly and to investigate any unusual client complaints or physiological changes. Prompt nursing attention can significantly decrease client complications and poor outcomes.

PRACTICE QUESTIONS

1. Jugular vein distension (JVD) is most prominent in which disorder?

   1. Varicose veins.

   2. Abdominal aortic aneurysm.

   3. Myocardial infarction (MI).

   4. Heart failure.

   Correct answer: **4.** Jugular vein distension due to elevated venous pressure indicates heart failure. Jugular vein distension isn't a symptom of varicose veins or abdominal aortic aneurysm. An MI can progress to heart failure if severe enough, but jugular vein distension is not a symptom of MI in and of itself.

2. Which symptom is most commonly associated with left-sided heart failure?

   1. Hypotension.

   2. Crackles.

   3. Arrhythmias.

   4. Vertigo.

Correct answer: 2. Crackles in the lungs are a classic sign of left-sided heart failure. This is due to fluid backing up into the pulmonary system. Hypertension, not hypotension, is associated with left-sided heart failure due to increased workload of the heart. Arrhythmias can be found in both left- and right-sided heart failure. Vertigo is not a symptom of left-sided heart failure.

3. Most abdominal aortic aneurysms are caused by:

   1. Pericarditis.

   2. Hypertension.

   3. Atherosclerosis.

   4. High output failure.

Correct answer: 3. Atherosclerosis accounts for 75% of all abdominal aortic aneurysms. The aortic wall weakens due to plaque buildup. Pericarditis, hypertension, and high-output failure are not directly responsible for abdominal aortic aneurysms.

4. The hereditary disease most closely linked to aneurysm is:

   1. Marfan's syndrome.

   2. Syphilis.

   3. Fibromyalgia.

   4. Systemic lupus erythematosus.

Correct answer: 1. Marfan's syndrome causes decreased elasticity and weakening of the aortic wall, which may lead to an aneurysm. Systemic lupus erythematosus, fibromyalgia, and syphilis aren't hereditary diseases.

5. Which invasive procedure is necessary for treating cardiomyopathy if medical treatments fail?

   1. Intra-aortic balloon pump (IABP).

   2. Heart transplantation.

   3. Pacemaker insertion.

   4. Cardiac catheterization.

Correct answer: 2. Damage to the heart muscle is irreversible. This means that if other medical treatments are not effective, a heart transplant is the next step for the client with cardiomyopathy. IABP is a temporary treatment that assists a failing heart. A pacemaker is used to make the heart beat in a more normal rhythm. Cardiac catheterization diagnoses coronary artery disease.

6. Which is the predominant cause of angina?

   1. Extreme cold temperatures.

   2. Decreased afterload.

   3. Decreased oxygen supply to the heart muscle.

   4. Increased preload.

   Correct answer: 3. Decreased oxygen supply to the heart muscle causes the pain associated with angina. Extreme cold temperatures are associated with Raynaud's disease. Decreased afterload causes low cardiac output. Increased preload is responsible for right-sided heart failure.

7. Common symptoms of hypertension are (select all that apply):

   1. Headache.

   2. Decreased urine output.

   3. Aphasia.

   4. Facial drooping.

   Correct answers: 1 & 2. High pressure in the arterioles of the brain can cause headache. Vasoconstriction and decreased kidney perfusion leads to decreased urine output. Aphasia and facial drooping are symptoms of stroke. Hypertension can lead to stroke, but symptoms of stroke are not initially associated with hypertension.

8. Which treatments may be used to eliminate varicose veins? Select all that apply.

   1. Hydrotherapy.

   2. Laser therapy.

   3. Intense exercise.

   4. Sclerotherapy.

   Correct answers: 2 & 4. Sclerotherapy uses small needles to inject a chemical solution into each varicose vein, causing the vein to close. Blood is rerouted to other veins. Laser therapy sends intense bursts of light on to the veins to seal them off, causing them to dissolve over time. Hydrotherapy and intense exercise do not eliminate varicose veins.

9. To relieve pain from thrombophlebitis:

    1. Apply heat to the affected area.

    2. Maintain bed rest at all times.

    3. Walk at least 45 minutes, 3 times a week.

    4. Elevate the affected leg.

Correct answer: 4. Leg elevation alleviates the pressure caused by thrombophlebitis and helps with venous return. Heat will dilate the vessels, pool blood in the area of the thrombus, and increase the risk of further thrombus formation. Venous stasis increases with bed rest and adds to the risk of thrombus formation. Exercise may be resumed once the clot has dissolved and the physician has granted permission for the client to exercise.

10. What is the most common complication of a myocardial infarction (MI)?

    1. Hepatomegaly.

    2. Endocarditis.

    3. Heart failure.

    4. Arrhythmia.

Correct answer: 4. The most common complication of an MI is an arrhythmia caused by a decrease in oxygen to the heart muscle. Heart failure is the second most common complication, because an MI interferes with the heart's pumping ability. Endocarditis and hepatomegaly are not complications of an MI.

References

1. Hurst M. *A Critical Thinking and Application NCLEX® Review.* Brookhaven, MS: Hurst Review Services; 2006:55.

2. Sanders AB, Cummins RO, Aufderheide TP, et al. *Advanced Cardiac Life Support. Emergency Cardiovascular Care Programs.* Dallas: American Heart Association; 1997–1999: chapter 3.

3. Chobonian AV, Bakris G, Black H, et al. *The Seventh Annual Report of the Joint National Committee on Prevention, Detection, Evaluation and Treatment of High Blood Pressure.* Washington, DC: National Institutes of Health; 2003:12.

4. McCance K, Huether S. *Pathophysiology: The Biological Basis for Disease in Adults and Children.* 4th ed. St. Louis: Mosby-Year Book; 2002:980–981,985,1023,1025.

5. Corwin EJ. The cardiovascular system. In: *Handbook of Pathophysiology.* 3rd ed. Philadelphia: Lippincott Williams & Wilkins; 2008:392–463.

6. Schilling McCann JA, ed. Cardiovascular disorders. In: *Just the Facts: Pathophysiology.* Ambler, PA: Lippincott Williams & Wilkins; 2005:1–47.

7. Schilling McCann JA, ed. Heart failure. In: *Nurse's 3 Minute Clinical Reference.* Springhouse, PA: Lippincott Williams & Wilkins; 2003:246–247.

8. Beers MH, ed. Heart failure. In: *Merck Manual of Medical Information.* 2nd home ed. New York: Pocket Books; 2003:150–158.

9. Schilling McCann JA, ed. Cardiomopathy. In: *Nurse's 3 Minute Clinical Reference.* Springhouse, PA: Lippincott Williams & Wilkins; 2003:112–115.

10. Beers MH, ed. Cardiomyopathy. In: *Merck Manual of Medical Information.* 2nd home ed. New York: Pocket Books; 2003:158–163.

11. Schilling McCann JA, ed. Mitral stenosis. In: *Nurse's 3 Minute Clinical Reference.* Springhouse, PA: Lippincott Williams & Wilkins; 2003:348–349.

12. Beers MH, ed. Heart valve disorders. In: *Merck Manual of Medical Information.* 2nd home ed. New York: Pocket Books; 2003:175–183.

13. Beers MH, ed. Heart and blood vessel disorders. In: *Merck Manual of Medical Information.* 2nd home ed. New York: Pocket Books; 2003:113–239.

Bibliography

Becker D, Franges EZ, Geiter H, et. al. *Critical Care Nursing Made Incredibly Easy.* Ambler, PA: Lippincott Williams & Wilkins; 2004.

Gasparis Vonfrolio L. *Enhancing Your Critical Care Skills.* Staten Island, NY: Education Enterprises; 1998.

Hurst M. *A Critical Thinking and Application NCLEX® Review.* Brookhaven, MS: Hurst Review Services; 2006.

Hurst Review Services. www.hurstreview.com.

McCance K, Huether S. *Pathophysiology: The Biological Basis for Disease in Adults and Children.* 4th ed. St. Louis: Mosby-Year Book; 2002.

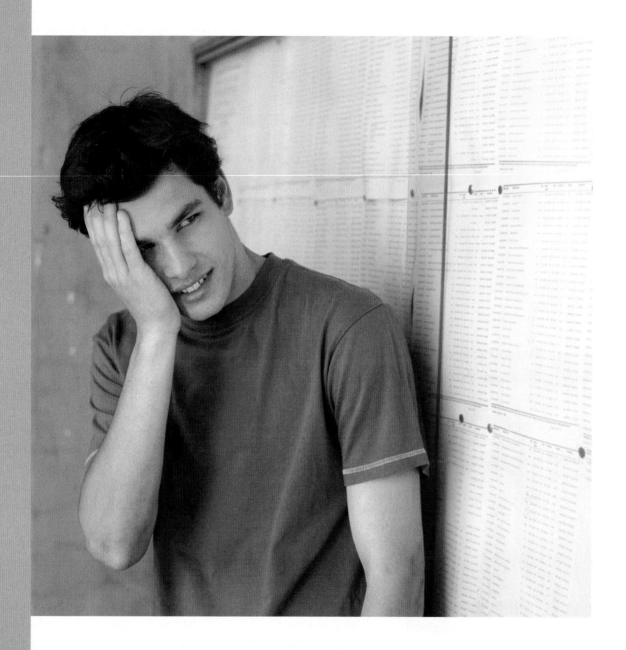

CHAPTER

7 Shock

OBJECTIVES

In this chapter, you'll review:

* The key concepts associated with cardiogenic and three forms of circulatory shock.
* The causes, signs and symptoms, and treatments for cardiogenic and circulatory shock.
* The complications associated with cardiogenic and circulatory shock.

LET'S GET THE NORMAL STUFF STRAIGHT FIRST

I'll bet you already have a mental picture of the "shocky" client: cold, clammy skin with a weak, thready pulse, tachycardia, and hypotension. But don't you need to know what kind of shock is in progress? Yes, you do! Because the treatment for shock is to quickly correct the underlying problem while trying to maintain circulation to keep vital organs and body tissues alive. You can't do this unless you understand which type of shock your client is experiencing.

Various types of shock can occur suddenly due to a number of different causes, but all pathology is directly related to problems within the cardiovascular space: either the heart itself or the vascular space. The vascular space is the network that allows blood to be moved throughout the body. The vascular space includes all of the blood vessels in the body: veins, venules, arteries, arterioles, capillaries. Does the vascular space also include the heart? Yes, it does! Remember, it is called the <u>cardio</u>vascular system. The heart is continuous with the vascular space and is a partner in circulation. The heart serves as the pump to support circulation, keeping the blood in the vascular space moving forward.

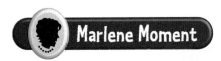

Marlene Moment

So now you've got to be a nurse and a detective? Yes! Snoop Dawg out the cause of shock to better understand the signs, symptoms, and treatments!

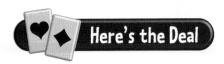

Here's the Deal

Shock is caused by either a pump problem or a problem with the blood circulating through the great vessels, lungs, or heart.

✚ What is shock?

Shock is classified as either circulatory or cardiogenic. Circulatory shock occurs when the vascular space becomes empty (volume depleted), too large (vasodilated) for the available volume, or obstructed. With cardiogenic shock, the heart ceases to effectively pump blood forward. With both forms of shock, circulation through the vascular network is impaired, the cardiac output bottoms out, and compensatory mechanisms immediately begin to try to restore circulation. The most common cause of cardiogenic shock is sudden, acute pump failure following myocardial infarction, which will be discussed later in this chapter. Circulatory shock (nonpump problems) is related to changes in the vascular space.

TYPES OF CIRCULATORY SHOCK

There are three types of circulatory shock: hypovolemic, obstructive, and distributive. The names of each type of shock give you a hint as to the underlying problem. But regardless of the cause of shock, the body tissues are not receiving adequate circulation. If shock is not treated promptly and aggressively in delivering oxygen and nutrients to the tissues, vital organs will develop irreversible damage. Circulatory collapse may be the immediate cause of death, but death can occur later due to organ failure as a result of poor perfusion during the time of shock.

✚ Classification of circulatory shock

Table 7-1 describes the categories of circulatory shock.

Table 7-1

Type of shock	Cause of shock	Examples of conditions leading to shock
Hypovolemic shock	Hemorrhagic/loss of whole blood from the vascular space	Massive trauma, disseminated intravascular coagulation (DIC), aortic aneurysm; intraoperative postoperative complications related to incision and ligation of arteries; obstetric causes related to the placenta or the fundus of the uterus: placental abruption, placenta previa, postpartum uterine atony When faced with obstetric problems . . . think bleeding first
	Intravascular dehydration due to loss of fluid from the vascular space	Polyuria, diarrhea, hyperglycemic hyperosmolar nonketotic (HHNK) coma, diabetes insipidus, addisonian crisis, removal of fluid accumulation via paracentesis or thoracentesis. With all of these conditions, the client is losing volume. By losing volume long enough from anywhere in the body, fluid volume deficit will eventually occur. The faster the loss of volume, the more life threatening the situation
	Intravascular volume loss due to massive fluid shifts and third-spacing of fluid	Burns, ascites, pleural effusion. With these conditions the volume may actually still be in the body, but not in the correct place (the vascular space). Since the fluid is not in the correct place, the body thinks it is in shock
Obstructive shock	Blood cannot be ejected from the left ventricle into systemic circulation because the heart is displaced or compressed	Cardiac tamponade, cardiac myxoma (heart tumor), mediastinal shift, diaphragmatic hernia or diaphragmatic rupture, pneumothorax. If the blood cannot physically get out of the heart to the rest of the body, the vascular space will be depleted. Therefore, the body thinks it is in shock, even though the blood is still in the body
Distributive shock	Loss of vasomotor tone due to interference with sympathetic nervous system function leads to neurogenic shock. Different conditions make the vascular space vasodilate. Prior to the vasodilation, there is adequate volume for the size of the vessels. When vasodilation occurrs, the vessels become larger. This makes the volume seem less to the body, so the body will think it's in shock	Spinal cord injury, dissection of the spinal cord; severe acute pain (this will stimulate the vagus nerve, which will make the heart rate drop; when this happens, not as much blood is being pumped out by the heart, so the vascular system thinks it's in shock). Brain injury, which alters the vasomotor center in the brainstem or sympathetic outflow to vessels; hypoxemia, insulin reaction, CNS depressants, and adverse effects of anesthetic agents[4,9]

(Continued)

Table 7-1. (*Continued*)

Type of shock	Cause of shock	Examples of conditions leading to shock
	Release of histamine-like substances in the blood, which cause vessels to dilate all over the body and induce anaphylactic shock. See the description above about how vasodilation affects volume	Severe allergic reactions to insect stings; foods such as nuts and shellfish; plants; medications such as penicillin; and contact with latex, which causes anaphylaxis (anaphylactic shock)[9]
	The presence of systemic inflammatory mediators elicits endotoxins, which produce generalized vasodilation and trigger septic shock. See the description above about how vasodilation affects volume	Most frequent cause: gram-negative bacteremia, and to a lesser extent gram-positive bacilli and fungi.[8] Urosepsis is a common systemic infection of the elderly, especially when incontinent or with indwelling catheter

Source: Created by author from References #1 to #4.

LET'S GET DOWN TO SPECIFICS

Hypovolemic shock is used as the prototype for all types of shock (with the exception of distributive or vasodilated shock) because of the common symptoms that characterize shock syndromes. Since the body cannot tell the difference among various clinical shock syndromes, only one set of mechanisms is initiated in an attempt to restore or maintain circulating volume regardless of the actual cause. The compensatory mechanisms triggered by shock syndromes really help the person in hypovolemic shock, because more volume and more pressure is what the person actually needs!

✚ Hypovolemic shock

Circulating blood volume must be adequate to maintain cardiac output. Anytime blood volume in the vascular space drops, stroke volume and cardiac output drop, causing an immediate drop in the systolic blood pressure. Systolic blood pressure is a direct reflection of cardiac output. If systolic blood pressure suddenly drops critically low, prompt aggressive action is required to restore perfusion to vital organs—heart, brain, lungs, and kidneys—before damage can occur. The body has a wonderful set of backup systems to compensate for fluid volume losses. These include increased vasomotor tonus and a volume of readily available blood and fluid that can be quickly shifted to the vascular space. A volume of blood is stored in the liver, and there is always pooled blood in the venous system that can be mobilized and delivered to central circulation very quickly if there is any sudden threat to the critical level of intravascular blood volume. Hopefully, this mechanism coupled with sympathetic stimulation (tachycardia and vasopressor effects) will initiate compensation to restore volume and blood pressure, thereby halting progression of shock while the underlying problem is being resolved.

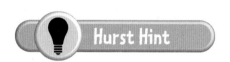

Less volume = less pressure.

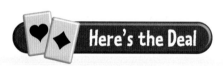

When you see the word "vasopressor," this means the vascular system is constricting down on less fluid. This will make it seem like there is more fluid in the vascular space since the vasoconstriction made the vascular space smaller. Remember: vasoconstriction = increased BP; vasodilation = decreased BP.

What is it?

Hypovolemic shock refers to a particular set of symptoms in reaction to the body's failed attempt to compensate for the acute loss of circulating blood volume.

OTHER THINGS YOU NEED TO KNOW . . .

- Whole blood can be lost from circulation during hemorrhage.

- The liquid portion of the blood (plasma) can be lost from circulation due to seepage out of the vascular space.

- Any injury to vessel walls, such as a burn injury, can increase capillary permeability (means vessels are leaking) and cause a fluid shift out of the vascular space.

- Vascular fluid deficit from extracellular fluid losses (vomiting, diarrhea, polyuria) can also lead to hypovolemic shock.

- Symptoms of shock occur because of rapid loss of circulating fluid volume. Did I say TOTAL fluid volume? NO! A person can have fluid volume that is not in the vascular space, and is therefore not available for circulation of oxygen and nutrients to the tissues and removal of metabolic waste products. When the gas tank is empty, can the vehicle continue to run? NO! Likewise, when the vascular space is empty, the vital organs of the body can no longer perform essential functions for sustaining life.

- Our bodies are optimized to maintain circulating fluid volume. This is programmed into every organ system. The heart responds to the problem of low circulating volume by speeding up (sympathetic stimulation) the heart rate to move the available blood volume around faster.

- When the kidneys sense low circulating volume, they immediately go into the mode of conserving fluid (reabsorbing) and the renin–angiotension system is activated for the vasopressor effect to raise blood pressure. Angiotensin II is a potent vasoconstrictor. Also, the renin–angiotensin system will cause aldosterone to be secreted, which makes the body retain sodium and water, therefore building the volume back up in the vascular space.

- The autonomic nervous system helps by clamping down on blood vessels to shunt blood away from organs with low oxygen consumption, allowing the scant available supply to be directed to the "vital" or most essential organs.

- Of the four vital organs—heart, brain, lungs, and kidneys—the kidneys are the first to be "voted off the island." Acute renal failure can occur after only 20 minutes of interrupted renal perfusion.

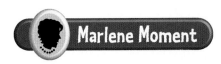

Marlene Moment

Think about it like this: While experiencing shock, would you rather have more blood going to your brain or to your skin? Would you rather have a dead brain and pretty skin or bad skin and a great brain?

What causes it and why

Table 7-2 gives an overview of the causes of shock and corresponding explanations.

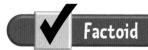

Factoid

Many times, with an intestinal obstruction. Fluid will leak out of vascular space into the lumen of the intestine causing a vascular volume deficit.

Table 7-2

Causes	Why
Dehydration	Excessive perspiration, severe diarrhea or vomiting, diabetes insipidus, adrenal insufficiency, diabetic ketoacidosis, diuresis, inadequate fluid intake; internal fluid shift
Intestinal obstruction	Internal fluid shift; excessive fluid shift when the material in the bowel cannot move past the obstruction
Hemorrhage	Trauma; loss of whole blood directly from the vascular space
Burns	Internal fluid shift; injury to vessel wall increases capillary leakage, causing a fluid shift out of the vascular space
Peritonitis	Internal fluid shift; inflammation or injury to vessel walls of peritoneum can cause bleeding and fluid shift out of the vascular space
Ascites	Internal fluid shift; excessive fluid shift between the membranes lining the abdomen and abdominal organs (the peritoneal cavity); fluid leaves vascular space and leaks into abdomen

Source: Created by author from References #1 to #3.

Signs and symptoms and why

Table 7-3 summarizes the signs and symptoms of shock.

Table 7-3

Signs and symptoms	Why
Early Shock (Adaptive Mode)	
Restlessness	Activation of sympathetic nervous system stimulation causes the release of epinephrine and norepinephrine (also called catecholamines, or stress hormones for fight or flight)
Apprehension, irritability	Cerebral hypoxia due to decrease in cardiac output and the sense of impending doom—that something is very wrong
Tachypnea	Beta receptors respond to cellular hypoxia to initiate bronchodilation[3]; helps get more air in
Bounding pulse (the heart is pumping <u>harder</u> to get what blood is left out to the vital organs)	Sympathetic stimulation has a direct effect on the myocardial cells to increase the force of contraction, causing adaptive efforts to combat early shock.[11] Beta receptors are responsible for the increased oxygen usage by the heart muscle in an attempt to adapt to correct shock states[3]
Thirst	A very basic compensatory mechanism for any condition of hemoconcentration to replace fluid volume. As vascular volume decreases, serum osmolarity increases and the thirst center in the

(Continued)

Table 7-3. (*Continued*)

Signs and symptoms	Why
	hypothalamus is activated. In addition to the thirst signal, the posterior pituitary gland releases antidiuretic hormone (ADH) for additional water conservation. The kidneys release angiotensin II, which has a direct effect on the hypothalamus as an added trigger to thirst[1]
Reduced urinary output	Kidneys sense low circulating volume and begin to reabsorb water, decreasing the amount of urine excreted to offset existing hypovolemia. Continued hypotension activates the renin–angiotension system, which signals the adrenals to secrete aldosterone to hold more salt and water, and then the pituitary gets into the picture with an increase in ADH to further conserve water[4]
Tachycardia (heart is pumping <u>faster</u> to get what little blood is left out to the vital organs)	Sympathetic stimulation has a direct action on the pacemaker of the heart to speed up the heart rate and increase the force of contraction
Narrowed pulse pressure (the difference in the systolic and diastolic blood pressure)	Sympathetic stimulation causes vasoconstriction, which causes the diastolic pressure to rise, but the systolic pressure, stays the same
	Advanced Shock
Pulse quality: weak, thready	Progressive fluid volume deficit results in a small vascular space, and coupled with the vasoconstriction from continued sympathetic stimulation, the pulse feels like a very small thread-like string of a vessel when palpated, and the low volume is reflected in the low pulse pressure exerted on the wall of the vessel. When oxygen is lacking, cellular metabolism shifts to the anaerobic mode, causing lactic acid to build up. The resultant acidosis depresses the myocardium. When the heart is depressed it doesn't pump as well
Skin changes: cool, pale, clammy	Fat, bone, and skin can better survive ischemia than organs with high oxygen consumption. Blood flow is therefore diverted away from the skin, as well as the GI tract and the liver, in an effort to direct more blood flow to the heart, brain, and lungs
Oliguria	As blood pressure drops in shock, renal perfusion decreases, therefore reducing the kidney functions of filtration and excretion
Hemoconcentration: elevated HCT, Hgb	Progressive fluid volume loss through intravascular dehydration leaves a concentration of solids (particles) within the vascular space, which in turn causes sluggish blood flow and can lead to tissue damage, which may trigger another potentially lethal complication of DIC (see Chapter 8)

(*Continued*)

Table 7-3. (*Continued*)

Signs and symptoms	Why
Hypotension	The hallmark of failed compensatory mechanisms is reflected in a decreased systolic blood pressure. The cause of the shock has not been corrected, the backup system can no longer hold the cardiac output steady, and the cardiac output decreases as reflected by the progressive decline in the systolic blood pressure
Late Shock	
Decreasing level of consciousness (LOC): apathy, confusion, stupor, finally coma	When the cardiac output falls below a critical level, the brain is no longer receiving adequate blood flow. Brain cells that require high levels of oxygen and glucose cannot continue normal functions of orientation, comprehension, responsiveness, and wakefulness
Shallow respirations	With progressive brain dysfunction due to critically insufficient perfusion of oxygen, the medulla oblongata of the brain (which normally regulates respirations) ceases to relay the life-saving message for the lungs to take in more oxygen
Oliguria/anuria	With continued lack of perfusion due to cardiac output, the kidneys can no longer function. Kidneys shut down secondary to continued loss of circulating volume and sluggish blood flow
Cardiac failure/circulatory collapse	End-stage onset of anaerobic metabolism produces acidosis, which depresses the heart muscle fibers

Source: Created by author from References #4 to #6.

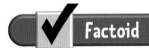

Factoid

When shock is due to a loss of whole blood, the fluid volume (plasma) and solids (RBCs, WBCs, and platelets) are reduced. Therefore, the HCT and Hgb will be low rather than high.

DERAILED   Remember the formula for cardiac output? CO = SV × HR. In advanced shock, hypotension results because compensatory mechanisms fail. When shock progresses beyond the point of no return, organ systems shut down due to prolonged ischemia. After the onset of late shock, the client cannot recover because of critical injury to vital organs. Blood pressure and perfusion must be restored BEFORE multiple-system organ failure occurs! What a train wreck! Shock not only derails the train . . . it destroys the engine and crushes all the cars.

Quickie tests and treatments

Tests:

- Serum hematocrit and hemoglobin: low.
- Serum red blood cell and platelet: low.
- Serum potassium, sodium, creatinine, and blood urea nitrogen: elevated.
- Urine specific gravity (greater than 1.020) and urine osmolality: elevated.
- pH: decreased.
- Occult blood test: positive.

- X-rays: help to identify internal bleeding sites.
- Gastroscopy: helps to identify internal bleeding sites.
- Invasive hemodynamic monitoring: reduced central venous pressure, right atrial pressure, pulmonary artery pressure, pulmonary artery wedge pressure (PAWP), and cardiac output.
- CT scan: helps detect internal bleeding.
- Abdominal (peritoneal) lavage (Fig. 7-1): helps detect abdominal/peritoneal bleeding.

Treatments:

- Treat the underlying cause(s).
- Maintenance of patent airway; preparation for intubation and mechanical intubation: prevent or manage respiratory distress.
- Supplemental oxygen: increase oxygenation.
- Pneumatic antishock garment: control internal and external hemorrhage by direct pressure.
- Isotonic IV fluid bolus: raise blood pressure.
- Fluids, such as normal saline or lactated Ringer's solution: to restore filling pressures.
- Packed red blood cells: restore blood loss and improve blood's oxygen-carrying capacity.
- Military antishock trousers (MAST): raise blood pressure.
- Plasma volume expanders and emergency transfusions may be indicated if the client's condition does not allow time for full type and cross-match procedures.
- Fluid resuscitation use of crystalloids, electrolyte solutions and colloids for fluid loss secondary to burn wounds.
- Fluid loss due to addisonian crisis or diabetes insipidus requires hormone replacement therapy as well as IV fluid volume replacement therapy.

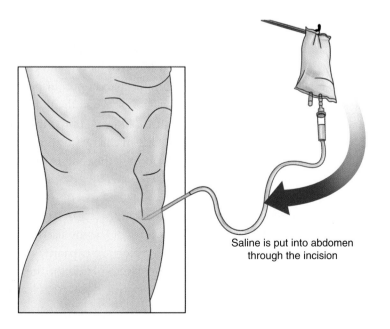

◄ Figure 7-1. Diagnostic peritoneal lavage.

Saline is put into abdomen through the incision

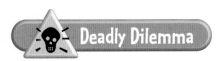

Deadly Dilemma

Once you see signs of shock, don't wait for the body to compensate, because compensatory mechanisms have already failed!

What can harm my client?

- Cardiac arrhythmias.
- Cardiac arrest.
- Organ failure.
- Adult respiratory distress syndrome (ARDS).
- Renal failure.
- Disseminated intravascular coagulation (DIC).

If I were your teacher, I would test you on . . .

- Causes and why.
- Signs and symptoms and why.
- Proper cardiovascular and respiratory assessment.
- Diagnostic tests.
- Medical management and nursing interventions.
- Proper IV insertion technique, monitoring, and management of complications.
- Fluids used to restore circulating volume.

✚ Circulatory shock: obstructive presentation

To understand circulatory shock, let's start with some basic anatomy and physiology first. The heart is anatomically placed in the center of the thorax between the lungs in the mediastinum. The heart is nestled in this snug space, moveable because it is hanging by the great vessels, surrounded and supported by the right and left lungs on either side and protected by the rigid, bony rib cage. The diaphragm closes off the thoracic cavity, which houses only the heart and lungs, keeping them separated from the abdominal cavity where all of the abdominal organs live.

Because the organs in the thoracic cavity fully occupy the available space, any changes in the size or position of the organs result in a full house within the cavity and <u>decreased</u> space for normal function. The chambers of the heart as well as the lung tissue experience rhythmic changes in size and position as they perform their respective functions. The chambers of the heart relax in diastole (ventricular filling of blood) and contract in systole to eject blood forward. The lungs expand upon inspiration and deflate with expiration of air. The available space in the thorax accommodates these changes in size and pressures, allowing both vital organs ample room to perform effective function. This all changes during obstructive circulatory shock, causing the organs to raise the roof and rock the house!

What is it?

Obstructive circulatory shock results in compression (squeezing) or displacement of the heart from the center of the mediastinum, causing decreased ventricular filling, decreased ejection capacity, and a drop in the cardiac output. Mechanical factors are to blame for the interference of the filling or emptying of the heart or great vessels that leads to systolic hypotension and poor perfusion.

What causes it and why

Table 7-4 summarizes the causes and associated explanations for obstructive circulatory shock.

Table 7-4

Causes	Why
Pulmonary embolism	Interference with ventricular emptying
Tension pneumothorax, cardiac tamponade, atrial tumor, or clot	Mechanical interference with ventricular filling
Diaphragmatic hernia (abdominal content moves up into thoracic cavity)	Not enough room in the thorax for the heart and lungs PLUS any abdominal organs; the heart is compressed by the extra pressure and ventricular filling is compromised, leading to decreased stroke volume and cardiac output and obstructed circulation
Cardiac tamponade, cardiac myxoma (heart tumor), mediastinal shift	Heart is displaced or compressed; blood cannot physically get out of the heart to the rest of the body, depleting the vascular space. Therefore, the body thinks it is in shock, even though the blood is still in the body

Source: Created by author from References #1 to #4.

Signs and symptoms and why

Table 7-5 gives an overview of the signs and symptoms of obstructive circulatory shock.

Table 7-5

Signs and symptoms	Why
Differences in Shock Presentation with Obstructive Shock	
Dyspnea, tachypnea	Remember that circulatory volume is normal in this form of circulatory shock! When blood flow through the lungs is compromised by a pulmonary embolus, air can't get into the lung for diffusion of oxygen into the blood
Distended neck veins	Increased pulmonary pressure causes backward pressure in the right heart. Elevated right heart pressure and elevated central venous pressure causes a backflow that engorges jugular veins
Systolic hypotension with decreased left ventricular stroke volume output	When the heart is displaced or compressed, the chambers cannot properly fill, and therefore cardiac output and systolic pressure decrease. During inspiration, the pressure of blood flowing into the right heart pushes against the intraventricular septum, creating internal pressure to add to the external pressure compressing the heart[9]

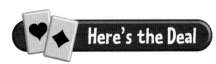

Here's the Deal

Any mechanical blockage to blood flow through the great veins, heart, or lungs can obstruct circulation and cause shock.

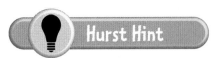

Hurst Hint

With a pulmonary embolus the pressure in the lungs increases. The heart has trouble pumping against the high pressure so cardiac output drops.

(Continued)

Table 7-5. (*Continued*)

Signs and symptoms	Why
Displaced trachea	Lung collapse due to air or blood in the pleural space on the affected side causes one-sided ventilation and a shift in the position of mediastinal structures: the trachea, esophagus, and heart. If the client has a right pneumothorax, everything will be displaced to the left side
Pulsus paradoxus	When the heart is being squeezed (compressed), the cardiac output falls. With inspiration, the lungs inflate and draw blood into the right heart, pushing the intraventricular septum to the left, increasing compression to the already compressed left chamber and the cardiac output falls further (think of this as a "double squeeze"). With each inspiration, the systolic pressure falls at least 10 mm Hg and rises 10 mm Hg with each expiration, reflecting a little better cardiac output with reduced internal pressure on the heart[9]
Muffled heart sounds	Heart sounds are muffled when auscultated through a mass in the cardiac muscle or a volume of blood or exudates in the pericardial sac
Central venous pressure (CVP)	Because the heart is being squeezed, the pressure inside of the heart is elevated and all chambers of the heart reflect increased pressures. When you squeeze an inflated balloon, what happens to the pressure inside the balloon? It goes up until the pressure becomes so great that the balloon pops. This is exactly the way the heart feels too as it is being squeezed externally with excess blood or fluid. Usually when the blood pressure is low, the CVP will also be low (and vice versa) except in the event of cardiac tamponade

Source: Created by author from References #5, #6, #8, and #9.

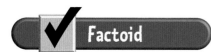

Factoid

Usually the CVP and the BP mirror each other except in cardiac tamponade!

CVP ⇧ BP ⇧ in fluid volume excess.

CVP ⇩ BP ⇩ in fluid volume deficit.

CVP ⇧ BP ⇩ in cardiac tamponade!

Quickie tests and treatments

Tests:

- Chest x-ray: identifies cardiac tamponade or pneumothorax.
- Echocardiography: identifies fluid accumulation in the pericardial sac.

Treatments:

- Maintain patent airway; preparation for intubation and mechanical ventilation: to prevent or manage respiratory distress.
- Supplemental oxygen: to increase oxygenation.
- Chest tubes with water seal and suction: promote re-expansion of the lung.
- Surgery: repair of diaphragmatic abnormalities or injuries.
- Pericardiocentesis: needle aspiration to remove excess blood or fluid from pericardial sac (Fig. 7-2).

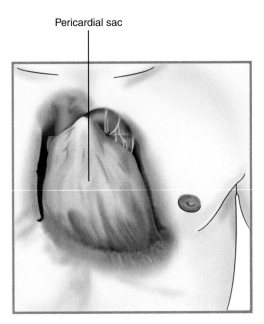

Pericardial sac

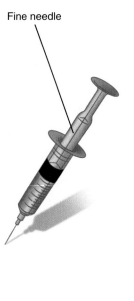

Fine needle

◀ Figure 7-2. Pericardial sac.

What can harm my client?

• Cardiac arrest.

• Fatal arrhythmia with pulseless electrical activity (PEA).

CASE IN POINT   Imagine you are with a client's family at the bedside. The cardiac monitor shows a sinus rhythm of 88, but you cannot feel a pulse. This is pulseless electrical activity. The family thinks PawPaw (grandpa) is still alive because they see the rhythm on the monitor. How would you handle this scenario?

1. Cut off the monitor.

2. Explain to the family that PawPaw is really gone.

3. Leave the room.

4. Call a code.

Let's see how you did:

1. Okay, if you cut off the monitor, the family will think you just killed PawPaw. Not nice. So you're a nurse who can work magic and you put the monitor back on. You just brought PawPaw back to life! NO!

2. The family will not understand what you are saying, as they are fixated on the monitor. They are going to sue you big time for providing inappropriate information. Besides, no one can be pronounced dead until they have flatlined.

3. Leave the room?! What a sweet, caring nurse you are!

4. You better call a code . . . and quick!

OTHER THINGS YOU NEED TO KNOW . . .   Imagine your patient has a beautiful, normal sinus rhythm on the monitor, but is dead as a post! This is WEIRD! While initiating CPR, review the 4 Hs and 2 Ts (see on the next page) that can be the problem. And always remember to consider hypoxia FIRST! PEA requires that the problem be corrected FAST to restore a pulse when the patient is clinically dead! Be on the lookout for:

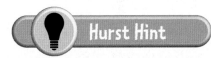

Hurst Hint

Pulseless electrical activity (PEA) is when the electrical heart conduction continues in the absence of a mechanical contraction of the heart; no pulse is generated.

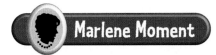

Marlene Moment

A client or family must be in the right frame of mind and **ready** to learn. Now is not the time to try and explain that just because PawPaw has a rhythm on the monitor he is really no longer with us. Okay?

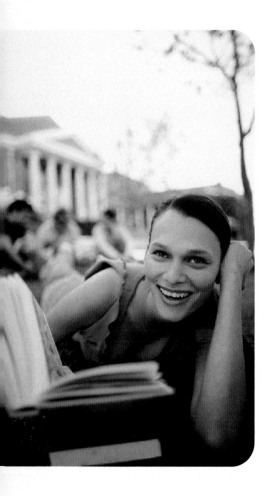

First the 4Hs:
- Hypoxia.
- Hypovolemia.
- Hypothermia.
- Hypokalemia.

Then the 2 Ts:
- Cardiac tamponade.
- Tension pneumothorax.

If I were your teacher, I would test you on . . .
- Causes and why.
- Signs and symptoms and why.
- Signs and symptoms and management of pneumothorax.
- Signs and symptoms and management of cardiac tamponade.
- Assessment and emergency care for PEA.
- Emergency measures indicated to relieve cardiac compression and/or mediastinal shift to restore effective cardiac output.
- Clinical data used to evaluate the effectiveness of interventions to relieve obstructive shock.

✚ Circulatory shock: distributive presentation

The size of the vascular system is directly related to vasomotor tone (vasoconstriction or vasodilation), which is under autonomic control. Vasodilation increases the size of the vascular system; if circulating volume remains the same, the effect will be lower blood pressure. Vaso-constriction decreases the size of the vascular system; if blood volume remains unchanged, higher systolic blood pressure is expected. Under autonomic nervous system regulation, a hot environment triggers vasodilation to bring more blood to the surface to promote cooling, whereas a cold environment results in vasoconstriction to shunt blood to prevent body heat from being lost to the environment.

Autoregulation and adaptive mechanisms produce changes in the vascular system in response to internal as well as external conditions (above) to maintain homeostasis and normotension. If circulating volume is lost for any reason, hypotension triggers sympathetic stimulation to produce vasoconstriction, which will rapidly raise the blood pressure. Primary or secondary hypertension with normal blood volume results in edema as a response to increased capillary pressure. Edema (interstitial space fluid) reduces volume in the vascular space when the size of the vessel is too small for the circulating volume. Normally changes of pressure in the circulatory system are affected by these two factors: the size of the blood vessel and the amount of fluid volume within the vascular space. Distributive shock is classified as anaphylactic, septic, or neurogenic in origin.

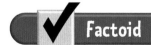

Factoid

The vessels clamp/squeeze down on vascular volume causing BP to go up.

What is it?

Distributive shock occurs when blood volume is normally displaced in the vasculature—for example, when blood pools in the peripheral blood vessels. This displacement of blood volume causes a relative hypovolemia because not enough blood returns to the heart, resulting in decreased tissue perfusion.

What causes it and why

Distributive shock can be caused by an impaired baroreceptor response, altered autonomic pathways (neurogenic shock), or the presence of substances in the blood that produce vasodilation (anaphylactic shock and septic shock). Table 7-6 summarizes distributive shock causes and rationales.

Table 7-6

Causes	Why
Severe allergic reactions to insect stings; foods such as nuts and shellfish; plants; medications such as penicillin; and contact with latex, which causes anaphylaxis (anaphylactic shock)[9]	Release of histamine-like substances in the blood, which cause vessels to dilate all over the body and induce anaphylactic shock
Most frequent cause: gram-negative bacteremia and to a lesser extent gram-positive bacilli and fungi.[8] Urosepsis is a common systemic infection of the elderly, especially when incontinent or with indwelling catheter	The presence of systemic inflammatory mediators elicits endotoxins, which produce generalized vasodilation and trigger septic shock
Spinal cord injury, dissection of the spinal cord; severe acute pain (this will stimulate the vagus nerve, which will make the heart rate drop; when this happens, not as much blood is being pumped out by the heart, so the vascular system thinks it's in shock). Brain injury, which alters the vasomotor center in the brainstem or sympathetic outflow to vessels; hypoxemia, insulin reaction, CNS depressants, and adverse effects of anesthetic agents[4,9]	Loss of vasomotor tone due to interference with sympathetic nervous system function leads to neurogenic shock. Different conditions make the vascular space vasodilate. Prior to the vasodilation, there is adequate volume for the size of the vessels. When vasodilation occurs, the vessels become larger. This makes the volume seem less to the body, so the body will think it's in shock

Source: Created by author from References #4, #8, and #9.

Signs and symptoms and why

Table 7-7 takes a look at the signs and symptoms of distributive shock.

Table 7-7

Signs and symptoms	Why
Distributive Shock Presentation	
Skin Sensations/Temperature	
Warm, pink, flushed skin	With septic shock, there is fever as well as vasodilation causing increased blood flow to the skin. Anaphylactic shock is characterized by generalized vasodilation, which brings more blood flow to the skin
Warm sensation, itching, burning, hives, angioedema	Histamine release (anaphylactic shock) causes allergic manifestations such as urticaria (hives) and increased capillary permeability, causing fluid to seep out of vessels
Normal skin color, dry to touch	In neurogenic shock, sympathetic pathways are disrupted, so pallor, clamminess, diaphoresis, and tachycardia will not be present
Vital Signs	
Systolic hypotension, normal pulse	In distributive shock, the blood volume is normal, but because of vasodilation, the vascular space has become too large for the normal circulating volume of blood, and peripheral pooling of blood causes a sudden drop in the blood pressure
Respiratory Symptoms	
Dyspnea, air hunger, wheezing, chest tightness, coughing	Histamine released in anaphylactic shock increases capillary permeability and leaky vessels cause laryngeal edema. The vascular smooth muscle response causes bronchospasm, which closes off the airway[9]

Source: Created by author from Reference #9.

✚ Anaphylactic shock

Anaphylactic shock is a type of distributive shock that involves the immune system. The body has a great system for protecting itself against foreign substances that get past the gatekeepers (physical and chemical barriers) and enter the body. Once inside, the inflammatory response is activated first, and then the immune system kicks in to defend the body against these invaders. The plasma antibody response is activated for the "seek and destroy" mission. Each of the five immunoglobulins (IgG, IgM, IgA, IgD, and IgE) is programmed to respond in a unique way. IgM and IgG attach to the invader to hopefully destroy the foreign substance. The immunoglobulin responder for most allergic reactions is IgE, which rides on the basophils in the plasma. Once IgE is activated by the presence of the offending agent, heparin and histamine are released.[7] This IgE response can be a good thing if the person has a parasite that needs to be destroyed.[4]

What is it?

Anaphylactic shock is a syndrome that occurs in persons who are hypersensitive to a particular allergen (also called an antigen). The person is said to have become "sensitized" to the allergen after repeated exposures causing the buildup of IgE immunoglobulins (antibodies). Chemicals are released into the blood, bind to the mast cells, and start the deadly cascade of complement factors that leads to damage of vessel walls, increased permeability, and leakage of fluid from the vascular space, resulting in hypovolemia and hypotension. Cardiac output falls, cardiac function deteriorates, and lung function is compromised by bronchospasm and laryngeal edema.[11]

What causes it and why

Systemic exposure to sensitizing agents:

- Chemicals (sulfobromophthalein sodium, sodium dehydrocholate, radiographic contrast media).
- Foods (legumes, nuts, berries, seafood, egg albumin).
- Drugs (penicillin, antibiotics, sulfonamides, local anesthetics).
- Enzymes.
- Hormones.
- Insect venom.
- Vaccinations.
- Allergen extracts.
- Serums (horse serum).
- Sulfite-containing food additives.

Signs and symptoms and why

Table 7-8 lists the signs and symptoms of anaphylactic shock.

Table 7-8

Signs and symptoms	Why
Sudden nasal congestion	Leakage of fluid into extracellular tissues due to increased capillary permeability
Flushed, moist skin	Blood vessels dilate, bringing increased blood flow to the surface[11]
Nervousness, anxiety, feeling of doom	Decreased cerebral blood flow secondary to a decrease in cardiac output
Red, itchy wheals (urticaria and pruritis)	Reaction to allergens
Tachypnea and crowing (stridor)	Bronchospasm and laryngeal edema obstruct the intake of oxygen on inspiration. Oxygen lack triggers more rapid breathing
Generalized edema	Leakage of fluid into extracellular tissues due to increased capillary permeability
Hypotension	Fluid shifting from the vascular space into the tissues results in a fluid volume deficit in the vascular space and a drop in blood pressure

Source: Created by author from Reference #11.

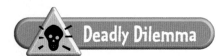

Deadly Dilemma

Bronchospasm and laryngeal edema are life threatening! Epinephrine STAT relaxes smooth muscles of the bronchus and vaso-constricts blood vessels to raise the BP![9,10]

Quickie tests and treatments

Tests:

- Determine the underlying cause: guides treatment and prevention.
- Skin testing: develops a specific antigen.

Treatments:

- Maintain a patent airway: maintain oxygenation.
- Cardiopulmonary resuscitation (CPR): treat cardiac arrest.
- Oxygen therapy: increase tissue perfusion.
- Tracheostomy or endotracheal intubation and mechanical ventilation: maintain patent airway.
- Epinephrine 1:1,000 aqueous solution (IM or subcutaneously if patient hasn't lost consciousness and is normotensive; IV if reaction is severe), repeat dosage every 5 to 20 minutes as needed: reverse bronchoconstriction and cause vasoconstriction.
- Corticosteroids: to reduce inflammatory reaction.
- Diphenhydramine (Benadryl) IV: to reduce allergic response.
- Vasopressors (norepinephrine, dopamine): to support blood pressure.
- Norepinephrine (Levophed): to restore blood pressure.
- Volume expanders: to maintain and restore circulating plasma volume.
- Dopamine (Dobutrex): to support blood pressure.
- Aminophylline (Truphylline): to dilate bronchi and reverse bronchospasm.

What can harm my client?

- Cardiopulmonary arrest.
- Vascular collapse.
- Immediate threat of death.

If I were your teacher, I would test you on . . .

- Causes and why.
- Signs and symptoms and why.
- Medication administration, monitoring, and side effects.
- CPR techniques.
- Monitoring and evaluating ventilator settings.
- Oxygen equipment and administration safety.
- Patient education regarding allergens.

✚ Septic shock

Septic shock is caused by widespread infection and is the most common type of circulatory shock. The very young and the very old are at greater risk for septic shock.[6]

What is it?

Septic shock is caused by an infection in the bloodstream (sepsis) in which blood pressure falls dangerously low and many organs malfunction because of inadequate blood flow.

What causes it and why

Table 7-9 summarizes causes and explanations for septic shock.

Table 7-9

Causes	Why
Sepsis caused by any pathogenic organism	Cytokines (substances made by immune system to fight infection) and toxins produced by bacteria cause blood vessels to dilate, which decreases blood pressure. Blood flow to the kidneys and brain is decreased. The heart works harder to fight the decreased blood flow, only to weaken it. The walls of the blood vessels leak, allowing fluid from the bloodstream into the tissues, causing swelling. This can develop in the lungs, causing respiratory distress
Clients with weakened immune systems (newborns; elderly; patients with AIDS, with cancer, or who are receiving chemotherapy; those who have chronic diseases like diabetes or cirrhosis)	Weakened immune system allows bacteria to take control of the immune system
Invasive tests, treatments, surgery, or trauma	Bacteria can find their way through the body due to the openings these create; bacteria can harbor on medical equipment and prosthesis in the client (e.g., a prosthetic hip)

Source: Created by author from References #5, #6, #9, #11, and #12.

Signs and symptoms and why

Septic shock's presentation is described in Table 7-10.

Table 7-10

Signs and symptoms	Why
Alteration in temperature: hyperthermia or hypothermia	Fever and a high white count may accompany the bacteremia in early shock, but hypothermia due to a decreasing basal metabolic rate in late shock[3] and low white count may be present in the immunosuppressed
Warm, flushed skin	Febrile conditions coupled with bacterial toxins in the blood cause excessive vasodilation[10]
Hypotension	Excessive systemic vasodilation reduces the pressure within the vascular space

(Continued)

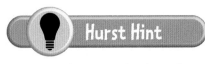

Hurst Hint

Hyperventilation may be the earliest sign of septic shock in the elderly!

Table 7-10. (*Continued*)

Signs and symptoms	Why
Confusion, behavioral changes	Decreased perfusion to brain tissues and toxins alter cerebral function
Hyperventilation (early shock) and hypoventilation (late shock)	Fast breathing occurs in response to cellular hypoxia and can result in respiratory alkalosis.[9] Lactic acidosis may result from hypoventilation when the respiratory center becomes depressed[4]

Source: Created by author from References #3, #4, #9, #10, and #12.

Quickie tests and treatments

Tests:

- Blood cultures: identifies causative organism.
- Complete blood count: evaluating for anemia, leukopenia, neutropenia, thrombocytopenia.
- Liver panel: BUN is elevated; creatinine is decreased.
- Prothrombin time (PT) and partial thromboplastin time (PTT): abnormal.
- Urine studies: increased specific gravity (more than 1.020), osmolality, and decreased sodium.
- Arterial blood gas: monitor for acidosis or alkalosis.
- Invasive hemodynamic monitoring: increased cardiac output and decreased systemic vascular resistance in warm phase; decreased cardiac output and increased systemic vascular resistance in cold phase.

Treatments:

- Antibiotic therapy: rids causative organism; broad-spectrum antibiotics are started immediately after blood is drawn and continued for 48 hours until culture reports are finalized.
- Inotropic and vasopressor drugs (dopamine, dobutamine, norepinephrine): improve perfusion and maintain blood pressure.
- Maintain airway, prepare for intubation and mechanical ventilation: prevent or manage respiratory distress.
- Supplemental oxygen: increases oxygenation.
- IV fluids, crystalloids, colloids, or blood products as necessary: to maintain intravascular volume.
- Monoclonal antibodies to tumor necrosis factor, endotoxin, and interleukin-1: to counteract septic shock mediators.

What can harm my client?

- Lethal arrhythmias.
- DIC.
- ARDS.
- Multisystem organ failure.
- Renal failure.
- GI ulcers.

If I were your teacher, I would test you on . . .

- Causes and why.
- Signs and symptoms and why.
- How septic shock affects elderly clients.
- The differences between colloids and crystalloids and how to administer each.
- Monitoring for acidosis and alkalosis.
- Interpreting laboratory values and evaluating treatments based on values.

✚ Neurogenic shock

What is it?

Neurogenic shock occurs when the sympathetic nervous system stops sending signals to the vessel walls, causing the vessels throughout the body to vasodilate (also called loss of sympathetic vascular tone) and the blood pressure to drop. This usually occurs when there is severe damage to the central nervous system, specifically the brain and spinal cord. It is most often seen after acute spinal cord injury due to blunt trauma—motor vehicle accidents (MVAs), falls, and sports injuries. The cervical spine area is the most commonly injured area. The higher the spinal cord injury, the more severe the neurogenic shock. With injuries to the brain, the function of the autonomic nervous system is decreased, which leads to vasodilation throughout all vessels. In other words, the spinal nervous system cannot control the diameter of the blood vessels. When the vasomotor center of the brain is injured, the sympathetic nervous system does not function properly, leading to systemic vasodilation. As a result, blood pools in the venous system, the amount of blood returning to the right side of the heart is decreased, and ultimately cardiac output drops and hypotension occurs.

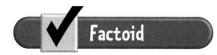

Factoid

When neurogenic shock is caused by a spinal cord injury, it is called spinal shock.

What causes it and why

The causes and associated reasons for neurogenic shock are given in Table 7-11.

Table 7-11

Causes	Why
General anesthesia	Interferes with the sympathetic nervous system, thus causing dilation
Brain injury	See "What is it?"
Decreased blood sugar	Brain does not function properly with low levels of glucose
Spinal anesthesia	May cause nerve damage
Spinal cord injury above the midthoracic region, usually T-5 or higher	See "What is it?"
Overdose on barbiturates	Causes damage to the brain

Source: Created by author from References #9 to #11.

SOMETHING ELSE YOU SHOULD KNOW . . . Neurogenic shock may be seen without a specific injury. If a client is experiencing severe pain, fright, or any excessive stimuli (shell or bomb shock), the nervous system may become overwhelmed. As a result, blood vessels dilate, heart rate slows, and BP falls. Next, the client will faint. If the head is placed lower than the rest of the body, this will usually relieve this type of shock.

Signs and symptoms and why

Table 7-12 lists signs and symptoms for neurogenic shock.

Table 7-12

Signs and symptoms	Why
Bradycardia	Sympathetic nervous system not functioning properly
Dry, warm skin	Vasodilation causes skin to be warm
Orthostatic hypotension	Vasodilation makes the vessels feel like they do not have enough volume (even though no volume has been lost). Less volume, less pressure
Fainting	When cardiac output decreases, not as much blood makes it to the brain
No sweating below the level of the injury	Sympathetic activity is blocked
Flaccid paralysis below level of injury	Blood vessel tone is lost below level of injury, causing general dilation of vessels
Poikilothermia	Body adopts the temperature of the local environment because the hypothalamus (major temperature regulator) does not function properly in an injured brain. Because of this, clients with spinal cord injuries have difficulty controlling and maintaining normal body temperatures
Priapism	Abnormal and prolonged erection of the penis; due to lesions in the central nervous system

Source: Created by author from References #9 to #11.

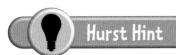

Hurst Hint

The signs and symptoms of neurogenic shock decrease when spinal cord edema lessens.

Quickie tests and treatments

Tests:

- Test for the underlying disorder.

Treatments:

- Secure airway: improves oxygenation.
- Protect the C-spine by positioning the client level; using a spine board: to prevent further damage.
- Oxygen by nonrebreather mask: to reoxygenate and reperfuse.
- Large-bore IV with normal saline at 1 to 2 L over 30 to 60 minutes: increases BP.
- Corticosteroids: decrease spinal cord edema.
- Vasopressors: improve perfusion and increase heart rate.
- Atropine: increases heart rate.
- Transcutaneous or transvenous pacing: controls bradycardia.

What can harm my client?

- Death.
- Fluid volume excess.
- Permanent spinal cord injury.
- Brain damage.

If I were your teacher, I would test you on . . .

- Causes and why.
- Signs and symptoms and why.
- Medication administration, monitoring, and side effects.
- Neurological assessment.
- Recognition and monitoring of fluid overload.
- Care of a trauma client.
- Care of the client with transcutaneous pacing.

ANOTHER SHOCK

The second major category of shock is cardiogenic. Let's take a brief anatomy and physiology lesson to further understand this type of shock. The heart is the pump for the body designed to maintain the flow of oxygenated blood first to itself, through the coronary arteries that branch right off the base of the aorta from the left heart, and then to all tissues of the body. The heart can do this job very effectively when there is an adequate blood volume, a strong and coordinated ventricular muscle, functional valves within the heart to keep blood moving forward, and a normal heart rate and rhythm. The size and tone of the vascular space—capillaries, veins, and arteries—provide the optimal pathway to get blood to the cells and back to the heart. Healthy tissues are able to take up the oxygen and nutrients from the blood for use at the cellular level. Blood pH within normal limits (7.35–7.45) also keeps the heart muscle happy. Now, keeping the heart happy is very important! "If Mama's not happy, ain't nobody happy!" Ever heard that truism? Well, if the heart is not happy—if it's damaged, suffering from a failing pump, has depressed myocardial fibers from acidosis, valves that leak, or experiences arrhythmias—nobody (meaning none of the other vital organs) is happy!

✚ Cardiogenic shock

What is it?

Cardiogenic shock, sometimes called pump failure, is a condition of diminished cardiac output that severely impairs tissue perfusion.

OTHER THINGS YOU SHOULD KNOW . . .   Cardiogenic shock can happen because of a damaged muscle, poor ventricular filling, or poor outflow from the heart.

- By the time you see your client's symptoms reflecting failing cardiac output (see previous hypovolemic shock symptoms), you can be sure that the body's compensating mechanisms have already failed. By this time, blood flow has already been diverted away from the organs with lesser needs for oxygen—skin, intestines—and diverted to vital organs—lungs, heart.

- As cardiogenic shock progresses, the vital organs begin to lose perfusion until the heart is no longer able to perfuse itself!

- The heart is not able to move blood forward at this point. The heart ordinarily likes to keep blood moving forward at all times. When more blood returns to the heart (increased preload) than the heart can effectively move forward, pressure builds up in the pulmonary circulation. The little capillary beds surrounding the alveoli get leaky, allowing fluid to pour into the interstitial space around the alveoli, and then fluid moves into the alveoli themselves, producing acute pulmonary edema.

- Cardiogenic shock following acute MI means that the heart is too damaged to effectively perfuse itself. When this happens, the heart cannot eject blood forward, and the ischemic heart muscle cannot continue to function effectively. In the presence of ischemia, the heart begins to beat erratically and cardiac output falls drastically.

What causes it and why

Table 7-13 summarizes the causes and associated reasons for cardiogenic shock.

Table 7-13

Cause	Why
Myocardial infarction	Damaged heart cannot eject blood and cardiac output drops suddenly. The systolic pressure falls as compensatory mechanisms fail, and because the heart operates under the "all or none law," the heart will do the best it can at any given moment under the existing circumstances, until finally the pump can no longer perfuse itself
Lethal ventricular arrhythmias	The patient in sustained ventricular tachycardia will rapidly become unstable. Systolic blood pressure (a direct measure of the cardiac output) will fall secondary to the rapid rate and reduced ventricular filling time. Ventricular tachycardia can progress to ventricular fibrillation at anytime due to myocardial hypoxia following acute MI[1]
End-stage congestive heart failure	Scarring of the myocardium from previous heart attacks, ventricular dilatation, and chronic myocardial ischemia lead to damage of the heart muscle. Any additional stressor can be the "straw that breaks the back" of the ailing pump! As a rule, scar tissue fills a hole left in the heart after leukocytes clear away the necrotic heart muscle following acute MI, but the scar tissue in the heart is not contractile tissue (it does not help pump, just goes along for the ride). Therefore, the wall motion of the heart muscle can become uncoordinated (the ventricular chambers are not pumping together in synchrony). The damaged pump cannot effectively pump blood forward, and pressure builds in pulmonary circuit as blood returning to the heart (preload) joins residual blood that has yet to leave the heart because the failing pump cannot overcome the arterial resistance (afterload) to keep blood moving forward

(Continued)

Table 7-13. (*Continued*)

Cause	Why
Cardiac tamponade (note that this is a heart problem, but is classified as obstructive shock because of how it obstructs circulation)	Myocardial infarction can cause necrosis all the way through the heart muscle (transmural). After the necrotic tissue is removed by leukocytosis, the ventricular wall becomes very thin and can blow out, allowing blood to accumulate in the pericardial sac compressing (squeezing) the heart so that it cannot adequately fill with blood and pump blood forward to perfuse vital organs. Endocarditis or myocarditis (inflammatory conditions) or nearby cancer cells can also cause stuff (exudates) to leak into the pericardial sac and compress the heart so it can't pump.[5] Fluid accumulates in space between the outside covering of the heart (the epicardium) and the myocardium (the muscle layer of the heart, called the pericardial sac). Tamponade means to apply external pressure to something, so when fluid builds up in the pericardial sac, it applies pressure on the heart, hindering incoming blood flow, so the heart cannot fill; therefore the cardiac output will drop dramatically, depending on how much fluid accumulates
Mediastinal shift	Note that this is a heart problem, but is classified in terms of what it does to the heart (obstructive shock) rather than where the problem originated. This shift will occur as pressure builds up in the pericardial sac and displaces the heart. For example, when a patient pulls a knife out of his right chest wall, the sucking chest wound collapses the right lung and the pressure displaces the heart to the left. The heart can't pump very well from under the left armpit!

Source: Created by author from References #1 and #5.

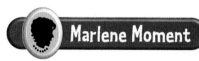

Signs and symptoms and why

Table 7-14 lists signs and symptoms of cardiogenic shock.

Table 7-14

Signs and symptoms	Why
Tachycardia	The heart beats faster due to sympathetic stimulation causing the heart muscle to require additional oxygen when the supply may already be compromised by infarction and necrosis in the muscle. The coronary vessels are perfused during diastole, and since diastole is shortened with tachycardia, there is decreased coronary artery perfusion as well as blood flow through the collateral vessels in the muscle wall[6]
Hypotension	Systolic pressure falls because the damaged heart muscle cannot effectively eject blood from its chambers
Cool, ashen skin	Vasoconstriction secondary to sympathetic stimulation brings less blood flow (warmth and color) to the skin
Diaphoresis	Sympathetic stimulation activates the sweat glands[8]
Cyanosis of lips and nail beds	Stagnation of blood in the capillary bed after available oxygen has been extracted

Source: Created by author from References #6 and #8.

Marlene Moment

When the client enters the ED with a machete sticking out of his side, do not pull out the penetrating object. Just tell the client to take two seats since that machete takes up so much room. NOT! Get him to the back at once!

Quickie tests and treatments

Tests:

- Serum enzymes: elevated creatinine kinase, lactate dehydrogenase indicating MI, ischemia, heart failure, or shock
- ABGs: metabolic and respiratory acidosis and hypoxia.
- Cardiac catheterization and echocardiography: reveal other conditions that can lead to pump dysfunction and failure like cardiac tamponade, pulmonary emboli, and hypovolemia.
- Electrocardiography: acute MI, ischemia, or ventricular aneurysm.
- Pulmonary artery pressure monitoring: increased PAWP shows ineffective ventricular pumping and peripheral vascular resistance.
- Invasive arterial pressure monitoring: systolic arterial pressure less than 80 mm Hg caused by impaired ventricular ejection.

Treatments:

- Maintenance of patent airway; preparation for intubation and mechanical ventilation: prevent or manage respiratory distress.
- Supplemental oxygen: to increase oxygenation.
- IV fluids, crystalloids, colloids, or blood products: to maintain vascular volume.
- Vasopressors: reduce left ventricle workload.
- Inotropics: increase heart contractility and cardiac output.
- Intra-aortic balloon pump (IABP) therapy: reduces left-ventricle workload by decreasing systemic vascular resistance.
- Coronary artery revascularization: restores coronary artery blood flow if cardiogenic shock is due to MI.
- Emergency surgery: to repair papillary muscle rupture or ventricular septal defect if either is cause of cardiogenic shock.
- Ventricular assist device: assists pumping action of heart when IABP and drug therapy fail.

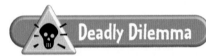

Deadly Dilemma

To combat shock, you must quickly and efficiently increase the oxygen supply and decrease the oxygen demand while reducing the workload on the heart.

What can harm my client?

- Multisystem organ failure.
- Death.

If I were your teacher, I would test you on . . .

- Causes and why.
- Signs and symptoms and why.
- Medication administration, monitoring, and side effects.
- Administration and monitoring of fluids and blood products.
- Priority nursing interventions to reduce workload on the heart and improve circulation.
- Proper assessment.
- Nursing steps to prepare the client for invasive and surgical procedures.

SUMMARY

This review of the pathophysiology of shock states will improve your nursing skills and care. You can now face your clients with confidence because of your ability to understand the causes, signs and symptoms, and WHY of shock states. You have also gained a better understanding of diagnostic tests, treatments, and possible client complications to monitor—each of these skills will lead to improved patient care and safety.

PRACTICE QUESTIONS

1. Which patient would the nurse monitor most closely for the development of hypovolemic shock?

   1. Adult male who has acute myocardial infarcton.

   2. A middle-aged patient in acute addisonian crisis.

   3. Elderly female following insertion of a central line.

   4. A young adult male who has a pulmonary embolism.

Correct answer: 2. The client in addisonian crisis has a deficit of aldosterone and is at risk for hypovolemia because sodium and water losses result in decreased circulatory volume. The acute MI patient (1) is prone to develop cardiogenic shock. The patient who had a central line inserted (3) could have the right atrium nicked, causing iatrogenic cardiac tamponade (circulatory shock, but obstructive type), and the young man (4) with the PE is at risk for obstruction to outflow from the heart (also obstructive type).

2. Which intervention would the nurse predict to be of least benefit for hypotension when the patient is in cardiogenic shock following acute myocardial infarction?

   1. Prompt, aggressive thrombolysis.

   2. Vasopressor agents (catecholamines).

   3. Vasodilating agents (such as the nitrates).

   4. Plasma volume replacement therapy.

Correct answer: 4. The hypotension accompanying acute MI is unrelated to a deficit of circulating volume. Replacing plasma volume is not indicated and will be harmful in that the increased preload would place more workload on to an already failing heart. For that reason vasopressor agents (3) are used cautiously to raise systolic blood pressure while carefully monitoring the effect of increased afterload. Options 1 and 2 are both indicated as standard treatment modalities to restore and maintain perfusion to the myocardium to improve contractility.

3. When assessing shock states, which type of shock would the nurse recognize as being different from all other classic presentations of shock?

   1. Burn shock.

   2. Septic shock.

   3. Hemorrhagic shock.

   4. Cardiogenic shock.

   Correct answer: 2. Septic shock is a form of distributive shock triggered by systemic inflammatory mediators which causes the person to be hypotensive due to vasodilation giving rise to warm flushed skin, rather than the classic presentation of cold and clammy skin as seen with vasoconstriction, the sympathetic response to (1) burn shock, (3) hemorrhagic shock, and (4) cardiogenic shock.

4. Following spinal anesthesia, a hypotensive mother and unborn baby are at risk for effects of distributive shock due to loss of sympathetic vasomotor tone. Which immediate nursing intervention is priority upon recognition of this shock state?

   1. Place the woman in a Trendelenburg position.

   2. Administer an IVF bolus of isotonic solution.

   3. Rotate tourniquets on both lower extremities.

   4. Lower the head of the bed and apply oxygen at 2 L/min.

   Correct answer: 2. When the vascular space is unusually large (due to vasodilation) administering the fluid bolus will add volume to improve cardiac output and raise the blood pressure to better perfuse the placenta and save the unborn baby from hypoxemia. Option 1 would further compromise fetal oxygenation by reducing chest expansion of the woman with pressure of a gravid (35-lb) uterus on the maternal diaphragm and forcing blood flow away from the uterus by gravity. Option 3 would also aggravate the problem by trapping maternal venous blood, keeping it out in the periphery and away from central circulation. Both legs could be raised and drained into central circulation for the effect of a physiological fluid bolus. Lowering the head of the bed (option 4) and option 1 could have the very dangerous effect of allowing the spinal anesthetic to migrate farther up the spinal canal and paralyze the woman's diaphragm. Oxygen at 2/L minute is ineffective for an obstetric emergency which requires 100% oxygen by tight-fitting face mask to salvage a fetus in distress.

5. Following the insertion of a central line, the nurse notes that the patient's CVP is elevated, yet the systolic blood pressure is steadily decreasing. Which first intervention is indicated?

   1. Notify the physician.

   2. Lower the head of the bed.

   3. Apply oxygen per nasal cannula.

   4. Hang the patient's legs in a dependent position.

Correct answer: 3. Iatrogenic cardiac tamponade should be suspected as a common site of bleeding in the right atrium after insertion of a central line. Oxygen is indicated when cardiac output is decreasing due to cardiac compression. Option 1, notifying the physician, is indicated after the immediate intervention of applying oxygen. (Rule: if there is something you can do first to help reduce a complication, do it!). Options 2 and 3: shifts in position to trap blood in the periphery or to get more blood to the brain do nothing to improve cardiac output or tissue oxygenation.

6. A post-MI patient shows signs and symptoms of early cardiogenic shock. Which nursing intervention takes priority?

   1. Administer oxygen per nasal cannula.

   2. Replace damp, diaphoretic gown and linens.

   3. Administer prescribed sedation for restlessness.

   4. Set up the intra-aortic balloon pump for immediate usage.

   Correct answer: 1. Administer oxygen. Maintaining a patent airway is priority. Option 2 is delaying treatment. Damp clothing never killed anybody! Option 3, administering sedation, even further depresses the central nervous system that is already depressed due to lack of oxygen. Option 4 is a bit premature for EARLY shock, which, if treated promptly, and aggressively may be reversed to restore effective circulation.

7. An unresponsive patient arrives in the ER wearing a medic-alert bracelet stating severe peanut allergy. Respiratory arrest and collapse occurred after ingestion of a chocolate candy-topped ice-cream dessert. Which immediate intervention is priority?

   1. Prepare to assist with endotracheal intubation.

   2. Administer 100% oxygen per nonrebreather face mask.

   3. Administer epinephrine and antihistamines as prescribed.

   4. Open additional IV access for a hypotonic IV fluid bolus.

   Correct answer: 3. Epinephrine and antihistamines are the only options to relieve the bronchospasm in anaphylactic shock. Other options for supplying oxygen may be ineffective due to closure of the airways. Fluid bolus (option 4) with a hydrating solution does not solve an oxygen problem.

8. An infant is delivered and with the birth cry develops cyanosis and marked dyspnea. Which nursing assessment would confirm obstructive shock?

   1. Concave abdomen.

   2. Mottled, splotchy extremities.

   3. High systolic blood pressure.

   4. High-pitched crowing sounds with respirations.

Correct answer: 1. Abdominal organs sucked upward into the thoracic cavity result in the concave appearance of the abdomen. Option 2: acrocyanosis is normal in the newborn. Option 3: systolic blood pressure will be low rather than high because the cardiac output falls when the heart is being compressed by crowding with abdominal organs. Option 4: high-pitched crowing is associated with bronchospasm. Ventilatory efforts will be shallow due to lack of room for lung expansion.

9. When the patient is in shock, which clinical parameter is used initially to evaluate the effectiveness of treatment?

   1. Urinary output.

   2. Pulse pressure.

   3. Systolic blood pressure.

   4. Skin color and temperature.

   Correct answer: 3. Blood pressure is the best evaluator of effectiveness of treatment. Option 1: urinary output may be compromised due to lack of renal perfusion. If acute renal failure has occurred, the urinary output cannot increase if the kidneys are not functioning. Option 2: pulse pressure normalizes only after systolic blood pressure begins to rise. Option 4: skin has a very low demand for oxygen during shock, and will perfuse only after all vital organs receive adequate circulation.

10. Which patient could the registered nurse safely assign to a licensed practical nurse?

    1. An elderly patient with diabetic ketoacidosis.

    2. An infant during the first 24 hours post major burn.

    3. A young adult who has hematuria from a kidney stone.

    4. A middle-aged woman with polyuria following sinus surgery.

    Correct answer: 3. A young adult who has hematuria from a kidney stone is stable in relation to the other clients. All other options involve patients who are unstable because of age extremes and/or fluid loss increasing the risk for the development of shock.

References

1. Corwin EJ. *Handbook of Pathophysiology*. 2nd ed. Philadelphia: Lippincott Williams & Wilkins; 2000:406–407.

2. Gutierrez KJ, Peterson PG. *Real World Nursing Survival Guide: Pathophysiology*. Philadelphia: Saunders; 2002:1–13.

3. Hogan MA, Hill K. *Pathophysiology: Reviews & Rationales*. Upper Saddle River, NJ: Prentice Hall Nursing; 2004:521–536.

4. Huether SE, McCance KL. *Understanding Pathophysiology*. 3rd ed. St. Louis: Mosby; 2004:689–700.

5. *Pathophysiology: A 2-in-1 Reference for Nurses*. Philadelphia: Lippincott Williams & Wilkins; 2005:139–156.

6. *Straight A's in Pathophysiology*. Philadelphia: Lippincott Williams & Wilkins; 2005:225–248.

7. *Expert LPN Guidelines: Pathophysiology*. Philadelphia: Lippincott Williams & Wilkins; 2007:236–241.

8. Porth CM. *Pathophysiology: Concepts of Altered Health States*. 6th ed. Philadelphia: Lippincott Williams & Wilkins; 2002:560–568.

9. Porth CM. *Essentials of Pathophysiology: Concepts of Altered Health States*. 2nd ed. Philadelphia: Lippincott Williams & Wilkins; 2007:430–437.

10. Beers MH. *Merck Manual of Medical Information*. 2nd home ed. Whitehouse Station, NJ: Merck; 2003:148–149;1118–1120.

11. Merkle CJ. *Handbook of Pathophysiology*. 2nd ed. Philadelphia: Lippincott Williams & Wilkins; 2005:315–347.

12. Torpy JM. New threats and old enemies: challenges for critical care medicine. *JAMA*. 2002; 287:1513–1515.

Bibliography

Hurst Review Services. www.hurstreview.com.

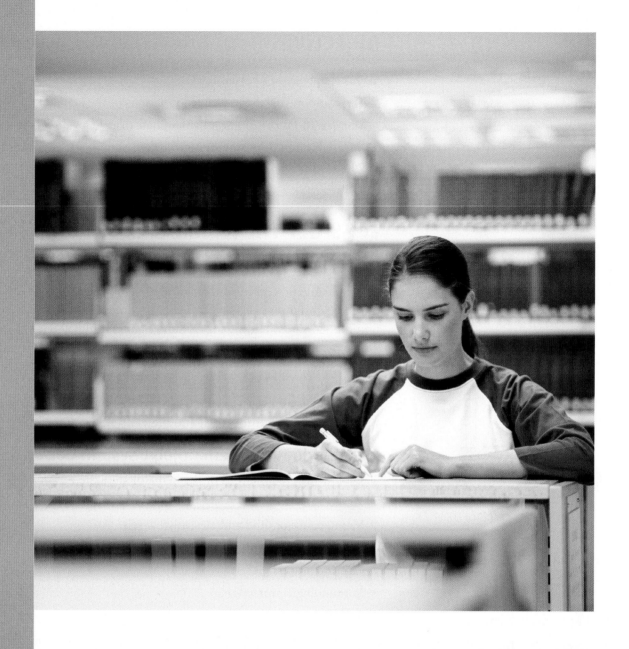

CHAPTER

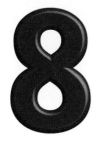 Hematology

OBJECTIVES

In this chapter, you'll review:

* The components and associated functions of the hematologic system.
* Manifestations of common hematologic disease processes.
* Information to help provide appropriate care for patients with hematologic disorders including diagnostic tests, treatments, and common complications.

LET'S GET THE NORMAL STUFF STRAIGHT FIRST

The hematologic system consists of plasma, proteins, cells, and a variety of other substances necessary to maintain homeostasis. Plasma is the liquid portion containing all substances, including clotting factors. Other materials found in plasma, which acts as a transport medium, include albumin, antibodies, hormones, carbon dioxide, electrolytes, oxygen, glucose, fats, amino acids, urea, creatine, and uric acid. The cellular portion of plasma consists of white blood cells (leukocytes), red blood cells (erythrocytes), and platelets (thrombocytes).

✚ What does the hematologic system do?

The following are functions of the hematologic system:

* Maintenance of pH.
* Maintenance of fluid and electrolyte levels.
* Temperature regulation.
* Clotting process.
* Immunologic protection.
* Transport of oxygen, other nutrients (glucose), and hormones.
* Waste removal (carbon dioxide and other waste products).

✚ What are the roles of the cellular portions?

Table 8-1 and Figure 8-1 provide an explanation of the cells carried in the blood including their functions and pertinent information.

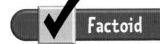

Factoid

Arterial blood has a pH of about 7.4, with a range of 7.35 to 7.45. Venous ranges are somewhat lower, at about 7.31 to 7.41. Maintenance of this range must occur in order for the body to preserve homeostasis.

Table 8-1

Cell	Normal limits (will vary slightly between laboratories)	Life span	Function
Red blood cells (erythrocytes)	About 5 million	120 days	Carry oxygen on hemoglobin molecule; definition of blood types
White blood cells (leukocytes)	About 4,500 to 10,000	Varies from hours to many months depending on type of leukocyte	Fight infection and allergic response
Platelets (thrombocytes)	Between 150,000 and 450,000	Approximately 10 days	Clotting

Source: Created by author from References #2, #3, #4, #6, and #7.

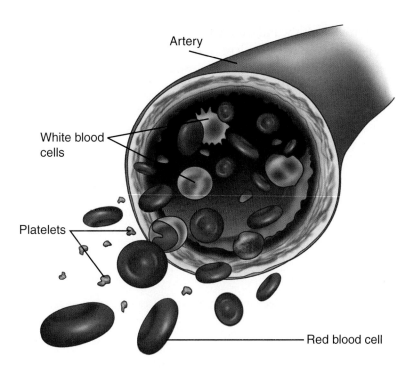

Artery

White blood cells

Platelets

Red blood cell

- Individuals who live at high altitudes have an increased number of erythrocytes to assist in carrying oxygen, since the air is thinner at high altitudes, thus making it more difficult to breathe.

- A white blood cell count under 500 is a serious problem. This is a setup for a patient to acquire an infection that she cannot fight due to a lack of WBC's. Levels over 30,000 can indicate disease processes such as leukemia or serious infectious processes.[7]

✚ What is a "differential count?"

White blood cells (leukocytes) are comprised of 5 different types of cells (Table 8-2). These cells are counted individually and recorded as percentages, which should total 100%. This is what we call the differential count. Each of these cells has separate duties. An increased number of bands or "stabs" on the differential count indicates an acute infection. Bands are immature neutrophils. "Segs," also known as polymorpho-nuclear neutrophil leukocytes, are the mature neutrophils.

When you look at the CBC, here are some things you need to be aware of (in terms of infectious processes)

- Look at your total WBC. Up or down? The total WBC rises with bacterial infection or viruses. However, the total can also drop if it is viral.

- Look at the lymphocyte count next. It usually rises in viral infections.

- Next, look at your neutrophil count. It is important to know that the neutrophil count may be listed as "segs", "bands" etc. If the neutrophil count is elevated, think "bacteria". Why? Because that is what they are responsible for.

- Next look to see if the "bands" are elevated. If so, you have got a serious infection going on. Why? Because remember, the "bands" are immature

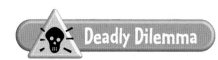

Deadly Dilemma

Patients who have neutropenia (decreased neutrophils) must be guarded closely against infection. Neutropenia may occur from radiation, chemotherapy, other drugs, infectious processes, and neoplasms. ***A neutropenic patient with a fever is a medical emergency.***[8]

neutrophils. If the infection is bad enough, the immune system is sending out the kids to fight. The "bands" SHOULD NOT be elevated with nonlifethreatening infections. This indicates overwhelming infection! This is called a LEFT SHIFT.

- Monocytes can rise with either type of infection but are not as important DIAGNOSTICALLY. Know that they will classically rise in mono and early on in the "flu".
- We won't talk about eosinophils or basophils here as they are not really significant in a basic assessment of CBC with respect to infections.

Please remember that interpreting a CBC requires an experienced health care provider. These are only the basics that you need to know.

Table 8-2

	Neutrophils	Eosinophils	Basophils	Monocytes	Lymphocytes
Functions	Biggest source of defense against bacteria	Respond to allergic reactions to fight inflammatory responses. Fight parasitic infections	Release heparin, histamine, bradykinin. Work to remove fat after eating high-fat meal	Remove debris, bacteria/viruses via macrophages. Important in chronic infections	Formation of antibodies. Immunity production. Have both B-cell and T-cell lymphocytes. Increase with viral illnesses
Normal Differential Count	50–70%	1–3%	0.4–1%	4–6%	25–35%

Source: Created by author from References #3, #4, and #7.

LET'S GET DOWN TO SPECIFICS

Let's get down to specific illnesses that may occur when the hematologic system malfunctions.

✚ Anemia

Anemia is one of the more common blood disorders and occurs in many forms.[1] Anemia occurs when there is a deficiency in the number of red blood cells or in the ability of the cells to actually carry oxygen. The end product of anemia is hypoxia because of the deprivation of oxygen. General causes include:

- Actual blood loss.
- Destruction of red blood cells.
- Manufacture of damaged red blood cells.

Table 8-3 lists common types of anemia and related information. Sickle cell anemia will be discussed separately.

Table 8-3

Type of anemia	Causes and why	Signs and symptoms and why	Effect on lab values	Quickie tests and treatment	What will harm my client?	If I were your teacher, I would test you on . . .
Vitamin B$_{12}$ Deficiency Anemia (same as pernicious must have vitamin B$_{12}$ to produce RBCs anemia)	• Lack of vitamin B$_{12}$ in the body due to decreased intake of foods from animals; especially seen in vegetarians who do not use dairy products or eat meat • Clients who have had gastric or ileal surgeries, which lead to malabsorbtion, e.g., partial gastrectomy (without B$_{12}$ you can't make proper RBCs). After gastrectomy not enough HCL in stomach + decreased intrinsic factor → without intrinsic factor, can't absorb oral B$_{12}$ in the stomach → can't make good red blood cells • Malabsorption diseases • There may be a genetic predisposition • Seems to be related to thyroid diseases • Age (the older you get, the less vitamin B$_{12}$ foods you take in) • The use of agents that block acid in the stomach has also been implicated. Lack of vitamin B$_{12}$ causes difficulties with cell division and the maturation process within the nucleus of the cell • Certain drugs and radiation can cause a decrease in vitamin B$_{12}$ absorption	• Weakness (when RBCs are decreased, tissue becomes hypoxic, so client feels weak) • Sore tongue (papillae of the tongue atrophy with decreased B$_{12}$; as tongue becomes inflamed, it becomes hard to eat, which decreases intake of B$_{12}$ even more • Numbness/tingling (paresthesia) in extremities, poor position sense (proprioception), poor coordination, positive Romberg and possibly a positive Babinski (without myelin nerves have impaired, impulse transmission). B$_{12}$ is needed for nerves to work correctly. It is also needed for myelin production • Pallor (due to hypoxia) • Jaundice of sclera (RBCs breaking down, releasing bilirubin)	• Serum vitamin B$_{12}$ level decreased (<0.1 μg/mL) • Schilling test (this is THE test for this type of anemia) • Low hemoglobin • Low hematocrit • Low RBC count • Bone marrow has increased megaloblasts; few normal RBCs • Gastric analysis (decreased or absent HCL)	• Increase intake of vitamin B$_{12}$ • Vitamin B$_{12}$ injections (given weekly at first for one month, then monthly for the remainder of life) • Iron replacement, folic acid replacement (both of these increase RBC quality and production) • Bed rest due to hypoxia • Blood transfusions depending on how low the hemoglobin is • If client is in heart failure, this will need to be treated as well	• Possible permanent CNS problems • Heart failure • Stomach cancer (without adequate HCL in stomach, bacteria can grow and normal cell division is affected)	• Pathophysiology • Causes and why • Signs and symptoms and why • Lab work changes • Proper dosing and administration of IM B$_{12}$ • How the Schilling test works • How heart failure is treated • Why the patient could get stomach cancer • Nursing interventions for clients receiving PO iron and folic acid • Administration of blood products

(Continued)

Table 8-3. (*Continued*)

Type of anemia	Causes and why	Signs and symptoms and why	Effect on lab values	Quickie tests and treatment	What will harm my client?	If I were your teacher, I would test you on . . .
		• Numerous GI complaints (mucous membranes of stomach shrink; decreased HCL production)				• Rule: Vitamin B_{12} deficiency—think nerve damage
		• Double (diplopia) or blurred vision (optic nerve shrinks)				
		• Hearing problems (otic nerve shrinks)				
		• ↓ taste				
		• Impotency (nerve damage)				
		• Incontineuce				
		• CNS changes (e.g., decreased memory, mood changes, due to nerve damage)				
		• Headache (brain needs oxygen; CO_2 could be building up)				
		• Irritability (brain needs oxygen)				
		• Cardiovascular changes (shortness of breath, increased pulse, arrhythmias, heart failure); heart is pumping harder to compensate for decreased oxygen in the body				

Folic Acid Deficiency Anemia

- A slow-developing disease; a megaloblastic anemia
- Patho in a nutshell: you must have folic acid to produce good RBCs
- Folic acid is a necessary component of DNA production and the development of red blood cells. The lack of folic acid causes a decrease in cell maturity and makes cell division difficult, resulting in decreased red blood cells
- Most people get plenty of folic acid in their regular diet

- Folic acid deficiency is caused by a lack of the vitamin folate. Ways this can occur are:
- Decreased dietary intake
- Malabsorption (may be due to intestinal disorder, e.g., Crohn's disease or from bowel surgery)
- Cooking food too much (heat destroys folic acid)
- Long-term drug therapy (e.g., antiseizure meds, hormones and methotrexate—decrease absorption of folic acid; also can prevent folic acid from being converted to its active form)
- Increased need in pregnancy (baby is growing rapidly)
- Drinking cow's milk (if it's straight from the cow, it's deficit in folate)
- Malnutrition as seen with alcoholics, geriatric population, and young women
- Tumors which battle for the use of the folic acid
- Drugs that interfere with folic acid absorption, e.g., methotrexate (Trexall), phenytion (Dilantin), phenobarbital (Luminal), triamterene (Dyrenium)
- Rapid growth during infancy, especially now that premature infants are surviving more

- Signs and symptoms are the same as with iron deficient anemia and folic acid deficient anemia
- However, there are no neurological symptoms with this type of anemia as the nerves are not affected

- Serum folic acid (folate) levels will be <4 mg/L
- Serum vitamin B_{12} levels decrease. The Schilling test will be done to make sure the client does not have vitamin B_{12} deficient anemia
- Macrocytosis with normal hemoglobin
- Decreased reticulocyte count
- Abnormal platelets
- Increased mean corpuscular volume

Marlene Moment

Stop milking your own cow and buy milk that has folate already in it. Why? It's very difficult to get the cow to take the folate due to GI upset. That's a joke!

- Supplementation of folic acid either oral or parenteral (oral give 400 μg per day)
- Provide diet rich in folic acid and vitamin B_{12}
- Identify the cause and treat
- Well-balanced diet
- Anyone planning to become pregnant should start taking a folic acid supplement at least 3 months prior to conception (400 mg per day)
- The FDA requires folate to be added to cereal products
- In severe disease, blood transfusions may be needed
- May try a round of vitamin B_{12} injections to see if client improves

- Maternal folic acid deficits are associated with neural tube defects in infants
- In adults folic acid deficit is associated with cardiovascular disease

- Pathophysiology
- Causes and why
- Signs and symptoms and why
- How the lab work will be affected
- Foods high in folic acid (green leafy vegetables, liver, citrus fruits, nuts and dried beans, broccoli, mushrooms, oatmeal, peanut butter, wheat germ, whole grain breads, bananas, and eggs)
- Identifying high-risk populations
- Performing a nutritional assessment

(continued)

Table 8-3. (Continued)

Type of anemia	Causes and why	Signs and symptoms and why	Effect on lab values	Quickie tests and treatment	What will harm my client?	If I were your teacher, I would test you on . . .
	• The RBCs produced in this condition are megaloblastic and have a very short lifespan • Folate = folic acid • Most folic acid is absorbed in the intestine • Pregnancy increases the need for folic acid by 5–10 times the norm			• Frequent rest periods • Teach client to report signs of hypoxia (shortness of breath, chest pain, or dizziness) • Explain importance of using commercial baby formulas • Explain to the client to keep taking supplements even when they begin to feel better • Avoid alcohol, nonherbal teas, and antacids, as these can impair vitamin B_{12} and iron absorption		

260

Aplastic Anemia

- Also called hypoplastic anemia
- Patho in a nutshell:
- There has been an injury to stem cells, causing a decrease in all blood elements (pancytopenia); erythrocytes, leukocytes, and thrombocytes may all be depressed
- Sometimes called bone marrow failure
- Can come on slowly or all of a sudden or at any age

- Suppression of bone marrow caused by radiation therapy, chemotherapy
- Drugs or chemicals, e.g., benzene, chloramphenicol (Chloromycetin); can occur one week after a drug is started
- Half of these anemias occur from drugs
- Infectious processes such as with viruses (e.g., hepatitis)
- Cancerous infiltration of bone marrow
- May be born with it
- Often the cause is unknown

- Weakness, fatigue, pallor (because of anemia)
- Petechiae and bruises (decreased platelets)
- Frequent infections (decreased neutrophils or leukocytes)
- Bleeding from GI tract, gums, nose, or vagina (decreased platelets)
- General signs of anemia: fever, infections, bleeding, heart failure

- Bone marrow biopsy shows pancytopenia
- Also may show a dry "tap" (no cells)
- Decreased platelets
- Decreased neutrophils
- Decreased lymphocytes
- Prolonged bleeding times
- Low reticulocyte count
- Large RBCs (macrocytic)
- Increased megakaryocytes (platelet precursors)

- Bone marrow or stem cell transplant
- Immunosuppressive therapy with lymphocyte immune globulin
- Red cell transfusions for anemia
- Platelet transfusions if needed
- Steroids to suppress the immune system's response to stem cell injury (which decreases all blood elements)
- Immunosupresive drugs such as chemotherapy drugs (cyclophosphamide, ocytoxin)
- Oxygen therapy if needed
- Splenectomy: suppresses immune response

- If due to a drug reaction, can be fatal as many times it is irreversible
- If client has bone marrow or stem cell transplant, may develop graft-versus-host disease, rejection, and infections
- Bleeding, infection, heart failure; most common complication is hemorrhage from mucous membranes

- Pathophysiology
- Causes and why
- Sign and symptoms and why
- Significance of lab work
- Care of a client undergoing a stem cell transplant
- Care of a client undergoing dialysis
- Care of a client undergoing a splenectomy
- Lab work
- The importance of preventing infection
- Importance of avoiding communicable diseases
- Bleeding precautions if client has low platelets
- Safety precautions to prevent falls and trauma (will bleed)
- Proper nutrition to fight infection
- Signs and symptoms of hemorrhage
- Importance of reporting infection immediately
- Administering blood and watching for reactions

(Continued)

Table 8-3. (*Continued*)

Type of anemia	Causes and why	Signs and symptoms and why	Effect on lab values	Quickie tests and treatment	What will harm my client?	If I were your teacher, I would test you on . . .
						• Teach parents to keep hazardous chemicals out of reach of children • Teach people working around radiation to take proper precautions and to wear a radiation detecting badge

Marlene Moment

Heinz bodies are not produced by the same company that makes Heinz Ketchup. Also, cats that eat onions will develop Heinz bodies. Weird, huh?

Type of anemia	Causes and why	Signs and symptoms and why	Effect on lab values	Quickie tests and treatment	What will harm my client?	If I were your teacher, I would test you on . . .
Glucose-6-Phosphate Deydrogenase Deficiency Anemia • Patho in a nutshell: • A sex-linked enzyme defect; the enzyme affected is G6PD • Specifically, it is decreased. This deficit causes a breakdown of RBCs when the client is exposed to various	• Hemolytic anemia that occurs when clients with the genetic predisposition respond to certain drugs, foods, or illnesses (i.e., infectious processes or diabetic ketoacidosis). Some of the drugs include antimalaria agents, NSAIDs, Primaquine phosphate, sulfonamides, nitrofurantoin (Furadantin), glibenclamide (Glyburide), salicylates, thiazide diuretics, quinine derivatives. Also fava beans and mothballs have been known to bring on an attack. These triggers cause oxidation to occur, resulting in damaged red blood cells • Other things that can cause a state of oxidative stress in the body are severe infections and certain foods. Any oxidative state in the body	• Many people never experience any signs or symptoms • No symptoms until client exposed to certain agents or until client develops a severe infection • Acute phase: anemia, jaundice (metabolism of HgB) • Paleness (anemia) • Jaundice (when RBCs break down, they release bilirubin which discolors the skin) • Weakness, dizziness, confusion, intolerance to physical activity, increased pulse (anemia)	• "Heinz bodies" present (appear as small round inclusions in the red cells; formed by damage to hemoglobin molecules through oxidations; also known as aggregates of protein seen in RBCs) • Liver enzymes (to rule out other causes of jaundice) • Coombs test (should be negative) • Thyroid-stimulating	• Treat the cause • Avoidance of triggers • Vaccinations (e.g., hepatitis A) to prevent potential illness • Blood transfusions • Dialysis (if kidneys are failing) • Splenectomy (to stop spleen from filtering out all RBCs) • Steroids to promote erythropoiesis: high doses of androgens increase erythropoietin production	• Rarely renal failure or death can occur after a severe hemolytic crisis metabolized hemoglobin is excreted by kidneys	• Pathophysiology • Causes and why • Signs and symptoms and why • Teach client to avoid situations or chemicals that can trigger the problem (e.g., fever, aspirin, vitamin K, fava beans, mothballs, diabetic ketoacidosis) • Usual signs and symptoms of anemia • Lab tests • Nursing care of client receiving an osmotic diuretic • Use of a bili light in a neonate

- triggers (infections, drugs)
- Mainly seen in African or Mediterranean races
- Mainly seen in males as it is transmitted X-linked trait (inherited deficiency on the X chromosome)
- Can cause a mild case in women
- G6PD is an enzyme that protects RBCs from toxic chemicals. Without this enzyme, red blood cells are likely to break down
- Is a hemolytic anemia
- G6PD deficiency is the most common enzyme deficiency in the world.

- damages enzymes, proteins (hemoglobin), and can cause electrolyte imbalances. This oxidative state also causes splenic sequestration of RBCs (makes the spleen want to filter out bad cells)
- Henna has been known to cause a hemolytic crisis in G6PD deficient infants

- Enlarged spleen (spleen is trying to filter out broken down RBCs)
- Enlarged liver due to infection
- Prolonged neonatal icterus (jaundice; RBCs are breaking down, releasing bilirubin)

- hormone (TSH) to increase enzyme production
- DNA testing for the gene or sequencing of the G6PD gene
- Beutler fluorescent spot test (a direct test for G6PD); can only be done several weeks after a hemolytic episode because it can give a false-positive result during active hemolysis
- Bite cells (this is when a macrophage in the spleen spots an RBC with a Heinz body; the macrophage removes a small piece of the membrane of the cell, leading to the characteristic "bite cells" . . . the macrophage took a bite out of the cell
- Abdominal pain (enlarged spleen and liver)
- Back pain (kidney involvement)

- Avoid drugs that trigger the problem
- Everyone should be screened for this deficiency prior to giving blood; can cause problems for recipient
- Hydrate during episodes of hemolysis (trying to prevent kidneys from getting clogged up from broken-down cells, as this can lead to acute tubular necrosis . . . renal failure)
- Osmotic diuretics (mannitol) to flush out kidneys; this will remove fragments of broken-down cells in kidneys which can lead to renal failure
- Can be diagnosed with a simple blood test
- Can measure G6PD enzyme activity between episodes
- Measure bilirubin during an episode

- Signs and symptoms of renal failure
- Administration of blood
- Care of the client undergoing spleen removal
- Side effects of steroids

(Continued)

Table 8-3. (*Continued*)

Type of anemia	Signs and symptoms and why	Causes and why	Effect on lab values	Quickie tests and treatment	What will harm my client?	If I were your teacher, I would test you on . . .
The major problem this deficiency causes is hemolytic anemia • G6PD is a major cause of mild to severe jaundice in newborns			• Decreased red blood cell count and hemoglobin (RBCs are breaking down) • Increased bilirubin (due to RBC breakdown; bilirubin is released into the bloodstream) • In severe and chronic forms or G6PD deficiency, clients can have gallstones or cataracts (etiology unknown) • Dark urine (bilirubin discoloring urine) • Elevated absolute reticulocyte count (reticulocytes are baby RBCs, which are forming to try and correct the anemia)	• The client will recover in about 8 days (prognosis is excellent) • Treating elevated bilirubin in newborns by exposing them to bright light has decreased the need for neonatal transfusions • Newborns likely to have G6PD deficiency need to be screened to make sure they won't be subjected to any triggers • Pregnant clients who live in areas where G6PD deficiency is high should avoid eating fava beans • Alternative treatments: vitamin E and folic acid (antioxidants); decrease hemolysis • Genetic counseling		

Marlene Moment

Fava beans go great with a nice glass of Chianti! (I wish I could make that sound that Hannibal Lecter made in the movie for you right now . . . .)

Iron Deficiency Anemia

- Patho in a nutshell:
- Deficiency of iron in the body. Without iron, proper RBCs cannot form. Without red blood cells, oxygen cannot be carried throughout the body
- Iron is necessary for the production of red blood cells and hemoglobin synthesis. Iron is released from old erythrocyte breakdown and can be used again, but some iron is always lost and must be replaced

- Causes of decreased iron:
- Low dietary intake (less than 1 mg per day). Examples: long-term breast feeding where iron has not been supplemented, bottle feeding in infants under stress from disease, any pediatric client experiencing rapid growth (need more iron)
- Lack of absorption. Examples: severe diarrhea (losing iron), partial or total gastrectomy no stomach . . . decreased iron absorption), celiac disease, pernicious anemia (decreased vitamin B_{12} absorption)
- Actual blood loss. Examples: anticoagulants, aspirin, steroids (can make you bleed)
- GI bleeding is the major cause of iron deficient anemia in males
- Heavy periods is the main cause of iron deficient anemia in females
- Hemorrhage or trauma
- Cancer (tumor can invade organs and make you bleed)
- Diseases that cause RBC breakdown
- An artificial heart valve or vena cava filter can cause RBC destruction as well

- Fatigue (decreased oxygen makes you tired)
- Weakness (decreased oxygen makes you tired)
- Tachycardia (heart rate increased to pump what few red blood cells are left around the body in an effort to help with oxygenation)
- Palpitations (heart needs oxygen too)
- Dyspnea (no oxygen)
- Orthopnea (no oxygen)
- Heart failure (the heart is working hard to pump oxygen, so it will eventually hypertrophy and fail if this goes uncontrolled)
- Pallor (poor oxygenation)
- Brittle, spoon-shaped nails (koilonychia; poor capillary circulation)
- Headache (lack of oxygen)
- Irritability (your brain needs oxygen)
- Forgetfulness (your brain needs oxygen)

- Serum iron (will be low)
- Serum ferritin (will be low)
- Visualization of irregular shape and size of red blood cells
- Hemoglobin level (in males it will be less than 12 g/dL; in females it will be less than 10 g/dL
- Hematocrit (in males it will be less than 47%; in females it will be less than 42%)
- RBC count (will be low)
- Red cells will be microcytic (small) and hypochromic (pale)
- Decreased mean corpuscular volume (measures size); cells will be small
- Mean corpuscular hemoglobin (decreased); this determines how much hemoglobin is present

- Stop blood loss
- Increase intake of iron: oral (treatment of choice) or parenteral iron supplements help hemoglobin regenerate
- Increase vitamin C (ascorbic acid increases iron absorption)
- Remember antacids decrease absorption
- Parenteral iron is good for those who won't take their iron orally; if you ever give iron IM, give it Z-track to prevent staining of the skin
- In pregnant clients or elderly clients with severe anemia, an infusion of iron dextran

- Depends on the cause (if caused by hemorrhage, could die from hypovolemic shock)

- Pathophysiology
- Causes and why
- Signs and symptoms and why
- Drug therapy used in treatment
- High-risk populations
- Iron needs with pregnancy
- Ways to help client conserve oxygen
- Pica
- Signs and symptoms of overdose of iron supplements
- Lab work
- How the heart is affected
- How vitamin C affects iron absorption (know high vitamin C foods)
- Major complaint with oral iron preparations are constipation and GI upset
- The best way to take an oral iron supplement is on an empty stomach for maximum absorption
- However, most people cannot do this due to GI upset. Therefore

(Continued)

Table 8-3. (Continued)

Type of anemia	Causes and why	Signs and symptoms and why	Effect on lab values	Quickie tests and treatment	What will harm my client?	If I were your teacher, I would test you on . . .
	• Pregnancy (fetus uses maternal iron stores) • Increased needs of body (i.e., fetus and mother; periods of growth for the infant, child, and adolescent) • Who gets it: premenopausal women, premature or low-birthweight infants, children, adolescent girls. Why? Usually a result of an improper diet	• Red sore tongue (atrophy of papillae on tongue) • Pica (craving to eat weird stuff such as clay, dirt, old ice in the freezer; the body is telling you that you are deficient in something) • Cheilosis (cracks in the corners of mouth, due to poor nutrition or vitamin deficit)	in the RBC as compared to its size • Iron stores are decreased or absent	may be given (some people are allergic to this)		we usually tell people to take this with food. Be aware that taking oral iron supplements with food decreases absorption by 40% • A regular diet provides the body with 12–15 mg per day of iron (only 5–10% of this is actually absorbed) • Ferritin (this is how iron is stored in the body) • Iron is excreted by the body at a rate of less than 1 mg per day. How? Urine sweat, bile, and feces • The female loses 0.5 mg or iron per day or may lose 15 mg per month during menses • Know your iron-rich foods • Know how to give a z-track

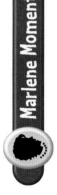

Marlene Moment

When I worked as a home health nurse, I had a little client who collected pans of clay from different parts of her property. She would send it to her relatives in Illinois, who in turn would send her clay from their property. These people had some serious pica problems, and yes, they were eating the clay . . . for real!

Marlene Moment

When I was little, I used to love to go to my Granny's house and scratch the ice out of her freezer and eat it. Come to think of it, I had pica, too. Yum. Yum!

✛ Sickle cell anemia

Sickle cell anemia (Fig. 8-2) is a genetically passed type of anemia. The hemoglobin (oxygen transporter) inside the RBC is defective so it does not carry oxygen well. This is why it is termed hemoglobinopathy. It is a defect in hemoglobin. In addition, the RBCs have a tendency to sickle. When the RBC sickles, it changes its shape. Think of a crescent moon or a C-shaped cell. These sickled cells cause three major problems:

Sickled cells, due to their shape, get tangled with each other very easily. When this occurs, little clots form in different parts of the body. These clots can cause severe pain, organ damage, infarction, and edema.

- Sickled cells cannot carry oxygen well. As a result the client is always a little hypoxic.
- Sickled cells are very fragile and rupture easily. Therefore, the client is always anemic.

Sickled cell

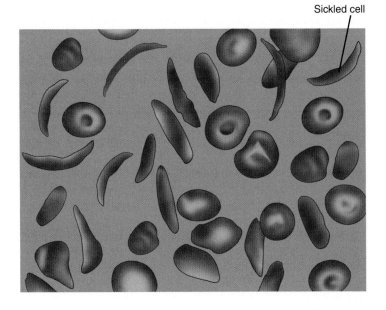

◄ Figure 8-2. Red blood cells, multiple sickle cells.

The sickling process is always occurring. However, there are certain stressors (triggers) which can cause the sickling process to accelerate. When the RBCs are sickling at a rapid rate, this is called a sickle cell crisis. We will review these stressors shortly. In addition, it is important to remember that this disease is not only known for its crisis, but a lifetime of chronic problems. Chronic problems include:

- Swollen joints: edema occurs where clots form
- Exertional dyspnea: RBCs hemolyze, decreasing oxygen
- Leg ulcers: clots occlude circulation causing irritation of tissue
- Fatigue: RBCs hemolyze decreasing oxygen

Sickled cells can go back to the normal shape with proper treatment, but many are filtered out by the spleen. Also, remember, sickled cells are very fragile, so they usually rupture and disintegrate.

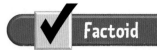

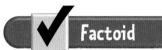

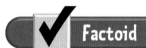

Sickle cell disease is most common in african americans, but is also seen in other populations: people from the mediterranean, middle easterners, east indians, south americans, central americans, and people from the caribbean.

There are several types of sickle cell diseases including sickle cell anemia, (hemoglobin SS disease), sickle hemoglobin C disease (SC), and sickle beta-plus thalassemia and sickle beta-zero thalassemia.

What causes it and why

Sickle cell disease is congenitally acquired. For the disease to be active, the patient must have 2 sickle cell genes. A client with one gene is considered a carrier. If both parents carry the sickle cell trait, offspring will have a 25% chance of inheriting the disease. Individuals with sickle cell trait have about 40% of their red blood cells affected. If a client with sickle cell disease has children, the children will at the very least carry the trait. When a person has the "trait," he carries one normal gene and one abnormal gene—the HbS gene, which can be passed down to offspring. The client with sickle cell trait has only minimal signs of the disease if any at all. This client may not ever know they have this problem until a serious illness develops or until the patient undergoes anesthesia. In those who have the disease, a large portion of their red blood cells are sickled. Table 8-4 summarizes the specifics of what is happening with the hemoglobin and the RBCs in sickle cell diseases.

Table 8-4

Causes	Why
Production of HbS (abnormal hemogloblin molecule) instead of HbA (normal hemoglobin molecule)	Hemogloblin molecule on the red blood cell carries a mutation
Red blood cell changes from biconcave to sickle shape	Red blood cells carrying HbS mutation deoxygenate, changing the shape of the red blood cells

Source: Created by author from References #2, #5, and #13.

Signs and symptoms and why

Symptoms usually do not present until after the age of 6 months (Table 8-5). Why? Because the increased amount of fetal hemoglobin protects the infant for this initial period of time. The severity of the symptoms depends on how much HbS is present in the bloodstream. Many of the symptoms listed below are only seen during an actual crisis.

Table 8-5

Signs and symptoms	Why
Increased pulse	Hypoxia
Enlarged heart	Heart works harder during hypoxia, causing enlargement
Fatigue, lethargy	Hypoxia
Shortness of breath	Hypoxia
Enlarged liver	Thickened blood slows flow; infarction of liver may occur, causing inflammation and edema
Jaundice, dark urine	Breakdown of RBCs causes release of bilirubin, which yellows the skin and darkens the urine. In dark-skinned clients, check the roof of the mouth for jaundice as well as the whites of eyes (sclera)
Intense pruritis	Jaundice (Fig. 8-3)
Swelling of joints	Clots form in joints, causing inflammation and hypoxia
Pain: most common	Pain may occur in chest, joints, abdomen, muscles, or bones due to poor circulation; sign of crisis from clots; results in hypoxia and ischemia in many parts of the body
Low-grade fever	Clots cause ischemia and inflammation, which leads to fever
Pallor	Anemia
Splenomegaly	Spleen working to filter broken-down cells
Heart murmur, S3	When heart works hard, additional heart sounds may occur

Source: Created by author from References #12 and #13.

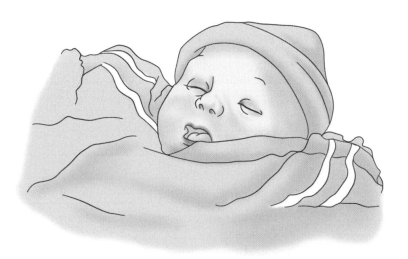

◀ Figure 8-3. Jaundice.
Note the yellow tint to skin.

TYPES OF CRISES   The major cause of a sickle cell crisis is infection. There are three main types of sickle cell disease crises that can occur (Table 8-6).

Table 8-6

Aplastic	Hemolytic	Vaso-occlusive
Also called a megaloblastic crisis. This type is associated with infections, usually viral, which depress the bone marrow significantly. This causes a decrease in red blood cell production. High-output congestive heart failure can be a response to this due to anemia. Usually seen between 8 and 24 months	This occurs when there is an increase in the destruction of red blood cells and the bone marrow cannot keep up with production to maintain a normal level. The sickling process itself can induce cell destruction involved in hemolysis. The liver is affected big time with this type of crisis	This is the most common of the complications. When cells become sickled, they cannot pass through vessels, especially the microcirculation. The vessels then become occluded and cellular and organ damage can take place. These occlusions can occur anywhere. Clients can present with a stroke or acute chest syndrome with a pulmonary infarction that causes atypical pneumonia. The acute chest syndrome is one of the leading causes of death for clients with sickle cell disease. Manifestations also occur depending on the extremity or organ that is occluded—liver, spleen, heart, kidneys, penis, or retina. Clients can present with pain and/or symptoms associated with osteomyelitis, pulmonary embolism, pneumonia, hepatomegaly, meningitis, stroke, cor pulmonale, priapism, and a host of others from either an acute insult or from chronic, repeated offenses This type of crisis is usually seen after 5 years of age

Source: Created by author from References #2, #5, and #13.

SICKLE CELL CRISIS TRIGGERS   The sickling process can be triggered by several different things. Different clients experience different triggers. Some clients have a higher tolerance for the disease, so they do not have as many acute sickling crises. Other clients may have a low tolerance, causing frequent bouts of the sickling process, requiring hospitalization.

SITUATIONS THAT PROMOTE/TRIGGER CRISIS   One of the major goals of care is to prevent a crisis (Table 8-7).

Table 8-7

Exacerbations	Why
Cold environment	Vasospasm
Physical exercise	Exertion
Dehydration	Decreased blood volume
Acidosis	Oxygen carried on the hemoglobin molecule drops off easier. In a patient with sickle cell disease, this decreases the amount of oxygen in the hemoglobin
Stress including things like menstruation, anxiety—basically any type of stress	Exact etiology unknown
Sleep	Decreased oxygen tension
Infection	Infection is stress on the body
Unpressurized aircraft	Hypoxia can occur at high altitudes; pressurization prevents this

Source: Created by author from References #2, #4, and #13.

Remember, any type of stress (as listed above) can precipitate a crisis especially infection and dehydration!

Quickie tests and treatments

Tests:

Tests that help to make the diagnosis of sickle cell disease are:

- Electrophoresis: designates the types of hemoglobin present.
- Complete blood count: determines the presence of anemia and elevated white count.
- Reticulocyte count: low with aplastic anemia crisis.
- Presence of sickled cells in a peripheral smear.
- Test for trait.
- X-ray: may show abnormal vertebral spine called a Lincoln Log, which looks like the corner of log cabin; skull x-rays may show "crew cut" look.

Treatments:

The goal is to stop the sickling process.

- Pain control with NSAIDs for moderate pain is used as well as oral opioids.
- Meperidine (Demerol) is not recommended for patients with chronic pain due to the possibility of seizures from the accumulation of normeperidine, a metabolite of meperidine (Demerol).
- Opioids like morphine or hydromorphone (Dilaudid) are the best drugs for pain relief; when clients are admitted in a crisis they usually receive IV opioids for the first 48 hours (routine IV or by patient-controlled analgesia). Some nurses worry about patient addiction, but this is rare. Do not be judgmental about your client's pain.
- IM injections should not be given, as circulation is impaired and the medication is not absorbed.
- Hydration with intravenous fluids: number one intervention needed to stop the sickling process; give 1.5 to 2 times the normal fluid needs; decreases thickness of blood; give normal saline IV; no caffeine drinks due to their diuretic effect. Another way to look at fluid replacement is like this: in an acute crisis, client needs 200 mL/hour of oral or IV fluid.
- Oxygen therapy: hyperoxygenates the RBCs that aren't sickled; oxygen needs to be nebulized to help prevent dehydration.
- Warmth treatments: warm compresses to affected joints to decrease inflammation, edema, pain.
- Exchange transfusions.
- RBC infusions: reverses anemia and hypovolemia; use sparingly, as iron overload can occur with too many infusions; too much iron can damage organs like the heart, liver, and all endocrine organs.
- Bone marrow transplant: must have an HLA-matched donor; may stop sickled cells from being produced; clients will have to be on immunosuppressive agents for the rest of their lives to prevent rejection.

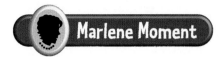

Marlene Moment

It would be mean to advise your client with sickle cell disease to go to the beach for vacation. Why? He will get dehydrated and go into a crisis. Don't be mean; you'll never get a nursing license like that!

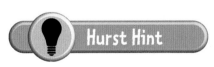

Hurst Hint

Erythrocyte is the term for RBC. Reticulocyte is the term for immature RBC. Normally, reticulocyte counts rise to compensate for anemia but with bone marrow failure they don't.

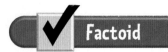

Clients with sickle cell disease usually do not have low iron levels.

- Cord blood stem cell transplant.
- Hydroxyurea (Droxia): decreases episodes of pain by increasing production of fetal hemoglobin; associated with development of leukemia; as this drug can cause birth defects, the client should use 2 forms of birth control.
- No pressure behind knees; no knee or hip flexion: increases formation of clots.
- Iron supplements: if required.
- Folic acid supplements: include a diet high in green leafy vegetables.
- Antibiotics: if infection is present.
- Strict sterile technique with procedures.
- Bed rest.
- Head of bed (HOB) raised: maximizes lung expansion; decreases cardiac workload.
- Assessment: cardiovascular, pulmonary system, skin, abdomen, musculoskeletal system, central nervous system, and psychosocial needs.
- Infection control: hand-washing; yearly flu shot for client; select patient roommates carefully; masks for visitors with respiratory infections. Sickle cell clients are at high risk for infection from organisms such as *Streptococcus pneumoniae* and *Haemophilus influenzae*.
- Monitor O_2 saturation by pulse oximetry.
- Monitor ABGs.

What can harm my client?

Sickle cell crises can be precipitated by many situations. Patients must be educated about sickle cell crises, how to avoid them, and how to manage them. Individuals with the potential for pregnancy (or males who carry the trait or have the disease) must be cautious regarding the use of hydroxyurea (Droxia), a cytotoxic agent that can adversely affect the fetus. Yes, even if the male takes it!

Other things that can harm the client are:

- Retinopathy: the tiny vessels in the retina get clots and cause death of the retina.
- Nephropathy: same thing happening in the kidney.
- Brain infarction: same thing happening in brain; stroke could occur.
- MI: see above; same thing happening in coronary arteries.
- Infection leading to gangrene: area affected is not getting oxygen, so tissue becomes infected and dies.
- Splenic sequestration: sudden accumulation of blood in the spleen; causes hypovolemic shock and death. A splenectomy may have to be performed.
- Aplastic crisis: bone marrow stops working.
- Avascular necrosis: especially of the long bones; due to vascular occlusion; hip replacement may be required.
- Priapism: penile vessels become obstructed; may lead to impotence; penile implant may be required.

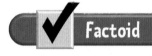

Priapism is a sustained prolonged and painful erection. This is a urological emergency.

If I were your teacher, I would test you on . . .

- Pathophysiology of sickle cell disease.
- Causes and management of sickle cell crises.
- Types of crises including signs and symptoms and factors that can exacerbate signs and symptoms.
- Infectious processes and the role of the spleen.
- Pain control.
- The role of hydroxyurea (Droxia).
- Importance of teaching patients to report fever or signs of infection at once (infection is a major cause of death).
- Importance of avoiding low oxygen and dehydration.
- Importance of avoiding activities requiring increased oxygen.
- Importance of genetic counseling.
- Importance of not wearing tight clothes that could obstruct circulation.
- Importance of taking care of teeth; going to the dentist is stressful and could trigger a crisis.
- Importance of telling practitioners of the disorder prior to any treatments or procedures.
- The effects of pregnancy can be life threatening; if the client already has organ damage, she should avoid pregnancy. Barrier methods of birth control are better for this client than oral contraceptives. Why? Because oral contraceptives make the blood thicker, especially if the client smokes.
- The importance of other family members getting genetic counseling.
- 50% of clients do not live past age 20; most clients don't live past age 50.

Pediatric implications:

- A sickle cell crisis in a child may be called "chest syndrome," causing severe chest pain and difficulty breathing.
- Children usually develop an enlarged spleen; by teenage years the spleen is dysfunctional due to atrophy.
- A child may have decreased growth due to hypoxia; a change in the growth curve occurs around age 7; puberty starts later than usual.
- Pediatric clients usually have a short torso and long arms, legs, fingers, and toes.
- Since children experience changes in the bones and bone marrow, it is common for them to have pain in the hands and feet, and they may need hip replacements.
- Young men may develop priapism (usually no lasting damage if caught early and dealt with).
- A sickle cell crisis in children may present with anemia, stomach pain, bone pain, and GI upset.
- Children 4 years and younger may be given penicillin prophylactically to prevent infection.

• Importance of keeping immunizations up to date: pneumococcal vaccine should be administered before age 2 with a booster shot at age 5.

✛ Thrombocytopenia

Thrombocytopenia is the most common cause of hemorrhagic disorders and may be congenital or acquired. The acquired form is more common, especially among the elderly. The survival rate of drug-induced thrombocytopenia is high if the drug is withdrawn in time.

What is it?

Thrombocytopenia is a decrease in circulating platelets. This is represented by a number less than 100,000/μL for platelets of the complete blood count. Platelets are necessary for the formation of clotting. There are four major reasons thrombocytopenia may occur.

1. A decrease in the production of platelets.
2. A decrease in the lifespan of platelets.
3. Blood pooling in the spleen.
4. Dilution of the bloodstream.

The specific cell that produces platelets is called a megakaryocyte. When these cells are decreased, platelet numbers are decreased.

TYPES OF THROMBOCYTOPENIA   Table 8-8 describes the types of thrombocytopenia.

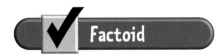

Note: the major drugs implicated in secondary thrombocytopenia are quinine, quinidine, some sulfa drugs, and heparin!

Table 8-8

Types of thrombocytopenia	Description
Idiopathic Thrombocytopenic Purpura (ITP)	A rare autoimmune disease that destroys the platelets via antibodies. It is seen in a chronic form in adults, more often in women. Acute ITP is mainly seen in children. Chronic ITP is mainly seen in adults. Platelets are covered with antibodies, so they don't look like themselves; therefore the spleen thinks they are something foreign, so the spleen gets rid of them. Splenectomy is usually performed. In ITP, the platelets clump together in small vessels → tissue ischemia occurs → renal failure, MI, stroke

If not diagnosed and treated quickly, the client usually dies in 3 months |
Thrombotic Thrombocytopenic Purpura (TTP)	This type of thrombocytopenia belongs in the category of abnormal distribution. Toxins released after bacterial invasion, as with *Escherichia coli*, produce damage to the endothelial lining of vessels, which causes widespread thrombosis. Sudden onset and can be fatal. The goal is to stop platelets from clumping together and to stop the autoimmune problem that could be occurring. Treatment includes FFP and plasmapheresis. Drugs, such as aspirin, can also be used to stop platelet aggregation
Secondary Thrombocytopenia	Due to a problem with platelet production; usually secondary to a drug; causes: medications (thiazides, aspirin, nonsteroidals, <u>sulfonamides</u>, Tagamet, Lanoxin, Lasix, heparin, morphine, Tegretol, and vitamins C and E,); spices (ginger, cloves, cumin, garlic, turmeric); infections (bacterial or viral); bone marrow disorders, chemotherapy; radiation therapy
Disordered Platelet Distribution	Occurs when numerous platelets are destroyed by the spleen; caused by lymphoma, portal hypertension, and hypothermia (as with heart surgery)

Source: Created by author from References #2, #4, and #14.

What causes it and why

There are 3 main reasons for thrombocytopenia to occur: a decreased production of platelets, an increased destruction of platelets, or an abnormality in the distribution of the platelets (Table 8-9).

Table 8-9

Causes	Why
Radiation therapy Chemotherapy Drugs such as quinidine Leukemia Aplastic anemia Drug toxicity	Antigen–antibody reaction sets up a response that lyses the platelets
Drugs such as antibiotics, sulfonamides, heparin, gold Autoimmune causes Disseminated intravascular coagulation (DIC) Cirrhosis Severe infection	Increased destruction of platelets outside the bone marrow; can cause platelets to aggregate
Splenomegaly	Splenomegaly is a cause of "abnormal distribution" of platelets. When splenomegaly occurs, an increased amount of platelets can be held in the spleen (up to 80% as opposed to the normal 30–40%), lowering the platelet count

Source: Created by author from References #2, #4, and #14.

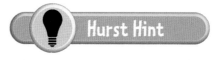

Abnormal/new bruising/bleeding may be the first sign of thrombocytopenia.

Signs and symptoms and why

Table 8-10 summarizes the signs and symptoms, and associated reasons, for thrombocytopenia. All symptoms are due to bleeding area resulting from low platelets.

Table 8-10

Signs and symptoms	Why or what
Petechiae	Tiny flat purple or red dots on the skin or mucous membranes. These are little hemorrhages in the tissue. Most common occurrence are on the chest, arms, and neck
Bleeding	Platelets are low, so blood can't clot. Bleeding may be seen in the form of nosebleeds (epistaxis), excessive menstrual bleeding, (menorrhagia), bleeding in the urine (hematuria), GI bleeding (indicated by blood in vomit or black, tarry stools [melena])
Oral blood blisters	Bleeding into the oral mucosa
Fatigue; weakness	Hemorrhage; blood moves from bloodstream into tissues
Purpura	Bleeding into tissue causing bruises. Most common places of occurrence are chest, arms, and neck
Ecchymosis (bruising)	Bleeding into the subcutaneous tissue causing flat or raised discolored areas of skin or mucous membranes

Source: Created by author from References #2, #4, and #14.

Quickie tests and treatments

The test for thrombocytopenia is simply a low platelet count. Other causes must be ruled out.

- Let's look at the lab values:

    Platelet count < 100,000/μL in adults.

    Increased PT and PTT. (This means it is taking longer for blood to clot.)

    Platelet antibody studies: shows why the platelet count is dropping.

    Platelet survival test: shows if thrombocytopenia is due to a platelet production problem or a platelet destruction problem.

- Bone marrow test: looks at the megakaryocytes.

Treatments for thrombocytopenia include: (Tx is totally dependent on cause.)

- IV gamma globulin and IV anti-Ro: prevent antibody-covered platelets from being destroyed.
- Platelet transfusions: transfused platelets are destroyed by the spleen just like the client's other platelets.
- Splenectomy: spleen is the major organ that removes platelets; if client doesn't respond to drugs, a splenectomy may be performed. Remember, that without the spleen, the client may be prone to infections.
- Cessation of drugs that could be causing thrombocytopenia.
- Corticosteroids and Imuran increase platelets; suppress immune system; therefore antiplatelet autoantibodies are decreased.
- Lithium carbonate (Eskalith)/folate: increases platelet production through stimulation of bone marrow.
- Blood product transfusion including platelets and fresh frozen plasma.
- Splenectomy (if it's gone, can't trap platelets.)
- Plasmapheresis: usually used for thrombotic thrombocytopenic purpura—removes plasma portion of blood and replaces it with fresh frozen plasma.
- Patient education: reduces the potential for bleeding by using stool softeners, drinking fluids to reduce the risk of constipation, using electric razors, and not using aspirin.

What can harm my client?

- Misdiagnosis due to subtle signs and symptoms of illness.
- Hemorrhage.
- Lack of patient education in assessing for bleeding problems.

If I were your teacher, I would test you on . . .

- What is it?
- Normal platelet count.
- Causes and why of thrombocytopenia.
- Differences between ITP and TTP.
- Signs and symptoms and why of thrombocytopenia.
- The importance of protecting from injury.

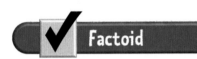

Factoid

An enlarged spleen may be an early sign of thrombocytopenia.

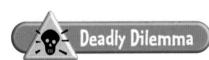

Deadly Dilemma

STOP! Treating thrombotic thrombocytopenic purpura (TTP) with platelets can be fatal! Proper diagnosis is imperative prior to treatment!

- Proper treatments including how they work.
- Bleeding or thrombocytopenic precautions.
- Medication administration and side effects.
- Monitoring for hematuria and other forms of bleeding.
- Safety measures for administering platelets.
- Recognition of transfusion reactions.

✚ Hemophilia and von Willebrand's disease

Hemophilia and von Willebrand's disease are classified as bleeding disorders versus clotting disorders. Hemophilia is an X-linked inherited recessive bleeding disorder. As a result, the client does not have enough clotting factors. With hemophilia A, the client does not have enough factor VIII. With hemophilia B, the client does not have enough factor IX. When these factors are absent, factor X cannot be activated. Factor X is the main enzyme that converts fibrinogen to fibrin. When factor X is not activated, a good clot cannot be formed and excessive bleeding occurs. Von Willebrand's disease is a hereditary problem seen mainly in females where the client has long bleeding times, poor platelet function, and a possible deficit of factor VIII. Von Willebrand factor is a protein that affects platelet function. It is found in plasma, platelets, and walls of blood vessels. If the factor is missing, malfunctioning platelets won't adhere to vessel walls at the injury site as they normally would; therefore, the bleeding won't stop as quick as it would normally. Von Willebrand protein also carries factor VIII so it is also possible that factor VIII could be diminished. That is the difference.

What is it?

Hemophilia and von Willebrand's disease are manifested by bleeding because of missing clotting factors. The severity of these diseases is variable.

What causes it and why

Table 8-11 gives the causes of von Willebrand's disease and hemophilia.

Table 8-11

	Cause	Why
Hemophilia A ("Classic Hemophilia")	Decrease in amount or functional ability of factor VIII	Factor X is not triggered in the clotting cascade due to decreased factor VIII, preventing fibrinogen from converting to fibrin, which produces a clot at the site of bleeding. Hemophilia A makes up 80% of all individuals who have hemophilia
Hemophilia B (Christmas Disease)	Decrease in amount or functional ability of factor IX	Factor X is not triggered in the clotting cascade due to decreased factor IX, preventing fibrinogen from converting to fibrin, which produces a clot at the site of bleeding
Von Willebrand's Disease	Defect in platelet function due to lack of von Willebrand's factor and decreased amount of factor VIII. This is an inherited autosomal dominant trait	Factor X is not triggered in the clotting cascade due to decreased factor VIII. Decreased von Willebrand's factor causes decreased platelet function

Source: Created by author from References #1 and #15.

OTHER THINGS YOU NEED TO KNOW . . . Hemophilia is passed congenitally as a recessive trait on the X chromosome. A mother who does not carry the gene and a father who has the disease will pass the mutation to daughters in the family (Table 8-12). A mother who carries the gene and a father who does not have the disease have a 50% chance of producing a son with the disease and a 50% chance of having a daughter who will be a carrier (Table 8-13). This is known as an X-linked recessive gene. The information for factors VIII and IX is carried on the X chromosome. The Y chromosome does not carry clotting factor information.

Table 8-12

		Unaffected mother	
		X	X
Affected Father	**+X**	**+X**X Female (carrier)	**+X**X Female (carrier)
	Y	XY Male	XY Male

All females will become carriers because of the X chromosome.
Source: Created by author from References #1 and #15.

Table 8-13

		Affected mother	
		+**X**	X
Unaffected Father	**X**	**+X**X Female (carrier)	XX Female
	Y	**+X**Y Male (hemophiliac)	XY Male

50% chance of a female who will be a carrier and a male with the disease.
Source: Created by author from References #1 and #15.

Signs and symptoms and why

Table 8-14 gives the signs and symptoms, and associated explanations, for hemophilia.

Table 8-14

Signs and symptoms	Why
Bleeding: spontaneous, excessive or prolonged bleeding, or associated with trauma, surgery, minor injury	No production of stable fibrin clot
Bruising	Subcutaneous or deep in the muscle; bleeding
Joint pain/deformity; edema; tenderness	Bleeding into joints (mainly weight-bearing joints)

(Continued)

Table 8-14. (*Continued*)

Signs and symptoms	Why
Hematuria; hematemesis	Bleeding from internal organs (kidney and GI tract)
Pain	Bleeding from internal organs
Shock	Loss of blood volume resulting in decreased blood pressure
Internal bleeding	Usually presents as pain in the abdomen, chest, or flank area
Excessive uterine bleeding (especially in von Willebrand's disease)	No production of stable fibrin clot
Epistaxis (nose bleeds)	No production of stable fibrin clot
Bleeding from gums	No production of stable fibrin clot

Source: Created by author from References #1 and #15.

Quickie tests and treatments

Laboratory studies may be used to diagnose and identify prenatal carriers. Diagnosis is made through laboratory tests such as:

- Bleeding time.
- Platelet counts.
- Prothrombin time (PT).
- Partial thromboplastin time (PTT).
- Factor VIII assay.
- Factor IX assay.

Treatments:

Hemphilia A and von Willebrand's disease:

- Factor VIII.
- Fresh frozen plasma.
- Cryoprecipitate or lyophilized factor VIII or IX: increases clotting factors.
- Desmopressin acetate (DDVAP): used in mild bleeding episodes; such as dental work or minor surgeries. It increases the amount of available factor VIII.
- Recombinant factor VIIa: new therapy used in both hemophilia A and B if factor VIII or IX is inhibited.[17]
- Amino caproic acid (Amicar): inhibits plasminogen activators during oral bleeding.

Hemophilia B AKA factor IX deficiency.

- Factor IX concentrate given during bleeding episodes.
- Factor IX.
- Antibody purified factor IX.

Gene therapy research is currently focusing on cloning the factor VIII and factor IX genes, which may provide new treatment regimens and cures for this disease.

Pediatric implications:

- Clothes should be padded on the knees and elbows.
- No contact sports.

What can harm my client?

- Hemorrhagic shock.
- Life- or limb-threatening crises.

If I were your teacher, I would test you on . . .

- Classifications of hemophilia including A, B, and von Willebrand's disease.
- X-linked recessive genes.
- Causes and why of hemophilia.
- Assessment, treatment, and monitoring complications associated with hemophilia.
- Administration and side effects of DDAVP.
- Monitoring for complications associated with blood product administration.
- Patient education to safeguard against, and manage, bleeding episodes.
- Patient education regarding dental prophylaxis and medical procedure safeguards.

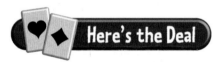

DIC starts with excessive clotting → clotting factors are depleted → excessive bleeding ensues.

✚ Disseminated intravascular coagulation (DIC)

What is it?

Disseminated intravascular coagulation (DIC) (also known as consumption coagulopathy and defibrination syndrome) is a secondary response to a primary insult. Anything can trigger this disorder in anyone. Simultaneous clotting and bleeding occur throughout the body with DIC. What happens is that small clots develop all over the bloodstream. Then all of the clotting factors and platelets get used up, making the client bleed from every available orifice or puncture site. There is an acute form of DIC and a more gradual, chronic form that manifests itself within the venous system including pulmonary embolism.

What causes it and why

The exact mechanism of action for DIC is not clearly understood; however, it is always precipitated by an initial disease process. Once clotting occurs, vessels become blocked and tissue and/or organ damage is present. The supply of clotting factors is then exhausted and bleeding ensues. Also, it is thought that a foreign protein can enter the bloodstream and cause vascular injury that triggers DIC. As the process continues, prothrombin is activated and thrombin is produced in excess. Thrombin is responsible for converting fibrinogen to fibrin. This causes fibrin clots to form in the tiny circulation (microcirculation). This entire process uses up almost all of the coagulation factors. Thrombin causes fibrin clots to dissolve, causing hemorrhage.

Primary insults include:

- Infections from any source: bacterial, viral, fungal, rickettsial, protozoans.
- Pregnancy issues: abruption placentae, fetal demise, pregnancy-induced hypertension, abortion, amniotic fluid embolism.
- Trauma.
- Burns.
- Emboli.
- Carcinomas.
- Heat stroke.
- Snakebites.
- Shock.
- Cardiac arrest.
- Necrotic situations.
- Blood transfusion reactions.
- Transplant rejection.
- Liver necrosis.
- Cirrhosis.
- Fat emboli.

Signs and symptoms and why

Signs and symptoms of DIC include both clotting and bleeding. Rapid clotting occludes small vessels; can cause necrosis as oxygen cannot get to where it needs to go; clotting factors are depleted and then hemorrhage occurs. Clotting tends to affect the kidneys, extremities, brain, lungs, glands, and GI tract (Table 8-15).

Table 8-15

Clotting
Dysrhythmias: clots in the coronary arteries prevent the heart from getting oxygen
Cyanotic, cold digits: clots in the circulation cause ischemia
Absent, unequal pulses: due to arterial clots
Hypoxia: clots in the lungs (pulmonary emboli)
Respiratory distress: decreased oxygenation
Diminished or absent breath sounds: clots in the lungs
Aphasia: clot in the brain

(Continued)

Table 8-15. (*Continued*)

Clotting
Unequal pupils: clot in the brain
Decreased urine output: clots in the renal circulation decrease kidney perfusion; usually less than 30 mL/hr; BUN >25 mg/dL increased; creatinine >1.3 mg/dL increased
Decreased bowel sounds: clots in GI tract that limit perfusion of bowel so bowels slow down
Necrotic extremities: clots in circulation lead to ischemia and necrosis
Confusion: clot in the brain
Pain to abdomen, chest, back: tissue hypoxia

Bleeding
Petechiae (ruptured tiny blood vessels)
Ecchymosis (bruising)
Epistaxis (nose bleed)
Gingival bleeding (bleeding from gums)
Gastrointestinal bleeding (may show up as nausea and vomiting)
Hematuria (blood in urine)
Hemoptysis (blood-stained sputum)
Venipuncture site bleeding
Wound bleeding
Signs of hypovolemic shock
Postpartum bleeding
Surgical site bleeding
Oozing from mucocutaneous sites

Source: Created by author from References #1 to #5.

Quickie tests and treatments

Tests:

- Hemoglobin/hematocrit: decreased due to bleeding.
- Prothrombin time: elevated as blood is taking longer to form a clot; greater than 15 seconds.
- Partial thromboplastin time: elevated as blood is taking longer to form a clot; greater than 60 seconds.
- Platelet levels: decreased as they have all been used up; less than 100,000/μL.
- Fibrin split products (D-dimer and fibrin degradation factor): elevated due to increased fibrinolysis.

- Fibrinogen level: decreased as all clotting factors have been used up; usually less than 150 mg/dL.
- Factor VIII levels: decreased in DIC as it is a clotting factor that has been used up.
- White blood cell count: should be assessed for diagnosis of infectious processes.

Treatment:

- Treat the underlying problem.
- Blood product transfusions.
- Fresh frozen plasma: replaces clotting factors.
- Cryoprecipitate: great source of fibrinogen and factors V, VII, and XIII.
- Platelets used if platelet count < 100,000/μL.
- Heparin makes your blood take longer to form a clot. This makes the liver think that it can stop putting out clotting factors; therefore the liver starts making more clotting factors to catch up but stores them instead of releasing them. Some think heparin gives the liver time to build up more clotting factors. If given in early stages, may prevent clotting in microcirculation (controversial).
- Studies are underway utilizing activated C-reactive protein.

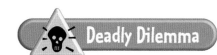

Deadly Dilemma

Heparin is not recommended in cases where the underlying pathology is central nervous system-related, involves hepatic processes, or concerns obstetrical events. The use of heparin with DIC is very controversial.

What can harm my client?

- Prognosis depends on how early DIC is detected.
- Hemorrhage.
- Venipuncture: use venous and arterial lines for blood draws and blood pressure monitoring.
- Manual blood pressure cuffs can cause petechiae and ecchymotic areas.

If I were your teacher, I would test you on . . .

- Pathophysiology of DIC.
- Causes and why of DIC.
- Signs and symptoms and why of DIC. (Especially early recognition.)
- Laboratory values.
- Treatment options.
- Controversial use of heparin.
- Client safety.
- Patient education.
- Importance of bed rest to prevent further injury and bleeding.
- Importance of watching for new bleeding site.
- Administration of blood and blood products.
- Signs and symptoms of shock.

- Recognition of high-risk clients.
- Signs and symptoms of renal failure.
- Psychosocial implications of client and family actually seeing bleeding.
- Care of pulmonary artery catheter in monitoring client's hemodynamic status.
- If client is pregnant: continuous fetal monitoring is indicated (watch for late decelerations, decreased variability, and bradycardia). Actions to take if these occur.
- Fluid resuscitation.
- Pad siderails to prevent injury and bleeding.
- Touch client gently to prevent bruising and dislodgment of clot.
- Importance of all staff members being aware of client's bleeding tendencies.
- Avoid as many needle-sticks as possible; hold pressure for at least 10 minutes after any puncture.

✚ Blood transfusion reactions

Several reactions to blood transfusions can occur. Blood typing and cross-matching is imperative prior to administration. In emergent situations, type-specific or universal donor blood can be used. The universal donor is O negative. Most institutions use O-negative blood exclusively for this purpose. O-positive blood can be given to males or females past child-bearing age.

What is blood typing?

ABO blood types include A, B, AB, and O. Each of these carries specific antigens and antibodies (Table 8-16). In addition, the Rhesus or Rh factor is determined for each of these blood types, which are either positive (present) or negative (absent).

Table 8-16

Blood group	Antigen	Antibody
A	A	Anti-B
B	B	Anti-A
AB	A and B	None
O	None	Anti-A and Anti-B

Source: Created by author from References #18 and #19.

Common reactions

Common reactions to blood product administration are listed in Table 8-17.

Table 8-17

Reaction	Cause	Signs and symptoms	Interventions
Acute hemolytic	• ABO incompatibility causes hemolysis—antibodies in the patient's system react against the "foreign" transfused cells • Wrong blood has been given!	• Quick onset—often after few drops of blood have infused • Fever • Chill • Dyspnea • Low back pain • Nausea • Pain at intravenous site • Hemoglobinemia • Oliguria • Renal failure • Tachycardia • Hypotension • Restlessness • Anxiety • Cardiovascular collapse • Chest tightness • DIC	• Stop the transfusion • Do not give even one more drop of blood • Start fresh bag of normal saline (with new tubing) at the insertion site • Collect blood sample from patient for blood bank and send the bag of blood back to the blood bank • Observe BUN and creatinine; get urine sample • Diuretics may be given • Dopamine can be used to increase renal flow • Keep urine output at 30–100 mL/hr • Check urine for hemolyzed RBCs
Febrile nonhemolytic	• Antibodies formed against transfused WBCs or platelets. Also may be related to cytokines that develop during storage of blood products	• Slower onset: 1–6 hours • Fever • Chilling • Malaise • May have dyspnea	• Stop the infusion • Hang new normal saline with new tubing at the insertion site • Must be differentiated from hemolytic reaction • Acetaminophen for fever • Patient may be premedicated prior to administration to ↓ occurrence of reaction • If high-risk patient, use leukocyte-filtered blood products
Allergic	• Reaction to plasma protein that is foreign to body	• Urticaria • Flushed appearance • Itching	• Stop infusion • Give anithistamines • Give steroids
Anaphylaxis	• Immune reaction to foreign products—anti-IgA antibodies present in patient—most common with blood products containing plasma • May occur with prior transfusions or multiple pregnancies	• Occurs immediately, often after few drops of blood have infused • Flushed appearance • Dyspnea • Bronchospasm • Edema • Chills • Chest pain • Abdominal pain • Hypotension	• Stop blood immediately • Start fresh normal saline with new tubing at the insertion site • Provide ABC support • Give intravenous volume • Administer epinephrine • Administer diphenhydramine • Administer corticosteroids

✔ **Factoid**

Back pain may be the first sign of acute hemolytic reaction as kidneys are getting clogged up from broken down cells.

(Continued)

Table 8-17. (*Continued*)

Reaction	Cause	Signs and symptoms	Interventions
		• Nausea • Vomiting • Diarrhea • Decreased LOC • Loss of consciousness	
Transfusion-related acute lung injury (TRALI)	• Seen with infusions of blood products containing plasma. Antileukocyte antibodies present in the donor blood react with leukocytes in the patient. This reaction activates complement, which then increases permeability in the vascular bed of the pulmonary system. Also, it is thought that inflammatory mediators collect during blood storage	• Dyspnea • Tachypnea • Rales/crackles • Fever • Chills • Hypotension • Pallor • Cyanosis • Tachycardia	• Support respiratory function • Monitor pulse oximetry • Administer oxygen—maintain pulse oximetry at or greater than 92% • Intubate if necessary (70–75% of patients require intubation)
Graft-versus-host disease	• Occurs when immunocompromised patient receives blood products containing lymphocytes, which create an immune response to the lymphoid tissue in the recipient. In normal circumstances, the donated lymphocytes are attacked and destroyed. The immunocompromised patient cannot perform that function	• Delayed reaction—may take 1 to several weeks to develop • Fever • Right upper quadrant pain associated with hepatitis • Rash • Nausea • Vomiting • Diarrhea • Decreased appetite	• Prevention by irradiating blood products that contain lymphocytes
Infectious	• Infections from donors can occur. Infections can also be introduced into the blood after acquisition—before or during administration	• Will vary depending on infection—can be bacterial or viral—some common processes that may be passed are HIV, hepatitis, cytomegalovirus, malaria	• Dependent on disease process

Table 8-17. (*Continued*)

Reaction	Cause	Signs and symptoms	Interventions
Overload (Fluid volume excess)	Transfusing large amounts of blood products to patients who also have underlying disease processes such as cardiac or pulmonary insults. The aged individual is also at risk for this	• Dyspnea • Respiratory distress • Cough • Pallor • Cyanosis • Rales/crackles • Pulmonary edema • Elevated central venous pressure	• Treat for pulmonary edema

Source: Created by author from References #3, #4, and #19.

More blood-related complications

More blood-related complications include:

- Hypothermia: infusion of cold blood.
- Acidosis: pH of stored blood.
- Alkalosis: citrate in stored blood.
- Hyperkalemia: breakdown of cells during storage increases release of potassium.
- Hypocalcemia: citrate in stored blood combines with calcium in patient leaving decreased amounts of unbound calcium.
- Loss of 2,3 DPG in stored blood causes hemoglobin molecule to hold on to oxygen. See Factoid. The longer the blood sits in the blood bank, the less 2,3 DPG there will be.

What can harm my client?

- Incorrect labeling of client blood specimens.
- Not checking blood products appropriately prior to administration.
- Not using 0.9% normal saline to infuse blood products.
- Not using filtered blood tubing and other filters as necessary.
- Infusing blood products too fast in the initial period of administration.
- Not observing the client closely for reactions while receiving blood products.
- Transfusing patients with underlying cardiac or pulmonary problems too quickly.
- Giving cold blood products: never attempt to warm blood products with a microwave! Use only approved warming devices.

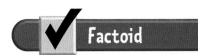
Factoid

2,3 DPG (diphosphoglycerate) is a substance found in RBCs that is responsible for controlling the movement of oxygen from the RBC to body tissues. Hemoglobin carries the oxygen and uses 2,3 DPG to control how much is released into the blood. Loss of 2,3 DPG results in less oxygen delivery.

If I were your teacher, I would test you on . . .

- Knowledge of ABO and Rh typing.
- Related physical assessment.
- Signs and symptoms and interventions for transfusion reactions.

- Understanding of basic pathophysiological background for transfusion reactions and complications.
- Patient safety.

✚ Polycythemia vera

Polycythemia vera is a rare disease that occurs more frequently in men than in women, and rarely in patients under 40 years old.[3]

What is it?

- Disease in which there is an increase in production of red blood cells.
- Increased hemoglobin levels are present.
- Plasma volume levels can be low or normal.

What causes it?

- Increased production by stem cells in the bone marrow.
- Causes highly viscous blood, decreased microcirculatory blood flow, and thrombotic episodes.

Signs and Symptoms

Decreased blood flow causing:

- Headache.
- Dizziness.
- Sensory deficits (vision, hearing).
- Chest pain.

Increased viscosity causing:

- Hypertension.
- Thromboses (major cause of mortality/morbidity).
- Shortness of breath, especially when lying flat.
- Splenomegaly.

Venous stasis causing:

- Ruddy appearance to face, especially the nose.
- Dusky appearance to lips and mucous membranes.
- Clubbing of the fingers.

Quickie tests and treatments

Tests:

- Complete blood count with differential.
- Hemoglobin and hematocrit.
- Serum iron.
- Vitamin B_{12} assay.
- Erythropoietin level.
- Bone-marrow biopsy.

Treatments:

- Therapeutic phlebotomy.
- Chemotherapy.
- Radiation therapy.
- Hydroxyurea (Droxia).
- Interferon-alfa.

What can harm my client?

- Misdiagnosis: symptoms may be absent in early stages.
- Not recognizing signs and symptoms of vascular occlusions, stroke, or heart attack, which can be caused by polycythemia vera and may not be recognized as the cause.

If I were your teacher, I would test you on . . .

- Blood cell levels in polycythemia vera.
- Causes and why of the disease process.
- Complications such as stroke and myocardial infarction.
- Diagnostics to identify the disease.
- Importance of bone-marrow biopsy in diagnosis.
- Rationale for therapeutic phlebotomy, chemotherapy, and radiation therapy as treatment.

SUMMARY

The hematologic system provides the body with the ability to fight infections, carry oxygen, and coagulate bleeding episodes. Understanding underlying pathophysiology of hematologic disease processes can help you assess, identify, and intervene appropriately for these patients. Many of these processes can be subtle but have life-threatening implications.

PRACTICE QUESTIONS

1. Which type of white blood cell is important in the immunologic process?

   1. Lymphocyte.
   2. Monocyte.
   3. Neutrophil.
   4. Eosinophil.

   Correct answer: 1. Lymphocytes are important in the development of antibodies. Monocytes assist in removal of bacteria and viruses. Neutrophils help to defend against bacteria, and eosinophils are important in allergic crises.

2. Lack of folic acid in a pregnant client's diet may cause which fetal problem?

   1. Dextrocardia.

   2. Cleft palate.

   3. Neural tube defects.

   4. Anencephaly.

   Correct answer: 3. Lack of folic acid during pregnancy can predispose a fetus to neural tube defects such as spina bifida. The other responses are not correct.

3. Which is a true statement regarding desmopressin acetate (DDAVP)?

   1. DDAVP is used to treat Christmas disease.

   2. DDAVP increases the number of erythrocytes.

   3. DDAVP increases the amount of white blood cells.

   4. DDAVP is used to stimulate the release of factor VIII.

   Correct answer: 4. DDAVP is a drug used to treat hemophilia A and von Willebrand's disease. It works in minor injuries to stimulate the release of factor VIII from von Willebrand's factor. DDAVP is not used in Christmas disease, which is hemophilia B and is a defect with factor IX. DDAVP does not increase red or white blood cells.

4. Hydroxyurea (Droxia) is a drug that is used to treat sickle cell disease by initiating the production of which type of hemoglobin?

   1. HbS.

   2. HbF.

   3. HbA.

   4. HbC.

   Correct answer: 2. Hydroxyurea (Droxia) is a cytotoxic drug that creates HbF, fetal hemoglobin that does not carry the sickling factor. HbS is the mutated form of hemoglobin implicated in sickle cell anemia. HbA is the mature form of hemoglobin which is normal. HbC is not a type of hemoglobin.

5. Idiopathic thrombocytopenic purpura is considered a(n):

   1. Autoimmune disease process.

   2. Platelet distribution problem.

   3. Decreased platelet production.

   4. Increased platelet production.

   Correct answer: 1. Idiopathic thrombocytopenic purpura is an autoimmune response. Types of platelet distribution problems are disseminated intravascular coagulation (DIC) or thrombotic thrombocytopenic purpura (TTP). Decreased platelet production occurs with chemotherapy or radiation therapy. Thrombocytopenia is a decrease in platelet production.

6. Which test is useful in the diagnosis of polycythemia vera?

1. Prothrombin time.

2. ABO typing.

3. Electrophoresis.

4. Bone-marrow biopsy.

Correct answer: 4. Bone-marrow biopsy is important in the diagnosis of poycythemia vera, since the disorder is a dysfunction of increased production of cells by the bone marrow. ABO typing is used with blood transfusions. Electrophoresis is utilized in sickle cell anemia to determine the specific type of hemoglobin that is present. Protime is useful in the diagnosis of disseminated intravascular coagulation (DIC).

7. If a client has blood type A, which antibodies are present?

1. Anti-A.

2. Anti-B.

3. Anti-A and anti-B.

4. None.

Correct answer: 2. Blood type A has anti-B antibodies. Blood type B has anti-A antibodies. Blood type AB has no antibodies present, and blood type O has both anti-A and anti-B antibodies.

8. Which may be found in a client with disseminated intravascular coagulation (DIC)?

1. Increased protime (PT).

2. Decreased partial thromboplastin time (PTT).

3. Increased fibrinogen.

4. Decreased fibrin degradation product.

Correct answer: 1. The prothrombin time in DIC is usually elevated, though it may remain within normal limits. The partial thromboplastin time is also increased. Fibrinogen is decreased because the supply has been exhausted. Fibrin degradation products are increased.

9. Immunocompromised clients are most likely to have which type of blood transfusion reaction?

1. Acute hemolytic.

2. Graft-versus-host disease.

3. Anaphylactic reaction.

4. Transfusion related acute lung injury.

Correct answer: 2. Immunocompromised clients are most likely to have a graft-versus-host disease process because the lymphoid tissue cannot respond appropriately by attacking and destroying infused lymphocytes. The other answers are blood transfusion reactions, but are not specific to immunocompromised patients.

10. A lack of 2,3 diphosphoglycerate (DPG) in stored blood creates a situation in which the hemoglobin molecule is unable to:

1. Let go of oxygen.

2. Accept oxygen.

3. Hold on to oxygen.

4. Create oxygen.

Correct answer: 1. DPG 2,3 is necessary to allow the hemoglobin molecule to let oxygen drop off and be used in the blood system. A lack of 2,3 DPG makes the hemoglobin molecule holds on to the oxygen or refuses to "let it go." DPG 2,3 has nothing to do with accepting or creating oxygen.

References

1. Carpenter DO. *Atlas of Pathophysiology*. Springhouse, PA: Springhouse; 2002.

2. Porth CM. *Essentials of Pathophysiology, Concepts of Altered Health States*. Philadelphia: Lippincott Williams & Wilkins; 2004.

3. Newberry L, Criddle LM. *Sheehy's Manual of Emergency Care*. 6th ed. Des Plaines, IL: Mosby; 2005.

4. Newberry L. *Sheehy's Emergency Nursing: Principles and Practice*. 5th ed. St. Louis: Mosby; 2003.

5. McCann JA. *Just the Facts: Pathophysiology*. Phildadelphia: Lippincott Williams & Wilkins; 2005.

6. *Effects on the Hematologic System*. Available at: www.rnceus.com/chem/heme.html. Accessed January 20, 2007.

7. *White Blood Cell Count (WBC) and Differential*. Available at: www.rnceus.com/cbc/cbcwbc.html. Accessed January 20, 2007.

8. Godwin JE, Braden CD. *Neutropenia*. Available at: www.emedincine.com/med/topic1640.htm. Accessed January 20, 2007.

9. Glucose-6-phosphate dehydrogenase deficiency. Available at: http://en.wikipedia.org/wiki/Glucose-6-phosphate_dehydrogenase_deficiency. Accessed January 20, 2007.

10. Johns Hopkins Medicine. *Types of Cancer: Aplastic Anemia*. Available at: www.hopkinskimmelcancercenter.org/cancerpes/aplastic-anemia.cfm?cnacerid=14. Accessed January 20, 2007.

11. Oh RC, Brown DL. *Vitamin B$_{12}$ Deficiency*. Available at: www.aafp.org/afp20030301/979.html. Accessed January 20, 2007.

12. Sickle Cell Society. *Information for Health Professionals*. Available at: www.sicklecellsociety.org/education/healthpr.htm. Accessed January 20, 2007.

13. Taher A, Kazzi Z. *Anemia: Sickle Cell*. Available at: www.emedicine.com/emerg/topic26.htm. Accessed January 20, 2007.

14. Symonette D, Hoffman E. *Thrombocytopenic Purpura*. Available at: www.emedicine.com/emerg/topic579.htm. Accessed January 20, 2007.

15. *Hemophilia Galaxy*. Available at: www.hemophiliagalaxy.com/general/
    encyclopedia.html. Accessed January 20, 2007.

16. National Hemophilia Foundation. *Future Therapies*. Available at:
    www.hemophilia.org/NHFweb/Mainpgs/MainNHF.aspx?menuid=
    202&contentid=384&prtname=bleeding. Accessed January 20, 2007.

17. Criddle LM. The trauma patient and recombinant factor VIIa.
    J Emerg Nurs. 2006;32:404–408.

18. *Blood Type*. Available at: http://en.wikipedia.org/wiki/Blood_type.
    Accessed January 20, 2007.

19. Karden E. *Transfusion Reactions*. Available at: http://emedicine.com/
    Emerg/topic603.htm. Accessed January 20, 2007.

Bibliography

Hurst Review Services. www.hurstreview.com.

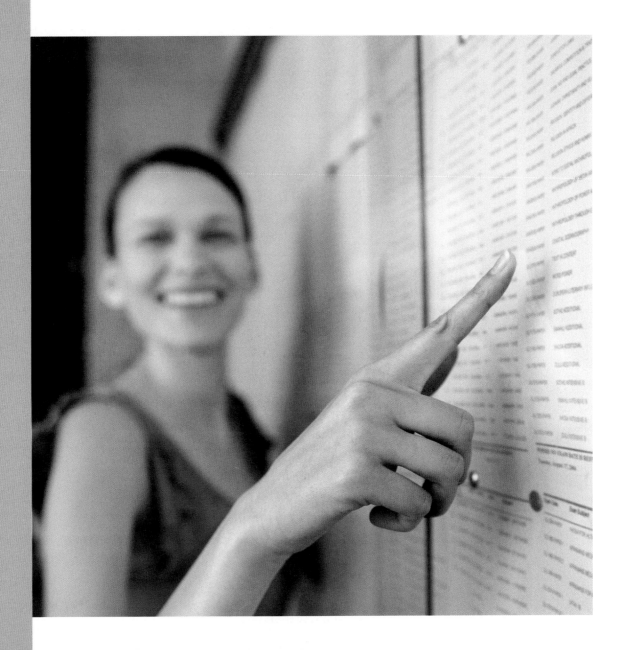

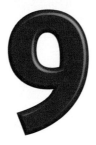

Nervous System

OBJECTIVES

In this chapter, you'll review:

* The function of the nervous system.
* The causes and signs and symptoms of, and the treatments for, nervous system disorders.
* The complications associated with nervous system disorders.

LET'S GET THE NORMAL STUFF STRAIGHT FIRST

The nervous system receives stimuli from the internal and external environment, interprets it, and integrates it into a selected response. The system is made up of two parts:

* Central nervous system (CNS).
* Peripheral nervous system.

✚ How does the nervous system work?

Let's break down the divisions further to help you better understand how they function together.

The central nervous system is divided into two parts:

* Brain, which controls many functions including mental, emotional, sensory, and motor functions (see "Brain structures and functions" later in this chapter).
* Spinal cord, which transmits messages from the spinal nerves to the brain and from the brain to the spinal nerves.

The peripheral nervous system is also divided into two parts (Fig. 9-1):

* Somatic nervous system, which consists of nerves that control voluntary body functions.
* Autonomic nervous system, which consists of nerves that regulate involuntary body functions.

▶ Figure 9-1. The nervous system. (From Saladin K. *Anatomy and Physiology: The Unity of Form and Function.* 4th ed. New York: McGraw-Hill 2007.)

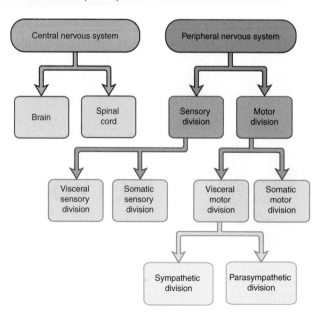

Brain structures and functions

Table 9-1 shows the different brain structures and their functions.

Table 9-1. Brain Structures and Functions

Structures	Functions
Cerebral cortex	Personality, judgment, thought, voluntary movement, language, reasoning, perception
Cerebellum	Movement, coordination, posture, balance
Medulla	Breathing, blood pressure, heart rate
Hypothalamus	Body temperature
Thalamus	Integration of emotions, maintenance of consciousness, sensory information, expression of recent memory
Hippocampus	Memory and learning
Basal ganglia	Integration of voluntary activity such as arm swinging and coordinating posture adjustments
Midbrain	Eye movements, body movements

Source: Created by author from Reference #1.

LET'S GET DOWN TO SPECIFICS

✚ Headache

What is it?

Headache is pain affecting the front, top, or sides of the head (Fig. 9-2). Often occurring in the middle of the day, the pain may have these characteristics:

- Mild to moderate.
- Constant.

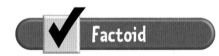

Factoid

The human brain weighs 1.3 to 1.4 kg (about 3 pounds); that's about 2% of your total body weight.

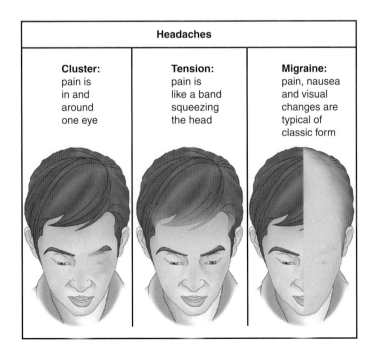

Headaches

Cluster: pain is in and around one eye

Tension: pain is like a band squeezing the head

Migraine: pain, nausea and visual changes are typical of classic form

◄ Figure 9-2. Types of headaches.

- Band-like pressure.
- Pressure or throbbing.

What causes it and why

Table 9-2 shows the causes of headache and why these causes occur.

Table 9-2

Causes	Why
Tension	Muscle tension from fatigue, emotional stress, or body position. Characteristics include mild to moderate pain that may be constant OR band-like pressure
Migraine	Constriction and then dilation of arteries to the brain. The pain is usually severe and throbbing in nature. Commonly unilateral, but can occur on both sides. Can be brought on by emotional upset, fatigue, nitrite- or tyramine-containing foods, or menstruation. May be related to the neurotransmitter serotonin
Cluster	Vasodilation that may be triggered by alcohol and tobacco. Most common in men, especially those who drink alcohol. A very common feature of the cluster headache is tearing of one eye. Pain is unilateral and is often described as a stabbing pain through one eye (knife-like or icepick). These headaches can be extremely severe and have been known to cause suicide
Symptom of serious illness	Underlying abnormality, such as arteritis, vascular abnormalities, subarachnoid hemorrhage, a brain lesion, bleeding, and disorders of the eyes, ears, sinus, or teeth
	Headaches due to intracranial masses or lesions usually present as dull and constant. Don't think that it's not a big deal just because its not severe. Approximately 1/3 of clients with brain tumor present with headache as their primary symptom
	Ocular or periocular pain usually accompanies a headache that has an ophthalmologic origin
	Sinus headaches usually have an accompanying tenderness overlying the skin and bone. This is known as maxillary or frontal sinus tenderness and is elicited by gentle percussion over these areas
Depression	Aches and pains are a common symptom of depression due to abnormality of serotonin in the brain. Certain neurotransmitters in the brain play a part in the interpretation of pain
Temporomandibular joint (TMJ) dysfunction	The TMJ is misaligned which triggers headache that is usually precipitated by chewing
Hypertension	Increased pressure can precipitate headache

Source: Created by author from Reference #2.

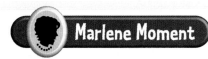

Marlene Moment

After retrieving a family friend from the middle of the floor one day, I drove him to the emergency department while he literally held his head, rocked back and forth, and banged it on the passenger side window because he was in such severe pain. I thought he might be psychotic or something but I soon found out he had a cluster headache including the typical feature of unilateral tearing.

Signs and symptoms and why

The signs and symptoms and rationales associated with headache are listed in Table 9-3.

Table 9-3

Signs and symptoms	Why
Pressure, pain, or a tight feeling in the temporal areas of the brain	Tight muscle fibers prevent or reduce blood flow to that area
Pain	Nervous system dysfunction or injury may trigger an inflammatory response
Nausea	Nervous system response or nervous system dysfunction
Headache pain with sensitivity to light (photophobia) and nausea	Response in brainstem causes reaction in the trigeminal nerve

Source: Created by author from Reference #1.

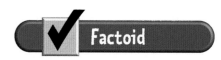

Factoid

About 23 million Americans suffer from a migraine each year.

Quickie tests and treatments

Tests:

- A thorough health history helps in making the diagnosis and determining the best treatment for headache.
- A physical examination with focus on the neurological exam.
- A skilled examiner can usually determine which type of headache the client is having OR determine the need for imaging studies such as CT or MRI if the neurological exam is abnormal.

Treatments include:

- Depends on the type of headache and whether it is acute or chronic.
- Quiet, dark room especially for migraines.
- Antiemetics such as phenergan if vomiting.
- Opiate analgesics.
- Meds like sumatriptan can be given to abort the headache but the cardiovascular risk must be weighed against the benefit. These are reserved for clients who are having two or more migraines per month. Ergot derivatives are also given to abort the headache but can also cause spontaneous abortion (miscarriage).
- Chronic migraines may be treated prophylactically with propranolol (beta-blocker), amitriptyline, clonidine, verapamil (calcium-channel blocker), cyproheptadine (Periactin), as well as various antidepressants.
- Opioid analgesics such as Demerol mixed with phenergan for severe attacks.
- Nonsteroidal, antiinflammatory drugs (NSAIDs) PO or IM such as Toradol, Decadron.

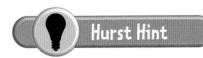

- Muscle relaxants (especially if precipitated by TMJ).
- Local measures such as heat, cold, or massage, especially if the pain affects the neck or upper back.

What can harm my client?

- Arteritis (vasculitis of medium- and large-sized vessels). Must be diagnosed rapidly to prevent permanent blindness. Treatment with prednisone and diagnosed by biopsy.
- Vascular abnormalities (aneurysms, etc.).
- Subarachnoid hemorrhage.
- Brain lesion.
- Bleeding.

If I were your teacher, I would test you on . . .

- Different types of headaches and defining features of each.
- Pain-control measures including meds.
- Key concepts of client education.
- Adverse effects of over-the-counter drugs.

Clinical application

If your client develops a headache (regardless of his reason for admission) and tells you he fell a few days ago, think "bleed" and notify the physician.

✚ Seizures

What are they?

A seizure is an abnormal electrical firing in the brain that interrupts normal function.

Epilepsy is a common condition in which unprovoked, recurrent seizures are caused by physiological changes.

TYPES OF SEIZURES   Seizures are classified as generalized seizures and partial seizures. Please see Table 9-4 for the types of seizures and their corresponding characteristics.

Table 9-4

Type	Characteristics
Absence seizure (also called petite mal seizure)	Generalized seizure
	Common in children
	Sudden onset
	Impaired responsiveness
	Eye fluttering or staring effect
	Duration less than 30 seconds

(Continued)

Table 9-4. (*Continued*)

Type	Characteristics
Generalized tonic clonic seizure (formerly called grand mal)	Generalized seizure Loss of consciousness followed by increased muscle tone Rhythmic muscle jerking
Myoclonic seizure	Generalized seizure Sudden muscle contractions Often occurs in limbs or face
Atonic seizure	Generalized seizure Called "drop attack" because person appears to drop the head, trunk, or limb and fall forward
Clonic seizure	Generalized seizure Loss of consciousness Sudden hypotonia Symmetrical jerking activity in the limb
Tonic seizure	Generalized seizure Sudden onset Increased tone Maintained in the muscles
Simple partial seizure	Partial seizure Does not produce an aura Sudden onset of cortical discharges that result in symptoms related to the area of the brain affected Symptoms may include an unusual taste in the mouth, vomiting, sweating, or facial twitching
Complex partial seizures	Partial seizure Cortical discharges that result in symptoms related to the area of the brain affected Altered level of consciousness
Status epilepticus	Consists of two consecutive seizures One continuous seizure that lasts greater than 30 minutes without a clearing in between. Medical emergency that can lead to brain damage and death Physiological changes occur during status epilepticus because of a release of epinephrine and norepinephrine Over time, progresses to maladaptive mechanisms, leading to permanent changes in the body

Source: Created by author from Reference #2.

What causes it and why

The cause of about 75% of seizure disorders is unknown. Table 9-5 shows the known causes of seizures and why these causes occur.

Table 9-5

Causes	Why
Idiopathic or constitutional	Unknown
Trauma	Damage to the dura mater
Abnormality in the brain	Tumor or other space-occupying lesion
Infectious diseases	Brain abscess, bacterial meningitis, herpes encephalitis, neurosyphilis, AIDS with concomitant infections with toxoplasmosis, cryptococcal meningitis, secondary viral encephalitis
Genetic factors, family history of seizures	Low threshold for stimuli that trigger seizures
Epilepsy	Abnormal neurons that fire spontaneously
Congenital abnormalities or perinatal injuries	Result in onset of seizures in infancy or childhood
Metabolic disorders	Alcohol or drug withdrawal Uremia hyperglycemia
Degenerative diseases	Alzheimer's

Source: Created by author from Reference #2.

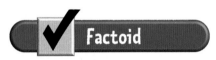

Alcohol and benzodiazepines (Xanax, Valium, etc.) are the only two types of drugs that can cause seizures and potential death during detoxification or withdrawal. Withdrawal from opiates, amphetamines, THC (pot), crack, cocaine, etc., will make the client miserable during detoxification but will not induce seizures.

Precipitating factors include:

- Lack of sleep (however, they do sometimes occur during sleep).
- Missed meals.
- Emotional stress or upset.
- Menstruation.
- Alcohol ingestion.
- Alcohol withdrawal.
- Fever.
- Infection.
- Flashing lights or flickering television (photosensitive epilepsy).
- Music.
- Reading.

Signs and symptoms and why

The following signs and symptoms and rationales associated with seizures are shown in Table 9-6.

Table 9-6

Signs and symptoms	Why
No aura and a loss of consciousness	Generalized seizures affect both sides of the brain
Aura, no loss of consciousness, motor or sensory effects	Simple partial seizures affect a specific area of the brain and the functions controlled by it
Aura, altered consciousness, and affective, behavioral, cognitive, or emotional effects	Complex partial seizures affect the temporal lobe
Continuous seizure activity without a return to consciousness	Repeated or continuous seizures (status epilepticus) exhaust the brain's neurons, causing them to stop working

Source: Created by author from Reference #2.

An aura is a phenomenon that occurs prior to a seizure. An aura may include a funny taste, smell, or staring. Some seizures are preceded by headache, mood changes, lethargy, jerking movements, etc. These are nonspecific changes and are not considered to be an actual aura.

Quickie tests and treatments

Tests:

- Obtain a complete description of the seizure and the events leading up to it. Obtain a complete history including past medical history, social and family history.
- MRI.
- Blood test for CBC, glucose, liver and kidney function.
- Electroencephalogram (EEG) confirms any electrical abnormality and the type and location of the seizure.

Treatments:

- Anticonvulsive drugs, including carbamazepine (Tegretol), phenobarbital, phenytoin (Dilantin), and valproic acid (Depakene) to prevent further attacks and may be discontinued after the client has been seizure free for 3 years. Drug levels must be monitored.
- Avoid situations that could be dangerous or life-threatening (bathing alone, driving, etc.).
- Surgery in which electrodes are inserted in brain tissue for a better evaluation of the source of the seizure.
- Vagal nerve stimulation.

What can harm my client?

- Brain damage (status epilepticus).
- Bodily injury.

If I were your teacher, I would test you on . . .

- Care of the client with status epilepticus.
- The types of seizures, with particular attention to the signs of status epilepticus.
- Types of anticonvulsant drugs that can be prescribed for your client.
- Client education regarding anticonvulsive drugs.
- Avoidance of triggers.
- Avoidance of potentially dangerous activities.
- Know that many of the drugs used require checking "blood levels" periodically.

✦ Guillain–Barré syndrome (acute idiopathic polyneuropathy)

What is it?

It is an inflammatory, demyelinating disease whose etiology is not completely understood but probably immunologic in origin. It affects people of any age, sex, or race and is characterized by extreme weakness and

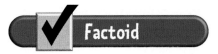

Factoid

Did you know that about 10% of people in the United States experience a single, unprovoked seizure in their lifetime?

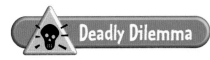

Deadly Dilemma

Status epilepticus is a medical emergency that can lead to further brain damage and death.

numbness or tingling in the extremities and a loss of movement or feeling in the upper body and face progressing to paralysis. There is an association with infections, vaccinations, and surgery. Most clients have good recovery but it may take months.

What causes it and why

The cause of Guillain–Barré syndrome is unknown, but in about 50% of cases, the onset follows the infections in Table 9-7.

Table 9-7

Causes	Why
Viral infection, bacterial infection, common cold, mononucleosis, hepatitis, gastrointestinal (GI) infection, inoculations	Pathogens in these infections, such as *Campylobacter jejuni* in GI infection, are thought to alter the immune system, causing T-lymphocytes to be sensitized to myelin and to trigger demyelination

Source: Created by author from Reference #2.

Signs and symptoms and why

The signs and symptoms and rationales associated with Guillain–Barré syndrome are shown in Table 9-8.

Table 9-8

Signs and symptoms	Why
Numbness	Nerve impulses slow down or cease
Tingling in fingers or toes	Nerve impulses slow down or cease
Mild difficulty in walking	With denervation, muscles atrophy
Complete paralysis of the extremities	With denervation, muscles atrophy

More on Signs/Symptoms

Weakness usually begins in the legs, then spreads to involve the arms and face. Respiratory muscles may be involved. Life-threatening complications can occur such as tachycardia, arrhythmias, and pulmonary dysfunction	

Source: Created by author from Reference #2.

Quickie tests and treatments

Guillain–Barré syndrome is difficult to diagnose because of the varied symptoms, but if symptoms occur uniformly across the body and progress rapidly, the diagnosis is made much easier.

Tests:

- Lumbar puncture cerebrospinal fluid (CSF) analysis (Fig. 9-3).
- Electromyography (EMG).
- Nerve conduction studies.

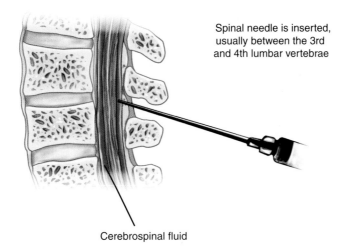

Spinal needle is inserted,
usually between the 3rd
and 4th lumbar vertebrae

◀ Figure 9-3. Lumbar puncture.

Cerebrospinal fluid

Treatments:

- Ventilatory support if indicated.
- Plasmapheresis in severe or rapidly declining cases.
- Immunoglobulin IV.
- Nutritional therapy.
- Treatment with prednisone is ineffective.

What can harm my client?

- Respiratory failure.
- Deep vein thrombosis and pulmonary emboli.
- Skin breakdown.
- Relapses.
- 10% to 20% of clients are left with residual disability.

If I were your teacher, I would test you on . . .

- Signs and symptoms of Guillain–Barré syndrome.
- Types of therapy for Guillain–Barré syndrome.
- Serious complications of Guillain–Barré syndrome.
- No flu shot if history of GBS!

✛ Alzheimer's disease

What is it?

This is a chronic, progressive, degenerative disease that affects clients over the age of 65, although it has been known to occur between the ages of 40 and 50. It is the most common form of dementia. Structural changes in the brain (Fig. 9-4) include accelerated decline in brain mass or weight with enlargement of the ventricles. Microscopic changes as well as chemical changes also take place. The degenerative changes result in a declining ability to cope with everyday life as brain cells die.

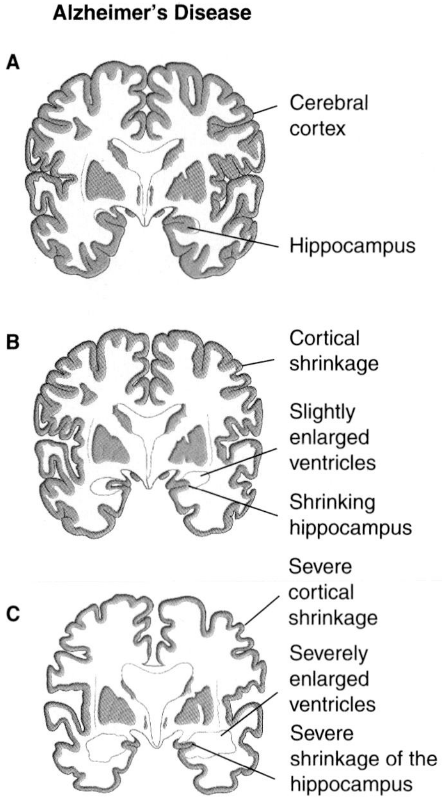

► Figure 9-4. The brain and Alzheimer's disease. **A.** Healthy brain. **B.** Mild Alzheimer's diseased brain. **C.** Severe Alzheimer's diseased brain.

Alzheimer's Disease

A
- Cerebral cortex
- Hippocampus

B
- Cortical shrinkage
- Slightly enlarged ventricles
- Shrinking hippocampus

C
- Severe cortical shrinkage
- Severely enlarged ventricles
- Severe shrinkage of the hippocampus

What causes it and why

The exact cause is unknown, but several factors contribute to the development of Alzheimer's disease as seen in Table 9-9. Age, however is the most important risk factor. AD is described as familial (inherited), sporadic (not related to genetics), early onset, and late onset. Early onset occurs prior to the age of 65. There have been cases as young as thirties and forties. Late onset occurs around 65 years and older.

Table 9-9

Causes	Why
Genetics—familial AD (FAD)	Certain genes (ApoE) mutate because they are defective, causing an excessive production of amyloid, which forms plaques in the brain. This type is related to early-onset AD. Most cases of early onset AD is associated with mutations in genes.
	Down syndrome is a risk factor for Alzheimer's (late onset) due to effect of apolipoprotein E on chromosome 19.
	There is currently ongoing research regarding genetics and AD.
Vascular degeneration	Exact mechanism is not understood. Leads to improperly functioning nerve cells.
Chemical imbalances	Reduced neurotransmitters in the brain (for whatever reason) are thought to be a factor in the development of AD, which leads to increased risk over time.
Family history	If one relative has Alzheimer's, then a familial component exists due to presence of gene mutations.

Source: Created by author from Reference #2.

LET'S GET SOMETHING STRAIGHT   Pick's disease is different from Alzheimer's. It is a rare form of dementia manifested by atrophy of the frontal and temporal areas of the brain. Pick bodies can be found in neurons. Average age of onset is 38, and it is more common in women than men. Clinical course usually begins with behavior symptoms such as loss of interest or concern progressing to hypotonia and eventual death. Remember, this is RARE.

Signs and symptoms and why

Alzheimer's disease has several familiar warning signs, as shown in Table 9-10.

Table 9-10

Signs and symptoms	Why
Short-term memory impairment is often the first sign	Decreased brain mass, enlarged ventricles, amyloid plaques, and decreased oxygenation of brain tissue lead to decreased cognitive function related to improperly functioning nerve cells
Language disturbance (can't find words to communicate—this is called scanning speech)	
Decline in motor skills	
Loss of abstract thought processes	
Visual processing impairment	
Repetitive actions	
Restlessness at night	
Incontinence, emaciation, irritability, and coma are late manifestations of the disease	

Source: Created by author from Reference #2.

CLINICAL APPLICATION   Asking the same question again and again, repeating the same story, forgetting how to perform activities of daily living, being unable to pay bills or balance one's checkbook, loss of the ability to sequence tasks (gets filter out for coffee, fills it up with coffee, but forgets to turn it on, or starts cooking and forgets about it and the house catches on fire), getting lost in familiar surroundings, misplacing objects, neglecting to bathe, wearing the same clothing again and again, relying on someone else to make decisions one previously made, not recognizing familiar places or people. In early stages they will have periods of complete mental lucidity (normal thought processes). Eventually they lose sense of time. Late stages result in lack of interest in food and they begin to lose weight. Depression is very common.

Quickie tests and treatments

Tests:

- No one test can determine if a person has Alzheimer's disease, but a blood test may be used to identify ApoE as a risk for dementia. Also, a newer skin test, Alzheimer's index, may be used to determine if early dementia results from Alzheimer's disease.

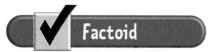

Factoid

The client can even get lost in her own home.

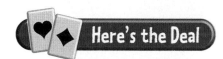

Here's the Deal

Many AD clients experience sundowning. This is when they become disoriented and begin to wander in the afternoon and evening time (worse on cloudy days).

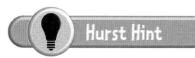

Hurst Hint

In late stages, they can't recognize close family members and eventually may not even recognize their own self in a mirror. This is why we do not place mirrors in AD clients' rooms. Seeing their own image in the mirror can precipitate violent behavior related to fear resulting in self-harm.

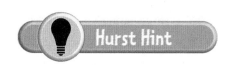

Hurst Hint

It would take air to make me lose interest in food!

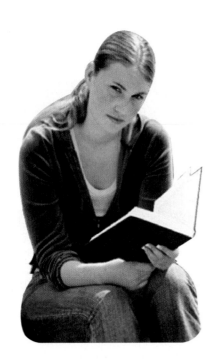

- Diagnosis can only be confirmed by examining brain tissue after death.
- Client history (must include family).
- CT, MRI, or SPECT (single-photon emission computed tomography).
- Neuropsychological.
- Mental status assessment.
- Blood tests for CBC, sed rate, chemistry panel, TSH, RPR (syphilis), urinalysis, B_{12}, folate, and HIV, part of a normal dementia workup. Remember, medical etiology is always ruled out when dealing with any type of psychiatric disorder.

Treatments:

- Cholinesterase inhibitors, such as donepezil (Acricept) for decreased memory.
- Selective serotonin reuptake inhibitors, such as sertraline (Zoloft) for depression.
- Antipsychotics, such as haloperidol (Haldol) for agitation.
- Hypnotics, such as zolpidem (Ambien) for difficulty sleeping.
- There is no cure for AD but we try to maximize what abilities they do have and prevent any further progression of the disease.
- Vitamin E may improve cognition.

Ways to prevent injury/harm:

- Put up any potentially dangerous chemicals. (I had a client who drank antifreeze by mistake thinking it was Gatorade).
- Fence the yard and lock rooms that contain unsafe items in them.
- Adjust the water heater to prevent burns.
- Replacing stove with microwave.
- Modify or apply safety devices over the controls on the stove.
- Labeling items may help in early stages of the disease but eventually this won't work.

What can harm my client?

- Unsafe behaviors (such as wandering out in the middle of the night or day)—they can't be left alone.
- Falls.
- Pain.
- Eating and swallowing difficulties.
- Infection.
- Malnutrition.
- Pressure ulcers.
- Compromised immune status related to wasting and malnutrition.

If I were your teacher, I would test you on . . .

- Warning signs of Alzheimer's disease (early manifestations).
- New tests to determine risks for dementia and treatment to slow progress of disease.

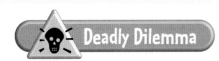

Aspiration pneumonia is a frequent cause of death due to swallowing difficulties later on in the disease.

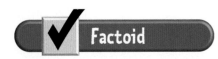

AD clients may live 8 to 10 years following diagnosis but some can actually live for up to 20.

- Common manifestations of the disease. (How do AD clients typically act? And what are they in danger of?)
- Shadow boxes are often used to help trigger memory or help the client recognize their room. A shadow box includes pictures from the past, etc.
- The nurse must consider the strain on the caregiver.

✛ Amyotrophic lateral sclerosis (ALS)

What is it?

A serious, rapidly progressive, debilitating, and fatal neurological disease, ALS (also called Lou Gehrig's disease) attacks the nerve cells that control voluntary muscles. There are no sensory or cognitive changes. Most people are diagnosed around the age of 40 to 50. It is most common in men in earlier age groups but after menopause, women are equally as affected. Problems with upper motor neurons cause weak muscles that are spastic with increased deep tendon reflexes (DTRs). Lower motor neuron problems cause flaccid muscles, weakness (paresis), paralysis, and wasting of muscle (atrophy).

What causes it and why

Table 9-11 shows the causes of ALS and why these causes occur.

Table 9-11

Causes	Why
Death of motor neurons that control the voluntary muscles of arms, legs, face, neck, and body	Motor neurons in the spinal cord and brainstem progressively degenerate may be familial or sporadic
Destruction of muscles that control the ability to talk, chew, swallow, and breathe	Dead neurons can't send signals to the muscles to activate them

Source: Created by author from Reference #2.

Signs and symptoms and why

The following signs and symptoms and rationales associated with ALS are found in Table 9-12. Signs and symptoms may vary according to the muscle group involved.

Table 9-12

Signs and symptoms	Why
Weakness in leg or hand	Muscle wasting, fasciculation caused by denervation
Clumsiness	
Difficulty swallowing and dysphagia	Atrophy of tongue and facial muscles
Slurring	↑ DTR's
Twitching in the arms	Muscle wasting
Extreme fatigue	

Source: Created by author from Reference #2.

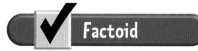

The most common motor neuron disease in the United States is ALS.

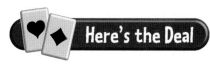

The major health problems seen with ALS are swallowing difficulties, communication problems, and loss of function of respiratory muscles.

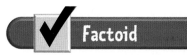

In ALS, the client's ability to see, hear, and feel as well as ability to think are unaffected.

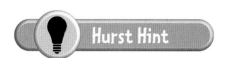

Paresis and twitching of muscles are commonly seen in the early stages. It usually travels from hands, shoulders, and arms to the legs over time.

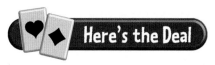

The symptoms of ALS may mimic other diseases such as stroke, carpal tunnel syndrome, and other neurological conditions, so these other disease processes must be excluded.

Quickie tests and treatments

Tests:

- Electromyography (EMG) gives information about what is happening with the muscles.
- There is no test to specifically diagnose ALS. Diagnosis is usually made by ruling out other conditions and by the signs/symptoms.

Treatments:

Treatment is geared toward:

- Making the client as comfortable and independent as possible.
- Slowing the progression of the disease.

The only drug approved for slowing the progression of ALS is riluzole (Rilutek). These other medications may also be used:

- The antibiotic minocycline (Minocin).
- The breast-cancer drug tamoxifen (Tamofen).
- The antioxidant coenzyme Q10.

The entire multidisciplinary team plays a key role in treating the client, using:

- Physical therapy.
- Speech therapy.
- Nutritional support.
- Respiratory therapy.

What can harm my client?

- Compromised respiration function—respiratory related death is usually what kills the client.
- Muscle wasting.
- Dysphagia.

If I were your teacher, I would test you on . . .

- The importance of using a multidisciplinary approach in caring for clients diagnosed with ALS.
- Side effects of the medications used in treatment of ALS.
- Coping strategies for families caring for an individual suffering from ALS.

✚ Multiple sclerosis (MS)

What is it?

A chronic, debilitating, progressive disease of the central nervous system. MS is characterized by demyelination of nerves of the central nervous system. MS usually appears between the ages of 20 and 50 and affects females more than males. An autoimmune response occurs as a result of a viral infection in a person who is susceptible genetically for MS. The inflammatory response sets in as T-cells, which were needed to fight infection, did not leave the CNS postinfection. Inflammation destroys myelin (which insulates nerves) and cells that produce myelin. The myelin sheaths that protect nerves normally are destroyed in a patchy manner. The patchy areas are called plaques. When the myelin is intact, the nerve impulses can move rapidly. However, in MS, the impulses are slow, distorted, and may become completely absent. The most commonly affected nerves are located in the following places: the white matter of the spinal cord, optic nerve, brainstem, cerebrum, and cerebellum.

MS can be classified in 4 ways:

1. Relapsing remitting: most common; acute attacks with either complete/partial recovery.

2. Primary progressive: steady debilitation; occasional episodes of improved health.

3. Secondary progressive: same as with relapsing remitting initially, but health significantly worsens even during remissions.

4. Progressive relapsing: steady debilitation coupled with periods of acute attacks.

What causes it and why

The definite cause of multiple sclerosis (MS) is unknown, but some researchers believe it is caused by the herpes virus or retrovirus, or some unknown antigen that triggers a reaction directed against the body's own tissue. The following tend to be associated with MS.

Table 9-13 shows the causes of MS and why these causes occur.

Table 9-13

Causes	Why
Heredity	Five percent of clients have a brother or sister who is affected, 15% have a close relative who is affected
Environment	Occurs mostly in clients who grow up in temperate climates; less likely to occur in those who grow up in tropical climates or near the equator
Inflammatory lesion	Inflammation causes deterioration and loss of axons, resulting in death of affected neurons
Infection	Refer to above information under "What is it?"

Source: Created by author from Reference #1.

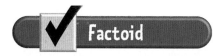

Remember there are many types of herpes viruses. Not just the one causing genital herpes!

Signs and symptoms and why

As different parts of the nervous system are affected, signs/symptoms will vary. There will be episodes of remissions and exacerbations (acute attacks). However, over time, the disease is progressive with inevitable loss of body function.

The following signs and symptoms and rationales associated with MS are shown in Table 9-14.

Table 9-14

Signs and symptoms	Why
Blurred vision, optic neuritis, double vision (diplopia), nystagmus	Inflammation of the optic nerve
Loss of muscle strength in extremities resulting in fatigue and weakness, clumsiness, tremor, uncoordinated eye movements, stiffness, unsteadiness, bowel and bladder changes, constipation	Demyelination of nerve fibers
Impaired reflexes (may increase, decrease, or may be normal)	Demyelination of nerves
Paresthesia—abnormal sensations including pain, burning, itching, numbness, tingling, prickling sensation	Damaged sensory nerve fibers
Mood swings, inappropriate giddiness, euphoria, depression, apathy, memory disturbances, decreased judgment, inattention	Demyelination in the brain
Difficulty articulating words (dysarthria)	Same

Source: Created by author from Reference #1.

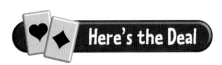

Factoid

The majority of clients with MS have problems associated with urination. These problems can also precipitate an acute attack.

Here's the Deal

The true cause of MS isn't understood. The treatment options delay the disease progression, but do not cure the disease. The MS client needs a comprehensive approach to lifelong disease management to optimize outcomes.

Quickie tests and treatments

No single test confirms MS, but a combination of tests may lead to a diagnosis.

Tests:

* Eye examination: optic nerve may be inflamed or unusually pale.
* Lumbar puncture: increased white blood cell count and protein CSF.
* MRI: detects areas of demyelination in the brain and spinal cord.

Treatments:

Because there is no cure, the goal is to delay the progression of the disease and treat symptoms accordingly to improve quality of life.

Medications used:

* Immunomodulators: interferon beta-1a (Avonex), interferon beta-1b (Betaseron), glatiramer acetate (Copaxone); slow progression of disease.
* Adrenalcorticosteroids: prednisone, adrenocorticotropic hormone (ACTH), methylprednisolone (Solu-Medrol); used to treat exacerbations and to prolong remissions.
* Muscle relaxants: baclofen, dantrolene, diazepam (Valium); relieve muscle spasms.
* Immunosuppressants: Imuran, Cytoxan; MS has an autoimmune component; as these drugs suppress the immune system, they may also suppress the disease.
* Anticholinergics: used for bladder spasms.
* Cholinergics: used to treat urinary retention associated with a flaccid bladder.

- Antidepressants: used in treatment of depression.
- Surgery for severe spasticity/deformity.
- Physical therapy.

The goals of management are to:
- Delay progression of disability.
- Treat relapses as effectively as possible.
- Manage the symptoms.
- Promote the best possible quality of life.

What can harm my client?

- Declining quality of life.
- Emotional instability.
- Sexual dysfunction.
- Immobility and pressure ulcers.
- Respiratory problems.
- Infections (bladder, lungs, possibly sepsis).
- Complications with being immobile.

If I were your teacher, I would test you on . . .

- Main goals of MS management.
- Ways to help clients manage symptoms and caregivers cope.
- Definition of MS.
- Causes and why.
- Signs/symptoms and why.
- Ways to manage symptoms associated with MS.
- Medications used in the treatment of MS.
- Complications.

✚ Myasthenia gravis

What is it?

Myasthenia gravis (MG) is a chronic autoimmune neuromuscular disease characterized by weakness of voluntary muscles. The major symptoms associated with MG are fatigue and severe weakness of the skeletal muscles. The client will experience times of complete remission but also have periods of exacerbation. The weakness associated with MG may affect only a few muscle groups (ocular muscles mainly). However, the condition may eventually affect all muscles. It is most common in women.

Causes and why

The underlying cause of myasthenia gravis is unknown. However, it is known that antibodies attach to the affected areas, impeding the muscle cells from receiving messages from the nerve cells (Table 9-15).

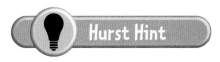

Hurst Hint

Rest or sleep may not relieve the extreme fatigue associated with MS.

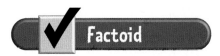

Factoid

The true cause of MS isn't understood, and the treatment options delay the disease progression but don't cure the disease. The MS client needs a comprehensive approach to lifelong disease management to optimize outcomes.

Table 9-15

Causes	Why
Decreased number of acetylcholine receptors	Acetylcholine (ACh) is a neurotransmitter found in the neuromuscular junction responsible for stimulation of muscles. Without it, the muscles will not be stimulated. Antibodies can destroy or change the neuromuscular junction, which will result in fewer acetylcholine receptors. Due to damage at the junction, there may be decreased ACh uptake as well
Thymus gland	The thymus gland is usually inactive after puberty; however, in MG it continues to produce antibodies for various reasons. These antibodies are responsible for initiating an autoimmune response

Source: Created by author from Reference #2.

Signs and symptoms and why

The signs and symptoms and rationales associated with myasthenia gravis are shown in Table 9-16. The signs/symptoms begin with the eyes, progressing to the face (speech and chewing problems) and then to the neck and on down to the lower limbs. Signs/symptoms and the severity may change from day to day.

Table 9-16

Signs and symptoms	Why
Vision changes such as double vision (diplopia), drooping of the eyelids (ptosis), difficulty keeping a steady gaze	Weakness of eyelid muscles and extraocular muscles
Difficulty swallowing, hoarseness, or a change in voice, drooling, inability to keep head from drooping	Weakness of proximal muscles of the neck
Weakness or paralysis, difficulty lifting objects, muscles that function best after rest	Weakness of proximal muscles of the shoulders and hips
Exhaustion of muscles of mastication (chewing muscles) leading to the need for a break during eating.	Muscle weakness
Abnormal appearance of expression (smile may look like a snarl or grimace)	Same
Voice is weak, muffled, and is nasal in quality	Same
Difficulty with fine motor movements (writing)	Seen early in disease

Source: Created by author from Reference #2.

What will exacerbate the symptoms? Any stress on the body (fever, overworking, heat); rest tends to relieve symptoms.

Quickie tests and treatments

Tests:

* Physical examination, which may be normal or reveal muscle weakness.
* Electromyography (EMG).

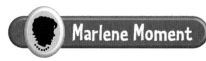

Marlene Moment

I had an encounter with a client one day. As an NP, he sat on the exam table with his chin on his chest during the entire visit. Turns out, he had MG.

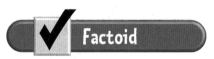

Factoid

MG is often associated with stress on the body (menses, pregnancy, infection). The diagnosis is often diagnosed when the client seeks treatment for signs/symptoms exacerbated by these things.

- Tensilon test—short-acting anticholinesterase. Client is considered to be positive for MG if muscle strength improves after injection of tensilon. This test is also used to differentiate between myasthenic crisis and cholinergic crisis. If crisis is myasthenic in nature, it will improve with tensilon. With cholinergic crisis there will be no improvement.
- Blood test for acetylcholine antibodies.
- CT to detect enlarged thymus.

Treatments:

There is no known cure for MG.

Therapy may include:

- Surgical removal of the thymus.
- Neostigmine (Prostigmin) to increase nerve impulses.
- Prednisone to decrease inflammation.
- Adjustments to the client's lifestyle with special attention to scheduled rest periods. Plasmapheresis to remove antibodies.
- Management of myasthenia crisis as needed.

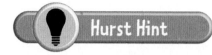

Teach the client to avoid heat exposure because, along with stress, it can aggravate symptoms of myasthenia gravis.

What can harm my client?

- Dysphagia.
- Aspiration.
- Respiratory distress.
- Myasthenic crisis—sudden onset of weakness that can cause respiratory complications as well as aspiration. It usually occurs when client has missed a dose of medication and blood level drops OR is precipitated by an infection. Look for signs of severe respiratory distress, anxiety, and impaired speech.
- Cholinergic crisis—seen when the client is taking too much of her anticholinergic medication. Look for severe muscle weakness and respiratory distress.
- Both types of crises are medical emergencies and may require mechanical ventilation.

If I were your teacher, I would test you on . . .

- Definition of MG.
- Causes and why.
- Symptoms of myasthenia gravis.
- Helping the client and family cope with lifestyle changes.
- Teaching the client about prescribed drugs and side effects.
- Importance of rest and minimizing fatigue.
- Cranial nerve assessment.
- Importance of respiratory assessment.

✚ Parkinson's disease

What is it?

Parkinson's disease is a progressive disorder of the CNS, affecting a person's movement, balance, and muscle control. It is more common in males with onset of symptoms typically between the ages of 40 and 70. The average age of onset is 60. Normally a system of checks and balances exists within the brain with regard to motor function. This is made possible through the actions of the neurotransmitters dopamine and acetylcholine (ACh). Neurons that produce ACh are responsible for transmitting excitatory messages and dopamine inhibits the functions of these neurons, which results in control over voluntary movement. If it were not for this system, you could not voluntarily pick up a pen or pencil and write your name. In PD there is a lack of dopamine, which results in loss of ability to refine or coordinate motor movements on a voluntary basis. Also, a lot of ACh-producing neurons are still active, which results in an imbalance between excitation and inhibitory neuronal activity. So, you don't have enough dopamine in relationship to your ACh. You've got too much excitement and not enough reversal of the excitement.

What causes it and why

The exact cause of Parkinson's disease is unknown, but there are several possible causes, as seen in Table 9-17.

Table 9-17

Causes	Why
Genetics	Certain autosomal dominant and recessive genes are linked to the disease. Some clients with PD have been found to have an extra copy of the gene alpha-synuclein (SNCA), which results in excessive buildup of protein in the brain
Endogenous toxins	The disease has developed after intoxication with carbon monoxide and other toxins
Environmental exposures to toxins	Endotoxins called lipopolysaccharides (LPSs) are in the air in agricultural and other industries. Other risk factors may include living in rural areas or near wood pulp mills and well water consumption
Medications	Interfere with or block the action of dopamine and other neurotransmitters
Viral infection	The disease has developed after infection with type A encephalitis
Structural brain disorders	Brain tumor, stroke, and head injury cause damage to the brain

Source: Created by author from Reference #2.

Signs and symptoms and why

The signs and symptoms vary according to the stage of disease. The stages range from stage I, which is the initial stage resulting in mild symptoms, to stage 5, which results in complete dependence on others for care.

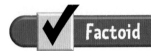
Factoid

Michael J. Fox (an actor who played on "Family Ties") developed PD in his thirties.

The signs and symptoms and rationales associated with Parkinson's disease are shown in Table 9-18.

Table 9-18

Signs and symptoms	Why
Stage 1—Initial	
Resting tremor with mild weakness, possibly unilateral (one sided)	Reduced production of dopamine and/or neurotransmitter imbalance. Emotional stress or fatigue increases tremor
Stage 2—Mild	
Bilateral symptoms with a mask-like facies (blunted or flat affect/no expression), and a slow shuffling gait	Neurotransmitter imbalance
Stage 3—Moderate	
All of the above symptoms with significant progression of gait disturbance and postural instability	Same
Stage 4—Severe Disability	
Akinesia (loss of movement/inability to initiate motor function) with rigidity. Rigidity can interfere with chewing and swallowing (involvement of pharyngeal muscles), resulting in malnutrition	Imbalance of neurotransmitters with eventual sustained muscle contraction
	Let's talk about rigidity for a moment: rigidity is the resistance to passive movement of the extremities. You may hear it referred to as "cogwheeling," which means a rhythmic interruption of the muscle (starting and stopping)
	Plastic rigidity is known as mildly restrictive movement
	Lead pipe rigidity is known as total resistance to movement
	The amount of rigidity will progress over time
Other Signs and Symptoms May Include	
Decreased sense of smell	Degeneration of brain cells in the areas involved in smell; difficulty sniffing
Drooling	Neurotransmitter imbalance. Ever notice how psychiatric clients on Haldol (alters chemical in the brain) often drool?
Dementia	Advanced disease with associated damage to the brain
Orthostatic hypotension and excessive perspiration	Baroreflex failure related to disease process once thought to be related to levodopa therapy

Source: Created by author from Reference #2.

Clinical application

When your father develops an unexplained "limp" followed by a slight tremor and forgetfulness, progressing to a shuffling "stooped over" or "forward-leaning" posture, you'd better be thinking about PD. These clients can become bed-bound and completely dependent within 1 year.

Quickie tests and treatments

Tests:

• There's no diagnostic test for Parkinson's disease. The diagnosis is based on the client's history and clinical observation after ruling out other disease processes.

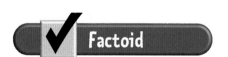
Factoid

By the time a client experiences symptoms of Parkinson's disease, as many as 90% of dopamine-producing cells have already been destroyed.

- CSF may show decreased dopamine levels, but again, it is usually just a diagnosis of exclusion because the features are so obvious in this disease.

Treatments:

Drug therapy includes the following:

- Dopaminergics, such as levodopa-carbidopa (Sinemet).
- Benzotropine (Cogentin).
- Monoamine oxidase inhibitors, such as selegiline (Eldepryl).
- Anticholinergics, such as trihexyphenidyl (Artane).
- Antihistamines, such diphenhydramine (Benadryl).
- Catechol-O-methyl transferase inhibitors, such as entacapone (Comtan).
- Surgery: medial pallidotomy results in destruction of cells in certain part of the brain, improving symptoms.
- Other therapy includes chronic deep brain (thalamus) stimulation (DBS): an implant is inserted under the skin to stimulate and disrupt the area of the brain that causes the disabling motor symptoms of Parkinson's disease. This can be effective when the client is unresponsive to medications.
- Brain tissue transplant is being researched/studied using fetal tissue with genetically engineered cells and animal cells. These are made in order to produce dopamine. Other ongoing research includes stem cell research. Please note there are many moral and ethical issues associated with this type of research. We only attempt to educate you regarding the latest.

Necessary therapy:

- Physical therapy with daily exercise including warm baths and massages to relax muscles.
- Occupational therapy to help with fine motor tasks.
- Speech therapy to help with speech and swallowing problems.
- Prevent constipation with high-fiber diet, increased water, implementing regular bowel regimen, and stool softeners or laxatives as prescribed.
- Emotional support.
- Community referrals such as home health, meals on wheels, transportation assistance, social services, etc. Consider this: some clients who develop PD may live alone; therefore, many changes are coming their way and fast. Realize this so you can offer support and be an advocate.
- Soothing music for relaxation.
- Assistive devices such as grab rails for tub/toilet/shower, raised toilet seat, and no throw rugs.

What can harm my client?

- Risks associated with brain surgery, such as stroke, confusion, attention problems, hemorrhage, and leakage of cerebral spinal fluid (CSF) around the implant device.
- Dementia.
- Depression.

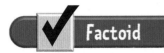

Currently, there is no known cure or prevention; however, it has been found that regular users of NSAIDs or at least two aspirin per day have a significantly lower risk for the development of PD than those who do not use them regularly. This reduction in risk registers in at 45%!

- Impaired communication.
- Immobility.
- Falls.
- Wounds related to incontinence and bed-bound status.
- Dysphagia and aspiration.
- Sleep disorders.
- Memory impairment.
- Abuse.

If I were your teacher, I would test you on . . .

- The role of dopamine and ACh in the development of Parkinson's disease.
- Signs/symptoms.
- Treatment.
- DBS surgery.
- Complications and/or what can harm my client.

✛ Stroke

What is it?

Stroke is an abrupt, dramatic neurological event caused by an interruption of blood flow to the brain. This disruption can either be ischemic or related to hemorrhage (aka hemorrhagic stroke). Ischemic stroke accounts for about 90% of all strokes, but hemorrhagic stroke is associated with a much higher fatality rate. The National Stroke Association is now referring to stroke as "brain attack."

In ischemic stroke, the most common type, a blood clot blocks arterial blood flow to part of the brain. The two types of ischemic stroke are:

- Embolic stroke (Fig. 9-5): an embolus is a group of emboli (aka group of clots). An embolus forms somewhere in the body (usually in the heart

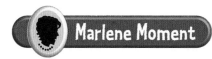

Marlene Moment

My grandmother used to call it an "attack" or a "spell." There is wisdom with age!

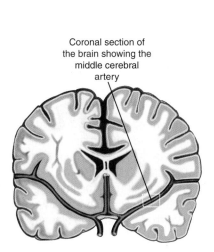

Coronal section of the brain showing the middle cerebral artery

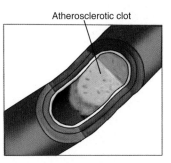

Atherosclerotic clot

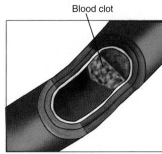

Blood clot

◀ Figure 9-5. Embolic ischemic stroke.

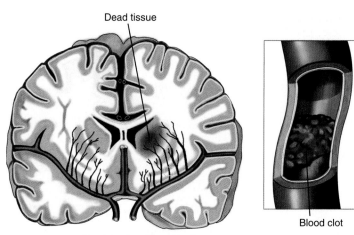

► Figure 9-6. Thrombotic ischemic stroke.

Dead tissue

Blood clot

Frontal cut-section of brain

or a large artery leading to the brain), travels to the brain, and blocks an artery, leading to a stroke.

- Thrombotic stroke (large vessel stroke; Fig. 9-6): thrombi are the most common cause of ischemic stroke. Thrombi usually form in atherosclerotic blood vessels. We will talk a little more about atherosclerosis in a minute.

In hemorrhagic stroke, a blood vessel bursts, spilling blood into the brain. This type can result from high blood pressure or an aneurysm, both of which weaken blood vessels.

Other types of stroke include small vessel strokes, which are also called lacunar infarcts. These are smaller infarcts that are typically located in smaller vessels deeper within the brain. They are commonly seen in chronic hypertension and diabetes. Since they are so small and due to the areas they typically affect, they usually do not cause defects such as apraxia or aphasia. They do cause motor and sensory hemiplegia as well as dysarthria (clumsiness, especially with the hands). The diagnosis is usually made clinically because even CT is not sensitive enough to detect tiny lacunar infarcts. MRI however can detect them.

What causes it and why

Table 9-19 shows the causes of stroke and why these causes occur.

Table 9-19

Causes	Why
Hypertension	Increased pressure weakens blood vessel walls leading to stroke
Atrial fibrillation	Irregular heartbeat can cause blood clot leading to stroke
Hyperlipidemia (increased lipids in the blood, i.e., cholesterol, triglycerides)	Hyperlipidemia is associated with the development of atherosclerosis. Atherosclerosis is actually a complex process, but in a nutshell it is an inflammation of the lining of arteries. It results in overgrowth and changes in the vascular smooth muscle cells. This all leads to plaque development. Well, LDL (the bad cholesterol) is instrumental in plaque development as it adheres to the arterial wall. Then the immune system gets involved by mounting up a response, and everything goes south from there, leading to plaque rupture. The ruptured plaque combined with clot-promoting elements in the blood leads to clot formation

(Continued)

Table 9-19. (*Continued*)

Causes	Why
Diabetes	Microvascular damage
Any coagulation disorder	Predisposes clients to clot formation
Alcohol abuse	Induces arrhythmias and altered ventricular function
	Induces hypertension
	Exacerbates already existing coagulation disorders
	Reduces cerebral flood flow
Cocaine	Causes ischemic and hemorrhagic strokes by causing vasospasm, increased activity of platelets, increased blood pressure, increased heart rate, temperature, and metabolic rate

Source: Created by author from Reference #1.

Signs and symptoms and why

The signs and symptoms and rationales associated with stroke are shown in Table 9-20.

Table 9-20

Signs and symptoms	Why
Sudden numbness or weakness of the face, arm or hand, or leg	Clot blocks an artery, blocking blood flow to part of the brain responsible for this area of the body
Sudden confusion	Same
Difficulty speaking or understanding including aphasia or dysarthria (slurred speech)	Same
Sudden trouble with vision in one or both eyes, double vision (diplopia), blindness, and/or tunnel vision	Same
Sudden difficulty walking, dizziness, or loss of balance and coordination	Same
Sudden severe headache, often referred to as the "worst headache of my life"	Blood vessel in the brain bursts

Source: Created by author from Reference #1.

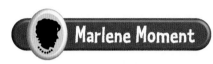

Marlene Moment

You didn't know all of this was taking place in your arteries while eating those greasy burgers with super-sized fries, did you?

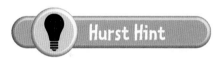

Hurst Hint

Risk factors that clients can control include obesity, smoking, lack of exercise, and hypertension. Risk factors that cannot be controlled include gender, race, genetic predisposition to develop diseases such as diabetes, sickle cell anemia, polycythemia, and blood dyscrasias.

Quickie tests and treatments

Tests:

- Immediate neurological exam. History and physical is often all that is needed to initially diagnose stroke. Follow-up studies are of course carried out in order to confirm the diagnosis.

- Blood work for CBC (high with major strokes due to compensation for lack of O_2 to the brain), possibly PT, PTT to establish baseline.

- Hemorrhagic stroke must be ruled out before intervention. Will usually begin with CT.
- Computed tomography (CT) scan, or MRI—it is important to note that often the CT will initially be negative until more progressive changes of ischemia that occur with time become apparent. The MRI is useful in this situation when the CT is negative initially but stroke is strongly suspected. The MRI will show changes much earlier than the CT.
- Carotid ultrasound (aka carotid dopplers) to determine the condition of the carotid arteries (degree of blockage, stenosis, etc.).
- CTA (CT angiography): identifies presence of cerebral hemorrhage, thus aiding in the search for the cause of the stroke (ischemia vs. hemorrhage).
- MRA (magnetic resonance angiography) to locate problems areas (decreased perfusion).
- SPECT (single-photon emission computed tomography): able to determine blood flow to certain regions of the brain.
- EKG, Holter monitor if cardiac etiology is suspected.
- Intracranial pressure (ICP) monitoring systems if indicated.

Treatment for ischemic stroke includes:

- Thrombolytic therapy (tissue plasminogen activator or tPA) per IV or catheter directed approach (if systemic therapy does not work)—dissolves the clot. Must be implemented within 6 hours of onset of symptoms after hemorrhagic etiology has been ruled out.
- Anticoagulation with antiplatelet drugs (heparin, coumadin, Lovenox, etc). Remember, a baseline PT and PTT are obtained prior to initiating heparin therapy, and approximately 8 hours after initiation as well as daily.
- Anticoagulants such as coumadin, low-molecular-weight heparin such as Lovenox, and antiplatelets such as Plavix can prevent recurrent stokes.
- Enteric-coated aspirin is often given for stroke prevention in high-risk clients but not in clients who have recently had a stroke. These clients are treated more aggressively.

Treatment for hemorrhagic stroke includes:

- Correction of airway compromise if indicated.
- Neurosurgical intervention.
- Therapy for blood pressure.
- Treatment for increased intracranial pressure.

The risk for the development of ICP is the greatest during the first 72 hours after ANY stroke. The Glasgow Coma Scale (GCS) is an assessment tool the nurse uses to perform neurological checks on the client with increased ICP. Remember, the first sign of increasing ICP is decreased LOC. There is controversy regarding whether the HOB should be elevated to 30 degrees or lower. The issues surrounding the controversy are centered on whether the flat bed helps to increase perfusion to the brain or the higher HOB which might decrease ICP. Follow your doctor's order because this may vary.

What can harm my client?

- Complications of tPA, especially in the presence of hemorrhage.
- Complications of anticoagulant therapy and antiplatelet therapy. These clients have high risk for bleeding.
- Increased ICP.
- Seizures.
- Residual deficits such as impaired mobility and sensation.
- Impaired communication and intellectual function.
- Potential for injury such as falls, decubitus ulcers.
- Swallowing difficulties leading to aspiration.
- Malnutrition related to neglecting to eat.
- Neglect from caregivers.
- Potential for abuse (vulnerable clients).

If I were your teacher, I would test you on . . .

- Symptoms of stroke.
- Causes and why.
- Risk factors.
- Importance of immediate intervention.
- Test and treatments.
- Complications or what could harm my client.

✚ Traumatic brain injury

What is it?

The brain is the most complex organ in the body with highly complex functions that enable us to think, interact in the environment as well as control virtually every aspect of the human body. Traumatic brain injury occurs due to a blow or external force applied to the head. Injury occurs at the site of impact as well as globally. This results in not only tissue damage but altered blood flow leading to changes in LOC, increased ICP, and even brain death.

OPEN HEAD INJURY   An open head injury is a severe blow to the head that breaks the skull (skull fracture). Once the skull is broken, the brain is vulnerable to injury and/or infection, which makes this type of injury very risky in terms of infection. The brain may actually be punctured by fragments of skull or the object that caused the injury in the first place such as a knife. It may result from a gunshot wound to the head or a high-speed car accident.

Types of skull fractures associated with open head injury:

- Linear fracture: simple, clean, or straight break of an area of the skull. Most common type.
- Depressed fracture: skull is pressed inward into the brain tissue.
- Open fracture: scalp is lacerated, which leads to direct opening to the brain tissue.
- Comminuted fracture: bone is pressed into brain tissue AND there are bone fragments involved.
- Basilar skull fracture: occurs at the base of the skull resulting in leakage of cerebrospinal fluid (CSF) from the nose or ears. The client is at risk for hemorrhage due to possible injury to the internal carotid artery, infection, and/or damage to the cranial nerves.

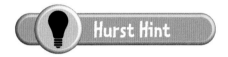

Open head injury—think, "risk for infection."

CLOSED HEAD INJURY   Let's get something straight: The brain is suspended in CSF normally, so when a forceful blow is delivered to the head, the brain can "bounce" around inside the skull. The brain can accelerate (speed up in motion or movement), then abruptly decelerate once it bounces off the skull. This is referred to *coup-contrecoup injury*. Let us explain: when the brain initially bumps into the skull as a result of a blow, it receives the *coup* injury. When it bounces back, the opposite side is injured. This is referred to as the *contrecoup* injury. This "bouncing around" results in damage to brain tissue, the cranial vault, blood vessels, and nerve tracts resulting in brain contusions and hematomas. This phenomenon is exactly why closed head injuries are classified as being the most serious type of injury when compared with open head injuries.

Types of closed head injuries:

- Concussion: brief interruption in brain activity with or without loss of consciousness.
- Diffuse axonal injury: diffuse (means widespread) injury to axons, the corpus callosum, white matter, and the brainstem. This one is bad. It is the cause of posttraumatic dementia as well as persistent vegetative states. This one is a prime example of the *coup-contrecoup* injury.
- Contusion: blunt trauma causes a bruise to the cortical surface of the brain resulting in permanent damage to the brain tissue. Bruised and necrotic tissue are eventually replaced with scar tissue and/or "crater."
- Hematoma: vascular bleeding. The type of hematoma is determined by the actual site of the bleeding vessels. Types of hematomas include epidural, subdural, and intracerebral hematomas.
  - Epidural: bleeding that occurs between the skull and the dura.
  - Subdural: bleeding between the dura and the subdural (arachnoid) space (Fig. 9-7).
  - Traumatic intracerebral: one or more hematomas. Occurs anywhere in the brain, but most common in the frontal or temporal lobes.

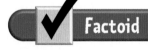

Intracerebral hematomas are very common in the elderly and the alcoholic due to fragility of blood vessels.

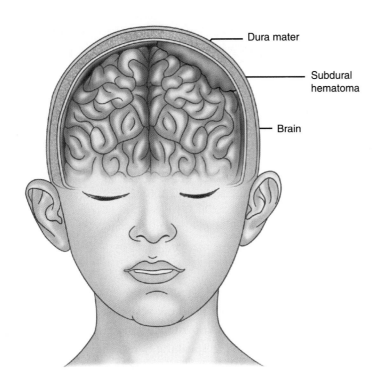

Dura mater

Subdural hematoma

Brain

◀ Figure 9-7. Subdural hematoma.

Signs and symptoms and why

Signs and symptoms are highly variable from client to client depending on the type and degree of injury but here are some of the most common ones.

The signs and symptoms and rationales associated with brain injury are found in Table 9-21.

Table 9-21

Signs and symptoms	Why
Alterations in sensory and motor function	Damaged brain tissue as a result of direct trauma with subsequent alterations in blood supply and oxygenation as well as damaged nerves and increased intracranial pressure
Altered LOC including confusion, delirium	Same. Deterioration of brain function leads to depressed states of consciousness
Stupor and/or coma	**Define time:** **Stupor:** unresponsiveness except in the presence of repeated vigorous stimuli **Comatose:** unarousable. No ability to respond to anything. However, the presence of reflex movements may be present. This is known as posturing (decortication and decerebration). The **Glasgow Coma Scale** is an assessment tool used to determine the level of consciousness or level/depth of coma. 15 is indicative of normal neurological function. 3 represents a deep coma **Decortication:** arms, wrists, and fingers are flexed and rotated inward toward the body. The legs will be flexed and the feet will be flexed and rotated inward. Everything flexes and points to the central portion or the "core" of the body. This is due to an interruption of the corticospinal pathway, hence, the term decorticate **Decerebration:** rigidity with extension and pronation of the arms and extension of the legs. Feet will be plantar-flexed. This posture is associated with brainstem involvement
Behavior changes including irritability, combativeness	Same. Sign of impending coma

(*Continued*)

Table 9-21. (*Continued*)

Signs and symptoms	Why
Alteration in respiratory function	**Forebrain injury**: Cheyne–Stokes (waxing and waning of the consistency of respirations with periods of apnea)
	Midbrain involvement: neurogenic hyperventilation where the rate may exceed 40 breaths per minute. This is due to the brain's loss of the ability to inhibit the inspiratory and expiratory centers of the brain
	Medulla involvement: ataxic respirations characterized by irregular or uncoordinated respirations
Abnormal eye movements	Brain death is identified by the loss of all brainstem reflex responses. These include pupillary, corneal, oculovestibular, oculocephalic, oropharyngeal, and respiratory. In addition, EEG and cerebral angiography help to confirm the diagnosis of brain death
Abnormal pupil reflexes	**Pupils:** uneven, unreactive, dilated, or constricted pupils represent brain injury

Source: Created by author from Reference #1.

Lets talk about the Doll's-head eye response: This is also known as the oculocephalic reflex. You know those baby dolls that you played with when you were little? (I'm speaking to girls here!) They gave them the eyes that move to make them look more like a normal person, right? If you have an unconscious client, you can test for doll's eyes by turning the head back and forth to check for movement. If the head is turned in one direction and the eyes remain in the opposite direction but eventually migrate back to midline, you have a positive doll's-eye reflex. That is good, because if you have to have a head injury, you want this response to be positive, because if it were negative, then your client would have a brainstem dysfunction, which is very bad. So, if the gaze remains constant and the eyes do not act like your baby doll's eyes did, then you really start to worry. If no doll's-eye reflex can be elicited, then the physician will perform the caloric test.

Oculovestibular reflex test (ice-water caloric test): cold water is instilled into the ear canal to elicit nystagmus (involuntary eye movements). If nystagmus is present, the client has some degree of brainstem function. Why? The auditory nerve, which is a cranial nerve arising from the brainstem, innervates the ear and causes a response when stimulated if there is brain function.

The above tests are used to identify brainstem reflex responses to help support the diagnosis of brain death.

Clinical application

You have a client who falls unconscious (possibly due to a heart irregularity) while practicing karate with her husband. CPR is delayed and there is difficulty with intubation when the ambulance arrives. The client suffers severe hypoxic brain injury. She has a negative doll's-eye response and a subsequent negative caloric test response. An EEG and cerebral angiogram confirm inactivity as well as absence of blood flow to the brain.

Quickie tests and treatments

Tests:

- Computed tomography (CT) scan.
- Magnetic resonance imaging (MRI).

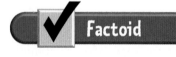

If there is a bilateral lesion at the ventrolateral medulla, complete apnea will occur, in which case a ventilator will be required.

- Positron emission tomography (PET).
- Evoked potential studies.
- Assess airway and breathing pattern.
- Assess vital signs.
- Neurological assessment.
- Eye assessment: changes in pupil size, irregularities, and reactivity to light indicate brain damage. The type of pupil change will depend on the area of the brain injured.

Treatment (depends on extent and location of injury):

- Surgery for emergency evacuation of collected blood if indicated or craniotomy.
- ICP monitoring.
- Hemodynamic and/or vital sign monitoring.
- Ventilatory support: may give IV opiates such as morphine or fentanyl to decrease agitation and control restlessness as well as possible pain.
- NMBAs (neuromuscular blocking agents) are used if the client is dangerously agitated. The agitation causes increased ICP. These drugs paralyze the client and are not given alone but in combination with sedatives. Think about it: your client has a head injury, is semi-conscious and agitated with increased ICP. You need to give NMBA. How do you think the client would feel if given without sedatives? This is very inhumane! Never do it! You also never give these agents to a client who is not provided ventilatory or respiratory assistance, because they suppress or paralyze the respiratory drive.
- Prevention/management of ICP: mannitol (osmotic diuretic) is used to treat cerebral edema by pulling off the excess fluid from the extra-cellular space of the edematous brain tissue. Administered IV.
- Barbiturates are also given for the control of ICP in that they decrease the metabolic demand on the brain.
- Fluids and electrolytes as indicated. Remember, diabetes incipidus (DI) and syndrome of inappropriate antidiuretic hormone secretion (SIADH)? The head trauma client is at risk for developing these due to injury or compression of the pituitary due to cerebral edema.
- Nutrition management.
- Seizure precautions/management.
- Neurochecks as ordered.
- Assessment for respiratory compromise.

Above all, these clients need emergency care in the field. Frequently, they need intensive care unit (ICU) care, so hemodynamic stability can be monitored. The goals are to protect the airway, control the ICP, and prepare the client for surgery to remove blood or ischemic tissue. Removing the nonvital tissue allows for brain expansion without causing further elevations of ICP.

What can harm my client?

- Increased ICP.
- Seizures.

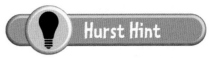

Hurst Hint

You may see a progression from one of these phases of respirations to the next as the injury begins to encompass more areas of the brain. Why? The full extent of the injury cannot be appreciated initially.

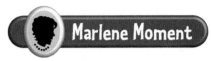

Marlene Moment

The oculovestibular test (ice-water calorics) is not something you go around performing on the night shift because you are bored looking for something to do! This is done by the physician and the client must be turned on their side with their head elevated before you leave the room in order to prevent aspiration from vomiting (nursing care).

- Brain death.
- Hyperthermia—due to injury or pressure of hypothalamus.
- You need to know that even slight changes in respirations, neurological status, and/or behavior can signal a problem.
- Decubitus ulcers.
- DI.
- SIADH.

If I were your teacher, I would test you on . . .

- Anatomy and physiology of the brain.
- Symptoms of increasing ICP.
- Importance of immediate intervention.
- Complications.
- How to care for a client after surgery.
- Community referrals may be in order—the client could have long-term residual damage, depending on the degree of injury.
- Do you administer neuromuscular blocking agents alone? What do you administer them with?
- Doll's-eye response (oculocephalic): brainstem reflex response.
- Caloric test (oculovestibular): brainstem reflex response—nursing care related to this test—elevate the HOB and turn the client to the side after the test prior to leaving the room to prevent aspiration from vomitus (this test can induce vomiting).

✚ Restless leg syndrome

What is it?

Restless leg syndrome is a neurological sensorimotor condition in which the legs have an extreme urge to move while sitting or lying down. This terribly unpleasant feeling tends to go away with walking or movement. The characteristic worsening of symptoms at nighttime leads to disruptions in sleep, which can cause excessive daytime sleepiness. The client usually reports that the symptoms are most severe during times when sitting still is necessary (having a hair cut, air travel, riding in car, lying in bed, watching a movie). Different clients may describe the restless leg sensation in different ways (see signs/symptoms given later). In rare cases, the arms may become involved as well.

What causes it and why

The exact cause of restless leg syndrome is unknown, but about 50% of cases appear to be genetic. Other possible factors associated with restless leg syndrome are listed in Table 9-22.

Table 9-22

Associated factors	Why
Pregnancy, obesity, smoking, iron deficient anemia, hypothyroidism, diabetes, vitamin deficiencies, kidney failure, certain drugs such as H_2-histamine blockers, antidepressants, antiemetics, calcium-channel blockers, caffeine, and alcohol	Not a cause but frequently associated with restless leg syndrome
Possible dopamine imbalance	Dopamine regulates the nerve cells that help control body movements
Neuropathy of nerve axons (as in diabetes)	Microvascular blood vessel changes/damage, resulting in nerve damage

Source: Created by author from References #1 and #2.

Signs and symptoms and why

The signs and symptoms and rationales associated with restless leg syndrome are found in Table 9-23.

Table 9-23

Signs and symptoms	Why
Burning sensation in the legs, tingling sensation in the legs, a creepy-crawly feeling in the legs	Etiology unknown
Tugging of the leg muscles, twitching of the legs, cramping in the leg muscles, painful legs	Etiology unknown

Source: Created by author from Reference #1.

Quickie tests and treatments

Tests:

The diagnosis of restless leg syndrome is based primarily on client history. Common questions asked to determine the presence of RLS are:

1. Have you ever experienced creepy-crawly sensations in your legs?

2. Are the sensations associated with an urge to move the legs?

3. Does movement help to relieve the symptoms?

4. When are you most bothered by these symptoms?

5. Do you have difficulty falling asleep or staying asleep?

6. Have you been told you move a lot during your sleep?

Polysomnography (sleep studies) may be used to rule out other disorders but is not necessary to confirm diagnosis. May be tested for other associated diseases.

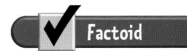

Factoid

Stress and pregnancy tend to increase RLS.

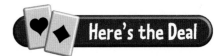

Here's the Deal

Some clients experience RLS for the first time in the 3rd trimester of pregnancy. RLS usually disappears postdelivery.

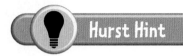

Treatments:

Drug therapy may include:

- Anti-Parkinson agents such as levodopa-carbidopa (Sinemet), Requip, and Mirapex.
- Magnesium supplements.
- Neurontin.
- Anticonvulsants, such as carbamazepine (Tegretol).
- Antianxiety drugs, such as lorazepam (Ativan).
- Opioids, such as oxycodone (Oxycontin).
- Muscle relaxants (baclofen).
- Long-acting benzodiazepines (Klonopin).
- Low caffeine.
- Warm or cold bath.
- Electric nerve stimulator.
- Acupuncture.
- Increase exercise (not close to bedtime).
- Decreased alcohol.
- Massage therapy.
- Relaxation such as yoga and/or meditation.

What can harm my client?

Chronic sleep disruption leading to depression, chronic pain, chronic fatigue, decreased productivity at work, and inability to participate in routine activities.

If I were your teacher, I would test you on . . .

- Definition.
- Symptoms of restless leg syndrome.
- Treatments for restless leg syndrome.
- Associated conditions.
- Techniques to promote sleep.

✚ Trigeminal neuralgia

What is it?

Trigeminal neuralgia is a chronic disease of the 5th cranial nerve (CN V). The disease causes pain over one side of the face that many times is described as feeling like electric shocks to extreme pain. The pain may be intermittent or continuous.

What causes it and why

The true cause of trigeminal neuralgia is unknown, but it is thought to be associated with certain disorders (Table 9-24).

Hurst Hint

Sometimes the medication that has worked well to relieve RLS stops working or the client's symptoms are beginning earlier in the day than they once did. This is treated by taking drug holidays, changing meds, or changing the time of day the med is taken.

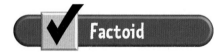

Factoid

The other names for trigeminal neuralgia are tic douloureux or glossopharyngeal neuralgia.

Table 9-24

Causes	Why
Flu-like illnesses	The exact mechanism is unknown, but inflammation of the nerve may be the cause
Trauma	Same
Infection	Same
Pressure on CN V	• Pressure due to a tumor which can inflame a nerve • Compression from an artery or vein could irritate the nerve as well due to structural abnormality
Multiple sclerosis	Due to demyelination of nerves

Source: Created by author from References #1 and #2.

Signs and symptoms and why

Table 9-25 gives the signs and symptoms of trigeminal neuralgia.

Table 9-25

Signs and symptoms	Why
Extreme, sudden, and/or severe facial pain (surface pain)	Irritation and/or inflammation of the nerve
Unilateral (nerve does not cross midline of face)	
Episodes are short-lived (few seconds to couple of minutes), can be recurrent, and can be variable from client to client (some may have many episodes while others have only a few)	
Knife-like or like electric shocks usually beginning on one side of the mouth moving toward the ear	
When the "trigger zone" is stimulated, pain occurs; trigger zones usually follow the path of a nerve	

Source: Created by author from References #1 and #2.

Quickie Tests and Treatments

Tests:

There is no single test to confirm the disease (the physician mainly bases diagnosis on symptoms reported by client; however, some testing may be initiated to rule out other conditions.

• CT scan.

• MRI.

• Neurological assessment.

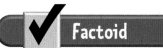

Factoid

The slightest of things can initiate an attack: swallowing, sneezing, talking, chewing, brushing teeth, touching the face in any way, change in temperature, or feeling breeze on the face.

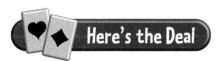

Here's the Deal

In an effort to decrease pain, the client may not eat, talk, or bathe, as the slightest of stimuli may precipitate an attack.

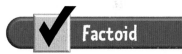

Factoid

Trigeminal neuralgia has periods of exacerbations and remission (may be free from pain for years). Over time, the client may complain of a dull ache even during times of remission.

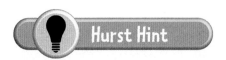

Hurst Hint

Many times clients may visit the dentist for pain relief, as they believe the pain is associated with a problem tooth. The dentist may remove a tooth/teeth and the pain persists; the client soon learns the pain is not related to dental problems.

Treatments:

- Tegretol is used for pain; if this does not give client relief, then other meds may be used such as Dilantin or Neurontin.
- Skeletal muscle relaxants may be used as well.
- The nerve may have to be surgically incised (rhizotomy).
- Nerve blocking with local anesthetics.

Nursing care:

- Help client identify triggers (hot/cold foods).
- Monitor weight and intake and output (I&O).
- Encourage client to chew on unaffected side.
- Do not rub eyes.
- Wear sunglasses.
- Regular dental checks as client may not be able to feel infection/caries.
- Use an electric razor.

What can harm my client?

- Problems associated with weight loss.
- Dehydration.
- Depression associated with chronic pain.

If I were your teacher, I would test you on . . .

- Definition.
- Causes and why.
- Signs/symptoms and why.
- Pain triggers.
- Pain relief.
- Care of the eyes.
- Importance of dental care.

✚ Bell's palsy

What is it?

Bell's palsy is a problem associated with the 7th cranial nerve (facial nerve) where unilateral paralysis of the face occurs. The facial nerve (which is mainly a motor nerve) is responsible for expression on one side of the face. The sensory part innervates the anterior two-thirds of the tongue. The majority of the clients with Bell's palsy recover without treatment. Many recover within a few weeks. The few clients who develop permanent facial paralysis usually are elderly or have other conditions as well (diabetes mellitus).

What causes it and why

No exact cause of Bell's palsy has been identified; however, some believe the herpes simplex virus is associated in some form. Odds are, it is the result of the inflammatory response.

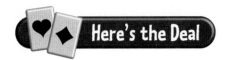

Here's the Deal

Bell's palsy is also called facial paralysis.

Signs and symptoms and why

Table 9-26

Signs and symptoms	Why
Sudden onset	Inflammation of the affected nerve *The "why" or rationale for all symptoms is the same*
Unilateral involvement	
Pain before paralysis (pain is usually behind the ear/along the jaw; pain may last 2 hours or 2 days prior to actual onset of paralysis; once this symptom begins, maximum paralysis usually occurs within 48 hours)	
Numbness or stiffening that changes the normal appearance of the face; process continues until the fade is asymmetrical; face droops on one side; unable to wrinkle forehead/close eye/pucker lips on affected side; unable to whistle	
Corneal reflex is absent on affected side	
Taste changes	
Increased lacrimal tearing on affected side	
Drooling from one side of mouth	

Source: Created by author from References #1 and #2.

Quickie tests and treatment

Tests:

- There are no specific tests for Bell's palsy.
- CN assessment.
- CT or MRI to rule out stroke, tumor, trauma.
- EMG (to assess nerve function).
- Diagnosis is based on presentation of symptoms.

Treatments:

- Acyclovir (to treat herpes infection).
- Prednisone (limits damage to nerve by decreasing inflammation).
- Physical therapy/facial exercises (helps maintain muscle tone).
- Moist heat, massage, and analgesics (decreases pain).
- Eye care: artificial tears for affected eye; wear sunglasses outside; patch eye at night (protects cornea from drying).
- Soft diet to limit chewing; no hot foods; inspect mouth carefully after eating (may not be able to feel food present).
- If Bell's palsy doesn't improve in 6 to 12 months, the client is a candidate for surgery. Surgery involves grafting another nerve to the facial nerve.

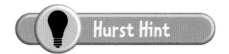

Hurst Hint

Clients with Bell's palsy usually are fearful they have had a stroke.

What can harm my client?

- Malnutrition.
- Dehydration.

- Facial contractures.
- Corneal ulcerations, inflammation of cornea, vision loss.
- Body image changes associated with facial paralysis.

If I were your teacher, I would test you on . . .

- Definition.
- Signs/symptoms and why.
- Causes and why.
- Treatments.
- Cranial nerve assessment.
- Eye/vision care.
- Pain relief measures.

✛ Meningitis

What is it?

The meninges (dura, archnoid, and pia mater) are the coverings surrounding the brain. The purpose of meninges is to protect the brain and spinal cord from invading organisms. Meningitis is inflammation of the meninges (specifically the pia mater, the arachnoid, and the subarachnoid space, which includes the CSF) caused by an invading organism (bacteria, viruses, fungi, etc). Infection and inflammation (caused by pathogens releasing toxins) can progress rapidly due to the circulating CSF around the brain and spinal cord. Actual brain damage may occur from the inflammation. WBCs rush to the subarachnoid space causing the CSF to become cloudy. The brain, spinal cord, and optic nerves can become infected as well. As a result, an increase in intracranial pressure is likely when the brain begins to respond to the pathogen. The invading organism and the increase in intracranial pressure can cause significant damage to the brain if not recognized and treated promptly. Meningitis is considered to be a major infection of the central nervous system and can be an acute or chronic condition.

People who live in close quarters (military personnel, students in dorms) are at high risk for contracting meningitis. Bacterial meningitis is usually caused by either *Streptococcus pneumoniae* (pneumococcal meningitis) or *Neisseria meningitidis* (meningococcal meningitis). *S. pneumoniae* is the major cause of bacterial meningitis in children.

The pathogens that cause meningitis are very attracted to the nervous system and must overcome many barriers to get there (invade the CNS). The pathogens usually colonize and multiply in the nasopharyngeal area, break into the bloodstream, and then break through the blood–brain barrier. In addition, the pathogen must be able to survive the body's natural immune response and the inflammatory response as well. These pathogens are very determined!

The major focus of this section will be on bacterial meningitis.

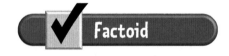
Factoid

Pneumococcal meningitis is mainly seen in the very old and the very young.

What causes it and why

Table 9-27

Causes	Why
Bacteria: *Neisseria meningitidis, Streptococcus pneumoniae*, meningococcus, *Haemophilus influenzae*, and *E. coli*	Are very attracted to the nervous system and are strong enough to overcome many barriers that normally protect this area
Anytime there is a break in the meninges (brain surgery, skull fractures, postcraniotomy), the risk of developing meningitis increases	A break in the meninges provides direct access for the pathogen to invade the CNS
Simple infections such as otitis media or sinusitis can increase the risk for developing meningitis as well	Any infection in close proximity to the CNS can invade the CNS if not treated promptly and completely. *S. pneumoniae* and *Staphylococcus aureus* are the major invading organisms
Anyone who is immunocompromised has an increased incidence of CNS infections	Can't fight infection
Potential IV line infection	Bacteria can enter bloodstream and then invade the CNS

Source: Created by author from References #1 and #2.

Signs and symptoms and why

Table 9-28

Signs and symptoms	Why
May begin with flu-like symptoms	Initial infection response
Headache that won't stop	Inflammation of meninges and possible beginning increased intracranial pressure; any sound makes headache worse
Fever, chills	Infection
Back, abdominal pain	Invasion of pathogen through spinal cord area
Nuchal rigidity (stiff neck)	Inflammation of meninges
Positive Brudzniski's sign (when neck flexed, hip and knee flex too)	Inflammation of meninges
Positive Kernig's sign (client cannot extend knee with hip flexed at 90-degree angle	Inflammation of meninges
Photophobia	Optic nerve affected; client will want lights to be out
Diplopia	Optic nerve affected; intracranial pressure
Signs of increased intracranial pressure (see complete review of IICP later in the chapter)	Cerebral edema; HOB elevated 30 degrees or as ordered by physician will help decrease ICP
Seizures	Increased intracranial pressure and inflammation/infection
Rash	A rash (petechial rash) may be seen in meningococcal meningitis over the skin and mucous membranes. The rash spreads rapidly

Source: Created by author from References #1 and #2.

Good fact to know:

Haemophilus influenzae meningitis has decreased significantly due to the *Haemophilus* B vaccine (HIB vaccine).

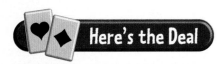

The older client may present with confusion instead of headache and fever.

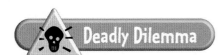

Bacterial meningitis must be treated promptly or death can occur within a few days.

Points to remember about viral meningitis:

- Symptoms basically the same as bacterial meningitis, but less severe; red, maculopapular rash may be seen in children.
- Usually appears after the mumps.
- Doesn't last as long as bacterial meningitis.
- Usually complete recovery.
- Treatment is aimed at alleviating client's symptoms (relief from fever, pain relief, no antibiotics, no isolation necessary).

Quickie tests and treatment

Tests:

- CBC (to assess white count).
- Blood cultures (to assist in determining the causative pathogen).
- Lumbar puncture for culture of CSF (THE test used for diagnosis); spinal fluid will be cloudy, have increased WBC count, increased protein, and decreased glucose (bacteria eating glucose).
- CT or MRI (helps rule out other problems).

Treatments:

- Respiratory isolation (until pathogen identified and for 24 hours AFTER antibiotics started).
- IV broad-spectrum antibiotics (to kill pathogen) until CSF cultures return; then give organism-specific antibiotic for 1 to 3 weeks.
- Corticosteroids (to control ICP; decreases cerebral edema).
- May require anticonvulsants for seizures.
- Antipyretics for relief of fever.
- Analgesics for pain (physician must be careful NOT to prescribe an analgesic, which could alter the neuro checks (opiates).
- Antiemetics for nausea/vomiting.
- Prevent dehydration.
- Frequent neuro checks.

What can harm my client?

- Damage to auditory nerve (CN VII); cochlear implant may be considered.
- Increased intracranial pressure.
- Brain tissue can die due to increased intracranial pressure and microthrombi than can develop in cerebral circulation.
- In children residual effects may be seen (learning problems, paresis, CN dysfunction, spasticity).
- Seizures.
- Severe increased intracranial pressure may cause herniation/compression of brainstem.
- Disseminated intravascular coagulation (DIC).

Other important points to remember

- Those who will be living in college dormitories or those entering the military should consider the vaccination for meningococcal meningitis. This bacteria can be transferred by drinking after an infected person, living in close proximity (they could innocently sneeze in your presence and you could become infected!), or even smoking after an infected person.
- If exposed to meningococcal meningitis, Rifampin is given prophylactically.

If I were your teacher, I would test you on . . .

- Definition.
- Causes and why.
- Signs/symptoms and why.
- Transmission.
- Isolation recommended.
- Increased intracranial pressure.
- Nursing care of someone with meningitis.
- Cranial nerve assessment.
- Neuro assessment.
- Vaccinations/prevention.
- Those at risk for becoming infected.

✚ Encephalitis

What is it?

An inflammation of the parenchyma of the brain or spinal cord due to infection. It is usually caused by a virus but may be caused by bacteria or fungi (Table 9-29). Examples of offending pathogens include herpes virus, arbovirus, rabies virus, flavivirus (West Nile encephalitis or Japanese encephalitis). The virus or organism invades the brain tissue and causes subsequent degeneration of the neurons. Certain viruses have a propensity for certain areas of the brain. Clients are usually more ill with encephalitis than with meningitis.

What causes it and why

Table 9-29

Causes	Why
Virus infection	Travels through the bloodstream to the CNS or travels along cranial nerves to the CNS
Meningitis infection	Travels from the meninges to the brain
Protozoan infection (amebic meningoencephalitis)	Found in warm fresh water and can enter through the nose of the client. These protozoa can also be found in decaying soil and vegetation

Source: Created by author from References #1 and #2.

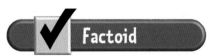
Factoid

Regarding protozoan infection: diagnosed by culture of CSF or biopsy. No effective treatment is available and incidence is increasing in North America.

Signs and Symptoms and why

Signs and symptoms (Table 9-30) are very close to those of meningitis. You may refer to that section for a review.

Table 9-30

Signs and symptoms	Why
Altered sensorium	Infected brain tissue
Seizures	Same
Fever, stiff neck, and headache	Same
May even develop aphasia, hemiparesis, or facial weakness	Same

Source: Created by author from References #1 and #2.

Quickie tests and treatments

Tests:

- Culture and Gram stain of CSF per lumbar puncture.
- All other tests are the same as for meningitis.

Treatments:

- Antiviral drugs such as acyclovir, when indicated.
- Incision and drainage (I&D) of brain abscess if indicated.
- Supportive management to prevent complications.
- Treatment for ICP if indicated related to cerebral edema. Refer to ICP section later in the chapter.
- If infection is related to bacteria, appropriate antibiotics will be given.

What can harm my client?

- The client can become comatose, with subsequent brain death.
- Complications from ICP.
- Decubitus ulcers with infection.
- Permanent neurological deficits.

If I were your teacher I would test you on . . .

- What is it?
- Know that it is very similar to meningitis but clients are generally more ill with encephalitis.
- Causes and why.
- Complications.
- Nursing care is the same as for meningitis!

✛ Intracranial pressure

What is it?

Normally throughout the day, intermittent increases occur according to our activity. For example, coughing, sneezing, lifting, or straining can precipitate an increase in ICP.

These intermittent increases are not harmful. Normal incracranial pressure is considered to be 15 mm Hg or below.

Three factors play a part in normal intracranial pressure:

- Brain tissue.
- Cerebrospinal fluid.
- Blood volume.

When one of these factors increases, something must decrease to keep the pressure within normal limits. This process is known as the Monro–Kellie hypothesis. Our brain can compensate for increases only to a certain point in the adult, as the skull is a rigid cavity. Babies can compensate a little easier than adults as they have sutures in the skull that can separate and allow for expansion as well as the presence of fontanels that can bulge when there is increased pressure.

Increased intracranial pressure (IICP) is prolonged, elevated pressure in the cranium leading to hypoxic brain tissue with permanent brain damage. Increased intracranial pressure is a medical emergency.

Our brain can compensate to a certain degree for IICP through the following mechanisms:

- Movement of CSF from intracranial area to the subarachnoid space.
- A certain amount of CSF can be reabsorbed via arachnoid villi in the ventricles of the brain.
- Displacement of cerebral blood volume (blood in the brain can be moved other places in the presence of IICP).

What causes it and why

Tables 9-31 and 9-32 give the causes, signs and symptoms, and associated reasons for intracranial pressure.

Table 9-31

Causes	Why
Tumor or abscess	Increased pressure
Hemorrhagic stroke	Bleeding increases ICP
Ischemic stroke	Hypoxia to the blood vessels can result in tissue damage and/or death with subsequent cerebral edema
Prolonged hypoxia for whatever reason	No oxygen transport to the brain
Traumatic head injury	Tissue damage, bleeding, cerebral edema
Excess CSF	Hydrocephalus (condition where the production of CSF is so rapid the arachnoid villi of the ventricles cannot reabsorb it fast enough)

Source: Created by author from References #1 and #2.

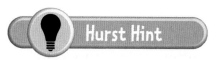

As a rule, we do not like to see bulging fontanels, but in the presence of increased intracranial pressure, this may not be such a bad thing (as the open fontanele gives the pressure a place to go outwardly instead of pressing inwardly into the brain).

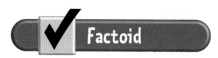

Cerebral edema is the most common cause of sustained IICP.

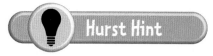

Think of IICP as intracranial hypertension.

Signs and symptoms and why

Table 9-32

Signs and symptoms	Why
Change in LOC	
subtle changes first, progressing to coma	The neurons of the cerebral cortex are VERY sensitive to a decreased oxygen level. This is why a change in LOC is the earliest sign of increased intracranial pressure
Disorientation to time initially, but then progresses to disorientation to place/person	Same
Other LOC changes that are manifested as behavior changes include:	
Restlessness	
Lethargy	
Personality changes	
Irritability	
Decreasing ability to follow commands	
Decreasing responsiveness to auditory stimuli	
Decreasing response to painful stimuli	
Subtle changes that may be difficult to connect with IICP	Same
Headache	
Vomiting	
Forced breathing	
Mental cloudiness	
Purposeless movements	
Changes in speech	
Changes in cranial nerve assessment	
Decreased gag reflex	
Decreased swallowing reflex	
Decreased corneal reflex	
Babinski+	
Seizures	
Posturing	
Decerebrate posturing	Brainstem injury
Decorticate posturing	Cerebral injury
Definition of these terms are found in the Traumatic Brain Injury (TBI) section	
Widening Pulse Pressure	Pressure on brainstem
Pulse Changes	Pressure on brainstem
	Bradycardia will convert to tachycardia as ICP increases
Changes in Pattern of Respiration	Pressure on brainstem
Tachypnea (early sign) manifested as rapid respirations	**Define time:**
Cheyne–Stokes respirations	**Cheyne–Stokes:** rate goes up and down. Depth goes up and down. Periods of apnea
Kussmaul respirations	**Kussmaul:** deep and gasping in nature

(Continued)

Table 9-32. (*Continued*)

Signs and symptoms	Why
Central neurogenic hyperventilation	**Central neurogenic hyperventilation:** sustained rapid, regular, and deep
Apneuistic breathing	**Apneuistic:** inspiration is prolonged ending with a pause. Expiration also may or may not end with a pause
Ataxic breathing	**Ataxic:** rate, pattern, and depth are all irregular. There are also irregular periods of apnea
If ICP increases rapidly, the client may stop breathing	
Hyperthermia, then Hypothermia	Pressure on brainstem
Hemiparesis/Hemiparesis on Contralateral Side (early sign)	Pressure on pyramidal tract
Projectile Vomiting	IICP triggers vomiting center in the brain
Cushing's Response (increased systolic BP, widening pulse pressure, bradycardia)	Alteration of the normal regulatory mechanism of the CNS
Vision Changes	Pressure on visual pathways and cranial nerves
An early sign of IICP. They include:	
Blurred vision	
Diplopia	
Decreased field of vision	

Source: Created by author from References #1 and #2.

DEFINE TIME   The pulse pressure is the difference in the systolic and diastolic BP.

Pupillary/eye signs and symptoms and why

The pupils/eyes are very important when studying the neurological system as they can provide some valuable clues as to what is going on with your client. Let's take a closer look (Table 9-33)!

Table 9-33

Signs and symptoms	Why
May begin as a sluggish response to light progressing to fixed	Pressure on optic and oculomotor nerves
	Changes will first be noted on ipsilateral side (same side as initial injury)
	Injury to the cranial nerve nuclei in the midbrain and pons
Fixed and dilated	Midbrain involvement
Pinpoint	Pontine involvement
Unilateral dilating pupil ipsilateral to part of brain damaged	Uncal herniation
Unequal with slow reaction to light	Uncal herniation

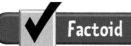

Factoid

The reticular activating system (RAS) is responsible for alertness and/or arousal. It is comprised of neurons that innervate the thalamus and upper brainstem. The axons of reticular neurons extend throughout the brainstem and spinal cord.

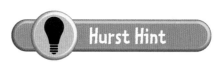

Hurst Hint

Cognition is more complex and is controlled by the cerebral hemisphere. It controls thought processes, memory, perception, problem-solving, and emotion.

(*Continued*)

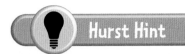

Hurst Hint

In test questions where the client has a history of something that could possibly increase intracranial pressure, do not delay getting the client medical help if she starts exhibiting signs/symptoms of IICP (change in LOC, personality change). Assume the worst! There is NO TIME to waste when ICP starts going up, as death can occur rapidly!

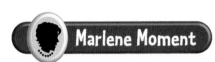

Marlene Moment

The use of painful stimuli should be a last resort when performing a neurological assessment. Please do not do a sternal rub on someone who is sitting up in the bed watching television. You are going to get fired!

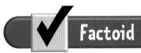

Factoid

The headache associated with IICP is most commonly seen in the morning (upon awakening) and with position changes (increases when lying down/decreases when sitting up).

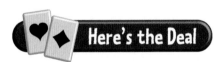

Here's the Deal

The oculocephalic and oculovestibular reflexes are methods that can be used to determine if the brainstem is intact. These include doll's-eyes and the ice-water calorics test discussed earlier in the chapter.

Table 9-33. (*Continued*)

Signs and symptoms	Why
Over time, the contralateral pupil (opposite side of injury) may become fixed and dilated	Uncal herniation
Fixed in midposition with no response to light	Brainstem herniation
Dysconjugate gaze (eyes not moving together)	Loss of normal function of oculomotor nerves
Random eye movements	Same
Ptosis	Drooping of the eyelid. This is an oculomotor dysfunction
Papilledema—may be a late sign	Optic nerve compression

Source: Created by author from References #1 and #2.

Quickie tests and treatments

Tests:

- CT scan to determine underlying cause of IICP.
- MRI to determine underlying cause of IICP (tumor, hydrocephalus, abscess, trauma, etc.).
- Lumbar puncture.
- Measurement of ICP.
- Complete neurological assessment.
- Blood test for glucose: rule out metabolic disturbance as a cause.
- Blood test for electrolytes: assess for metabolic disturbances (SIADH, etc.).
- Serum osmolality: osmolality states are associated with coma. We like to keep serum osmolality slightly elevated in order to help pull off excess intracellular fluid into the vascular system.
- ABGs to assess acid–base balance and oxygen status. Hyperventilation (per ventilator) with slight respiratory alkalosis helps to minimize cerebral vasodilation, which helps to keep ICP down or from rising further.

Treatments:

- Monitor neurological status/LOC continuously.
- Monitor respiratory status continuously as well as breath sounds. Monitor airway and ventilator settings/readings. Ventilatory care.
- Surgery (to repair injury, to stop bleeding or whatever cause might be).
- Mannitol (an osmotic diuretic to decrease ICP).
- Loop diuretics (lasix; to promote diuresis; to treat fluid volume excess caused by mannitol).
- Corticosteroids (to control cerebral edema). These are controversial with respect to their effectiveness as well as their propensity to cause gastritis and GI ulcers, increased blood sugar, and hemorrhage.

- Barbiturate-induced coma (to decrease cerebral metabolism; to decrease movement of client). This is used in severe cases when the IICP is refractory to first-line therapy.
- Monitor and treat temperature changes accordingly (antipyretics/hypothermia blanket).
- Anticonvulsants for seizures such as phenytoin.
- Calcium-channel blockers: calcium can further injure damaged brain tissue. Blockers prevent vasospasm and reduce ischemia.
- Elevate HOB (to decrease ICP).
- Mechanical ventilation (may require Pavulon for neuromuscular paralysis).
- Prevent peptic ulcer disease (client is highly stressed; may need H_2 antagonist or proton pump inhibitor).
- Monitor vital signs closely (mean arterial pressure must be maintained at a certain level to ensure cerebral perfusion).
- Monitor hydration status by close observation of I&O.
- Monitor kidney function and electrolytes continuously.
- Quiet environment (noise increases ICP).
- ICP monitor: offers a continous assessment of ICP. The type of monitor you will see will likely vary from one institution to the other.
- Cerebral perfusion pressure can be calculated (difference between MAP and ICP). This helps to monitor and treat cerebral perfusion deficits in order to prevent further ischemia.
- Keep close care of ICP monitoring device to prevent infection.
- Skin care with prevention and/or treatment of any breakdown.
- Do not give phenytoin with dextrose solutions due to precipation and give IV very slowly.

What can harm my client?

- Seizures.
- IICP if not controlled can lead to rapid death.
- Do not give mannitol with blood.
- Rebound headaches can occur if any meds are discontinued abruptly.
- Skin breakdown.
- SIADH.
- DI.
- Infection from invasive monitoring devices.
- Pneumonia.

If I were your teacher, I would test you on . . .

- Neurological assessment.
- Signs/symptoms and why.
- Causes and why.
- Medications used to treat ICP.

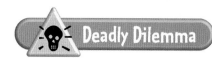

Deadly Dilemma

Brain herniation (displacement of brain tissue to another area, which causes damage and pressure to other areas of the brain). There are several types of herniation depending on the location.

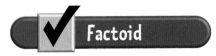

Factoid

Oxygenating the client prior to suctioning will help guard against IICP during suctioning.

- Nursing interventions to control ICP.
- Care of an intracranial pressure monitor.
- Care of the client on the ventilator.
- Limit suctioning (increases ICP).
- Space nursing interventions (activity increases ICP).
- Decrease fluid intake (a small amount of dehydration decreases cerebral edema)
- Complications of IICP.

✚ Spinal cord injury

What is it?

An injury to the spinal cord via trauma by external force. These injuries usually occur as a result of motor vehicle crashes, diving, trampoline accidents, etc. The spinal cord is injured when the cord undergoes abnormal motions of acceleration and deceleration. There are several types of movements that the spinal cord can become injured by. They include hyperflexion (bending forward), hyperextension (bending backward), axial loading (compression of the cord, as when landing on your head—ever heard of a compression fracture?), and rotation (turning of the head too far either way). All of this leads to soft-tissue injury, fractures of bones of the spinal column, torn ligaments and muscles, or an actual penetration of the cord itself. The cord is rarely severed. The spinal cord can also be injured by penetrating objects such as a bullet or a knife. The injury is identified by the level of injury and by complete/ incomplete depth of injury. For example, level C5 is an injury at the 5th cervical vertebrae. That is the level. The cord injury may be complete or incomplete. If it is complete, motor and sensory pathways are damaged and/or transected. This will result in permanent loss of motor and sensory function below the level of injury. In our example, the loss of function would be from C5 down. Incomplete injuries are categorized by syndromes. Each syndrome has its own characteristic deficits depending on the type of injury and the location of the injury to the cord, but the deficits will still be from the level of the injury down. The focus of this section will be on actual spinal cord injuries rather than disc herniations, pulled and/or torn muscles, etc. The main things you need to know are the deficits associated with the level of injury as well as the nursing care and complications these clients frequently endure.

What causes it and why

The initial injury causes damage to the gray matter of the cord but the hemorrhaging, edema, and ischemia will extend to involve a larger area of injury, eventually affecting the entire gray matter of the cord. This explains why the extent of sensory/motor deficits remains to be seen right after an injury. It is sometimes days before we realize the magnitude of the injury. Have you ever heard of clients who could still move their legs right after an accident but later were paralyzed from the waist down? This is one answer. Another is that the client with a spinal cord injury must be carefully moved and transported in order to avoid further damage to the cord. This is why you see the big white collars on clients with possible neck injuries—to prevent any further injury to the cervical spine. We have established that it is usually an accident that causes the injury, but the following (Table 9-34) are internal causes as a result of the accident.

Table 9-34

Causes	Why
Contusion	Accidents such as car crashes, diving, falls (commonly related to trampolines and construction work)
Concussion	Same
Laceration	Same or may be from penetrating object
Transection	Same or may be from penetrating object
Hemorrhage	Bleeding from trauma
Blood vessel damage to vessels that supply the cord	Related to the trauma
Fractured bones can damage	Bone fragments can be a penetrating object the cord

Source: Created by author from References #1 and #2.

Signs and symptoms and why

The signs and symptoms (Table 9-35) vary according to the level and depth of injury.

Table 9-35

Signs and symptoms	Why
Areflexia (loss of reflex function)—characterized by low pulse, low BP, paralysis and weakness of muscles, loss of sensation/feeling, bowel/bladder dysfunction, loss of ability to perspire	Initial response to spinal cord injury characterized by temporary loss of reflex function below the level of injury. The cord does not function at all because it has been separated from communication with the brain. Parasympathetic responses including bradycardia and hypotension will ensue. This will end and some of the reflex function may return. This is one reason why you see clients regain some function months later after their initial injury
Neurogenic shock resulting in cardiovascular changes such as orthostatic hypotension and bradycardia	Brainstem cannot regulate reflexes
Respiratory dysfunction	Loss of innervation to the diaphragm (C1–C4 injury) with the inability to breathe on one's own
Hypothermia	Brainstem not functioning properly
Paralytic ileus	Loss of reflex function
Urinary retention, incontinence	Loss of reflex function
Thrombophlebitis	Decreased peripheral resistance, loss of muscle function/movement
Paralysis with muscle spasms **Paraplegia:** paralysis of the lower portion of the body with lower trunk involvement **Quadriplegia:** aka tetraplegia, is paralysis or impaired function of all four limbs, trunk, and pelvic organs	Upper and lower motor neurons pathways in the brain are affected

Source: Created by author from References #1 and #2.

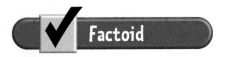

Factoid

Ever heard the term *incomplete quad*? This is a term used to describe a client with quadriplegia who may have some minimal function of the arms or trunk.

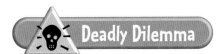

Deadly Dilemma

Autonomic dysreflexia is over-activity of the sympathetic nervous system due to lack of ability of higher centers to control the auto-nomic nervous system. With a stimulus such as a full bladder or lying on a hard object, the sympa-thetic nervous system (SNS) is excessively stimulated. As a result, there is excessive vasoconstriction with subsequent hypertension, bradycardia, sweating, and severe headache. The stimulus must be removed. This is a medical emergency.

Quickie tests and treatments

Tests:

* X-ray, CT, MRI of the spine to locate the injury as well as the extent of damage.
* EMG (electromyography) may help to locate the level.
* ABGs to determine oxygenation status and/or acid base balance.
* See the TBI section earlier in the chapter for other tests that may be performed in the presence of head injury.

Treatments:

* Oxygen if injury is at thoracic level.
* Nasogastric (NG) tube to prevent paralytic ileus.
* Foley catheter to prevent bladder distention.
* Invasive monitoring devices in order to monitor cardiovascular status.
* Methylprednisolone administered within 8 hours of injury helps to prevent further ischemia by reducing edema.
* Opiate antagonists such as nalmefene might promote blood flow to the spinal cord.
* Vasopressors to treat bradycardia due to spinal shock.
* Muscle relaxant to help with spasms.
* Analgesics to reduce pain.
* Surgery to stabilize the spine from further injury—cervical traction may be initiated using Gardner–Wells tongs and halo external fixation device.
* Surgery to remove bone fragments or hematoma, decompression laminectomy, spinal fusion, metal rods, etc.
* H_2 antagonists to prevent GI stress ulcer.
* Anticoagulants to prevent clot formation.
* Stool softeners to prevent constipation and to initiate bowel program.

What can harm my client?

* If the halo external fixation device becomes loose, the spinal cord could be injured further.
* Pulling on the halo ring.
* Respiratory compromise, depending on the level of injury.
* Cardiovascular compromise related to spinal shock.
* Autonomic dysreflexia—complications arising from elevated blood pressure.
* Decubitus ulcers requiring surgery and grafting.
* Pneumonia.
* Infection.

If I were your teacher, I would test you on . . .

- What is it?
- Signs and symptoms and why.
- Causes and why.
- Nursing care.
- Complications.
- Autonomic dysreflexia.

SUMMARY

Millions of Americans of all age groups are affected by neurological diseases. This review of the causes, signs and symptoms, tests, and treatments for key neurological disorders will help prepare you to meet the challenges of caring for these clients.

PRACTICE QUESTIONS

1. Which are the two main parts of the nervous system?

1. Central nervous system (CNS) and peripheral nervous system.

2. Brain and spinal cord.

3. Somatic nervous system and autonomic nervous system.

4. Brain and CNS.

Correct answer: 1. The two main parts of the nervous system are the CNS and peripheral nervous system. The brain and spinal cord are the main parts of the CNS. The somatic nervous system and autonomic nervous system are the main parts of the peripheral nervous system.

2. Which of the following brain structures controls body temperature?

1. Hypothalamus.

2. Medulla.

3. Hippocampus.

4. Cerebellum.

Correct answer: 1. The hypothalamus controls body temperature. The medulla controls breathing, blood pressure, and heart rate. The hippocampus controls memory and learning. And the cerebellum controls movement, coordination, posture, and balance.

3. Which of the following are symptoms of headache? Select all that apply.

1. Sensitivity to light.

2. Nausea.

3. Pain down one arm or leg.

4. Pressure.

Correct answers: 1, 2, & 4. Symptoms of headache include sensitivity to light (photophobia), nausea, and pressure in the temporal areas. Stroke may cause pain down one arm or leg.

4. Which of the following may be used to treat seizures? Select all that apply.

  1. Carbamazepine (Tegretol).

  2. Riluzole (Rilutek).

  3. Phenytoin (Dilantin).

  4. Temporal lobectomy.

Correct answers: 1, 3, & 4. Carbamazepine (Tegretol) and phenytoin (Dilantin) are commonly used anticonvulsants. Temporal lobectomy is a surgical intervention that may be indicated for seizures. Riluzole (Rilutek) is approved for amyotrophic lateral sclerosis (ALS).

5. Which of the following is a chronic, debilitating disease of the central nervous system (CNS) that is characterized by myelin destruction?

  1. Parkinson's disease.

  2. Myasthenia gravis.

  3. Multiple sclerosis.

  4. Pick's disease.

Correct answer: 3. Multiple sclerosis is a debilitating, progressive disease that is characterized by myelin destruction. Parkinson's disease is a progressive disorder of the CNS that affects movement, balance, and muscle control. Myasthenia gravis is an autoimmune disease characterized by weakness of voluntary muscles. Pick's disease is a brain disorder characterized by progressive dementia.

6. Vision changes, such as double vision, difficulty maintaining a steady gaze, and eyelid drooping are symptoms of which disease?

  1. Parkinson's disease.

  2. Myasthenia gravis.

  3. ALS.

  4. Lou Gehrig's disease.

Correct answer: 2. Myasthenia gravis causes weakness of eyelid muscles and extraocular muscles, resulting in vision changes. Symptoms of Parkinson's disease include resting tremor, muscle rigidity, and loss of autonomic movement. Symptoms of ALS include leg or hand weakness, clumsiness, difficulty swallowing, slurring, twitching in the arms, and extreme fatigue. Lou Gehrig's disease is another name for ALS.

7. Which of the following may cause trigeminal neuralgia?

   1. Hypertension.

   2. Multiple sclerosis.

   3. Diabetes.

   4. Atrial fibrillation.

Correct answer: 2. Multiple sclerosis is one cause of trigeminal neuralgia. Hypertension, diabetes, and atrial fibrillation may cause stroke, not trigeminal neuralgia.

8. Which of the following are symptoms of stroke? Select all that apply.

   1. Sudden numbness or weakness of the face, arm, or leg.

   2. Sudden confusion.

   3. Optic neuritis.

   4. Changes in bowel function.

Correct answers: 1 & 2. Sudden numbness or weakness of the face, arm, or leg and sudden confusion are symptoms of stroke. Optic neuritis and changes in bowel function are symptoms of multiple sclerosis, not stroke.

9. Which test would a physician order to determine if facial weakness results from Bell's palsy?

   1. Blood tests to rule out diseases, such as Lyme disease, HIV, and syphilis.

   2. Lumbar puncture.

   3. Nerve conduction studies.

   4. Electroencephalogram (EEG).

Correct answer: 1. A physician may order blood tests to rule out other causes of facial weakness. A physician might order a lumbar puncture or nerve conduction studies to determine if a client has Guillain–Barré syndrome. A physician may order an EEG to determine if a client has a seizure disorder.

10. A physician may order electromyography (EMG) to diagnose which of the following?

   1. Guillain–Barré syndrome.

   2. Pick's disease.

   3. Parkinson's disease.

   4. Spinal cord injury.

Correct answer: 1. EMG may be used to diagnose Guillain–Barré syndrome, ALS, and myasthenia gravis. Pick's disease can only be diagnosed by a postmortem exam of the brain. There's no diagnostic test for Parkinson's disease; the diagnosis is based on the history and clinical observation. Tests for spinal cord injury include computed tomography (CT) scan and magnetic resonance imaging (MRI).

References

1. Bader MK, Littlejohns LR. *AANN Core Curriculum for Neuroscience Nursing*. 4th ed. St. Louis: Elsevier; 2004.

2. Lewis SL, Heithemper MM, Dirksen SR, et al. *Medical-Surgical Nursing: Assessment and Management of Clinical Problems*. 7th ed. St. Louis: Mosby Elsevier; 2007.

3. Mayo Foundation for Medical Education and Research. 1998–2007. Available at: www.mayo.edu. Accessed July 6, 2007.

4. Medifocus. *MediFocus Guidebook on Parkinson's Disease*. Available at: www.medifocus.com/parkinsons-disease.php?a=a&assoc=pcosa. Accessed July 6, 2007.

5. Solomon D. Bell's palsy and other VII lesions. In: RW Evans, ed. *Saunders Manual of Neurologic Practice*. Philadelphia: Saunders; 2003:348–352.

Bibliography

Hurst Review Services. www.hurstreview.com.

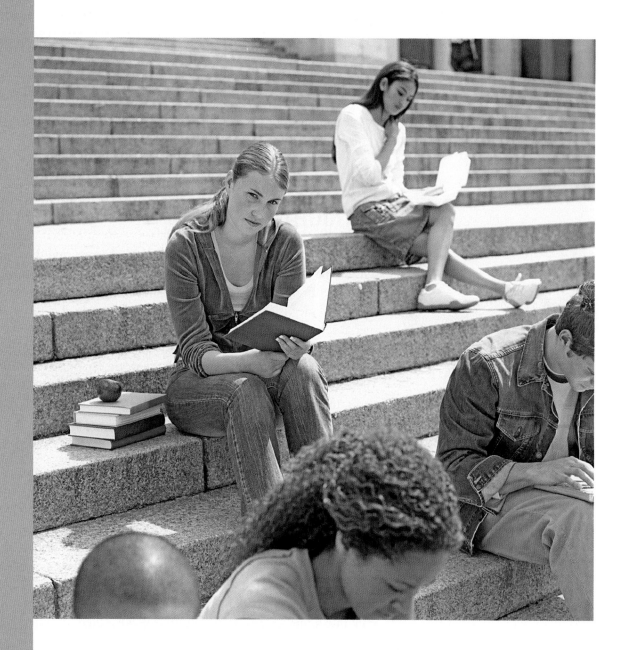

CHAPTER

10 Sensory System

OBJECTIVES

In this chapter, you'll review:

- The sensory organs and their related functions.
- The causes, signs and symptoms, and treatments for sensory disorders.
- The complications and client education associated with sensory system disorders.

LET'S GET THE NORMAL STUFF STRAIGHT FIRST

The sensory system is composed of the general senses and the special senses. The general senses control a person's body temperature, sense of proprioception, tactile sensation, and ability to feel pain. The special senses include vision, hearing, touch, smell, and taste. It is through the special senses that a person is able to interact with the environment.[1] These special senses provide a person with the ability to enjoy life more fully, for it is through these senses that the world can be better appreciated. These senses also provide a means for safety in an environment full of perils. In this section, we will first learn how the sensory organs normally function and then we will examine some pathologic disorders of these organs. So, let's begin with the eyes (Fig. 10-1).

✚ Vision

The eyes are complex organs that provide a person with the ability to interact with the environment. When functioning properly, the eyes provide us with the ability to distinguish color, shape, and depth—in other words, vision. Not only do the eyes provide vision for us as an excellent way to interact with the world around us, vision also gives us a means to protect ourselves from danger. Without the ability to see, a person may walk into a busy intersection or tumble down a flight of stairs. Without

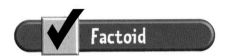

Factoid

Proprioception is the body's ability to tell what position the body is in. For example, proprioception is a person's ability to tell if he is lying down or sitting up.

▶ Figure 10-1. Anatomy of the eye. (From Saladin K. *Anatomy and Physiology: The Unity of Form and Function.* 4th ed. New York: McGraw-Hill; 2007.)

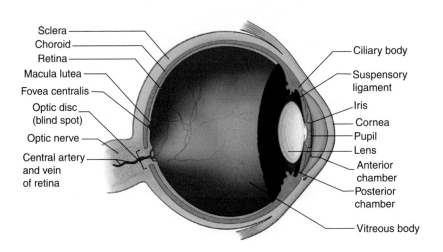

Sclera
Choroid
Retina
Macula lutea
Fovea centralis
Optic disc (blind spot)
Optic nerve
Central artery and vein of retina

Ciliary body
Suspensory ligament
Iris
Cornea
Pupil
Lens
Anterior chamber
Posterior chamber
Vitreous body

vision, you would not be able to read this pathophysiology book, play a game on your computer, view a sunset, or watch your favorite television show. Now, let's understand exactly how the normal eye works to provide us with vision.

Eye anatomy and physiology

The eye wall is made up of three layers. The outermost layer of the eye wall, known as the sclera, is thick tissue that is white in color until it reaches the cornea, where it becomes translucent. The cornea allows light to enter the eye. The middle layer of the eye wall is the choroid, which is heavily pigmented so that light allowed in by the cornea does not scatter randomly throughout the eye. The part of the choroid lying directly behind the cornea is known as the iris. Depending on the genetic makeup of a person, the color of the iris may be blue, green, brown, or hazel. Light passes from the cornea into the eye through a round opening, the pupil, found in the center of the iris. Smooth muscle attached to the pupil will change the size of the pupil in order to allow for varying degrees of light. If a person enters a room with dim light, the pupil size will enlarge, or dilate, so that more light can be let into the eye. If that person walks out into the sunlight, the pupil will constrict to decrease the amount of light entering the eye. The same principle applies to a camera. When you want to take a picture in the sunlight, the camera lens gets smaller. When you take a picture indoors, the lens widens and you need a flash of extra light. Located immediately behind the iris and the pupil is the lens, which is a flexible, biconvex crystal structure that focuses light on to the retina. The lens divides the anterior chamber of the eye into the aqueous chamber and the vitreous chamber.

The aqueous chamber is filled with aqueous humor, which provides nutrients to the lens and the cornea. It is the pressure of the aqueous chamber that the ophthalmologist measures in order to detect glaucoma. A gel-like substance known as vitreous humor fills the vitreous chamber to keep the eyeball formed.

The retina, the innermost layer of the eye wall, contains millions of cones and rods. The cones and rods convert light into nerve impulses. Cones, found predominately in the center of the retina, relay information to the brain about color and detail of objects. Rods are predominately located around the retina's periphery and are responsible for transmitting peripheral and dim light vision to the brain for interpretation.

In each eye, toward the back of the retina, lies the optic disc. This area of the retina cannot respond to light stimulation since no cones or rods are located here—thus, many call the optic disc the blind spot. The optic disc is the beginning of the optic nerve, or cranial nerve II. There are well over a million nerve cells in each optic nerve. You may wonder why we do not notice this blind spot since it is found in both eyes. The reason we do not normally notice the blind spot is because the blind spot of the right eye corresponds with a part of the seeing retina in the left eye. And the blind spot of the left eye corresponds with a part of the seeing retina in the right eye. The optic nerve leaves the eyeball at the optic disc and runs to the optic chiasm, just below and in front of the pituitary gland.

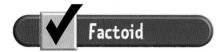

Factoid

The direct light reflex is when the pupil constricts in response to light. The consensual reflex is when you shine light in one eye and the OTHER pupil constricts.

The optic nerve fibers that began on the inside, or nasal, half of the retina cross over to the other side. Optic nerve fibers that began on the outside, or temporal side, of the retina do not cross over. Now the fibers become optic tracts, passing through the thalamus, and then advancing to the visual cortex located in the occipital lobe at the back of the brain. The visual cortex is what interprets the nerve impulses and changes it into a picture we can understand.[1]

So let's look at how we are able to see a tree (Fig. 10-2).

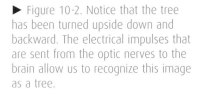

▶ Figure 10-2. Notice that the tree has been turned upside down and backward. The electrical impulses that are sent from the optic nerves to the brain allow us to recognize this image as a tree.

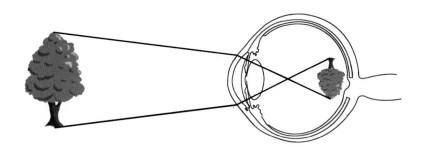

Light waves from a tree enter the cornea of the eye, where the cornea bends the waves. From the cornea, the light waves travel through the pupil, and then through the lens, where the light waves are further bent. At the back of the lens, the light wave image turns upside down and backward. The light progresses through the vitreous humor to the macula of the retina. The macula is located in a small central area of the retina and provides the best vision of any other retina location. In the retina, the light impulses are changed into electrical impulses that can be sent through to the optic nerve. The electrical impulses follow the optic nerve tracts to the occipital cortex of the brain, where they are interpreted by the brain as an image we recognize as a tree.

So, now that you understand how the eye works, let's look at what can happen to the eye that can impair vision.

LET'S GET DOWN TO SPECIFICS

✚ Cataracts

What are they?

Do you remember reading about the lens earlier in the chapter? The lens is located immediately behind the iris and the pupil. The lens divides the anterior chamber of the eye into the aqueous chamber and the vitreous chamber. The lens is a flexible, biconvex, crystal structure that focuses light on to the retina. Imagine a diamond. What is its most common quality? A diamond is clear. You can see through it if the clarity is good. Wouldn't you agree that the lens of the eye should be crystal clear? Yes, so light can pass through the lens, right? So what happens when the lens is not clear?

Cataracts develop on the lens of the eye (Fig. 10-3). The lens is made up of water and protein, which is arranged in a very exact manner so that the lens remains clear. The lens must be clear so that light can pass through it. Unfortunately, as a person ages, protein found on the lens can clump together. This clumping clouds the lens. This clouding is the cataract, which gets larger and more cloudy over time. The cloudiness of the lens leads to a decrease in light passing through the lens. In addition to becoming cloudy, the lens of the eye becomes increasingly harder. Think about it. The lens is normally flexible so that light can be directed to the retina. With a lens that is much less flexible, light scatters across the back of the eye rather than being focused on to the retina. The result is blurring of vision and difficulty seeing. One other thing to keep in mind about cataracts is that there is a decreased ability of the person to distinguish green and blue colors.[1]

Normal, clear lens

Lens clouded by cataract

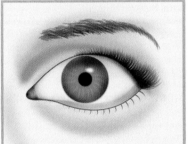
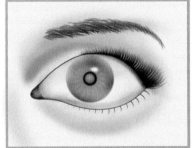

◀ Figure 10-3. Cataract.

Would you like to see what this would be like? Get a pair of inexpensive or toy glasses. Apply a thin layer of petroleum jelly over the lens, then put them on and try to walk around or tie your shoes. Look at a light. What do you see? What do you experience? How do you think you would feel if you couldn't take off those glasses when you were tired of experimenting with them?

There are three types of cataracts you should be aware of:

1. A nuclear cataract begins to form in the center of the lens and is caused by natural changes occurring with aging.

2. A cortical cataract begins at the cortex of the lens and moves into the center of the lens. Diabetics are most often those who develop a cortical cataract.

3. A subcapsular cataract starts at the back of the lens. People who have diabetes, or take a lot of steroids, are prone to this form of cataract.[2]

What causes them and why

No one knows for sure why a person's eye lens begins to change as we age. We do know that there are things that can contribute to the formation of cataracts, such as diabetes, medications, trauma, and exposure to ultraviolet light.

Table 10-1 shows the causes and explanations for cataracts.

Table 10-1

Causes	Why
Traumatic cataracts	Blunt injury to the eye, penetrating injury to the eye, intraocular foreign body, radiation exposure or therapy, and chronic sunlight exposure
Aging (also called senile cataract)	The lens becomes harder (from water loss) and cloudy. A yellow-brown pigment accumulates because protein within the lens breaks down
Nutritional deficiencies	Decrease in vitamin C, protein can lead to cataract formation. Poor nutrition, obesity
Toxic cataracts	High doses of corticosteroids can damage the lens. Other medications can be toxic including phenothiazine derivatives, miotic agents, and some chemotherapy drugs. Cigarette smoke can also be toxic to the lens
Associated cataracts	Diabetes mellitus, hypothyroidism, and Down syndrome are all affiliated with increased risk for cataract development

Source: Created by the author from References #1, #6, #7, and #10.

Signs and symptoms and why

Table 10-2 shows the signs and symptoms and associated reasons for cataracts.

Table 10-2

Signs and symptoms	Why
Increased glare and painless, blurred vision	With a lens that is much less flexible, light scatters across the back of the eye rather than being focused on to the retina. This causes sensitivity to light and blurring of vision
Decreased vision	The cloudiness of the lens leads to a decrease in light passing through, dimming vision
Decreased color perception	Decreased ability to distinguish green, blue, and yellow colors. The macula is located in a small central area of the retina and contains cells called cones and rods. Cones are responsible for central vision and color vision. Rods are responsible for seeing shades of gray
Absence of red reflex and presence of white pupil	Opacity of lens

Source: Created by the author from References #1, #6, #7, and #10.

Quickie tests and treatments

Tests:

- Slit-lamp examination: enables examiner to view lens opacity under magnification.
- Tonometry: measures intraocular pressure (IOP) to help rule out other disease processes.

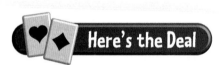

Hurst Hint

The client with cataracts has difficulty focusing. The fancy word for "focusing" is accommodation.

Here's the Deal

In cataracts, CENTRAL vision is lost. When two little white things (cataracts) sit on top of the pupil, straight ahead vision is obscured.

Factoid

Age-related cataracts are painless and usually not associated with any redness of the eye.

- Ophthalmoscopic examination: rules out diseases of the retina.
- Perimetry: determines the extent of vision throughout the visual field, which is usually normal with cataracts.
- Ophthalmoscopic exam and funduscopic exam: sometimes used interchangeably—either way, the examiner uses an ophthalmoscope to view the internal and external structures of the eye. The fundus of ANY organ is considered to be the larger portion of the organ such as the inside, the top, the bottom, the base, etc. In this case it is the inner part of the eye!

Treatments:

- Surgical removal especially if bilateral, one eye at the time. This is done under local anesthesia with preoperative eye drops. PO meds are given to decrease intraocular pressure (IOP).
- Intraocular lens implants may be implanted at the time of surgery to help restore distance vision.
- Minimize IOP after surgery by providing proper positioning. No lifting, stooping, bending, lifting, or straining. Teach the client to avoid rapid movements. Assist the client to lie on the unaffected side with HOB at 30 degrees.

What can harm my client?

Cataracts will not kill your client! Thank goodness, right? Right. However, you do need to worry about your client's safety and quality of life. So, the key here is education in order to promote safety. With diminished vision, a person is at greater risk for encountering home and environmental hazards. Prior to cataract removal, a client is at greater risk for:

- Falls.
- Accidents related to operating hazardous machinery, such as driving a car.
- Pain related to procedures and surgery.
- Degeneration of the cornea.
- Malpositioning or dislocation of the lens.
- Blindness.
- Infection after surgery.
- Increased intraocular pressure after surgery.

If I were your teacher, I would test you on . . .

- What is a cataract?
- All aspects of client education.
- Safety measures needed to protect the client from hazards.
- Education of clients should include:
  1. Promoting regular eye exams, since this is the key to early detection.
  2. Individuals over the age of 65 should have an eye exam at least every other year.

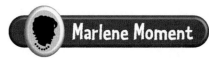

Marlene Moment

When and if you had to perform an ophthalmic exam during skills lab, I know you faked it and said, "Yes, I see the retina and possibly some AV nicking." Yea, right!

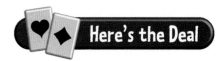

Here's the Deal

Postop, it is very important to decrease stress on the surgical area (suture line). To achieve this, the client must be positioned on the back or unoperative side.

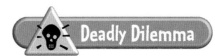

Deadly Dilemma

Well, it's not really deadly, but the client should report ANY decrease in vision and increase in severe pain postoperatively. Some discomfort is expected, but not severe pain.

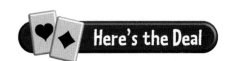

Here's the Deal

Atropine drops can be given postop to decrease inflammation. You better apply pressure on the inner canthus of the eye for one minute to prevent systemic absorption or the client's heart rate will go up, up, up!

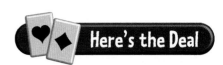

Here's the Deal

If you administer atropine eye drops, don't freak out when the pupil dilates! This is a normal response.

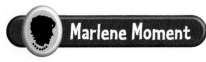

- Teach the following to clients at risk for cataract development:
  1. **Don't smoke.** Smoking produces free radicals, increasing the risk of cataract development.
  2. **Eat a balanced diet.** Plenty of fruits and vegetables should be encouraged.
  3. **Protect the eyes from the ultraviolet light coming from the sun.** Whenever possible, wear sunglasses when outdoors. Sunglasses also reduce glare.
  4. **Take care of other health problems.** Clients with other disorders such as diabetes can prevent or slow cataract formation if clients follow their treatment plan.
  5. **Use a magnifying glass to read.**
  6. **Improve home lighting.** Halogen lights or 100- to 150-watt incandescent light bulbs work better for providing enough light to see.
  7. **Limit night driving.** Night driving can be hazardous, since vision is more impaired with decreased light.

✚ Glaucoma

First, understand that the optic nerve is really a bundle of over a million nerve fibers that connect the retina to the brain. The retina is made up of special light-sensitive tissue that is located at the back of the eye. In order for a person to have good vision, the optic nerve must be healthy.

The lens divides the anterior chamber of the eye into the aqueous chamber and the vitreous chamber. The aqueous chamber is filled with aqueous humor, which provides nutrients to the lens and the cornea. It is the pressure of the aqueous chamber that the ophthalmologist measures in order to detect glaucoma. Normal intraocular pressure ranges from 12 to 20 mm Hg.

In order to maintain a normal intraocular pressure, the ciliary body found in the posterior chamber secretes aqueous humor, which then flows through the pupil into the anterior chamber. Once in the anterior chamber, some of the aqueous humor is reabsorbed through the trabecular network and drains into a channel called Schlemm's canal. The fluid then flows into the bloodstream. Any changes in secretion, circulation, or resorption can lead to glaucoma.

What is it?

Rather than a single eye disorder, glaucoma has been identified as a group of conditions. Glaucoma, the leading cause of vision loss, most commonly develops from a slow increase in intraocular pressure (IOP) within the aqueous chamber. As pressure builds up, ischemia (lack of oxygen to the tissue) occurs. If left untreated, an increase in IOP can result in pressure on the retina and optic nerve. The subsequent damage of the eye's optic nerve will result in vision loss, starting with peripheral vision. It can progress to total blindness. Would you like to experience loss of peripheral vision? Try this. Get two empty toilet paper rolls. Put one up to each of your eyes and then walk around a room you are not familiar with. What happened? Did you bump into the furniture? Can you see how dangerous this could be to an individual? The good news is that if it is treated early, serious vision loss can be averted.

Glaucoma is characterized as open angle or closed angle. It is either a primary or a secondary disorder.

• Glaucoma is said to be primary if there is no definitive cause of the glaucoma. In other words, the patient has no pre-existing condition of the eye or pre-existing disease that would have caused the glaucoma.

• Glaucoma is termed secondary if it occurs because of another condition, such as ocular trauma, prolonged use of steroids, tumors, or an inflammatory process of the eye.

Next, let's get open-angle and closed-angle glaucoma straight in our minds.

The most common form of glaucoma is primary open-angle glaucoma.

• Although the etiology is not clear, it is believed that there is an impairment of aqueous humor flow through the trabecular network, which leads to an increase in intraocular pressure.

• Most commonly seen in the 6th decade of life, open-angle glaucoma develops gradually without giving any warning signs.

• The bad thing about this type of glaucoma, is that the individual ends up with permanent vision damage since there are no early warning signs. The key is regular screening for increasing intraocular pressure.

Closed-angle glaucoma (angle-closure glaucoma) is considered a medical emergency because vision loss can occur within 24 hours of symptoms.

• Closed-angle glaucoma results when the pupil and lateral cornea angle narrow to a point where there is a decrease in aqueous humor flow out of the anterior chamber.

• When an individual has closed-angle glaucoma, pupil dilation can be dangerous due to the sudden increase in intraocular pressure. Immediate treatment is required.

• Keep in mind what causes the pupils to dilate. Darkness, stress, excitement, and medications can cause the pupils to dilate. Specific medications you need to be aware of are antihistamines, tricyclic antidepressants, as well as dilating eyedrops.

So who is at risk for glaucoma? Although anyone can develop glaucoma, African Americans over the age of 40 are at greater risk than the general population. Other high-risk clients include individuals over the age of 60, Americans of Mexican decent, or those with a family history of glaucoma.

What causes it and why

Table 10-3 explores the causes of glaucoma and the reasons behind them.

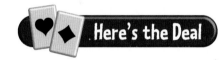

To put it simply, glaucoma is when the aqueous humor can't circulate like it needs to, so it builds up and makes the pressure go up (more volume, more pressure).

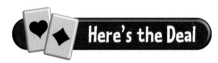

When a client presents with closed-angle glaucoma expect complaints of a sudden onset of severe pain, a red eye, and vision problems. This is very dangerous, as the retinal artery could be compressed!

Table 10-3

Causes	Why
Age	Age, especially after age 60, is the number one risk factor for the formation of glaucoma. African American risk starts rising after the age of 40
Race	Those of African American, Mexican-American, or Asian-American descent are at greater risk than Caucasians to develop glaucoma. Glaucoma is much more likely to cause permanent blindness in these groups. The reasons for these differences aren't clear
Family history of glaucoma	A family history of glaucoma puts a person at a greater risk for developing glaucoma. It is thought that glaucoma may have a genetic link. That means that there might be a defect in one or several genes that could lead to a person being more susceptible to glaucoma development
Medical conditions	There are several diseases that can contribute to the development of glaucoma. These include diabetes, uncontrolled hypertension, heart disease, and hypothyroidism. Regular coffee ingestion has also been implicated in slightly increasing a person's intraocular pressure
Physical injuries	Eye trauma, especially if severe, can cause an increase in eye pressure. The lens of the eye can also become dislocated, which can result in closing the drainage angle
Near-sightedness	Near-sightedness causes objects in the distance to look fuzzy. This increases the risk of developing glaucoma
Corticosteroid use	Prolonged use of corticosteroids increases a person's risk for developing secondary glaucoma
Eye abnormalities	There are some structural abnormalities of the eye that can lead to secondary glaucoma. Pigmentary glaucoma, one example, is caused by the back of the iris releasing pigment granules that block the trabecular meshwork[3]

Source: Created by author from References #1, #3, #9, and #11.

Signs and symptoms and why

When glaucoma begins to develop, the client may not experience symptoms. There is no pain and vision is still normal early on. However, as glaucoma progresses, peripheral vision diminishes and without treatment, blindness can result. Table 10-4 explores the signs and symptoms and associated reasons for glaucoma.

Table 10-4

Signs and symptoms	Why
Open-Angle Glaucoma	
No symptoms	In the beginning of glaucoma development, the fluid buildup is slow, and as with any other part of the body, it can compensate for a little while. So the individual may not even be aware that a problem has started with an increase in IOP that will eventually lead to optic nerve damage
Loss of peripheral vision	As IOP continues to increase, the optic nerve becomes affected. This pressure compresses on the optic nerve and a decrease in oxygen supply occurs. Nerve damage results if left untreated. Eventually, the person loses peripheral vision
Tunnel vision and eventually blindness	As glaucoma persists, more pressure is exerted on the optic nerve to the point that tunnel vision occurs. Remember putting the toilet paper rolls over your eyes? That is tunnel vision. Total death of the optic nerve causes blindness. Keep in mind, glaucoma can occur in one or both eyes
Acute Closed-Angle Glaucoma	
Sudden, severe eye pain	Increased intraocular pressure occurs suddenly, causing a sudden onset in eye pain. The eye does not have time to compensate when pressure goes up rapidly. This most often occurs when the person is sitting in a dark room, which causes the eyes to dilate. The angle diminishes, thus diminishing or occluding the flow of aqueous humor
Blurred vision	It is the buildup of pressure within the eye and around the optic nerve that causes vision to become blurred
Halos around lights	Again, it is the buildup of pressure within the eye and around the optic nerve that causes the person to see halos
Nausea and vomiting	Severe pain can stimulate the vomiting center
Hard eye to palpation	Increased pressure from fluid

Source: Created by author from References #1, #3, #9, and #11.

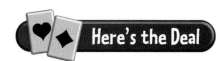

Here's the Deal

Pretend to look through the hole of a cardboard paper towel holder; this will give you an idea of how a decrease in peripheral vision feels.

Quickie tests and treatments

Tests:

- Ophthalmoscopic examination shows "cupping" of the optic disc. Atrophy may also be notable. The disc gets wider and deeper and changes color to white or gray.

- Measurement of visual field.

- Tonometry: measures IOP. Can be done by using air-puff tonometer. This is the less expensive way most commonly seen in the optometrist's office. It is great for screening large volumes of clients. The Goldman's

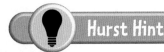

Hurst Hint

When performing a physical assessment, be sure and ask the client if they have had any eye surgeries, as this could alter the shape and appearance of the pupil/eye.

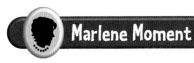

Marlene Moment

Have you ever had that blast of air blown into your eye that made you jump a mile high? "Now don't worry this is just a PUFF of air into your eye to check the pressure." Yeah, right!

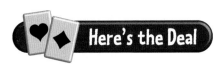

Here's the Deal

Glaucoma that occurs all of a sudden requires immediate treatment to decrease the intraocular pressure. Emergency surgery will probably be performed, but mannitol (osmotic diuretic) may be given as well to pull fluid out of the intraocular area.

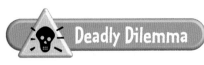

Deadly Dilemma

Never give atropine to someone with glaucoma. The pupil will dilate and aqueous humor cannot flow out properly. As a result, the intraocular pressure goes even higher!

applanation tonometer is used with a slit lamp, is very expensive, and is the standard way skilled ophthalmologists diagnose glaucoma. This is why you have the air blown into your eye at some clinics and not at others.

- Tonography: useful for measuring IOP.
- Gonioscopy: aids in determining drainage in the anterior chamber.

Treatments:

- Drugs that reduce IOP. They work by constricting the pupil so the ciliary muscle is contracted, which facilitates drainage of aqueous humor. These are "miotics." A few examples include atropine sulfate (Isopto Atropine) and pilocarpine hydrochloride (Salagen). Miotics can cause blurred vision for 1 to 2 hours as well as pupil constriction with difficulty seeing in low lighting.
- Drugs also work to reduce IOP by reducing the production of aqueous humor. A few examples include Xalatan, Travatan, Lumigan, and Rescula.
- Topical beta-blockers are also used, such as Apotimop, Timoptic, and Betagan. They don't cause pupil constriction.
- Laser surgery to control IOP.
- Surgery to create a drainage channel.

What can harm my client?

- Glaucoma will not kill your client; however, it can greatly alter your patient's quality of life.
- With diminished vision or blindness, a person is at greater risk for encountering home and environmental hazards.
- Operating hazardous machinery, such as driving a car, can put the patient at risk for an automobile accident.
- Remember, the person with glaucoma does not have peripheral vision. So, the key here is education in order to promote safety.
- Infection after surgery.
- Choroids hemorrhage or detachment after surgery as evidenced by eye pain, decreased vision, and changes in vital signs.
- Never give atropine to anyone with glaucoma.

If I were your teacher, I would test you on . . .

- What is it?
- Causes and why.
- Signs and symptoms and why.
- Treatment.
- Complications.
- Client education, including:

1. Promoting regular eye exams, since this is the key to early detection. Ophthalmologists recommend routine eye checkups every two to four years after age 40 and every one to two years after age 65.

African-Americans, who are at a much higher risk for glaucoma, should have routine eye exams every three to five years from age 20 to 29, and every two to four years after age 30.

2. Teach individuals at risk for glaucoma development to be alert for signs or symptoms of an acute angle-closure glaucoma attack. Signs and symptoms include severe headache or eye pain, nausea, blurred vision, or halos around lights. Emergency care is needed if any of these occur.

3. Clients at risk should understand that there is no proven method to prevent glaucoma.

4. Once diagnosed with glaucoma, it is important for the patient to understand the importance of taking glaucoma medication every day exactly as prescribed in order to reduce intraocular pressure.

Other recommended educational points to teach your client about are:

- **Maintain a healthy diet.** Fruits and vegetables provide important nutrients for the eyes, which include vitamins A, C, and E; zinc; and copper. Limit caffeine intake.

- **Exercise regularly.** Exercising three times a week may decrease intraocular pressure for the person who has open-angle glaucoma. The other forms of glaucoma, however, are not generally affected by exercise. Stress in patients who do yoga and other exercises that put the head in a dependent position might actually increase intraocular pressure.

- **Avoid stress.** Stress can precipitate an acute attack of closed-angle glaucoma. Teach your patient relaxation techniques such as relaxation and biofeedback.

- **Wear proper eye protection.** Eye trauma can increase intraocular pressure. Stress the importance of eye safety when playing sports or when using tools and machinery. Wearing safety goggles can prevent eye injury.

✚ Diabetic retinopathy

Do you recall what the function of the retina is? Let's review: the retina, which is the innermost layer of the eye wall, houses millions of cones and rods. Their function is to convert light into nerve impulses. Cones, found predominately in the center of the retina, relay information to the brain about color and detail of objects. Rods are predominately located around the retina's periphery and are responsible for transmitting peripheral and dim light vision to the brain for interpretation.

Toward the back of the retina lies the optic disc, which is the beginning of the optic nerve, or cranial nerve II. There are well over a million nerve cells in each optic nerve. The optic nerve leaves the eyeball at the optic disc and runs to the optic chiasm, just below and in front of the pituitary gland. The optic nerve fibers that began on the inside, or nasal half of the retina cross over to the other side. Optic nerve fibers that began on the outside, or temporal side of the retina do not cross over. Now the fibers become optic tracts, passing through the thalamus, and then

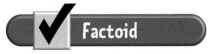

Factoid

Pilocarpine is a miotic drug that constricts the pupil, allowing aqueous humor to flow outwardly (intraocular pressure drops). Mydriatics are drugs that cause dilation of the pupil.

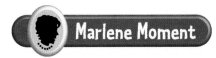

Marlene Moment

Before you call the neurologist about a client's fixed and dilated right pupil, be sure to find out if any surgery has been done!

advancing to the visual cortex located in the occipital lobe at the back of the brain. The visual cortex is what interprets the nerve impulses and changes it into a picture we can understand.[4]

What is it?

Diabetes can lead to a variety of complications that affect other systems within the body, including the eyes. Uncontrolled diabetes can lead to the most common diabetic eye disease, diabetic retinopathy. How does diabetic retinopathy develop? Basically, it develops because of changes in the blood vessels of the retina.

One of two things can happen to diabetics with diabetic retinopathy. One, the blood vessels may swell and leak fluid. Or, two, development of new blood vessels may grow on the surface of the retina. Remember, the retina is light-sensitive tissue found at the back of the eye. If the retina becomes unhealthy, then good vision cannot occur. Diabetic retinopathy progresses from no effect on vision to total vision loss in both eyes.

There are four stages of diabetic retinopathy:

1. Mild nonproliferative: earliest stage of diabetic retinopathy. At this stage, microaneurysms develop within the tiny blood vessels of the retina. Remember, an aneurysm is a very small outpouching with thinning, of a blood vessel.

2. Moderate nonproliferative: begins when some of the retina's blood vessels become blocked.

3. Severe nonproliferative: develops as more and more blood vessels become blocked. The retina is unable to get nourishment from this lack of blood supply. In order to compensate for this lack of blood supply, the body starts to grow new blood vessels for the retina.

4. Proliferative: The retina is continually signaling the brain to make new blood vessels so that it can receive proper nourishment. But, like new vessels grown anywhere, they are not as good as the originals were. These vessels are known as collateral circulation and are thinner and more fragile. They do not grow as a normal vessel would. They grow along the retina and along the surface of the vitreous gel inside the eye. If these vessels leak, severe vision loss and blindness can occur.

What causes it and why

Table 10-5 shows the causes and associated reasons for diabetic retinopathy.

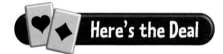

Here's the Deal

Diabetes has a serious effect on any vessel in the body. The retina is very vascular; therefore all diabetics should have a full eye exam yearly.

Table 10-5

Causes	Why
Diabetes	The longer someone has diabetes, the more likely she will be to get diabetic retinopathy
Type I	A person who has any type of diabetes is unable to utilize glucose (sugar) properly
Type II	Although a certain amount of glucose is necessary in the blood to provide energy to body
Gestational diabetes	cells, too much glucose will actually damage the blood vessels found throughout the body, including the tiny vessels found in the eyes. This damage leads to the four stages of diabetic retinopathy. Severity of retinopathy depends on level of glucose control

Source: Created by the author from References #1, #6, and #11.

Signs and symptoms and why

Unfortunately, there are no symptoms in the early stages of diabetic retinopathy. But the key is **NOT** to wait for symptoms to occur. All diabetics should have a comprehensive dilated eye exam at least once a year.

Table 10-6 shows the signs and symptoms and explanations for diabetic retinopathy.

Table 10-6

Signs and symptoms	Why
Blurred vision Poor night vision Difficulty adjusting from bright light to dim light	These may occur when the macula, which is the part of the retina that provides sharp central vision, begins to swell from leaking fluid. This condition is called macular edema
Vision loss Blindness	If new blood vessels grow on the surface of the retina, they can bleed into the eye and block vision
Floaters (spots in front of one's eyes) "Spiders," "cobwebs," or tiny specks floating in the person's vision Dark streaks or a red film that blocks vision	At first, the person will see a few specks of blood, or spots, "floating" in their line of vision. The person should seek medical attention immediately! A serious bleed may be occurring. Keep in mind that these hemorrhages tend to happen more than once, and often during sleep

Source: Created by the author from References #1, #6, and #11.

Quickie tests and treatments

Test:

- Full funduscopic exam by ophthalmologist for full visualization of retina.

Treatments:

- Laser therapy to stop bleeding from microaneurysms.
- Vitrectomy if retinal detachment is a possibility.

What can harm my client?

- Diabetic retinopathy will not kill your client; however, diabetes can.
- Just as with any other eye disorder we are discussing in this chapter, your client's quality of life can be greatly affected.
- Diminished vision, no matter what the cause, will place a person at a greater risk for encountering home and environmental hazards.
- Operating hazardous machinery, such as driving a car, can put the client at risk for an accident.
- Remember, the person with diabetic retinopathy will experience blurred vision, as well as poor night vision.
- No weight lifting or other strenuous exercise prior to laser therapy in order to prevent vitreous hemorrhage.
- The key here is education in order to promote safety, and prevent the deterioration of vision from occurring.

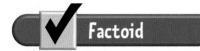

Factoid

Hypertensive retinopathy is damage to the retina due to damaged blood vessels related to sustained hypertension. This ultimately results in decreased vision.

If I were your teacher, I would test you on . . .

- What is it?
- Causes and progression of diabetic retinopathy.
- Education of clients, including:
  1. Diabetic clients should see an ophthalmologist to have their eyes dilated once a year.
  2. Emphasize the importance of controlling blood glucose levels. This can slow the progression of diabetic retinopathy.
  3. Good blood pressure can also reduce the risk for progression of the disease.

✚ Macular degeneration

Let's go back to the retina for a minute. The macula, which provides for normal central vision, is found in a small central area of the retina. The macula is made up of densely packed light-sensitive cones and rods. The cones are essential for central vision and for color vision. The rods enable an individual to see shades of gray.

It is important to understand that the choroid is an underlying layer of blood vessels that nourishes the cones and rods of the retina. The outermost surface of the retina consists of a layer of tissue that is called the retinal pigment epithelium (RPE). The RPE is a vital passageway for nutrients to go from the choroid to the retina. It also helps to remove waste products from the retina to the choroid.

What is it?

Macular degeneration is an age-related, chronic disorder of the eye (Fig. 10-4). It occurs when tissue in the macula deteriorates. Macular degeneration causes blurred central vision. It can also cause a blind spot in the center of an individual's visual field. The disease usually develops gradually, but can advance rapidly, leading to severe vision loss in one or both eyes. Any damage caused by macular degeneration is irreversible, but early detection and treatment may help reduce the extent of vision loss.

▶ Figure 10-4. Macular degeneration. **A.** Normal retina. **B.** "Wet" macular degeneration. **C.** "Dry" macular degeneration.

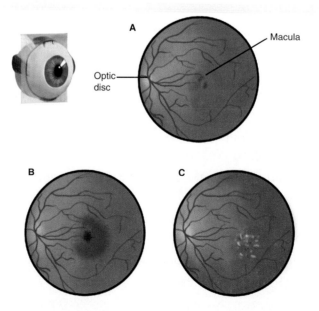

Several types of macular degeneration can occur:

1. Dry (atrophic) macular degeneration is the most common form, which commonly affects one eye first, eventually involving both. It occurs when the retinal pigment epithelium (RPE) cells begin to atrophy. Pigment is lost, so the normally uniform red color of the macula looks mottled. Fat deposits, called drusen, can be seen under the light sensing cells of the retina. Dry macular degeneration onset occurs over several years.

2. Wet macular degeneration only accounts for about 15% of all cases; however, this type is more likely to lead to severe vision loss. Wet macular degeneration develops when new blood vessels, called choroidal neovascularizations (CNVs), grow from the choroid underneath the macular portion of the retina. Unfortunately, these vessels leak fluid or blood, causing central vision to become blurry. In almost every case, wet macular degeneration started out as dry macular degeneration, and signs of this can be observed, such as drusen and mottled pigmentation of the retina. The individual will see wavy or crooked lines rather than straight lines when this occurs. In addition, what should be straight lines in your sight become wavy or crooked, and blank spots appear in your field of vision. With wet macular degeneration, loss of eyesight is usually rapid and severe. Onset is usually over several weeks to days.

3. One other form of macular degeneration exists, which is actually considered a type of wet macular degeneration. It is called retinal pigment epithelial detachment, which occurs when fluid leaks from the choroid under the RPE even though no abnormal blood vessels have started to grow. The fluid collects under the retinal pigment epithelium, looking like a blister under the macula. This kind of macular degeneration causes similar symptoms to typical wet macular degeneration; however, vision can remain relatively stable for months or years before it deteriorates.

What causes it and why

Researchers don't know the exact causes of macular degeneration, but they have identified some contributing factors, as seen in Table 10-7.

Table 10-7

Causes	Why
Age	Macular degeneration is the leading cause of severe vision loss for people over 60 in the United States
	As a person ages, the RPE may start to deteriorate, which leads to loss of pigment. This sets off a chain of events. First, the nutritional and waste-removing cycles are interrupted between the retina and the choroid. Waste deposits form. Unable to receive proper nutrients, the light-sensitive cells of the macula are damaged. These damaged cells cannot send normal signals through the optic nerve to the brain, so vision becomes blurred
Family history of macular degeneration	Chances of a person developing macular degeneration increases if family members also developed this disease. Researchers have been able to identify several genes they believe are associated with macular degeneration
Race	Although the reason is unclear, macular degeneration is more common in Caucasians than it is in other racial groups

(Continued)

Table 10-7. (*Continued*)

Causes	Why
Sex	Women are more prone to the development of macular degeneration than men. The primary reason for this is because women tend to live longer than men, thus are more likely to experience severe vision loss from the disease
Cigarette smoking	Exposure to cigarette smoke doubles a person's risk of developing macular degeneration. Cigarette smoke damages tissue by causing vasoconstriction, which decreases oxygen supply
Obesity	Obesity increases the chance that the early stages of macular degeneration will progress more rapidly to the more severe form
Light-colored eyes	People with light-colored eyes appear to be at greater risk than do those with darker eyes
Low levels of nutrients	Low blood levels of zinc and the antioxidant vitamins A, C, and E have been implicated in cell damage. It is believed that antioxidants may protect cells from oxygen damage. Lack of antioxidants may prove to be partially responsible for the effects of aging and for the development of diseases such as macular degeneration
Cardiovascular diseases	High blood pressure, stroke, angina, and heart attack all contribute to vessel damage and a decrease in blood supply to other organs of the body, including the eyes. Lack of oxygen leads to tissue damage

Source: Created by author from References #1, #11, and #12.

Signs and symptoms and why

Table 10-8 explores the signs and symptoms and associated reasons for macular degeneration.

Table 10-8

Signs and symptoms	Why
Dry Macular Degeneration	
Difficulty seeing or reading in low light Increasing blurriness of printed words A decrease in the brightness of colors Difficulty recognizing faces Gradual increase in haziness of overall vision Blind spot in the center of visual field Profound decrease in central visual acuity	All of these symptoms are caused by atrophy of the retinal pigment epithelium (RPE) cells. Remember, pigment is lost, and fat deposits, called drusen, form under the retinal cells. The macula, which is necessary for central vision, gradually loses its oxygen supply, making central vision difficult, and later impossible
Wet Macular Degeneration	
Visual distortions: straight lines look wavy; a street sign looks crooked; objects seem smaller and farther away than they actually are A decrease in or loss of central vision Central blurry spot	With wet macular degeneration, these symptoms may appear, and progress rapidly. Symptoms occur because of the new, weaker blood vessels that have developed under the macular part of the retina. The new vessels leak fluid or blood, causing central vision to become blurry
Visual Hallucinations	
	Some individuals with macular degeneration experience visual hallucinations as their vision loss increases. Hallucinations typically seen include unusual patterns or geometric shapes. They might see animals or frightening faces. Keep in mind that these individuals do not have a psychiatric disorder, but rather a visual disorder that is causing the hallucinations. The name for these hallucinations is Charles Bonnet syndrome

Source: Created by author from References #1, #11, and #12.

Quickie tests and treatments

Test:

- Full ophthalmoscopic/funduscopic examination.

Treatments:

- No cure.
- Disease is progressive, but may be slowed by increasing antioxidants and lutein and zeaxanthin, which are both carotenoids.
- Offer psychosocial support.
- Wet macular degeneration: the fluid and/or blood does sometimes resorb but not always. If not, laser therapy can be performed to "seal" leaking retinal/macular blood vessels.
- Teach.
    1. Large-print books to assist with reading.
    2. No driving. Instead, use a friend, family member, or public transportation.
    3. Availability of community organizations to those in need.
    4. Availability of support systems.

What can harm my client?

No, macular degeneration will not kill your client. It also will not cause total blindness, since it affects central but not peripheral vision. However, loss of central vision can decrease the person's quality of life. Patients with macular degeneration have difficulty reading, driving, recognizing people's faces, and doing detailed work. There is no cure and no treatment. A referral to community organizations such as a local chapter of the Lions club for assistance with adaptive devices/equipment is helpful.

If I were your teacher, I would test you on . . .

It is important for you to understand the disease process and how it will affect the client. Again, patient education is always important. Knowledge is power, and it is the nurse who is often in the best position to empower the patient. So, what is important to teach the client? Education of clients should include:

1. Eating foods containing antioxidants, such as green, leafy vegetables and fruits. It is believed that antioxidants promote good retinal health. Dietary supplement of antioxidants, zinc, and copper are thought to prevent oxidative damage to tissue, such as the retina.

2. Taking daily supplements of vitamin C, vitamin E, and beta-carotene. Studies have found that for people with moderate to advanced macular degeneration, taking these supplements has been effective in reducing the risk of further vision loss and may even prevent it altogether.

3. Recommending regular consumption of fish. The omega-3 fatty acids found in fish can result in a decreased risk of macular degeneration.

4. Wearing sunglasses that block out harmful ultraviolet light. Lenses that are orange, yellow or amber-tinted are better at filtering out ultraviolet and blue light. These glasses protect the surface of the eyes.

5. Encouraging smoking cessation, since smokers are more likely to develop macular degeneration than nonsmokers.

6. Educating the patient regarding the management of any other diseases, such as hypertension or angina. Emphasize the importance of taking medication.

7. Obtaining regular eye examinations for early detection of macular degeneration. It is recommended that after the age of 40 a person should get an eye exam every two to four years. After age 65, eye exams should be received every one to two years. Anyone with a family history of macular degeneration should have an eye exam yearly.

8. Teaching patients how to adjust to decreased central vision and avoiding potential hazards:

   - **Use caution when driving.** Do not drive at night, in heavy traffic or in bad weather.

   - **When possible use alternate transportation.** Use public transportation, such as buses, shuttles, or volunteers, or ask family members to help.

   - **Don't drive alone.**

   - **Get good glasses.** Correct glasses can assist vision. Keep an extra pair handy in case of loss or breakage.

   - **Use magnifiers.** Magnifying glasses will assist with reading and detailed work. Large-print books and magazines can also make reading easier.

   - **Have proper light in the home.** This will help prevent falls and will assist in activities such as reading.

   - **Remove home hazards.** Eliminate throw rugs and anything else which can create a fall hazard.

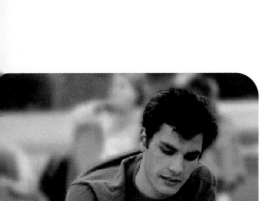

✚ Retinal detachment

Remember, the retina is the light-sensitive area of tissue found inside the eye. It is the retina that sends messages through the optic nerve to the brain for interpretation.

What is it?

Retinal detachment is the separation of the retina from its supporting layers (epithelium). After the retina detaches, it is pulled from its normal position. A delay in treatment can lead to permanent vision loss. There are three types of retinal detachment:

1. Rhegmatogenous: a tear in the retina following mechanical force lets fluid (vitreous) accumulate under the retina. This causes separation from the retinal pigment epithelium, which provides nourishment to the retina. This is the most common type of retinal detachment.

2. Tractional: develops after scar tissue (bands of fibrous tissue) forms on the surface of the retina. As this scar tissue contracts, it causes the retina to separate from the retinal pigment epithelium.

3. Exudative: inflammatory disorders, systemic disease, ocular tumors, or eye trauma causes fluid to collect in the area under the retina.

What causes it and why

Table 10-9 shows the causes and explanations for retinal detachment.

Table 10-9

Causes	Why
Tears or hole in the retina	Tears or holes (which can occur from aging or trauma) in the retina allow fluid to leak under the retina. This causes a separation or tear of the retina from the underlying tissues
Trauma	Trauma can cause a tear in the retina, which leads to leaking of fluid and subsequent retinal detachment
Uncontrolled diabetes	It can damage the vessels around the retina and can lead to tears
Previous eye surgery	Scar tissue formation
Family history of retinal detachment	Family history of inflammatory disease or systemic disease can predispose the client

Source: Created by the author from References #1, #6, #8, and #11.

Signs and symptoms and why

Table 10-10 shows the signs and symptoms and associated reasons for retinal detachment.

Table 10-10

Signs and symptoms	Why
Floaters (floating dark spots) and/or bright flashes of light (photopsia)	May occur when the macula begins to swell from leaking fluid and subsequent retinal detachment
The appearance of a curtain over the field of vision	During a detachment, bleeding from small retinal blood vessels may cloud the interior of the eye, which is normally filled with vitreous fluid. Central vision becomes severely affected if the macula, the part of the retina responsible for fine vision, becomes detached. Visual field loss corresponds to area of detachment
Blurred vision	May occur when the macula begins to swell from leaking fluid and subsequent retinal detachment
Blindness in part of the visual field in one eye. They have areas of BLANK vision!	Retinal detachment. The components of the retina convert light into nerve impulses that are transmitted to the brain for interpretation

Source: Created by the author from References #1, #6, #8, and #11.

Quickie tests and treatments

Test:

● Full ophthalmoscopic examination by ophthalmologist.

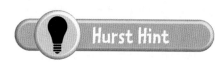

Here's the Deal

The retina lines the intraocular area. If someone gets hit in the head (football, MVA, fighting) the retina could become "unstuck" in one spot.

Hurst Hint

There is an area of the retina that is "unstuck" and it is floating around in the aqueous humor. If the detached part of the retina floats behind the pupil, no light can get in; then it can float up and out of the way and the client gets a flash of light.

Treatments:

- If detachment is suspected, place an eye patch over affected eye to reduce movement, which could cause further tearing or detachment. Restrict activity to prevent further tearing and to decrease the risk for fluid accumulation under the retina.

- Cryotherapy (freezing), photocoagulation (laser) therapy, or diathermy (high-frequency current) therapy are all used to close a tear or hole in the retina PRIOR to separation, which will reduce the risk for detachment. These techniques bind the retina and the choroids together at the break.

- Surgery under general anesthesia to reattach the retina to supporting structures. A common procedure is called the scleral buckling procedure. A piece of silicone is placed against the sclera, which is held in place by an encircling band. It keeps the retina in contact with the choroids and sclera to promote reattachment. Fluid under the retina is drained.

- Also, gas or silicone oil can be placed inside the eye, which floats up against the retina to hold it in place until healed.

- Topical drugs may be given prior to surgery to inhibit pupil constriction and accommodation.

- After surgery, if gas or oil was used, place the client on his/her abdomen to facilitate floating of the gas or oil against the retina. The client should lie with head turned—affected eye up. The client can also sit on side of bed with head lying over bedside table in the same fashion.

- Bathroom privileges can be resumed after fully awake.

- Give antiemetics and analgesics for nausea and pain. It is very important for this client not to vomit after surgery. The anesthesia may be causing the nausea, or it could be a complication of the surgery as well as the pain. Report this to the surgeon immediately.

- Monitor vital signs with particular attention to blood pressure and temperature. Blood pressure can increase intraocular pressure. Increased temperature can indicate infection.

- Observe the patch and shield for any drainage.

- Avoid any activities that would increase intraocular pressure (e.g., bending, stooping, lifting, coughing, and vomiting).

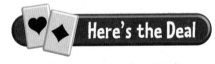

Here's the Deal

The client may be ordered to lie in a certain position for several weeks until the retina falls back into place. Since detachments can occur in different places in different clients, the position will vary.

What can harm my client?

Although not life threatening, a retinal detachment is a medical emergency. Anyone experiencing the symptoms of a retinal detachment should see an eye care professional immediately. It does not take long for permanent vision loss to occur.

If I were your teacher, I would test you on . . .

It is important for you to understand that retinal detachment is a medical emergency and that prompt treatment is necessary to prevent permanent visual loss. Client education should include:

- Emphasizing the importance of using protective eye wear to prevent eye trauma.
- How to control blood sugar levels for the diabetic client.
- Importance of yearly eye examination if at risk for retinal detachment.
- Preop care of the client with suspected retinal detachment.
- Postop care of the client with surgery to reattach the retina.
- Signs and symptoms to report to physician.
- Complications of surgery.

✚ Eye trauma

This section provides an overview of different kinds of eye trauma.

✚ Hyphema

What is it?

Hyphema is hemorrhage in the anterior globe of the eye.

What causes it and why

Hyphema is due to force from trauma.

Signs and symptoms and why

Signs and symptoms of hyphema include pain, photophobia (light sensitivity), and increased intraocular pressure—all related to hemorrhage.

Quickie tests and treatments

Test:

- Diagnosis is confirmed by client history and physical exam.

Treatments:

- Bed rest in semi-Fowler's position to promote gravity—keeps hyphema away from the center of the cornea. Bathroom privileges only.
- No sudden eye movements for about 5 days. No TV and no reading. Both restrictions are implemented to reduce bleeding.
- Patch and shield are worn for protection.
- Hyphema usually resolves within 5 to 7 days.
- Interior chamber paracentesis.
- Topical steroids.
- Cycloplegics.

What can harm my client?

- Rebleeding, leading to further damage to the eye (increased IOP) including the retina, with subsequent vision damage.
- Infection related to procedures.

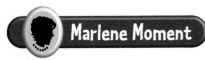

Marlene Moment

If a client comes into the emergency department with an object sticking out of the eye, please do not place a pressure dressing over the site! Also, a good rule of thumb is as follows: anytime a client presents to the ED with something sticking out of him (and it doesn't matter where or what it is), leave it for the physician to remove!

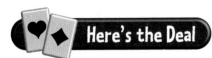

Here's the Deal

A car battery blows up in a client's face and his eyes are burning terribly. Hey! Don't wait for a physician's order. Go ahead and skip checking the vital signs and for allergies, as a part of your nursing assessment. The eyes must be irrigated at once to prevent blindness!

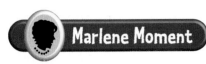

Marlene Moment

Children (and adults too) have even been known to superglue their eye shut. Now how does an adult manage that?! My friend knows (and she's a nurse).

If I were your teacher, I would test you on . . .

- Signs and symptoms and why.
- Treatment.
- Complications.
- Client safety.

+ Foreign body

What is it?

Foreign bodies (FBs) are often seen in the emergency department and may include eyelashes, dirt, bugs, glass, metal shavings, etc. It must be determined whether the FB has actually penetrated the eye or not. Sometimes there will be a simple corneal abrasion, but injury may be more extensive. If extensive damage is determined, an ophthalmological referral is in order. In simple cases, the FB will be removed by the physician or nurse practitioner in this setting, but there are some things you need to know in order to provide good care. FB in the eye is more common in men than women, due to recreational and work activities.

What causes it and why?

Table 10-11 explores the causes and why of foreign body.

Table 10-11

Causes	Why?
Riding ATVs	Particles from the air (bugs, dirt, other debris) or ground land in the eye
Welding or other work involving metal shavings (penetrating injury)	Sparks igniting
Children playing in the sand (they commonly throw sand into each other's faces)	
BBs (penetrating injury)	It is important to remember that accidents happen everyday
Bullets (penetrating injury)	
Glass (penetrating injury)	
Chemicals such as paint, gas, or cleaning fluids (these are foreign substances rather than foreign bodies)	Explosions, splashes, etc.

Source: Created by the author from References #1 and #11.

Signs and symptoms and why

Table 10-12 explores the signs and symptoms and explanations for foreign bodies.

Table 10-12

Signs and symptoms	Why
Pain	All related to presence of FB in eye
Increased tearing	
Photophobia	
Blurred vision	
Itching (leading to rubbing the eye causing a corneal abrasion)	Allergic reaction

Source: Created by the author from References #1 and #11.

Quickie tests and treatments

Tests:

- The physician or nurse practitioner in the emergency department setting will do a full eye exam to determine if an ocular injury is present.
- Visual acuity per Snellen chart.

Treatments:

- The primary care provider will remove any FBs after instilling a topical anesthetic (numbing drops) so the client can handle it! Be the advocate, have the numbing drops ready for the doc so the client will not jump up and run out of the room when she attempts to remove the FB! If the FB is embedded too deep, it will require surgical removal.
- Occular irrigation (done by the nurse per physican order after degree of damage is assessed and/or FB is removed).
- Next, to determine if a corneal laceration is present, the provider will stain the eye with fluorescein stain and shine a fluorescent light into the eye to visualize the laceration. Simple corneal lacerations require topical antibiotics in the form of drops or ointment. Sometimes a shield is placed over the eye just for comfort, but this is usually not necessary. Corneal abrasions usually heal very rapidly and are of no consequence.
- Tetanus booster.
- In the event of a foreign substance such as chemicals, copious irrigation is required.
- In the event of burns (thermal injury), apply sterile dressings and administer analgesics as ordered until the need for further care has been determined. Always leave fluid blebs intact with burns.
- You may be required as a nurse to contact poison control if working in the ED to obtain more information on how to handle certain chemical burns of the eye.

What can harm my client?

- Lack of timely management.
- Penetrating injury.
- Corneal laceration.

- Burns.
- Infection leading to further damage and vision loss.

If I were your teacher, I would test you on . . .

- I want you to understand the importance of timely management in the event of a serious eye injury. Do not leave this client waiting in the ED waiting room for 4 hours, because until the client is examined, the extent of damage is unknown. I don't care how busy ya'll are, get someone to take a look at this client expeditiously. Don't be responsible for the loss of someone's vision!
- What is a FB?
- How does FB injury occur?
- What do you need to know as a NURSE in this situation (importance of time management, poison control, etc.).
- Technique for proper ocular irrigation.
- Complications.
- How to take care of a client postop eye surgery.

Other serious eye injuries that are considered medical emergencies include lacerations and perforations of the globe, ruptured globe, and burns from chemicals or heat (thermal). Lacerations, perforations, and ruptured globes will likely require surgery. CT and MRI may be performed to determine the condition of the orbit.

CASE IN POINT   Your client enters the ED waiting room and states her eye is hurting and she is having trouble seeing. She elaborates further, telling you that she is on chemotherapy and commonly leaves her contact lens in place for extended periods of time. Think severe infection related to immunosuppression from chemotherapy. The infection is probably related to a corneal abrasion from the extended wear of the contact lens. Further assessment may reveal copious drainage and color changes of the eye. This client should be admitted immediately and given aggressive treatment under the supervision of an ophthalmologist in order to save her eye. You may need to instill drops every 5 minutes.

✚ Contusion

What is it?

The eye is subsequently pushed back into the socket where it is compressed, which leads to soft-tissue injury and even possible rupture.

What causes it and why

A contusion is due to a blow from a blunt object (a ball, a fist, etc.).

Signs and symptoms and why

Table 10-13 shows the signs and symptoms and explanations for eye contusion.

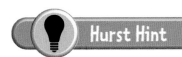

Hurst Hint

Some general principles for eye surgeries are as follows: have the client lie on the unaffected side or on his back; no straining with bowel movements; no vomiting, coughing, sneezing, or bending, as these can increase intraocular pressure.

Table 10-13

Signs and symptoms	Why
Edema of eyelids with pain, photophobia, and diplopia	Inflammation from trauma
Subconjunctival hemorrhage	Bleeding
Corneal edema	Inflammation from trauma
Hyphema	Bleeding
Periorbital ecchymosis "black eye"	Bleeding into the soft tissues

Source: Created by the author from References #1 and #12.

Quickie tests and treatments

Test:

- Eye contusion is confirmed by client history and physical exam.

Treatments:

- Ice needs to be applied immediately.
- Thorough eye exam by experienced provider to rule out more serious injury such as retinal detachment.

What can harm my client?

- Ruptured globe.
- Retinal detachment or any other serious eye injury related to the blow.
- Consider this: did this occur due to a violent act? You will find that you will be involved in more "situations" as a nurse than you ever dreamed. You need to know your hospital policy on reporting domestic and/or other forms of violent acts.

If I were your teacher, I would test you on . . .

- Signs and symptoms and why.
- Treatment.
- Complications.
- Importance of reporting domestic abuse and violent acts.

✚ Hearing

Let's look at the normal anatomy and physiology of the ear first (Fig. 10-5). The ear is divided into three different parts: the external ear, the middle ear, and the inner ear. The external ear consists of the pinna. The pinna is the part of the ear that you can see, and it collects sound and directs it into the outer ear canal. The ear canal transmits sounds to the eardrum or tympanic membrane (TM).

▶ Figure 10-5. Internal anatomy of the ear. (From Saladin K. *Anatomy and Physiology: The Unity of Form and Function.* 4th ed. New York: McGraw-Hill; 2007.)

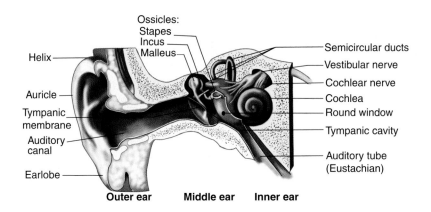

The tympanic membrane, a very thin membrane, is the beginning of the middle ear. When sound waves hit the tympanic membrane, it begins to vibrate. This vibration causes three tiny bones in the middle ear to vibrate as well. These three tiny bones are called the malleus (hammer), incus (anvil), and stapes (stirrup). From there, the vibrations travel to the inner ear. The eustachian tube connects the back of the nasopharynx to the middle ear. Why? The eustachian tube keeps pressure within the middle ear equal to the pressure in the outside atmosphere. It also allows normal drainage, as well as abnormal secretion drainage from the middle ear to the nasopharynx.

Sound vibration travels from the malleus, incus, and stapes to the inner ear. The inner ear is divided into the cochlea, the vestibule, and the auditory nerve. The cochlea is a spiral-shaped, fluid-filled structure that is lined with cilia. The cilia cause an electrical nerve impulse to form and then travel to the auditory nerve. From the auditory nerve, the impulse travels to the brain, where it is interpreted as sound. The vestibule or the semicircular canals are three loops of fluid-filled tubes that are attached to the cochlea in the inner ear. They help us maintain our sense of balance.

✚ Ménière's disease

The vestibule of the inner ear consists of three semicircular canals. These canals are loops of fluid-filled tubes that are attached to the cochlea. The purpose of these semicircular canals, in conjunction with cranial nerve VIII, is to maintain our sense of balance and sense of body position.

What is it?

Ménière's disease, an abnormality of the inner ear, leads to hearing loss, primarily in one ear.

What causes it and why

Even though about 100,000 people per year develop Ménière's disease, the exact cause is unknown. There is also no known cure for Ménière's disease. Table 10-14 shows the causes and reasons behind them for Ménière's disease.

Table 10-14

Causes	Why
Swelling of the endolymphatic sac	The endolymphic sac controls the filtration and excretion of fluid in the semi-circular canals. Swelling will decrease the ability of the sac to excrete excess fluid
Otitis media	Middle ear infections can cause scar tissue, which can prevent filtration and excretion of fluid in the semicircular canals
Head injury	Head injury leads to increased intracranial pressure, which can lead to increased pressure in the inner ear
Viral illness such as respiratory infection	Upper respiratory infections can carry the disease through the eustachian tube to the middle ear. This can lead to damage of the semicircular canals
Use of medication such as aspirin	Aspirin overdose can lead to damage to the semicircular canals

Source: Created by the author from References #1, #4, #11, and #12.

Signs and symptoms and why

The symptoms of Ménière's disease occur suddenly and can be as frequent as daily or as infrequently as once a year. It is important to remember that all of these symptoms are unpredictable. Typically, the attack is characterized by a combination of vertigo, tinnitus, and hearing loss lasting several hours. People experience these discomforts at varying frequencies, durations, and intensities. Some may feel slight vertigo a few times a year. Others may be occasionally disturbed by intense, uncontrollable tinnitus while sleeping. Ménière's disease sufferers may also notice a hearing loss and feel unsteady all day long for prolonged periods. Table 10-15 shows the signs and symptoms and explanations for Ménière's disease.

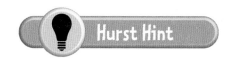

Hurst Hint

When talking to someone with Ménière's disease, stand directly in front of them. Any movement of the head can precipitate an attack.

Table 10-15

Signs and symptoms	Why
Vertigo	Often the most debilitating symptom of Ménière's disease. Vertigo is an abnormal sensation of movement of the environment. It can be episodic, lasting for minutes or hours. Movement makes it worse. It is caused by the inability of fluid to filter and leave the semicircular canals
Dizziness	Sensation that the individual is moving rather than the environment
Tinnitus	Ear noises, a loss of hearing, or a full feeling or pressure in the affected ear
Other occasional symptoms of Ménière's disease include headaches, abdominal discomfort, and diarrhea. A person's hearing tends to recover between attacks but over time becomes worse	Excessive fluid in the semicircular canals, generalized fluid excess in vascular space
Hearing loss in one ear	Low-frequency noises lost first
Nausea, vomiting	Vertigo attacks can lead to severe nausea, vomiting, and sweating (may be profuse) and often come with little or no warning
Nystagmus	Uncontrollable eye movements[5]

Source: Created by the author from References #1, #4, #11, and #12.

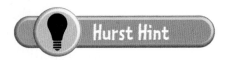

Hurst Hint

ENG—more sophisticated type of calorie test which assesses vestibular function.

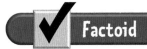

Factoid

Clients who have undergone a labyrinthectomy can have vertigo, unsteadiness, and dizziness for 48 hours postop. I'll bet the client is ticked off when they wake up, because this is why they had the surgery in the first place!

Quickie tests and treatments

Tests:

- Caloric test/electronystagmography (ENG) to differentiate Ménière's disease from an intracranial lesion—warm fluid is instilled into the ear canal, which precipitates an attack in those with the disease. Simple dizziness will occur in those who do not have the disease. Acoustic neuroma clients will have no reaction.
- Audiogram will show sensorineural hearing loss.
- CT scan, MRI to rule out acoustic neuroma.

Treatments:

- Treatment is focused on lowering the pressure within the endolymphatic sac and on treating symptoms.
- Client can keep a diary of attacks.
- Antihistamines, anticholinergics, and diuretics are used in an attempt to lower endolymphatic pressure by reducing the amount of endolymphatic fluid.
- Streptomycin or gentamycin are sometimes given to selectively destroy vestibular apparatus for excessive intolerable vertigo.
- Antiemetics such as phenergan for nausea and vomiting.
- Surgery: endolymphatic sac decompression, endolymphatic subarachnoid or mastoid shunt to relieve symptoms without destroying function. This is a conservative surgical approach. More aggressive surgeries include labyrinthectomy if attacks interfere with activities of daily living (ADLs). This results in complete deafness in the affected ear. Another surgery is vestibular nerve neurectomy.
- Low-salt diet reduces fluid retention.
- For severe symptoms of dizziness, vertigo, nausea and vomiting, the doctor may prescribe a sedative, benzodiazepines, and antiemetics.
- Surgery on the labyrinth, endolymphatic sac, or the vestibular nerve may be required if symptoms are severe and do not respond to other treatment.
- Hearing aids may be necessary if hearing loss becomes severe.

What can harm my client?

No, your client won't die if they have Ménière's disease. However, your patient is at risk for injury due to the vertigo and subsequent loss of hearing. Patients have difficulty hearing, walking, and driving. Any sudden head movement can lead to these symptoms. Complications include irreversible hearing loss and depression related to decreased quality of life.

If I were your teacher, I would test you on . . .

- Causes and why.
- Signs and symptoms and why.
- Treatment and complications.

● Client education and safety, including:

1. Teach the patient to avoid sudden movements that may aggravate symptoms.

2. They may need assistance with walking due to a loss of balance.

3. Rest needs to be emphasized during severe episodes, with gradual increase of activity.

4. During episodes, the patient should avoid bright lights, TV, and reading, which may make symptoms worse.

5. Avoid hazardous activities such as driving, operating heavy machinery, climbing, and similar activities until one week after symptoms disappear.

6. Physical therapy may be useful in order to assist the patient in becoming acclimated to various positions.

✚ Otitis media

What is it?

Otitis media (OM) is an infection or inflammation of the middle ear. Most of the time this inflammation begins as an infection, such as a sore throat, cold, or other respiratory or breathing problem. This infection can spread fairly easily to the middle ear. Children are much more prone to the development of otitis media, and the majority of children will experience at least one episode of otitis media by their third birthday. Although otitis media is primarily a disease of infants and young children, it can also affect adults.[6]

What causes it and why

Table 10-16 shows the causes and explanations behind them for otitis media.

Table 10-16

Causes	Why
Bacterial or viral infection of the throat, oro-pharynx, respiratory system.	The eustachian tubes are open to the oro-pharynx and are shorter in the infant and young children. Bacteria and viruses can travel more easily to the inner ear, causing inflammation and infection

Source: Created by the author from References #1 and #11.

Signs and symptoms and why

Otitis media is often difficult to detect because most children affected by this disorder do not yet have sufficient speech and language skills to tell someone what is bothering them. Table 10-17 shows the signs and symptoms and explanations for otitis media.

Table 10-17

Signs and symptoms	Why
Severe pain	Pain develops from fluid pressure on the nerves
Although the hearing loss caused by otitis media is usually temporary, untreated otitis media may lead to permanent hearing impairment	Persistent fluid in the middle ear as well as chronic otitis media can reduce a child's hearing at a time that is critical for speech and language development. Children who have early hearing impairment from frequent ear infections are likely to have speech and language disabilities
	Unresponsiveness to quiet sounds, or other signs of hearing difficulty such as sitting too close to the TV or being inattentive, may be early signs of hearing loss
Unusual irritability	Due to the pain
Difficulty sleeping	Due to ear pain
Tugging at ear	Pain that results may cause the child to tug at the affected ear. This is a common sign for children
Fever	Inflammation causes fever to develop
Fluid draining from the ear	Fluid buildup behind the eardrum can cause rupture of the eardrum and fluid can then drain from the ear. Pain is usually relieved at this point; however, there is now a bigger opening for infection to enter the middle and inner ear
Loss of balance	Fluid affects the cochlea and thus the balance of the child

Source: Created by the author from References #1 and #11.

Quickie tests and treatments

Tests:

- Examination with otoscope will show inflamed or bulging tympanic membrane without normal visible bony landmarks.
- Tympanometry: tells if the tympanic membrane is moving or not (normally it should have mobility).

Treatments:

- Most middle ear infections are self-limited and will resolve spontaneously.
- Treat any underlying allergies that could predispose the client to recurrent infections. Allergies lead to conducive conditions for bacterial overgrowth.
- PE (pressure equalizing) tubes.
- Adenoidectomy.
- Antibiotics [amoxicillin (Augmentin), cephalosporins].

What can harm my client?

The development of meningitis can kill your client. An untreated infection can travel from the middle ear to the nearby parts of the head, including the brain. Prompt treatment is necessary to prevent the spread of infection.

Another danger for infants and small children is the development of a high fever, which can lead to febrile seizures. Prompt fever control is vital for management of fever. Typically Tylenol and ibuprofen are alternated to bring fever down. Tepid sponge bath may be necessary to bring fever down.

- Hearing loss.
- Mastoiditis.
- Perforation of the TM.
- Delayed speech and language development.

If I were your teacher, I would test you on . . .

- What is it?
- Causes and why.
- Signs and symptoms and why.
- Complications.
- Children who are cared for in group settings have more ear infections.
- Children who live with adults who smoke cigarettes are more prone to ear infections.
- The best prevention is to educate parents about making sure that their child avoids contact with sick children and environmental tobacco smoke.
- Infants should not nurse from a bottle while lying down, since that can precipitate the development of otitis media.
- Breast-fed infants tend to have fewer ear infections.

✛ Mastoiditis

What is it?

Mastoiditis is an infection, generally bacterial, of the mastoid bone of the skull commonly affecting children. Usually mastoiditis develops after acute otitis media. The infection spreads from the ear to the mastoid bone of the skull. The mastoid is the bony bump off the base of the skull, located just behind the ear slightly above the level of the earlobe. This bone is made up of air cells that communicate with the middle ear. If the air cells fill with an infection, the mastoid structure may deteriorate. Mastoiditis is classified as either acute or subacute.

What causes it and why

Table 10-18 shows the causes and explanations for matoiditis.

Table 10-18

Causes	Why
The bacteria that cause mastoiditis are those most commonly associated with acute otitis media. They include the following bacteria: • *Streptococcus pneumoniae* • *Haemophilus influenzae* • *Moraxella catarrhalis* • *Staphylococcus aureus* • *Pseuodomonas aeruginosa* • *Klebsiella* • *Escherichia coli* • *Proteus* • *Prevotella* • *Fusobacterium* • *Porphyromonas* • *Bacteroides*	Acute mastoiditis occurs after an incidence of otitis media and involves the development of an abscess behind the ear. Subacute mastoiditis is a chronic form of the disease typically seen when otitis media is not treated fully with antibiotics

Source: Created by author from References #1 and #11.

Signs and symptoms and why

Table 10-19 shows the signs and symptoms of mastoiditis and the reasons behind them.

Table 10-19

Signs and symptoms	Why
Increasing earache Pain behind the ear Redness and swelling behind the ear	The eardrum is inflamed with swelling of the ear canal wall. Swelling of nerves, which transmits pain to brain
Fever, may be high or spike	Inflammation causes fever to develop
Drainage from the ear	Fluid buildup behind the eardrum can cause rupture of the eardrum, and fluid can then drain from the ear. Pain is usually relieved at this point; however, there is now a bigger opening for infection to enter the middle and inner ear

Source: Created by author from References #1 and #11.

Quickie tests and treatments

Tests:

• No diagnostic test, but may be manifested by inflamed tissue in the scalp or over the mastoid process.

• Otoscopic exam reveals red, dull, immobile eardrum.

• Lymph nodes behind the ear are usually swollen and tender.

• Diagnosis is usually made by clinical exam.

Treatments:

- IV antibiotics to prevent spread.
- Culture any ear drainage.
- Mastoidectomy if no response to antibiotics.

What can harm my client?

Before the use of **antibiotics**, mastoiditis was one of the leading causes of death in children. As of early in the 2000s, it is relatively uncommon and is a much less dangerous disorder.

- Damage to cranial nerves VI and VII, causing neuromuscular deficits of the face.
- Vertigo.
- Meningitis.
- Brain abscess.
- Chronic purulent OM.
- Wound infection with subsequent complications.

If I were your teacher, I would test you on . . .

Prompt and complete treatment of all ear infections reduces the risk of developing mastoiditis.

Mastoiditis is curable with treatment but may be hard to treat and may recur. Ear pain is a common complaint from children, but parents should suspect serious ear infection if the ear area is red and swollen. Mastoiditis often causes the ear to be sticking out at an angle. Parents should be aware that ear infections are very common in children, especially those younger than 2 years of age.

- What is it?
- Signs and symptoms and why.
- Causes and why.
- Treatments and complications.

Quickie review of sensory perception disturbances and related causes

Table 10-20 outlines the different perception disturbances.

Table 10-20

Disease processes such as	
Multiple sclerosis	Damage to the myelin sheath of the white matter of the CNS. The myelin is responsible for electrochemical transmission of nerve impulses between the brain, spinal cord, and the rest of the body. Sensoriperceptual manifestations involve motor function, dizziness, aphasia, hearing loss, vision changes, diminished sensitivity to pain, decreased temperature perception or paresthesia (tingling, burning, etc., of the extremities)

(Continued)

Table 10-20. (*Continued*)

Disease processes such as	
Diabetes	Decreased peripheral sensation, paresthesias (numbness, tingling, burning, etc.), vision changes
Spinal cord injuries	Partial or total paralysis with loss of function of major motor, fine motor, sensation, reflexes, and bowel and bladder control. Worst-case scenario is when the client loses the ability to breath on his own. Complications include loss of muscle tone with atrophy, pressure ulcers, etc.
Stroke	Visual or spatial perceptual disturbances including depth and distance perception as well as right and left or up and down discrimination. Other deficits include unilateral neglect, vision changes in one or both eyes (hemianopsia), all related to right hemisphere damage
	Left hemisphere damage results in memory deficits, apraxia (inability to perform previous motor skills/commands). Patients usually move very slowly and demonstrate fear and excessive caution when trying to perform tasks
	Expressive or receptive aphasia occur as a result of damage to other areas of the brain, such as the frontal lobe or the temporoparietal lobe
	Physical therapy is imperative for stroke clients in order to assist them with all perceptual deficits such as depth and proprioception, neglect syndrome, and major motor skills, etc.
	Nursing care involves teaching your client to use both sides of the body when dressing, washing, etc. Remind the client to turn his/her head in order to experience a more full visual field while eating
	Speech therapy will be needed for language deficits and swallowing problems
	OT will be needed for assistance with fine-motor skills
Head trauma	Traumatic brain injury resulting in neurological changes, such as amnesia; behavior changes, such as confusion, combativeness (temporary or permanent); vision and papillary changes; motor deficits; hearing deficits; etc., depending on the extent and location of brain injury
Sensorineural hearing loss	Defect in the cochlea, CN VIII, or the brain. May be the result of sustained exposure to loud noises, such as machinery or music (watch those rock concerts!). Sometimes the hearing loss is profound and requires the use of hearing aids
Burns	Disturbed sensory perception including visual (periorbital edema or ulcerations), auditory, and tactile deficits
Guillain–Barré syndrome	Immune system destroys myelin (autoimmune) sheath surrounding axons impairing nerve conduction leading to weakness, paresthesia, and paralysis. Can involve everything including speech, vision, breathing, etc.
Raynaud's phenomenon	Cold, painful, and pale to bluish-colored fingers related to arteriolar vasoconstriction. Unusual sensitivity to cold, autoimmune problems, or emotional stress are thought to play a role in the etiology of the syndrome

Source: Created by author from References #1, #11, and #12.

Quickie cranial nerve (CN) overview

There are 12 of them, and their primary functions are outlined in Table 10-21.

Table 10-21

Nerve	Function
CN I—olfactory nerve	Sense of smell
CN II—optic nerve	Visual acuity and visual fields
CN III—oculomotor	Responsible for pupillary function and movements of extraocular eye muscles
CN IV—trochlear	Eye movement
CN V—trigeminal	Motor and sensory function of the face
CN VI—abducens	Eye movement
CN VII—facial	Motor function of the face
CN VIII—acoustic	Sense of hearing and vestibular function
CN IX—glossopharyngeal	IX and X are tested together. They are responsible for the gag reflex and movements of the uvula and palate
CN X—vagus	Same as CN IX
CN XI—spinal accessory	Responsible for sternocleidomastoid and upper trapezius muscles
CN XII—hypoglossal	Motor function of the tongue

Source: Created by author from References #1, #11, and #12.

SUMMARY

The nurse's understanding of sensory illnesses is paramount to client safety and improved health. Knowledge of sensory illnesses enables the nurse to develop an appropriate plan of care and advocacy for clients.

PRACTICE QUESTIONS

1. A 63-year-old male client comes to the clinic with blurring vision and inability to see well in the sunlight. The nurse suspects the client is experiencing symptoms of:

   1. Glaucoma.

   2. Cataract.

   3. Retinal detachment.

   4. Macular degeneration.

   Correct answer: 2. Cataracts are characterized by painless, blurred, decreased vision with increased glare and decreased color perception.

2. A client diagnosed with asthma takes large doses of glucocorticoids. The nurse should teach the client to:

1. Monitor for signs of hypoglycemia.

2. Engage in routine hearing assessments.

3. Increase protein in the diet.

4. Engage in regular eye examinations.

Correct answer: 4. Glucocorticoids can cause changes to the eye. Clients who take large doses of glucocorticoids should engage in regular eye examinations.

3. A nurse educates a client about glaucoma on the basis of an intraocular pressure finding greater than:

1. 5 mm Hg.

2. 10 mm Hg.

3. 15 mm Hg.

4. 20 mm Hg.

Correct answer: 4. Normal intraocular pressure ranges from 12 to 20 mm Hg.

4. A client with a history of glaucoma arrives at the clinic for a physical examination. While performing the eye exam, the nurse makes sure to check the client's:

1. Peripheral vision.

2. Central vision.

3. Papillary response.

4. Blind spot.

Correct answer: 1. When glaucoma begins to develop, the client may not experience symptoms. There is no pain and vision is still normal at this point. However, as glaucoma progresses, peripheral vision diminishes and without treatment, blindness can result.

5. One goal of diabetic teaching to a client by a nurse should include:

1. Monitoring of eyes every 3 years by an ophthalmologist.

2. Treating mastoid infections to avoid mastoiditis.

3. Monitoring glucose levels to avoid diabetic retinopathy.

4. Monitoring yearly hearing exams for the development of Ménière's disease.

Correct answer: 3. Too much glucose can damage the tiny blood vessels found in the eyes. This damage leads to the four stages of diabetic retinopathy.

6. Six hours after playing a game of touch football, a 24-year-old male arrives at the emergency department with complaints of floaters in his field of vision. The nurse's priority intervention is to:

1. Perform a visual acuity exam.

2. Start an IV of lactated Ringer's.

3. Flush the eye with copious amounts of normal saline.

4. Prepare the patient for emergency surgery.

Correct answer: 4. Floaters in the field of vision are an indicator of retinal detachment, which requires emergency surgery. A delay in treatment can lead to permanent vision loss.

7. A client is admitted to the medical unit with a diagnosis of a severe episode of Ménière's disease. Which of the following orders should the nurse question?

1. Ambulate hallway independently.

2. Low-sodium diet.

3. Hydrochlorothiazide, one tablet every morning.

4. Phenergan 12.5 mg IVP prn n/v.

Correct answer: 1. Clients diagnosed with Ménière's disease experience vertigo and dizziness, making ambulation a safety risk.

8. A mother of a 2-year-old tells a nurse the child has been pulling at his/her ear for the last 2 days while running a fever. On exam, the nurse notes the child's vital signs: blood pressure 92/48 mm Hg, heart rate 104 beats/minute, respiratory rate 24 breaths/minute, temperature 102.9°F. The nurse's priority intervention should be to:

1. Administer ear drops for the client's pain.

2. Administer acetaminophen (Tylenol) for fever.

3. Notify the physician of the client's blood pressure.

4. Listen to the client's lungs.

Correct answer: 2. The nurse should control the client's fever prior to implementing other nursing interventions.

9. A nurse notes purulent drainage from the right ear of a 14-month-old diagnosed with otitis media. The nurse should:

1. Insert a cotton ball into the right ear to absorb drainage.

2. Document the drainage in the nurse's notes.

3. Prepare for emergency tympanectomy.

4. Irrigate the ear with warm saline.

Correct answer: 2. The nurse should monitor the drainage from the client's ear and document the findings in the nurse's notes. Should the client develop a fever or should the drainage become purulent, further action will be required.

10. While teaching a group of senior citizens about common eye disorders, a nurse explains that macular degeneration results in:

1. Auditory hallucinations.

2. Proprioception.

3. Nystagmus.

4. Blurring of central vision.

Correct answer: 4. A common symptom of macular degeneration is blurring of central vision.

References

1. Huether SE. Pain, temperature, sleep, and sensory function. In: Huether SE, McCance KL, eds. *Understanding Pathophysiology*. 3rd ed. St. Louis: Mosby; 2004:329–353.

2. Montgomery TM. *Anatomy, Physiology and Pathology of the Human Eye*. www.tedmontgomery.com/the_eye/overview.html. 1998–2006.

3. Mayo Foundation for Medical Education and Research. *Glaucoma*. www.mayoclinic.com/health/glaucoma/DS00283. 2006.

4. National Institutes of Health. *Ménière's Disease*. www.nlm.nih.gov/medlineplus/ency/article/000702.htm. 2006.

5. Gates GA. Cost-effectiveness considerations in otitis media treatment. *Otolaryngol Head Neck Surg*. 1996;114:525–530.

6. Lee J, Bailey G, Thompson V. *All About Vision*. Access Media Group, LLC. http://www.allaboutvision.com/conditions/cataracts.html: 2007.

7. Mayo Foundation for Medical Education and Research. *Cataracts*. http://www.mayoclinic.com/health/cataracts/. 2007.

8. National Institutes of Health. *Retinal Detachment*. www.nlm.nih.gov/medlineplus/ency/article/001027.html. 2007.

9. National Eye Institute. *Glaucoma*. www.nei.nih.gov/health/glaucoma/glaucoma. 2006.

10. National Institute of Aging. *Cataracts*. http://nihseniorhealth.gov/cataract/toc.html. 2005.

11. Sackett C. Assessment and management of patients with eye and vision disorders. In: Smelzer B, Bare BG, eds. *Brunner & Suddarth's Textbook of Medical-Surgical Nursing*. 10th ed. Philadelphia: Lippincott; 2004:1747–1788.

12. Smith D. Eye, ear, nose, and throat health problems. In: Hogan M, Hill K, eds. *Pathophysiology: Reviews and Rationales*. Upper Saddle River, NJ: Prentice Hall; 2004:201–231.

Bibliography

Hurst Review Services. www.hurstreview.com.

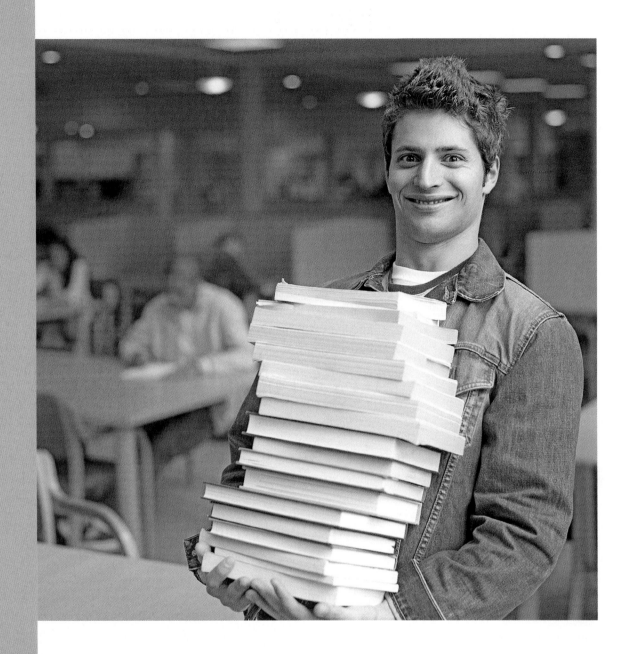

11 Musculoskeletal System

OBJECTIVES

In this chapter, you'll review:

- The general musculoskeletal system structure and function.
- Diseases and injuries that can occur within the musculoskeletal system.
- The causes, proper assessment, and treatment of these injuries and complications.

LET'S GET THE NORMAL STUFF STRAIGHT FIRST

The musculoskeletal system is the main system that sustains our body and enables us to remain mobile. Bones support and move the body while protecting the internal organs. Muscles also help move the body and respond independently of neural or hormonal stimulation or in response to neural stimulation. Diseases or injuries to the muscles or bones make movement difficult or painful. If cardiac or respiratory muscles are destroyed, life is impossible.[1]

LET'S GET DOWN TO SPECIFICS

Specific diseases or injuries to the musculoskeletal system may affect bones, muscles, tendons, ligaments, joints, and cartilage. Because the musculoskeletal system serves as the body's main line of defense against external forces, injuries are common and may result in permanent disability. Osteoarthritis, a common immune disorder that affects the joints, is discussed in Chapter 3.

✚ Carpal tunnel syndrome
What is it?

Carpal tunnel syndrome is a painful compression of the median nerve as it passes through the wrist (Fig. 11-1). Carpal tunnel syndrome is most common in women ages 30 to 60 years.[2] Tables 11-1 and 11-2 give the causes, signs, and symptoms associated with carpal tunnel syndrome.

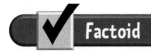

Factoid

Carpal tunnel syndrome is the most common nerve entrapment syndrome. The carpal tunnel is the canal in which the median nerve passes. If the canal is narrowed for any reason, the nerve will be affected.

▶ Figure 11-1. Carpal tunnel syndrome.

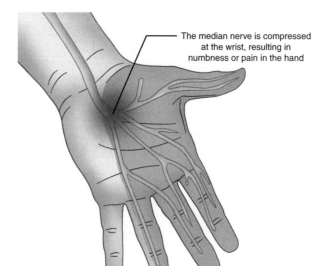

The median nerve is compressed at the wrist, resulting in numbness or pain in the hand

What causes it and why

Table 11-1

Causes	Why
Congenital predisposition	Carpal tunnel passage is smaller in some people than others
Trauma or injury to the wrist	Damage to the median nerve or the surrounding structures which ultimately affects the nerve
Overactive pituitary gland	Hormone imbalance increases pressure to the median nerve (joint inflammation)
Hypothyroidism	Hormone imbalance results in increased pressure to the median nerve (joint inflammation)
Rheumatoid arthritis	Joint inflammation increases pressure to the median nerve
Mechanical problems in wrist joint	Leads to joint inflammation, which increases pressure to the median nerve
Work-related stress	Repetitive wrist motions that cause excessive flexion or extension: typing on keyboard, turning screwdriver, and prolonged exposure to vibrations (operating jackhammer) (over use)
Fluid retention during pregnancy or menopause	Fluid causes further pressure to the median nerve
Development of cyst or tumor within canal	Pressure of cyst or tumor compresses the median nerve further
Obesity	Extra subcutaneous tissue adds pressure to the median nerve
Gout	Buildup of uric acid causes median nerve inflammation
Familial	Sometimes CTS runs in families and there is no known reason for the cause

Source: Created by author from References #2 to #4.

Signs and symptoms and why

Table 11-2

Signs and symptoms	Why
Weakness, pain, burning, numbness over the thumb, index finger, middle finger, and radial half of 4th finger	Nerve compression
Inability to clench hand into fist	Nerve compression
Possible pain, burning, and tingling in the arm and shoulder	Nerve compression radiates up the arm
Atrophy of muscles in hand on the thumb side (thenar atrophy)	Muscle atrophy is related to inability to use this muscle because there is a problem with the nerve that supplies it. Therefore, the problem is related to pain as well as to conduction.
Worsening of symptoms at night and in the morning	Vasodilation and venous stasis due to lack of movement

Source: Created by author from References #2 to #4.

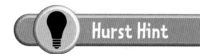

Factoid

Carpal tunnel syndrome is very common during pregnancy.

Hurst Hint

Signs and symptoms of carpal tunnel syndrome may occur in both hands, not just the dominant one, because the less dominant hand picks up the slack that the dominant hand is creating due to immobility.[3]

Quickie tests and treatments

Tests:

- Nerve conduction study: rules out other possible causes.
- Electromyography: median nerve motor conduction delay of more than 5 milliseconds.
- Digital electrical stimulation: median nerve compression by measuring length and intensity of stimulation from fingers to median nerve in wrist.[3]
- Compression tests:
  1. Positive Tinel's sign: tapping the nerve area causes tingling that radiates to the wrist.
  2. Positive Phalen's test: backs of hands held together for 60 seconds with wrists flexed at 90 degrees (fingers down); tingling or burning in area of median nerve.[2–4]

Treatments:

- Splinting wrist for 1 to 2 weeks: to rest hand.
- Correction of any underlying disorder: rheumatoid arthritis, gout, etc.
- Administering NSAIDs: to relieve pain and inflammation.
- Injection of carpal tunnel with hydrocortisone and lidocaine: significant but temporary relief of symptoms.
- Occupational therapy: prevent recurrence of symptoms.
- Surgical decompression of the nerve: relieves compression of nerve.
- Neurolysis: freeing median nerve from inflammatory adhesions. [2–4]

What can harm my client?

- Delayed treatment.
- Ignoring complaints of tingling and burning.
- Allowed continued wrist activity.
- Neural ischemia.
- Permanent nerve damage with loss of movement and sensation (thenar atrophy).

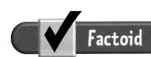

Factoid

If thenar atrophy is severe, full recovery may not occur.

If I were your teacher, I would test you on . . .

- Patient referral for occupation counseling if job change is needed.
- Medication administration and possible side effects.
- Preop and postop nursing care.
- Patient teaching regarding splint application and care, exercises, and medication regimen.
- Proper nursing assessment of affected hand and limb.
- Causes and why of carpal tunnel syndrome.
- Signs and symptoms and why of carpal tunnel syndrome.

* How to perform compression tests as part of nursing assessment.
* Know that thenar atrophy is a very important complication to watch for.

✚ Osteomyelitis

What is it?

Osteomyelitis is an acute infection of the bone caused by bacteria, although fungi and viruses may play a role (Fig. 11-2). Osteomyelitis can be very difficult to treat. Patients who are at high risk for osteomyelitis are the poorly nourished, elderly, or obese.[5] Tables 11-3 and 11-4 give the causes, signs, and symptoms associated with osteomyelitis.

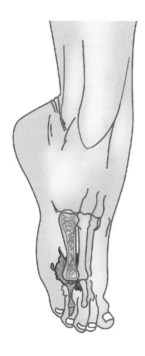

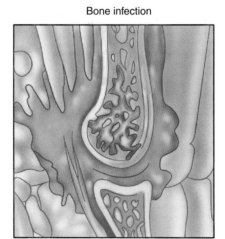

Bone infection

◀ Figure 11-2. Osteomyelitis.

What causes it and why

Table 11-3

Causes	Why
Trauma, surgery	Contaminants introduced directly to bone, where they settle, causing infection, abscess, and bone necrosis
Acute infection originating elsewhere in the body	Contaminated blood flows to the bone or surrounding tissue, where it settles and produces an abscess cutting off blood supply to the bone
Staphylococcus aureus; major cause of osteomyelitis	Microorganisms proliferate, produce cell death, and spread through the bone shaft, causing increased inflammation and destruction of bone cells

(Continued)

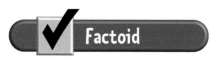

Factoid

When organisms enter the body, they can migrate to the vertebrae in adults or to the ends of arms and leg bones in children.

Table 11-3. (*Continued*)

Causes	Why
Puncture injury to soft tissue or bone (animal bite, stepping on nail with bare feet, misplaced intramuscular injection) with contaminated or nonsterile needle	Causes opening to body where bacteria, fungi, or virus may enter and travel to bone
Infection in adjacent bone or soft tissue	Contaminants from adjacent areas spread to nearby bone and soft tissue
Kidney dialysis	The access site is a portal of entry for microorganisms to travel to bones
IV drug users	Nonsterile needles are a source of contamination
Skin infections in patients with vascular insufficiency	Lack of oxygenated blood supply to area with penetration to bones
Artificial joints, surgical metal implants	Bacteria or fungi tend to migrate at the artificial joint or implant, and then are carried to the bone

Source: Created by author from References #1 and #5 to #8.

Signs and symptoms and why

Table 11-4

Signs and symptoms	Why
Chills, fever, malaise	Bacteremia
Pain on movement of the infected extremity	Irritation of the bone and surrounding area
Loss of movement	Pain in the area of infection
Localized tenderness, redness, edema	Bone inflammation
Nausea and anorexia	Due to pain and malaise
Drainage of pus through the skin	Opening forms through infected bone to the skin surface allowing pus to drain. Sometimes referred to as sinus tract
Tachycardia	Pain, infection, septicemia

Source: Created by author from References #1 and #5 to #8.

Quickie tests and treatments

Tests:

- Complete blood count: white blood cells (WBC) elevated; elevated sedimentation rate (ESR).
- Blood and wound drainage cultures: to identify appropriate antibiotic therapy.
- MRI: extent of infection.
- CT scan: extent of infection.
- Bone scan: indicates areas of infection.

- X-ray: soft-tissue swelling, irregular decalcification, bone necrosis, new bone formation.
- Bone tissue aspiration: organism identification.
- Joint fluid aspiration: organism identification.

Treatments:

- Antibiotic therapy: for *Staphylococcus aureus* and other bacteria; around the clock IV dosing for 3 to 6 weeks, then oral dosing for up to 3 months.
- Antifungal medications: for infections caused by fungus.
- Analgesics: for pain.
- Bed rest: promotes healing.
- Immobilization of affected area: cast or traction to promote healing.
- Surgery: to drain abscesses and stabilize bones, remove infected artificial joints, amputation for chronic and unrelieved symptoms, debridement.
- Sequestrectomy: removal of dead bone.[1,5–8]

What can harm my client?

- Delayed treatment.
- Possible amputation.
- Septicemia.
- Repeat infection.
- Further injury to the affected area.

If I were your teacher, I would test you on . . .

- What is it?
- Causes.
- Signs and symptoms.
- Possible physical assessment findings.
- Patient teaching regarding infection control, wound site care, and importance of follow-up examinations.
- Medication administration and monitoring for effectiveness.
- Causes of osteomyelitis and why.
- Signs and symptoms of osteomyelitis and why.
- Pre- and postop patient care.
- Monitoring for complications.
- Care of the patient in a cast and traction.

✛ Osteoporosis

What is it?

Osteoporosis is a metabolic bone disorder that results in the loss of bone mass due to the rate of bone resorption exceeding the rate of bone formation (Fig. 11-3). This decrease in bone density causes bones to become porous and brittle, which leads to easy bone fractures. Tables 11-5 and 11-6 give the causes, signs and symptoms, and the associated reasons for osteoporosis.

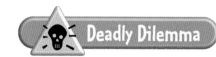

Deadly Dilemma

Bone infections are more difficult to treat than soft-tissue infections because the infected bone and corresponding immune responses become walled off, thus resisting antibiotics.[5]

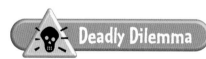

Deadly Dilemma

Osteomyelitis is a very serious condition and can be very difficult to treat. Many clients end up with a PICC line for months which interferes with quality of life significantly. Osteomyelitis can lead to death.

▶ Figure 11-3. Osteoporosis.

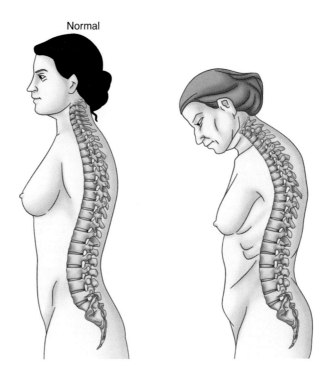

Normal

What causes it and why

Table 11-5

Causes	Why
Inadequate calcium and vitamin D intake during young adulthood	Young adults drink caffeine drinks instead of milk. Milk has vitamins A and D and calcium needed for bone growth and support
Rapid bone loss postmenopause	• Low estrogen levels (hysterectomy) • Intake of caffeine and nicotine • Lack of weight-bearing exercises
Family history	Predisposes to low bone mass
Prolonged steroid therapy	Interferes with glucose utilization and causes breakdown of protein, which forms the matrix of the bone
Prolonged heparin therapy	Increases collagen breakdown
Osteogenesis imperfecta	Imperfectly formed bones break easily
Immobility or disuse of bone	Bones need stress for bone maintenance
Medications: aluminum-containing antacids, corticosteroids, anticonvulsants, barbiturates	Affect the body's use and metabolism of calcium
Breast-feeding women	Bone density decreases during breast-feeding but returns to normal after weaning

(Continued)

Table 11-5. (*Continued*)

Causes	Why
Age	Decrease in hormones and weight-bearing activity
Nutritional deficit: protein, calcium, vitamins C and D	Makes bones soft, thin, and brittle
Excessive intake of caffeine, nicotine, and alcohol	Worsen pre-existing osteoporosis; reduces bone remodeling
Bone tumors	Impair new bone formation
Diseases like chronic kidney failure, liver disease, and hormonal disorders	Cause hormone changes that affect bone density and bone loss
Rheumatoid arthritis	Causes generalized bone loss
Nutritional abnormalities: anorexia nervosa, scurvy, lactose intolerance, malabsorption	Reduces nutrients needed for bone remodeling
Sedentary lifestyle	Disuse of bones and muscles
Even when mild, overtime (low calcium)	Calcium needed for bone growth and support
Declining gonadal adrenal function in males	Hormone changes affect bone density and loss

Source: Created by author from References #1, #5, and #9 to #12.

Signs and symptoms and why

Table 11-6

Signs and symptoms	Why
Kyphosis of thoracic spine (called "dowager's hump") see Figure 11-3	Several vertebral fractures causing excess curvature of thoracic spine
Loss of height	Bones collapse or fracture
Fracture(s): back, hip, wrist	Weakened bones; hormonal imbalance; fractures heal slowly
Pain; tenderness	Can be sudden and associated with bending or lifting; back pain associated with vertebral collapse; worse when patient stands or walks; muscles may become tender
Immobility	Change in posture; pain; weakened muscles
Change in breathing pattern	Stooped posture; pain; weakened muscles
Deformity	Immobility due to pain; bone collapse or fracture
Decreased exercise tolerance	Pain; immobility
Markedly aged appearance	Body structure changes/deformity; pain
Muscle spasm	Muscle strain due to weakened muscles; body structure changes/deformity

Source: Created by author from References #1, #5, and #9 to #12.

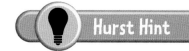

Hurst Hint

Remember, estrogen helps to maintain the integrity of the bone.

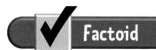

Factoid

As people age into their 70s and 80s, osteoporosis becomes a common disease.[1]

Fractures due to osteoporosis

Table 11-7 gives the details of fractures due to osteoporosis.

Table 11-7

Fracture site	Number per year	Treatment
Vertebral body	700,000	External bracing; nonosteoporotic (NO) would require internal fixation
Hip	300,000	Immobility, possible internal fixation
Wrist	200,000	Cast or brace

Source: Created by author from Reference #1.

Quickie tests and treatments

Tests:

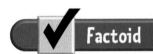

Factoid

Parathyroid hormone controls bone formation and the excretion of calcium and phosphorus, so lets make sure its not the parathyroid.

- Dual energy x-ray absorptiometry (DEXA): detects bone mass and bone density loss.
- Quantitative computed tomography (QCT): measures bone density.
- X-rays: identify suspected fractures.
- Quantitative ultrasound (QUS): shows injured or diseased areas.
- Blood tests: measure calcium, phosphorus, and alkaline levels; elevated parathyroid hormone. Remember, calcium and phosphorus have an inverse relationship.
- Bone biopsy: shows thin, porous bone.

Treatments:

- Physical therapy: slows bone loss.
- Moderate weight-bearing exercises: slow bone loss.
- Supportive devices (back brace, wrist splint): maintain function.
- Surgery: hip replacement; open reduction, and internal fixation for femur fractures.
- Hormone replacement therapy (estrogen and progesterone): slows bone loss and prevents fractures. Remember, estrogen helps to maintain bone.
- Analgesics: relieve pain.
- Local heat: relieves pain.
- Calcium and vitamin D supplements: promote normal bone metabolism.
- Calcitonin (Calcimar): reduces bone resorption and slow loss of bone mass.
- Bisphosphonates (etidronate [Didronel]): increase bone density and restore lost bone.
- Fluoride (alendronate [Fosamax]): stimulates bone formation.
- Diet rich in vitamin C, calcium, and protein: supports skeletal metabolism.

- Smoking cessation.
- Teriparatide (synthetic parathyroid hormone): builds bone and increases bone density.
- Testosterone therapy for men: reduces osteoporosis.
- AMG-162 (monoclonal antibody): inhibits bone resorption; in phase 3 clinical trials.
- Vertebroplasty and kyphoplasty: repair collapsed vertebra.

What can harm my client?

- Unsafe environment (floor rugs, lamp cords) leads to falls.
- Fractures of hips, shoulder, pelvis, etc.
- Postop surgical infection.
- Immobility.
- Compression fractures of the vertebrae.

If I were your teacher, I would test you on . . .

- Complete assessment of a patient who complains of "getting shorter." (Due to kyphosis and compression fractures.)
- Patient education regarding diet and exercise.
- Prevention education to family members. (To help provide proper care for elderly clients with osteoporosis.)
- Pre- and postop monitoring and nursing care. (Remember, fractures can be the cause of fat embolism.)
- Medication administration, monitoring, and possible side effects.
- Diagnostic tests, related patient education, and patient care.
- Fracture management and related patient education.
- Risk factors and causes of osteoporosis and why.
- Signs and symptoms of osteoporosis and why.

✚ Paget's disease

What is it?

Paget's disease, also known as osteitis deformans, is a chronic condition in which areas of the bone undergo slow and progressive abnormal turnover (see Factoid), resulting in areas of enlarged and softened bone. The skull, femur, tibia, pelvis, clavicle, humerus, and vertebrae are most commonly affected. The condition is most common in men after the age of 40.[13] It can be mild with no symptoms (Table 11-8) or severe.

What causes it and why

The cause of Paget's disease is unknown, and most patients never know they have it. Patients are typically misdiagnosed with arthritis or skeletal changes due to old age prior to a diagnosis of Paget's disease. There is evidence of family tendency, or possibly a viral infection contracted in childhood could cause a dormant skeletal infection that could later cause Paget's disease.[15]

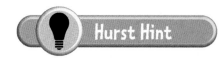

Hurst Hint

Clients should be encouraged to reach a calcium intake of 1500 milligrams and 400 to 800 units of vitamin D daily.

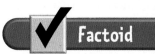

Factoid

"Turnover" is the term used to describe the normal breaking down and building of bone by osteoclasts and osteoblasts.

Signs and symptoms and why

Table 11-8

Signs and symptoms	Why
Severe, persistent pain worsened by weight-bearing activities	Bowing of legs causes malalignment of the hip, knee, and ankle joints, which causes arthritis, back, and joint pain; nerve compression causes pain
Cranial enlargement	Chronic bone inflammation; increased breaking down and rebuilding of bone in the area
Barrel-shaped chest	Chest and trunk flexes on to the legs to maintain balance
Asymmetric bowing of the tibia and femur	Chronic bone inflammation softens the bones, causing them to bend
Kyphosis	Several vertebral fractures, causing excess curvature of thoracic spine
Pathological fractures	Diseased bones are highly vascular and structurally weak
Waddling gait	Bowed femurs and tibiae
Muscle weakness	Bone structural changes and deformity weaken surrounding muscles; hypercalcemia
Immobility	Abnormal bone formation impinging on the spine
Loss of height	Deformities of the femurs, tibias, and fibulas
Warmth and tenderness over affected areas	Increased blood supply through affected bones
Paraplegia	Nerve compression from thickened bones
Blindness	Cranial nerve compression from thickened cranium
Hearing loss, tinnitus	Cranial nerve compression from thickened cranium; enlarged skull bones damage fragile inner-ear bones
Vertigo	Hearing loss and tinnitus; equilibrium off balance
Osteoarthritis	Bowing of legs causes malalignment of the hip, knee, and ankle joints, which causes arthritis; distortion of joints leads to osteoarthritis
Heart failure	Increased vascular bed and metabolic demands. Extra workload on heart
Small, triangular appearing face	Cranium enlarges making face appear smaller
Headaches	Cranial nerve compression from thickened cranium

Source: Created by author from References #1, #5, and #13 to #15.

Quickie tests and treatments

Tests:

- X-ray: shows bone deformity, expansion, and increased bone density.

- Blood tests: elevated serum alkaline phosphatase (enzyme involved in bone cell formation); anemia.

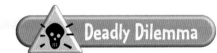

Factoid

Hypercalcemia: Some signs and symptoms associated with hypercalcemia are high blood pressure, muscle weakness, mild bowel disturbances, fatigue, weakness, anorexia, and renal calculi (stones).

Deadly Dilemma

Heart failure is a rare complication secondary to increased blood flow through the bone. This puts extra burden on the heart.

- Urine tests: elevated 24-hour urine hydroxyproline level (chemical involved in increased bone replacement).
- Bone biopsy: rules out infection or tumor; shows characteristic mosaic pattern of bone tissue.
- Bone scan: indicates which bones are affected.

Treatments:

- Calcitonin: slows rate of bone breakdown.
- Aspirin, acetaminophen, NSAIDs: reduce pain and inflammation.
- Heel lifts/walking aids: make walking easier.
- Physical therapy: improves mobility.
- Fractures: managed according to location.
- Hearing aid/sign language/lip reading: communication for hearing impaired.
- Surgery: relieves pinched nerves, replaces arthritic joints, reduces pathological fractures, corrects secondary deformities.
- Bisphosphonates (etidronate [Didronel]): slow progression of disease; given before surgery to prevent or reduce bleeding during surgery; treat pain; slow progression of weakness or paralysis in people who can't have surgery; prevent arthritis, further hearing loss, further bone deformity.
- Bed rest: should be avoided except when sleeping at night to prevent hypercalcemia.
- Treat hypercalcemia: IV fluids and diuretics.
- Dietary intake of calcium and vitamin D: incorporates calcium into the bone that is being remodeled rapidly to make it stronger.
- Calcium and vitamin D supplements: as above.

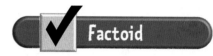

Asymptomatic clients do not need treatment. In those who do, bisphosphonates are the treatment of choice.

What can harm my client?

- Falls leading to fractures.
- Side effects from medications.
- Immobility from bone deformities.
- Emotional lack of self-esteem.
- Paralysis if not treated promptly.
- Heart failure (rare).
- Sometimes the affected bone will develop cancer. (<1% of clients)

If I were your teacher, I would test you on . . .

- What is it?
- Causes and why?
- Signs and symptoms.
- Complete physical assessment with emphasis on neurovascular component.
- Administration, monitoring, and possible side effects of medications.

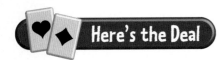

Body image changes can be a source of self esteem problems. Always be sensitive to these issues.

- Psychosocial strategies to help client cope with body image changes. (Kyphosis, bowed femurs/legs)
- Patient education regarding the disease and possible progression.
- Devices to promote client independence: hearing aids, walker, heel lifts.
- Care of the patient undergoing diagnostic tests; purpose of diagnostic tests.
- Patient education regarding pain relief, safety, medication side effects, and bed rest.

✚ Scoliosis

What is it?

Scoliosis is an abnormal lateral curvature of the spine, which is very common, especially among adolescent girls (Fig. 11-4). However, scoliosis does affect boys too Tables 11-9 and 11-10 give the causes, signs and symptoms and the associated reasons for scoliosis.

▶ Figure 11-4. Scoliosis. (Beers MH, ed. Bone Disorders: Scoliosis. In: *The Merck Manual of Medical Information* Home Edition. 2nd ed. New York, NY: Pocket Books. 2003:1603–1604.)

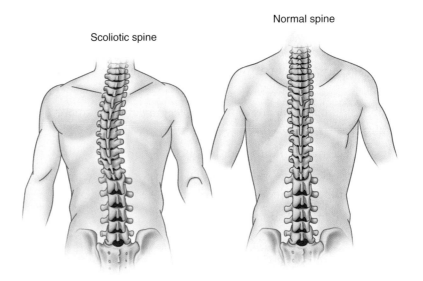

What causes it and why

Table 11-9

Causes	Why
Congenital deformity (birth defect)	Etiology unknown
Neuromuscular disease: cerebral palsy, muscular dystrophy, polio, or spinal muscular atrophy	Muscles deteriorate around the spine; spine does not receive adequate support and begins to curve
Leg-length discrepancy	Imbalance causing asymmetrical growth in spine
Paraspinal inflammation	Edema causes stress on the spine causing it to curve
Trauma	Acute disc disease; vertebral fractures

(Continued)

Table 11-9. (*Continued*)

Causes	Why
Age	Degenerative scoliosis found in older people with osteoporosis and degenerative joint disease of the spine
Imbalance in muscles around vertebrae	Causes spinal distortion with growth
High arches in feet	Alters balance and causes the spine and surrounding muscles to compensate
Coordination problems	Asymmetrical growth in the spine
Stress fractures in young athletes	Hormones affect bone growth
Tumors, growths, or other small abnormalities on the spinal column	Add stress to the spinal column and surrounding tissues, interfere with bone growth
Spinal cord injury or disease (spina bifida)	Affects vertebrae growth and growth pattern

Source: Created by author from References #1, #5, #16, and #17.

Signs and symptoms and why

Table 11-10

Signs and symptoms	Why
Shortness of breath	Curve in thoracic area impedes gas exchange; can lead to deformed and damaged lungs
Fatigue, back pain	Muscles pull on the spine, causing pain; pain causes fatigue
Prominent scapula, hip, breast, or anterior rib cage on convex side	Vertebrae rotate, forming the convex part of the curve; rotation causes prominence along thoracic spine
Asymmetry of thoracic cage and misalignment of spinal vertebrae when client bends over	Rotation and curvature of the spine
One shoulder higher than the other; clothes do not hang straight; waistline asymmetry	Curvature of the spine
Unevenness in height of iliac crest	One leg shorter than the other
Kyphosis	Rotation causes prominence along thoracic spine
Reduced pulmonary function	With thoracic curve exceeding 60 degrees; compresses lungs
Cor pulmonale in middle age. (Right sided heart failure)	With thoracic curve exceeding 80 degrees; pulmonary hypertension leads to cor pulmonale because right side of heart has to work against increased pressure
GI disturbance	Thoracic or lumbar deformity

Source: Created by author from References #1, #5, #16, and #17.

Quickie tests and treatment

Tests:

- Complete physical assessment from front, back, and side: detects curvature.
- X-rays: determine degree of curvature and flexibility of spine.
- Bone growth studies: determine skeletal maturity.
- Pulmonary function test (PFT): for thoracic curves greater than 60 degrees.

Treatments:

- No vigorous sports or diving.
- Prescribed exercise regimen.
- Surgery: posterior spinal fusion and internal stabilization (rods and spinal hardware).
- Casting/braces/splints: maintain proper spinal alignment. (Also known as orthotics)
- NSAIDs: relieve pain and decrease inflammation.

What can harm my client?

- Trauma.
- Untreated scoliosis can cause significant deformity.
- Thoracic curve greater than 60 degrees may cause cardiopulmonary compromise.
- Lumbar area may cause debilitating back pain.
- Neurological impingement could cause permanent disability if not treated immediately.

If I were your teacher, I would test you on . . .

- Complete neurovascular assessment.
- Proper body alignment.
- Patient education regarding the disease process.
- Patient education regarding respiratory distress.
- Pre- and postop patient care.
- Psychosocial measures to encourage ADLs.
- Addressing body image disturbance.
- Monitor pain and administer medications accordingly.
- Proper care of cast and monitoring of patient in cast.
- Monitor for skin breakdown.

✚ Bone fracture

What is it?

A bone fracture is a break in a bone, usually accompanied by injury to the surrounding tissue.[18] Table 11-11 gives the causes for fracture.

Deadly Dilemma

Monitor for signs of cast syndrome: nausea, abdominal pressure, vague abdominal pain, which may result from hyperextension of the spine.[17] (See treatment.)

Hurst Hint

No matter what, do not let your client insert a coat hanger or a soft, sterile cotton swab into the cast to relieve an itch. The correct protocol is to use a cool hair dryer or apply ice over the cast to the area that itches.

Marlene Moment

When I worked in the ED, for some reason I always became nauseous when a client's fractured foot pointed backward.

What causes it and why

Table 11-11

Causes	Why
Trauma: direct blows, crushing forces, sudden twisting motions, extreme muscle contractions	Bone is subjected to stress greater than it can absorb
Pathological	Weak bones from osteoporosis, bone tumor, cancer, infection, skeletal disease
Stress	Bones not able to adapt to added pressure; increased activity level; bones may be weak

Source: Created by author from References #1 and #18 to #21.

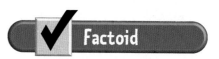

TYPES OF FRACTURE   Figures 11-5 and 11-6 show the types of fracture. Tables 11-12 and 11-13 show the types, signs and symptoms, and associated reasons for fractures.

Factoid

Fractures resulting from even minor falls are the most common cause of disability in the elderly. They rarely regain the same level of functioning they had before the fall.

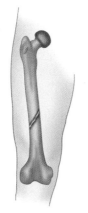
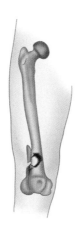
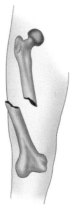

Nondisplaced and simple

Comminuted and closed

Compound or open

◀ Figure 11-5. Types of fractures (1).

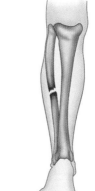
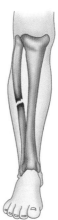

Greenstick (incomplete)

Simple

◀ Figure 11-6. Types of fractures (2).

Table 11-12

Type of fracture	Description
Closed	Skin remains intact. There are several types of closed fractures
Open (compound)	The fractured bone segment breaks through the skin; high risk for infection
Aligned (nondisplaced)	The bone remains in anatomical position
Displaced	Bone is not in anatomical position
Simple	The single fracture line separates the bone
Comminuted	The fracture site consists of multiple pieces of broken bone. Related to high impact with trauma or osteoporosis
Incomplete	The fracture line passes through only one side of the bone and does not go through the bone completely. For example, greenstick

Source: Created by author from References #1 and #5.

Signs and symptoms and why

Table 11-13

Signs and symptoms	Why
Swelling at site of injury	Soft-tissue edema caused by hemorrhage into muscles and joints
Joint dislocation	Force of trauma
Pain	Continuous and increases in severity until bone fragments are immobilized; muscle spasm
Loss of function	Pain; integrity of bones and surrounding tissue is compromised
Deformity	Displacement, angulation, or rotation of the fragments in a fracture; soft-tissue swelling
Shortening	Contraction of muscles above and below site of fracture
Crepitus	Rubbing of bone fragments against each other
Bruising	Bleeding into the tissues
Abnormal position of extremity	Force of trauma impacts alignment
Limited range of motion; immobility	Pain, misalignment of bone, swelling of tissues
Bone protruding through skin	Open fracture
Impaired sensation; tingling	Nerve impingement or damage
Hypotension	Large amount of blood moves from the bloodstream into the surrounding tissues
Loss of distal pulse	Compartment syndrome

Source: Created by author from References #1 and #18 to #21.

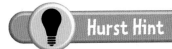

Hurst Hint

The fracture line may be transverse, oblique, spiral, comminuted, or segmental.

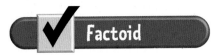

Factoid

Greenstick fractures occur in children only.

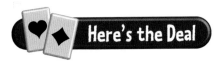

Here's the Deal

The terms used to describe the status of alignment of the bone are nondisplacement, displacement, and angulation.

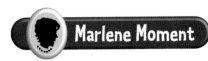

Marlene Moment

If a bone protrudes through the skin, something is really wrong, needing further investigation.

Quickie tests and treatments

Tests:

- X-rays: of affected area including a nonaffected joint.
- Bone scan: reveals stress fracture.
- CT scan: shows fine details of fractured joint; reveals fractures that are hidden by overlying bone.
- MRI: shows soft-tissue damage around bone, tendons, and ligaments, and evidence of cancer.

Treatments:

- RICE:

  Rest: promotes healing.

  Immobilization: cast, splint, sling, traction to minimize damage and allow for repair.

  Compression: to reduce swelling.

  Elevation: to level of heart to limit swelling.
- Surgery: for open fractures; joint replacement; bone grafting.
- Wound care: for open fractures.
- Realignment (reduction): recovers normal positioning and range of motion.
- Acetaminophen: pain control; no NSAIDs or aspirin—can worsen bleeding.
- Ice: controls pain and swelling.
- TED (antiembolism) hose: control swelling.
- If compartment syndrome: removing or loosening anything that constricts limb; emergency surgery (fasciotomy) to open constricting tissue; amputation if necessary.
- Prevent pulmonary embolism: heparin, warfarin (Coumadin), low-molecular-weight heparin (Lovenox) reduce potential for blood clot. (When indicated)
- Partial weight bearing: stimulates bone growth and density.
- Physical therapy: improves range of motion, mobility.
- Diet rich in vitamins C, A, D, calcium, and protein: supports bone growth and metabolism.

What can harm my client?

- Pneumonia: if extended bed rest.
- Venous thrombosis related to immobility and pooling of blood.
- Pressure sores: if extended bed rest.
- Social isolation/depression.
- Pulmonary embolus.
- Compartment syndrome.
- Fat embolism syndrome.

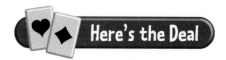

Compartment syndrome results when the muscle swells extensively beneath its fibrous covering. The fibrous covering places the muscle in its own compartment so when excessive swelling occurs, blood flow is compromised. Ultimately the muscle may die from lack of oxygen rich blood. Its like a heart attack, just not in the heart. The end result is that the muscle is permanently damaged or dead.

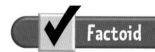

Always consider pulmonary embolism as a complication of fracture related surgeries.

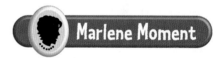

If your client is ever on Coumadin therapy, please teach her not to eat the antidote, green leafy veggies (vitamin K), because a clot may develop and death can occur!

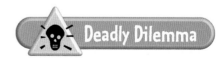

Fat embolism syndrome is very serious and can be fatal. It must be detected and treated early!

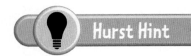

The emboli in the bloodstream travel and lodge in the capillaries and arterioles of the lung. Chest x-ray shows scattered infiltrates as a result.

FAT EMBOLISM SYNDROME   A fat embolus may occur after the break of a bone—especially a long bone. Fat is released into the circulatory system from the bone marrow, which can cause acute respiratory distress syndrome (ARDS) and respiratory failure.

- Clients at high risk are those with multiple fractures, hypovolemic shock, multiple traumas, and those who experienced a prolonged time between injury and treatment.
- Diagnostic tests show serum fat macroglobulemia and chest x-ray shows "snowstorm appearance."
- Signs and symptoms include dyspnea, tachypnea, confusion, drowsiness, petechial rash (head, neck, chest), tachycardia, hypotension, and jaundice.
- Treatments are oxygen therapy, mechanical ventilation, and corticosteroids.
- Prevention includes oxygen therapy, adequate immobilization of the fracture prior to transport, fluid homeostasis, and early operative fixation of long bone fractures.

If I were your teacher, I would test you on . . .

- The signs and symptoms of compartment syndrome.
- Patient education regarding cast care and proper positioning of injured extremity.
- Patient education regarding activity and weight bearing.
- Neurovascular (sensory, blood supply) assessment of injured extremity.
- Treatments and nursing care of clients with fractures.
- Medications and possible side effects.
- Pre- and postop care of surgical clients.
- Definition and treatments for fat embolism syndrome.
- Assessment and treatment of deep vein thrombosis.
- Assessment and treatment of pulmonary embolism.

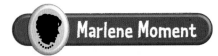

When performing a neurovascular assessment on an extremity, skip checking the level of consciousness (LOC). You don't have an LOC in your leg!

✚ Amputation

What is it?

Amputation is the removal of a body part, usually a part of or the entire extremity.[21]

What causes it and why

Table 11-14 gives the reasons or causes that may precipitate the need for amputation.

Table 11-14

Causes	Why
Peripheral vascular disease	Complication of diseases such as diabetes mellitus, where high sugar levels cause narrowing of peripheral blood vessels, decreasing blood flow to the area
Gas gangrene	Infection causes tissue death of extremity. Can even be caused by PVD due to lack of adequate blood flow
Trauma: crushing injuries, burns, frostbite, electrical burns	Damage to bone, nerves, and surrounding soft tissues
Congenital deformities	Etiology unknown
Chronic osteomyelitis	Infection causes tissue and bone death
Malignant tumor	Damage to the bone and surrounding soft tissues

Source: Created by author from References #1, #21, and #22.

Table 11-15 shows the signs and symptoms of the causes given in Table 11-14. These may precipitate the need for an amputation. Table 11-16 gives the details of amputation levels.

Signs and symptoms and why

Table 11-15

Signs and symptoms	Why
Necrotic areas on extremity	Poor blood flow due to trauma or infection
Pain, numbness, tingling	Nerve damage, nerve sensitivity, lack of adequate blood supply
Pale, cool extremity with very weak pulse	Poor blood flow to the extremity, may be related to PVD of the extremity

Source: Created by author from References #1, #21, and #22.

✓ **Factoid**

Peripheral vascular disease accounts for most amputations of the lower extremities.

AMPUTATION LEVEL

Table 11-16

Amputation level	Description
Symes	Slightly proximal to the ankle
BKA	Below the knee
KD	Knee disarticulation
AKA	Above the knee
HD	Hip disarticulation
HP	Hemipelvectomy
HC	Hemicorporectomy
BE	Below the elbow
AE	Above the elbow
SD	Shoulder disarticulation

Source: Created by author from References #21 and #22.

Quickie tests and treatments

Tests:

- X-ray: determines extent of bone damage.
- CT scan: determines extent of soft tissue damage.
- Bone scan: detects bone degeneration, inflammation, or tumor.
- MRI: identifies nerve damage.

Treatments:

- Elevate the limb: decreases swelling.
- Analgesics: decrease pain and inflammation.
- Wrap stump with compression bandages: decreases swelling, protects stump.
- Cast care: if rigid cast is implicated.
- Maintain proper body alignment: prevents contractures. Continuous flexion will lead to contractures. This is one reason why it should be elevated.
- Physical therapy: improves range of motion.
- Ambulation: stimulates blood flow to stump. (Gravity)
- Wound care: prevents infection.
- Prosthesis: improves coordination, movement.

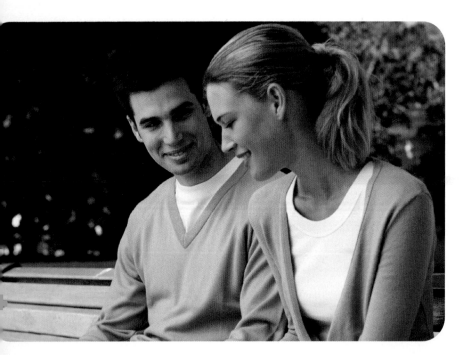

What can harm my client?

- Flexion contractures. When a limb stays flexed at a joint, a contracture will develop.
- Pressure sore at amputation site from prosthesis pressure.
- Wound dehiscence or infection. Dehiscence is opening the incision site again!
- Excessive edema due to improper wound dressing.
- Bone overgrowth.
- Phantom pain.

PHANTOM PAIN Phantom pain is an abnormal sensation(s) felt in a limb (or other amputated body part), which is no longer a part of the body. This is different from stump pain, which is pain that occurs in the remaining body stump. Phantom pain is caused by a malfunction in the brain and nervous system leading to the perception that the body part still exists.

- Signs and symptoms of phantom pain are feelings of abnormal sensations, heat, cold, touch, and pain.

- Treatment is difficult, but may include antiseizure medications, antidepressants, local anesthetics, and opioids.
- Nerve blocks, spinal cord stimulation, hypnosis, biofeedback, and distraction may also be useful.

A client's complaint of phantom pain must always be taken seriously and never questioned.

If I were your teacher, I would test you on . . .

- Vascular assessment.
- Proper dressing application to amputation site.
- Patient education regarding ambulation options.
- Emotional support and client coping strategies.
- Medications and possible side affects.
- Pre- and postop care of the surgical client.
- Patient education regarding prosthesis care and phantom pain.

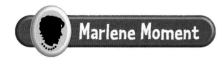

Marlene Moment

When your client experiences phantom pain, please don't tell them, "Your leg can't hurt; it's been burned in the hospital incinerator."

SUMMARY

In this chapter you have reviewed the key musculoskeletal diseases and injuries, their causes, signs and symptoms, and treatments. Always remember to assess your clients thoroughly and to investigate any unusual client complaints for physiological changes. Prompt nursing attention can significantly decrease client complications and poor outcomes.

PRACTICE QUESTIONS

1. The nerve that is compressed by the transverse carpal ligament is the:

   1. Radial nerve.

   2. Ulnar nerve.

   3. Median nerve.

   4. Musculocutaneous nerve.

   Correct answer: 3. The carpal bones and transverse carpal ligament form the carpal tunnel. Inflammation of the tendon that passes through the carpal tunnel causes compression and edema of the median nerve.

2. Carpal tunnel syndrome is caused by (select all that apply):

   1. Wrist injury.

   2. Systemic disease.

   3. Repetitive pronation and supination.

   4. Menopause.

Correct answers: 1, 2, & 4. Carpal tunnel syndrome is caused by wrist injury, systemic disease—such as rheumatoid arthritis—and fluid retention during pregnancy and menopause. It is also caused by repetitive flexion and extension of the wrist, not pronation and supination.

3. The major cause of osteomyelitis is:

1. Virus.

2. Protozoa.

3. Fungi.

4. Bacteria.

Correct answer: 4. The major cause of osteomyelitis is *Staphylococcus aureus*, a bacteria. Viruses and fungi can also contribute to osteomyelitis, but they are not considered the major cause.

4. The signs and symptoms of osteomyelitis include (select all that apply):

1. Pain with motion.

2. Warmth.

3. Fever.

4. Anorexia.

Correct answers: 1, 2, 3, & 4. Pain with motion, warmth, fever, and anorexia are all signs and symptoms of osteomyelitis.

5. The most frequent fracture site in a client with osteoporosis is:

1. Knee.

2. Vertebral body.

3. Wrist.

4. Hip.

Correct answer: 2. Approximately 700,000 vertebral fractures occur each year due to osteoporosis, making this the most frequent fracture site in clients with the disease. The hip is the second most common site, followed by the wrist. The knee is not a common site for osteoporosis.

6. What is the action of Teriparatide (synthetic parathyroid hormone) in the treatment of osteoporosis? Select all that apply.

1. Stimulates bone formation.

2. Increases bone density.

3. Reduces bone resorption.

4. Restores lost bone.

Correct answers: 1 & 2. Teriparatide (synthetic parathyroid hormone) builds bone and increases bone density in the treatment of osteoporosis. Calcitonin (Calcimar) reduces bone resorption and slows loss of bone mass. Bisphosphonates (etidronate [Didronel]) increase bone density and restore lost bone. Fluoride (alendronate [Fosamax]) stimulates bone formation.

7. Paget's disease is a disorder that:

1. Is possibly caused by a childhood viral disease.

2. Mainly affects menopausal women.

3. Has no family tendency.

4. Affects only the long bones.

Correct answer: 1. There is evidence of family tendency or possibility that a viral infection contracted in childhood could cause a dormant skeletal infection that could later cause Paget's disease. The skull, femur, tibia, pelvis, clavicle, humerus, and vertebrae are most commonly affected. The condition is most common in men after the age of 40.

8. Scoliosis is caused by (select all that apply):

1. High arches in the feet.

2. Leg length discrepancy.

3. Unilateral muscle strength.

4. Traumatic injury.

Correct answers: 1, 2, & 4. Scoliosis is caused by many factors, including high arches in the feet, leg length discrepancy, and traumatic injury, which impact the spine's growth and position.

9. Compartment syndrome is characterized by:

1. Yellow and blue hematoma in the area of the fracture.

2. Open wound in the area of the fracture.

3. Excessive swelling and pressure in the area of the fracture.

4. Petechial rash in the area of the fracture.

Correct answer: 3. Compartment syndrome is nerve and blood vessel damage or destruction due to excessive swelling and pressure in the area of the fracture. This decreases blood flow and oxygen to the muscle and surrounding areas, leading to tissue death. Hematomas and open wounds (in open fractures) may appear in the area of the fracture, but are not characteristic of compartment syndrome. Dyspnea, tachypnea, confusion, drowsiness, petechial rash (head, neck, chest), tachycardia, hypotension, and jaundice are characteristic of fat embolism syndrome.

10. Most amputations of the lower extremities are due to:

1. Gangrene.

2. Tumors.

3. Trauma.

4. Peripheral vascular disease.

Correct answer: 4. Peripheral vascular disease accounts for most amputations of the lower extremities. Trauma accounts for most amputations in young people. Gangrene and tumors do contribute to the need for amputation, but they are not the most common causes.

References

1. Corwin EJ. The musculoskeletal system. In: *Handbook of Pathophysiology*. 3rd ed. Philadelphia: Lippincott Williams & Wilkins; 2008:280–316.

2. Beers MH, ed. Carpal tunnel syndrome. In: Beers MH, ed. *The Merck Manual of Medical Information*. 2nd home ed. New York: Pocket Books; 2003:398–399.

3. Carpal tunnel syndrome. In: Schilling McCann JA, ed. *Nurse's 3 Minute Clinical Reference*. Springhouse, PA: Lippincott Williams & Wilkins; 2003:116–117.

4. Carpal tunnel syndrome. In: Schilling McCann JA, ed. *Just the Facts: Pathophysiology*. Ambler, PA: Lippincott Williams & Wilkins; 2005: 152–153.

5. Smeltzer SC, Bare BG. Management of patients with musculoskeletal disorders. In: *Brunner & Suddarth's Textbook of Medical-Surgical Nursing*. 10th ed. Philadelphia: Lippincott Williams & Wilkins; 2004: 2000–2074.

6. Osteomyelitis. In: Beers MH, ed. *The Merck Manual of Medical Information*. 2nd home ed. New York: Pocket Books; 2003:364–365.

7. Crutchlow EM, Dudac PJ, MacAvoy S, et al. Osteomyelitis. In: *Quick Look Nursing: Pathophysiology*. Thorofare, NJ: Slack; 2002: 250–251.

8. Osteomyelitis. In: Schilling McCann JA, ed. *Nurse's 3 Minute Clinical Reference*. Springhouse, PA: Lippincott Williams & Wilkins; 2003: 378–379.

9. Osteoporosis. In: Schilling McCann JA, ed. *Just the Facts: Pathophysiology*. Ambler, PA: Lippincott Williams & Wilkins; 2005:159–161.

10. Osteoporosis. In: Beers MH, ed. *The Merck Manual of Medical Information*. 2nd home ed. New York: Pocket Books; 2003:343–346.

11. Crutchlow EM, Dudac PJ, MacAvoy S, et al. Osteoporosis. In: *Quick Look Nursing: Pathophysiology*. Thorofare, NJ: Slack; 2002:249–251.

12. Osteoporosis. In: Schilling McCann JA, ed. *Nurse's 3 Minute Clinical Reference*. Springhouse, PA: Lippincott Williams & Wilkins; 2003: 380–381.

13. Paget's Disease. In: Beers MH, ed. *The Merck Manual of Medical Information*. 2nd home ed. New York: Pocket Books; 2003:346–348.

14. Crutchlow EM, Dudac PJ, MacAvoy S, et al. Paget's disease. In: *Quick Look Nursing: Pathophysiology*. Thorofare, NJ: Slack; 2002:250.

15. Paget's Disease. In: Schilling McCann JA, ed. *Nurse's 3 Minute Clinical Reference*. Springhouse, PA: Lippincott Williams & Wilkins; 2003: 390–391.

16. Bone Disorders: Scoliosis. In: Beers MH, ed. *The Merck Manual of Medical Information*. 2nd home ed. New York: Pocket Books; 2003:1603–1604.

17. Scoliosis. In: Schilling McCann JA, ed. *Nurse's 3 Minute Clinical Reference*. Springhouse, PA: Lippincott Williams & Wilkins; 2003: 512–513.

18. Fractures. In: Beers MH, ed. *The Merck Manual of Medical Information*. 2nd home ed. New York: Pocket Books; 2003:348–359.

19. Crutchlow EM, Dudac PJ, MacAvoy S, et al. Bone physiology. In: *Quick Look Nursing: Pathophysiology*. Thorofare, NJ: Slack; 2002: 246–248.

20. Hip fracture. In: Schilling McCann JA, ed. *Nurse's 3 Minute Clinical Reference*. Springhouse, PA: Lippincott Williams & Wilkins; 2003:268–269.

21. Smeltzer SC, Bare BG. Management of patients with musculoskeletal trauma. In: *Brunner & Suddarth's Textbook of Medical-Surgical Nursing*. 10th ed. Philadelphia: Lippincott Williams & Wilkins; 2004:2075–2111.

22. Amputation. In: Schilling McCann JA, ed. *Nurse's 3 Minute Clinical Reference*. Springhouse, PA: Lippincott Williams & Wilkins; 2003:613.

Bibliography

Carmona RH. *2004 Surgeon General's Report on Bone Health and Osteoporosis*. Washington, DC: Department of Health and Human Services; 2004.

Lewis S, Heitkemper MM, Cirksen SR. *Medical Surgical Nursing: Assessment and Management of Clinical Problems*. 6th ed. St. Louis: Mosby; 2004.

National Association of Orthopedic Nurses. *Core Curriculum for Orthopedic Nurses*. 5th ed. Upper Saddle River, NJ: Pearson; 2006.

Porth CM. *Pathophysiology: Concepts of Altered Health States*. 7th ed. Springhouse, PA: Lippincott Williams & Wilkins; 2005.

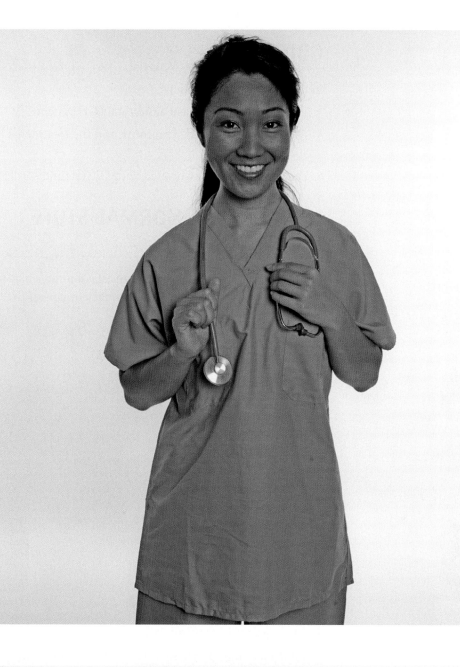

12 Gastrointestinal System

OBJECTIVES

In this chapter, you'll review:

- The function of the gastrointestinal (GI) system.
- The causes, signs, and symptoms, and the treatments for GI system disorders.
- The complications associated with GI system disorders.

LET'S GET THE NORMAL STUFF STRAIGHT FIRST

The gastrointestinal (GI) system consists of a muscular tube that extends from the mouth to the anus. The primary organs of the GI system include the:

- Oral cavity (mouth).
- Throat (pharynx).
- Esophagus.
- Stomach.
- Small intestine.
- Large intestine.
- Rectum.
- Anus.

The accessory organs of digestion include the:

- Liver.
- Gallbladder.
- Pancreas.

Specifically, the GI system:

- Aids ingestion, mastication, and salivation of food in the oral cavity.
- Transports and digests food material from the oral cavity through the esophagus into the stomach and small intestine.
- Absorbs nutrients in the small intestine that are transported by the bloodstream to the liver for metabolism.
- Reabsorbs water from digested food and eliminates indigestible material (chyme) in the large intestine.
- Stores chyme in the rectum for defecation through the anal canal.[1,2]

The accessory organs of digestion are not actual sites of digestion:

- The liver produces digestive secretions (bile).
- The gallbladder stores bile for use in the small intestine.
- The pancreas produces digestive enzymes.

✛ Which organ does what?

To better understand the disorders of the GI system (Fig. 12-1), you need a better understanding of the normal function of the organs, as seen in Table 12-1.

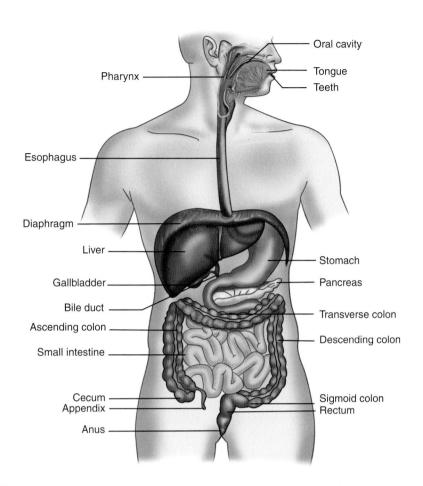

◀ Figure 12-1. The digestive system. (From Saladin K. *Anatomy and Physiology: The Unity of Form and Function*. 4th ed. New York: McGraw-Hill; 2007.)

Labels in figure:
Oral cavity
Tongue
Teeth
Pharynx
Esophagus
Diaphragm
Liver
Gallbladder
Bile duct
Ascending colon
Small intestine
Cecum
Appendix
Anus
Stomach
Pancreas
Transverse colon
Descending colon
Sigmoid colon
Rectum

Table 12-1

Segment	Organ	Functions
Upper GI system	Oral cavity (mouth), including: • Buccal mucosa • Lips • Tongue • Hard and soft palate • Teeth • Salivary glands	Mechanical digestion, chewing (mastication) Production of saliva, which moistens food for swallowing Start of carbohydrate breakdown
	Throat	Transport of food from oral cavity, which begins voluntarily and continues involuntarily
	Esophagus	Movement of food from throat to stomach by peristalsis, which is a rhythmic smooth muscle contraction (peristaltic wave) caused by stretching of smooth muscles as food enters the esophagus Prevention of a backflow of stomach contents done by the lower esophageal sphincter (located at the end of the esophagus)

(Continued)

Table 12-1. (*Continued*)

Segment	Organ	Functions
	Stomach	Reservoir for digestion by gastric secretion and mechanical movement of smooth muscles Consists of: • Cardia (holding area for food in the top of stomach) • Fundus (upper left part of stomach) • Body (holding area for food and the main area of stomach) • Antrum (lower stomach, where food mixes with gastric juices and chyme is formed) Substances (gastric juices) produced in stomach: • Mucus • Hydrochloric acid (converts pepsinogen to pepsin, which breaks down proteins) • Pepsinogen (precursor to pepsin, which is a digestive enzyme) Pyloric sphincter regulates passage of contents from stomach into small intestine
Lower GI system	Small intestine (longest portion of GI tract—16 to 19 feet in adults) Consists of: • Duodenum (first 12 inches) • Jejunum (8 feet) • Ileum (8 to 12 feet)	Completion of digestion Absorption of nutrients by slow propulsion (churning), which increases contact with intestinal wall and enzymes Pancreatic enzymes and bile enter through sphincter of Oddi
	Large intestine (5 to 6 feet long) Consists of: • Cecum (junction of small and large intestine. Attached to the cecum is a blind pouch known as the appendix) • Ascending colon • Transverse colon • Descending colon • Sigmoid colon (empties into the rectum)	Resorption of water Passage of indigestible material to rectum The large intestine contains needed bacteria that further digest materials and produce substances such as vitamin K

(*Continued*)

Table 12-1. (*Continued*)

Segment	Organ	Functions
	Rectum	Holds fecal material until an urge to defecate occurs
	Anus	Opening through which stool leaves the body. Anal sphincter provides closure of anus
Accessory organs	Liver (has many important functions not related to digestion)	Production of bile (breaks down fat) Processing of absorbed nutrients before circulation throughout body Storage of some minerals and vitamins
	Gallbladder	Storage and concentration of bile until its release is triggered by food entering the duodenum
	Pancreas	Produces digestive enzymes and hormones Digestive enzymes: ● Amylase-carbohydrate digestion ● Lipase-fat digestion ● Trypsin-protein digestion Hormones: ● Glucagon ● Insulin ● Somatostatin

Source: Created by author from References #1 to #3.

✚ How does the GI system work?

Mechanical digestion is accomplished by chewing food in the mouth and by the action of the three smooth muscle layers of the stomach. The secretion of gastric juices, acids, and pancreatic enzymes accomplishes chemical digestion. Movement of food material through the GI system is by one-way, wave-like smooth muscle motility of the esophagus and peristalsis of the stomach and intestines. Passage of food material into the next organ and prevention of backup is controlled by reflexes (swallowing and defecation), relaxation and closure of sphincters (esophageal and pyloric), and valves (ileocecal).

Effects of aging

Aging can significantly affect the GI system. The elderly may have reduced taste sensation, difficulty chewing from poor dental health, and reduced motility and muscle tone of the esophagus and intestines. Absorption of nutrients such as folic acid, iron, and calcium commonly decreases.[2] Decreased lactase levels often lead to an intolerance of dairy products. Constipation, a common problem in the elderly, can result from decreased motility or as a side effect of some prescription drugs. The elderly are at

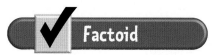

Factoid

If a client has a defective lower esophageal sphincter, stomach contents can more easily go backward into the esophagus, as in gastroesophageal reflux disease (GERD).

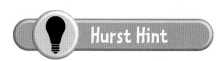

Hurst Hint

The pyloric sphincter is located in the lower RIGHT side of the stomach. This is why we turn clients on their right side during tube feeding to help the stomach empty completely after the feeding.

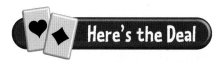

Here's the Deal

You need to know all the parts of the small and large intestines. When you study ileostomies and colostomies, you will have to know where in the intestinal tract the ostomy has been placed.

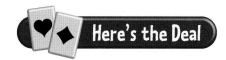

Here's the Deal

The small intestine is the major organ of absorption.

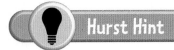

Hurst Hint

The longer the intestinal contents remain in the intestines, the more water is reabsorbed from the contents, leaving the stool more formed. If someone has a hyperactive intestinal tract (irritable bowel), the contents move through more rapidly, leaving less time for water to be reabsorbed and leaving the stool more liquid.

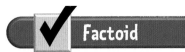

Factoid

The liver is important in drug metabolism and breakdown. The older the liver gets, the less it is able to do what it is supposed to do, so elderly clients should receive lower doses of medications.

increased risk of toxicity from drugs because of decreased enzyme activity in the liver, which depresses drug metabolism.

+ GI diseases and disorders

GI diseases and disorders typically:

* Cause distinctive, localized pain.
* Are exacerbated by certain factors.
* Disturb normal activity (frequency, motility).
* Vary in severity.

Table 12-2 shows the locations of GI diseases and disorders.

Table 12-2

Upper GI tract	Lower GI tract	Liver, gallbladder, and pancreas
Stomatitis	Polyps	Viral hepatitis
Gastritis	Hemorrhoids	Cholecystitis
Gastroenteritis	Dumping syndrome	Pancreatitis
Gastroesophageal reflux disease (GERD) (Fig. 12-2)	Hernia (inguinal, femoral, umbilical, incisional)	
Hiatal hernia	Intestinal obstruction	
Peptic ulcer	Appendicitis	
Achalasia (see define time)	Peritonitis	
	Crohn's disease	
	Ulcerative colitis	
	Irritable bowel syndrome	
	Diverticulitis	

Source: Created by author from References #3 to #5.

▶ Figure 12-2. Gastroesophageal reflux disease. **A.** Normally the lower esophageal sphincter is closed. **B.** If the lower esophageal sphincter does not close properly, the gastric contents can move backward into the esophagus.

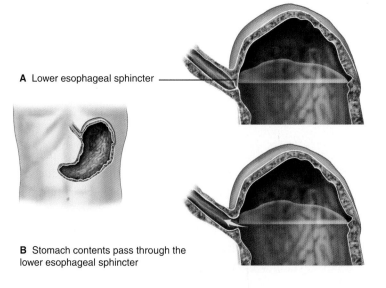

A Lower esophageal sphincter

B Stomach contents pass through the lower esophageal sphincter

LET'S GET DOWN TO SPECIFICS

✚ Aspiration

What is it?

Aspiration is the unintentional inhalation of foreign substances into the throat or lungs during inspiration. Most commonly, oral or gastric contents are aspirated.

What causes it and why

Table 12-3 shows the causes of aspiration and why those causes occur.

Table 12-3

Causes	Why
Gastroesophageal reflux disease (GERD)	The esophageal sphincter does not close properly, so stomach contents can easily go up into the esophagus and mouth or into the lungs
Narrowing of esophagus	Different circumstances (prolonged GERD) can cause the esophagus to narrow in spots. Such narrowing makes it difficult for food to pass as it's supposed to. A client usually needs to have the esophagus dilated
Swallowing dysfunction (dysphagia)	Difficulty swallowing increases the risk of choking on secretions from the mouth and stomach. If you can't swallow properly, food can come back into the throat and possibly the lungs. Dysphagia can result from anatomical, neurological, or physiological defects. It is common after a stroke
Hiatal hernia: a protrusion of a portion of the stomach above the diaphragm and into the esophagus; can cause gastroesophageal reflux and increase the risk of aspiration	When part of the stomach is pushed up into the thoracic cavity, increased pressure tends to push food up into the esophagus. Anytime abdominal pressure is increased, as with hiatal hernia, reflux is a strong possibility. When gastric contents are refluxed into the esophagus and throat, there is an increased likelihood of these contents moving into the lungs
Neurological disease: can alter normal GI processes and increase the risk of aspiration. Conditions such as stroke, head injury, and neuromuscular and seizure disorders should be monitored closely for swallowing dysfunction	• Stroke: affected nerves can affect movement (peristalsis) of food down into the stomach. Cranial nerves IX and X (swallowing impairment), cranial nerve IX (absent gag reflex), cranial nerve XII (impaired tongue movement) • Seizures: during a seizure, copious secretions can accumulate in the oropharynx because the client has lost control of the swallowing mechanism temporarily. This is why suction must be

(Continued)

Table 12-3. (*Continued*)

Causes	Why
	kept at bedside of client with history of seizures and why you must also turn clients on their side during a seizure (so the secretions will drain out of the mouth)
	• Guillain–Barré syndrome: the paralysis associated with this condition can move up to the thoracic region, paralyzing the esophageal muscles and leading to swallowing difficulty or an inability to swallow (secretions accumulate in the mouth)
	• Head injury: injuries to the brain lead to increased pressures (increased intracranial pressure) because the skull cannot expand to accommodate the increase of contents (blood or swollen brain). Increased pressures can damage or destroy the brain's ability to function properly. As pressures increase, vomiting and seizure activity can occur, which can also lead to aspiration. Long-term damage to cranial nerves IX, X, and XII increase the risk of aspiration
	• Parkinson's disease: this condition causes drooling, and choking can occur because of muscle rigidity in the face and throat. Aspiration is a major end-of-life concern; aspiration pneumonia is a common cause of death
Structural anomaly: An anomaly is a variation from the normal anatomy and can occur in any body system. Certain anomalies in primary organs of the GI system can decrease the ability to begin and complete the digestive process. Conditions such as cleft palate and esophageal atresia increase the overall risk of aspiration • Cleft palate is a split in the roof of the mouth that opens into the nose • Esophageal atresia is a congenital disorder in which the esophagus is not attached to the stomach. In most cases, a tracheoesophageal fistula (abnormal connection between the esophagus and trachea) is also present, allowing food to travel directly into the lungs	• Cleft palate: the baby is born with an opening in the palate so when the baby swallows, the formula can go up into places it shouldn't. The baby will cough and choke, and milk will bubble out of the nose • Esophageal atresia: the baby swallows, but the milk or formula cannot go where it needs to, so it bubbles back up into the oropharynx or travels through the tracheoesophageal fistula, and the baby aspirates

(*Continued*)

Table 12-3. (*Continued*)

Causes	Why
Impaired gag reflex	An intact gag reflex prevents unwanted food and other substances from entering the throat. An impaired reflex leads to an inability to ensure correct food passage Damage to cranial nerve IX (glossopharyngeal) or cranial nerve X (vagus) can lead to an absent gag reflex
Enteral feeding: Nutrition provided through a feeding tube such as a nasogastric (NG) tube (tube inserted through the nose into the stomach) or a tube surgically placed in the stomach or jejunum	Anytime nutrition is being given through an nasogastric (NG) tube, there is a risk that the tube may accidentally be moved from the stomach into the esophagus or throat, causing the feedings to enter the lungs If feedings are given too quickly or the amount is too much for the stomach, vomiting may occur, and gastric contents can enter the lungs

Source: Created by author from References #4, #5, and #9.

Signs and symptoms and why

A latent period (a period of no signs or symptoms) may occur between aspiration and the onset of symptoms. Most clients begin experiencing symptoms within 2 hours of aspiration, if not immediately. Table 12-4 shows the signs and symptoms and rationales associated with aspiration.

Table 12-4

Signs and symptoms	Why
Coughing	Response of body to rid lungs of gastric contents
Increased respiratory rate	Hypoxia develops because lungs are filled with stomach contents. Adequate gas exchange cannot occur, so the body's oxygen needs are not met
Shortness of breath	Hypoxia
Fever, chills	Gastric contents in lungs cause inflammation, leading to microbial growth and pneumonia
Increased sputum	Gastric contents enter the lungs, and the tissues become inflamed. Inflammation increases sputum production. Sputum may become purulent as infection develops from the increased growth of bacteria
Apnea, cyanotic episodes	Hypoxia
Wheezing, crackles	Gastric contents accumulate in lung fields
Sore throat, hoarseness	Reflux of gastric contents causes throat irritation

Source: Created by author from References #5, #7, and #9.

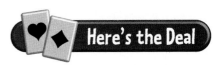

A large abdomen is one cause of hiatal hernia. A large abdomen causes excessive abdominal pressure, which tends to push stomach contents back up.

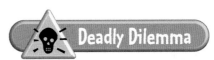

When caring for a newborn, it is VERY important to watch the first feeding closely and to ensure it is sterile water or breast milk (which is sterile). The baby could have a congenital anomaly (cleft palate) and could aspirate. If so, we want the aspirated contents to be sterile to prevent infection.

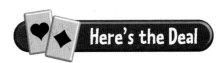

Remember that checking a client's gag reflex is one of the MOST IMPORTANT assessments you can perform.

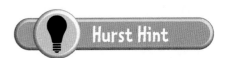

Stay with a client with dysphagia who is eating. ALWAYS assist the client yourself. DO NOT delegate feeding to assistive personnel.

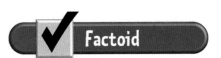

Damage to cranial nerve IX (glossopharyngeal), cranial nerve X (vagus), and cranial nerve XII (hypoglossal) poses the greatest risk of aspiration.

Quickie tests and treatments

The tests for aspiration include:

- Chest x-ray.

- Pulse oximetry: determine oxygenation status and the ability of oxygen to enter bloodstream.

- Upper GI studies: detect hiatal hernia, GERD, and other disorders that increase risk of aspiration.

- Swallowing studies: determine swallowing dysfunction.

- Esophageal manometry: measures pressures in the lower esophageal sphincter and identifies abnormal muscle contractions in the esophagus. Increased pressures in the esophagus can lead to more gastric reflux, which can increase the risk of aspiration.

Treatment of aspiration consists of managing the conditions that increase the risk of aspiration and treating the underlying cause:

- If the client has a history of seizures, always have suction equipment at bedside. During a seizure, position the client on the side to decrease risk of aspiration.

- Clients at risk for aspiration should have the head of the bed (HOB) elevated at least 45 degrees while eating and should remain at this angle for 30 minutes to an hour (to keep food down).

- Avoid having the client lie flat for 1 to 2 hours after meals.

- Consuming small, frequent meals may decrease risk of distention and vomiting.

- Avoid spicy foods, fatty foods (if GERD exists), and foods that are difficult to chew and swallow.

- For clients with an impaired gag reflex or damage to cranial nerve IX or X, liquids should be thickened. This can be done by using commercial powders such as Thick-it. Thicker foods (such as puddings) are less likely to be aspirated than liquids such as tea or water.

- Structural anomalies require surgical correction, but take care to prevent aspiration before surgery.

- A registered dietitian (RD) is often consulted to assess the client, determine the appropriate diet (thickening agents for liquids), and teach the client and family ways to avoid aspiration.

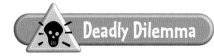

Ideal pulse oximetry readings are 95% to 100%. Readings below 90% should be reported, if previous readings have been normal. Remember, readings below 80% are life-threatening.

TUBE FEEDINGS   For permanent impairment of the gag reflex and other chronic neurological conditions that lead to an inability to consume nutrients without aspiration, feeding tubes may be used. These tubes can be placed through the nasal cavity into the stomach (nasogastric tube) or directly into the stomach or small intestine (percutaneous endoscopic gastrostomy [PEG] or percutaneous endoscopic jejunostomy [PEJ]) by surgical placement. Remember, even with feeding tubes, there is a risk of aspiration due to coughing, vomiting gastric contents, reflux or the tube could become dislodged.

- Initial tube placement should be confirmed by x-ray before administering feedings. A pH check of aspirant is the preferred ongoing placement verification method. Gastric pH ranges from 0 to 4.0; intestinal pH from 7.0 to 8.0; lung pH is greater than 6.0.

- Secure the tube with tape or an attachment device. Provide daily skin care and resecure the tube.

- Residual volumes (amount of feeding remaining in the stomach) should be checked every 4 hours and recorded. Refer to physician orders for acceptable residual amounts and interventions for excessive amounts (slow or stop feedings). You don't want to keep pushing tube feeding into the stomach, if the client has a large residual. An increased residual means the stomach is not emptying as quickly as it normally would.

- Never allow a client with a feeding tube to lie supine (flat on his back). Maintain the head of the bed at an elevation of 30 to 45 degrees.

- If vomiting occurs, turn off the tube feeding and place the client on her side. Suction the oropharyngeal cavity and assess the client for signs of aspiration (crackles, increased respiratory rate, and cyanosis).

- Be very diligent in checking tube placement, especially if you have an active client. Always stop tube feedings when repositioning clients in bed (pulling client up in bed). Check placement prior to resuming feeding.

ANTIBIOTIC THERAPY   Gastric contents in the lungs are a breeding ground for bacteria. Aspiration pneumonia commonly occurs and requires treatment with antibiotics.

What can harm my client?

- Aspiration pneumonia: poor oxygenation and permanent lung damage can occur.

- Chronic lung disease or bronchitis from repeated aspiration: scarring of lung tissue can lead to an increased risk of infection and decreased function of the lung tissues.

- Pulmonary fibrosis: repeated damage from aspiration can lead to microscopic injury. Air sacs in the lungs are replaced by fibrotic tissue, and scarring occurs. This leads to a decreased ability of the tissue to transfer oxygen to the blood.

If I were your teacher, I would test you on . . .

- Definition of aspiration.

- Causes of aspiration and the rationales.

- Signs and symptoms and the rationales.

- Client education for reflux management (foods to avoid, need for weight loss if obese, smoking cessation, elevation of head of bed, importance of not eating 2 to 3 hours before bedtime, importance of eating smaller frequent meals).

- Assessment of gag reflex (stimulate the back of the throat with a tongue depressor and elevation of palate, and gag should occur).

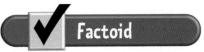

Factoid

The traditional method of confirming tube placement by auscultation is no longer considered reliable. This method involved instilling 20 to 30 mL of air into the nasogastric tube while listening with a stethoscope over the epigastic area of the stomach. A "whooshing" sound confirmed correct placement.

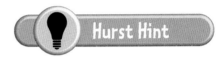

Hurst Hint

Any client at risk for aspiration should have suction equipment readily available.

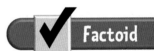

Factoid

Several years ago a few drops of blue food coloring was placed in tube feedings. Suctioning of blue-tinged sputum caused nurses to cringe, as aspiration of tube feeding into the lungs was the likely cause. The use of food coloring was stopped because of possible carcinogenesis problems with excessive use, but you may still hear experienced nurses talk about this practice.

- Nasogastric tube placement, verification, management.
- Seizure management to prevent aspiration.
- Recognizing signs of aspiration.
- Positioning of client to prevent aspiration. When client is receiving tube feeding, keep head elevated at 45 degrees; for an intermittent tube feeding, elevate head of bed, turn client on right side, and keep in this position for at least 30 to 45 minutes.
- Delegation of care for client who has dysphagia.
- Foods that are least likely to be aspirated with dysphagia client.
- Cranial nerves involved in swallowing.
- Pre- and posttest nursing management.
- Tracheostomy (an opening in the trachea used to maintain an airway). Evaluate swallowing ability, elevate head at least 45 degrees for at least 30 minutes after eating, deflate cuff completely or partially if possible during feedings (cuff on the tube is used to help seal airway from gastric secretions, but can interfere with the passage of food into the esophagus), avoid thin liquids, and have client chew slowly and dry swallow (no liquid with food) after each bite.

✚ Stomatitis

What is it?

Stomatitis is an inflammation of the mucous membranes of the mouth, involving the cheeks, gums, tongue, lips, and roof or floor of the mouth, and affecting all age groups. The two primary types of stomatitis are aphthous (also called a canker sore) and herpes simplex virus type 1 (also called a cold sore).

What causes it and why

Table 12-5 shows the causes of stomatitis and why these causes occur.

Table 12-5

Causes	Why
Trauma to mucous membranes	Poorly fitted dentures, biting of cheeks, jagged teeth, and hard bristled toothbrushes can traumatize the soft tissue of the mouth and lead to inflammation
Irritation	Hot beverages or foods can burn the mouth. Chronic mouth breathing can dry the soft tissues
	Excessive use of alcohol or tobacco products can irritate the mucosal lining and lead to stomatitis
	Sensitivity to toothpaste (e.g., toothpaste with cinnamon), mouthwash, or lipstick can irritate soft tissues of the mouth
Herpes simplex: viral infection of the mouth	Herpetic infections (cold sores) can occur by direct contact with someone infected with herpes virus; contact includes kissing and oral sex

(Continued)

Table 12-5. (*Continued*)

Causes	Why
HIV and AIDS: the human immunodeficiency virus progressively destroys the white blood cells, specifically the CD4 lymphocytes. Acquired immunodeficiency syndrome (AIDS) is the most severe form of HIV and is usually associated with a CD4 count of less than 200	HIV and AIDS clients have a compromised ability to defend the body from infection, so a fungal infection of the mouth can occur
Gonorrhea: a sexually transmitted disease that infects the lining of the urethra, cervix, rectum	A person who has oral sex with a partner with gonorrhea can develop an infection of the throat (gonococcal pharyngitis)
Measles: rubeola is a contagious viral infection that is spread through the air. It is characterized by a rash that begins around the ears and neck and extends to the trunk and extremities	A person with measles develops tiny white spots (Koplik spots) in the mouth before the rash appears. These areas may become irritated and inflamed
Leukemia: leukemias are cancers affecting the development of white blood cells. The body is unable to produce an adequate number of normal blood cells	A person with leukemia may experience bleeding gums from decreased platelets and infection from decreased white blood cells (WBC). Clients undergoing chemotherapy are at greater risk of developing fungal infections of the mouth because of the decreased ability to fight infection
Vitamin C deficiency (scurvy): ascorbic acid (vitamin C) is vital in forming bone and connective tissue	The gums turn purple, swell, and break open. Inflammation and open sores appear in the mouth
Fungal infection: *Candida albicans* (candidiasis) is an overgrowth of fungi	Fungal infections (such as thrush) can occur when normal flora that prevents fungal infection is destroyed by prolonged antibiotic use, radiation, chemotherapy, or immunocompromised systems

Source: Created by author from References #5, #8, and #9.

Signs and symptoms and why

Table 12-6 shows the signs and symptoms and rationales associated with stomatitis.

Table 12-6

Signs and symptoms	Why
Pain	Irritation of sores or inflamed areas can occur with contact from food, beverages, and oral care
Ulcerations, lesions	Ulcerations and lesions occur from irritation and inflammation. The appearance of the lesions varies according to the cause • Aphthous: small, white, shallow, painful ulcer lasting up to 2 weeks • Herpes simplex: painful cold sore on lips, cheeks, tongue, gums, or palate lasting several days. Can be a blister • Infective lesions can have pus-filled pockets (abscesses) • White plaque-like fungal lesions on tongue and cheeks
Swollen lymph nodes	Can occur with severe aphthous sores left untreated as inflammation and infection extend beyond oral cavity

Source: Created by author from References #5 to #7.

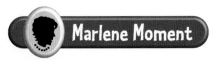

Many of you have heard of vitamin C deficiency occurring in sailors who have little access to vitamin C rich foods, such as oranges. Recall the teeth and gums of those pirates pictured in books and movies. YUCK!

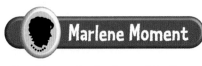

No chips and salsa for awhile if you have stomatitis.

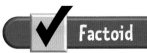

Medications like viscous lidocaine numb the throat and can impair swallowing. If these medications are prescribed, monitor the client closely for choking and aspiration.

Quickie test and treatments

The client history should include:

- Nutritional deficiencies.
- Use of dentures.
- Oral hygiene practices.
- Recent antibiotic use.
- History of other diseases that increase the risk of developing oral sores.
- Recent change in mouthwash, toothpaste, or lipstick.
- Excessive use of alcohol or tobacco.
- Onset of the problem.

Physical examination includes an assessment of sores and surrounding tissues. A physician, dentist, or advanced practice nurse identifies the type of stomatitis.

Tests for stomatitis include:

- Complete blood count to determine if an infection is present.
- Culture of scrapings of the lining of the mouth to identify the infectious agent.

Treatment of stomatitis includes:

- Good oral hygiene to prevent buildup of food particles that can lead to growth of infectious agents and an inflammation of the mucous lining.
- Appropriate dental care, including use of soft-bristle brushes, Toothette, and gauze to prevent injury to the mucous lining. Rough brushing of the gums should be avoided. Jagged teeth and poorly fitting dentures should be corrected by a dentist.
- Irritating foods and beverages, such as spicy foods, should be avoided while sores are present. Hot foods and drinks that can burn the mouth and sharp-edged foods, such as tortilla chips and nuts, should also be avoided.
- Topical anesthetics may be used to decrease the pain of stomatitis. Benzocaine anesthetics (Anbesol), camphor phenol, or 2% viscous lidocaine mouthwash may be used.
- Oral medications may be prescribed if the sores are from an infectious process: acyclovir for herpes simplex, tetracycline and corticosteroid rinses and tablets for recurrent aphthous ulcers, and nystatin oral suspension for fungal infections (swish and swallow).

What can harm my client?

- Herpes simplex virus types 1 and 2 are contagious infections that can be transmitted through direct contact until the sore is completely crusted over.
- Pain may prevent the client from eating or drinking, increasing the risk of dehydration. Cool liquids should be offered frequently as well as foods that can easily be swallowed (puddings, Jello).

● Oral hygiene with strong mouthwash can increase pain. Banging the toothbrush against the gums and tongue can further irritate mucous membranes.

● Review adverse reactions to prescribed medications with your client.

If I were your teacher, I would test you on . . .

● Definition of stomatitis.

● Causes of stomatitis and rationales.

● Signs and symptoms and rationales.

● Client assessment, including predisposing illnesses, medications, and oral hygiene habits.

● Client education regarding lifestyle changes for prevention, reduction of frequency, and symptom management.

● Oral hygiene interventions.

● Use of oral anesthetic and monitoring for complications.

● Commonly prescribed drugs.

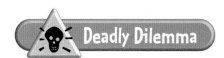

Deadly Dilemma

Young children and those with an impaired gag reflex or a swallowing dysfunction should not be given anesthetics such as viscous lidocaine, which can numb the throat and lead to choking!

✚ Gastritis

What is it?

Gastritis is a group of conditions characterized by inflammation of the stomach lining that can be acute (lasting only a few days) or chronic. Irritation of the stomach lining can lead to mucosal bleeding, edema, and erosion.

What causes it and why

Table 12-7 shows the causes of gastritis and why these causes occur.

Table 12-7

Causes	Why
Infection	*Helicobacter pylori* penetrates the mucosal layer of the gastric lining, leading to inflammation. Immunocompromised clients (those with AIDS or undergoing chemotherapy) may develop viral or fungal gastritis because of a decreased ability to fight infections
Irritation from medications, alcohol, food, and corrosive substances	Medications such as aspirin, BC powders, corticosteroids, and nonsteroidal antiinflammatory drugs (NSAIDs) can injure the stomach lining and lead to gastritis
	Excessive alcohol consumption and continual intake of certain foods such as spicy, highly seasoned foods can wear away at the stomach lining and lead to gastritis
	Accidental or intentional ingestion of corrosive substances leads to inflammation and destruction of the stomach lining
Stress	Sudden illnesses or injuries can lead to stress gastritis (due to hypersecretion of stomach acid). On admission to the hospital, many clients are given medications, such as omeprazole (Prilosec) to help prevent this type of gastritis
Radiation	Radiation administered to the lower chest or abdomen can irritate the lining of the stomach and lead to inflammation
Gastrectomy (partial or full removal of the stomach)	Inflammation can occur where tissue is sewn back together

Source: Created by author from References #7 to #9.

Signs and symptoms and why

Gastritis typically causes no symptoms. When symptoms do occur, they vary greatly based on the underlying cause of the inflammation. Table 12-8 shows the signs and symptoms and rationales associated with gastritis.

Table 12-8

Signs and symptoms	Why
Pain or discomfort	Rapid onset of epigastric pain as inflammation or necrosis of the gastric mucosa occurs Chronic gastritis pain may be relieved by ingestion of food
Dyspepsia (heartburn)	Commonly occurs from the erosion of the stomach lining
Gnawing or burning aches in upper abdomen	Inflammation of the stomach lining from acids, infection, or medication can cause a burning sensation in the gastric area
Nausea and vomiting	Nausea and vomiting can occur anytime the stomach lining is damaged by erosion
Loss of appetite (anorexia)	Indigestion, pain, and fullness decrease the desire to consume food because food intake may aggravate other symptoms
Bloating, belching	Increased acid production can cause indigestion, which leads to bloating and belching
Weight loss	Weight loss can occur from anorexia
Bleeding	Prolonged irritation of the stomach lining can lead to bleeding that appears as hematemesis (vomiting blood) or melena (passing black, tarry stools) Persistent bleeding can lead to anemia

Source: Created by author from References #5 to #7.

Quickie tests and treatments

The tests for gastritis include:

- Esophagogastroduodenoscopy (EGD) to check for inflammation of the gastric area and confirm the diagnosis. A biopsy sample determines the specific type of gastritis.

- Blood tests to check for anemia if bleeding is present and to detect *Helicobacter pylori.*

- Urea breath test to check for *H. pylori.*

- Stool tests to check for blood and *H. pylori* in the digestive tract.

Treatment of gastritis varies, depending on underlying cause and the degree of symptoms. Antacids and drugs that decrease acid production may be used:

- Proton-pump inhibitors—such as omeprazole (Prilosec), lansoprazole (Prevacid), esomeprazole (Nexium), and pantoprazole (Protonix)—to inhibit gastric acid formation.

- H$_2$-receptor blockers—such as nizatidine (Axid), ranitidine (Zantac), and famotidine (Pepcid)—to inhibit gastric acid secretion.
- Antacids—such as aluminum magnesium combinations (Mylanta, Maalox)—to neutralize existing gastric acid.
- Mucosal barrier fortifiers—such as sucralfate (Carafate) to protect the mucosal barrier.

Infection with *H. pylori* requires a 2-week course with three drugs. The most common combinations are bismuth subsalicylate (Pepto-Bismol) or a proton-pump inhibitor and metronidazole (Flagyl) and tetracycline (Achromycin) or clarithromycin (Biaxin) and amoxicillin (Amoxil).

Lifestyle changes include avoiding aspirin and NSAIDs, which irritate the stomach lining; avoiding foods that aggravate the condition, such as spicy, hot foods and fatty foods; and eliminating or decreasing alcohol consumption and tobacco use.

If conservative measures are unsuccessful or major bleeding occurs, surgery may be needed.

What can harm my client?

- Symptoms can be easily confused with those of myocardial infarction.
- Chronic gastritis can lead to ulcers, risk for stomach cancer, and risk of stomach-wall perforation requiring immediate surgery.
- Failure to complete antibiotic regimen can cause resistant strains to develop.
- Failure to complete prescribed course of treatment can lead to chronic irritation.

If I were your teacher, I would test you on . . .

- Definition of gastritis.
- Common signs and symptoms of gastritis and those requiring immediate attention.
- Causes of gastritis and rationales.
- Clients at risk for developing gastritis.
- Treatment of *H. pylori*.
- Client education stressing importance of medication regimen and lifestyle changes.[6,7,10]

✛ Gastroenteritis

What is it?

Gastroenteritis (better known as the stomach flu) is an inflammation of the GI tract. Although gastroenteritis can occur at any age, infants and older adults are at risk of having more severe symptoms.

What causes it and why

Table 12-9 shows the causes of gastroenteritis and why those causes occur.

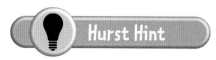

Be aware that clients undergoing major surgeries, suffering from severe burns, or being cared for in an intensive care setting are at increased risk of developing stress gastritis. Many physicians order medication to prevent complications of gastritis.

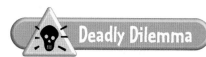

Life-threatening hemorrhage can occur as a result of gastritis. Carefully monitor vital signs and report new or increased hematemesis or melena. Hemorrhage can lead to intravascular volume depletion and shock!

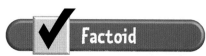

Gastroenteritis in less industrialized countries is a significant cause of death among the very young and old.

Table 12-9

Causes	Why
Pathogens: • Parasitic organisms (*Entamoeba histolytica* and *Cryptosporidium* and *Giardia* species) • Bacterial organisms (*Escherichia coli*, *Vibrio cholerae*, and *Campylobacter*, *Salmonella*, and *Shigella* species) • Viral organisms (astroviruses, Norwalk virus, rotaviruses) Chemical toxins (lead, arsenic, mercury, poisonous mushroom, exotic seafood)	Direct contact: • Infected person passes organism to another person • Unwashed or inadequately washed hands after a bowel movement • Diaper changes (in a daycare) without cleaning between infants • Use of dirty eating utensils (glasses, plates, silverware) Food: • Undercooked food that has been left out too long, or unpasteurized liquids can be sources of bacterial contamination Water: • (Water contaminated with infected stool of animals or people is ingested

Source: Created by author from Reference #5.

Signs and symptoms and why

Table 12-10 shows the signs and symptoms and rationales associated with gastroenteritis.

Table 12-10

Signs and symptoms	Why
Diarrhea (hallmark symptom of gastroenteritis)	Infected large intestine looses the ability to retain fluids, leading to diarrhea Diarrhea may resolve in 24 hours or last as long as 7 to 10 days, depending on the underlying cause
Nausea and vomiting	These defense mechanisms try to rid the body of invading agent
Abdominal cramps	As the lining of the GI system becomes inflamed, abdominal cramping occurs
Loss of appetite	Appetite loss is common as the other symptoms of GI inflammation occur
Fever and chills	Body's compensatory reaction to infection
Dehydration	From prolonged diarrhea accompanied by elevated temperature, nausea, and vomiting. Disturbances in fluid and electrolyte balances require fluid replacement
Weakness, fatigue	Prolonged nausea, vomiting, and diarrhea can lead to water and electrolyte imbalances that can cause extreme weakness

Source: Created by author from References #4 and #5.

Quickie tests and treatments

The client history should include:

- Onset of symptoms.

- Recent travel, especially to another country and tropical regions. Traveler's diarrhea is a common problem during visits to countries with poor sanitation.

- History of foods consumed. Consumption of foods with mayonnaise at a recent family reunion or undercooked foods or seafood should be explored.

Laboratory studies include:

- Stool culture to identify organism responsible for symptoms.

- Blood tests to evaluate cause and potential problems (if symptoms are severe or persist). If client is dehydrated, tests may include chemistry profile to assess potassium, sodium, and other electrolyte levels.

- GI studies to determine the presence of underlying disease (if the symptoms persist).

Treatments:

- Replacing fluids and electrolytes is the most important treatment. Fluid intake should continue, even if vomiting occurs. The amount consumed depends on the client's age.

- Avoid carbonated, caffeinated, and high-sugar drinks, which can increase diarrhea. Any beverage with a lot of particles, such as high-sugar drinks, can cause an osmotic pull of fluid into the intestines, which would increase diarrhea.

- First, use clear liquids with electrolytes (Pedialyte), then use clear broths and gelatin.

- Oral rehydration therapy (such as Pedialyte, Resol) may be needed for infants, children, and older adults.

- If vomiting and diarrhea persist or an inability to consume fluids occurs, IV fluids (fluids given through a vein) may be administered. Generally, hypotonic IV fluids are ordered and may include a potassium supplement if serum potassium level is low.

- Diet should progress, as tolerated. As the symptoms begin to subside, bland foods (cream soups, crackers, toast, rice, yogurt, custards) can be introduced into the diet. Spicy foods, dairy products, vegetables, fruits, high-sugar foods, and alcohol should be avoided for the first 2 to 3 days.

- Antibiotics may be ordered, if the infecting agent is bacterial. Often antibiotics are not used because they can cause further diarrhea and lead to antibiotic-resistant organisms.

- Antiparasitics may be ordered, if the infecting agent is parasitic.

- Antidiarrheals are not recommended because they can prolong the effects of the infection by preventing elimination of the organism.

- If severe vomiting occurs, suppositories or injectable medications may be ordered to decrease episodes of vomiting.

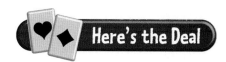

It may not be smart to immediately encourage medications to stop diarrhea because the body may be trying to get rid of the bacteria. But you must be very worried about the client becoming dehydrated.

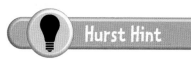

Signs and symptoms of dehydration include dry mucous membranes, poor skin turgor, decreased blood pressure, oliguria (urine output less than 30 mL/h), increased thirst, and weakness. Careful monitoring is imperative because fluid and electrolyte imbalances can occur quickly in the presence of diarrhea.

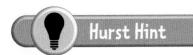

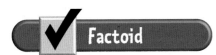

Caffeine increases GI motility and should be avoided!

- Skin irritation can occur from frequent diarrhea stools. Cleansing should include use of a washcloth with warm water. **PAT THE AREA**; avoid wiping. Barrier creams and ointments may prevent further irritation. Witch hazel compresses (Tucks) may be indicated to relieve discomfort.

What can harm my client?

- Dehydration is the greatest concern. Monitor your client for signs of dehydration, including decreased urination to less than 30 mL/h (oliguria), dark concentrated urine, decreased blood pressure, dry skin and mucous membranes, extreme thirst, weakness, sunken cheeks or eyes, low potassium and sodium levels, and elevated BUN (blood urea nitrogen) levels. Assess infants for sunken fontanels, the separations in the skull that are present at birth.
- Lack of knowledge of transmission of gastroenteritis can lead to spread of organisms. Education should include the importance of hand-washing after going to the bathroom and when handling food, cleaning areas used to prepare raw meat and eggs with disinfectant, and avoiding raw or improperly cooked meat and eggs.
- Traveling brings concerns about contracting gastroenteritis. When traveling (especially to other countries), clients should drink bottled water and other beverages from original container without using a straw. Avoiding raw meat, fruit, and vegetables is encouraged. If visiting an area with poor sanitation, clients should not use water from tap to brush teeth or clean dishes and avoid eating utensils and ice cubes.

If I were your teacher, I would test you on . . .
- Definition of gastroenteritis.
- Causes of gastroenteritis.
- Transmission of organisms.
- Signs, prevention, and treatment of dehydration.
- Lab values related to dehydration.
- Prevention of gastroenteritis.
- Standard precautions.

✚ Gastroesophageal reflux disease (GERD)
What is it?
GERD is a condition in which gastric contents reflux (move backward) into the esophagus.

What causes it and why
Table 12-11 shows the causes of GERD and why those causes occur.

GERD is a condition of gastric acid moving into the wrong place (primarily up into the esophagus and mouth), as compared to the stomach's hypersecretion of gastric acid, which leaks into surrounding tissues.

Table 12-11

Causes	Why
Insufficient closure of lower esophageal sphincter (LES)	Because pressure in the abdominal cavity is greater that the thoracic cavity, gastric contents are pushed through the weakened sphincter, causing burning in the esophagus and mouth Common causes include pregnancy and obesity
Gastric distention	The lower esophageal sphincter closes properly, but excessively high pressures in the abdominal cavity lead to gastric reflux into the esophagus. Distention may result from consumption of large meals, pregnancy, obesity, or clothing that binds abdomen
Hiatal hernia (protrusion of part of the stomach into the esophagus)	As pressure pushes part of the stomach into the esophagus, reflux of stomach contents begin to irritate the esophageal lining
Lifestyle	Smoking can weaken the LES and lead to reflux Dietary factors (including high-fat diet; increased intake of caffeine, chocolate, alcohol, and spicy foods; and excessively large meals) can lead to GERD
Medications	NSAIDs and some drugs to treat cardiovascular conditions (nitrates, calcium-channel blockers) place a person at risk for developing GERD

Source: Created by author from References #4, #6, and #7.

Signs and symptoms and why

Table 12-12 shows the signs and symptoms and rationales associated with GERD.

Table 12-12

Signs and symptoms	Why
Dyspepsia (heartburn)	Acid irritation of esophageal tissue Normal esophagus pH is 7.0, and stomach pH is 4.0. Repeated exposure to high pH leads to a burning sensation in the throat that can radiate into the chest Dyspepsia may become more intense when bending and lying flat
Regurgitation (may be described as bitter or sour tasting)	Warm food particles and fluid travel up the esophagus into the pharynx due to an inability of the LES to prevent backflow
Hypersalivation	Salivary glands increase saliva in response to reflux
Nausea	Prolonged reflux into the esophagus can lead to nausea. This is common in the morning

(Continued)

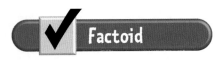

GERD pain can be experienced as burning, or pain that radiates to the neck, throat, and face.

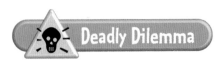

Regurgitation when a person is lying down increases the risk of aspiration. An increased respiratory rate and crackles in the lung fields may indicate aspiration.

Table 12-12. (*Continued*)

Signs and symptoms	Why
Pain	Caused by acid irritation of the mucosal lining Usually occurs 30 minutes after meals or when lying down at night
Hoarseness, throat clearing or sore throat	Acid irritation and backflow of gastric contents (irritates the throat)
Dysphagia (difficulty swallowing)	Scarring from long-term exposure to acid irritation (scarring can cause narrowing in esophagus)
Odynophagia (painful swallowing)	From spasms in the esophagus caused by irritation of tissue
Coughing	Irritation of the phrenic nerve

Source: Created by author from References #4, #6, and #7.

Quickie tests and treatments

Tests for GERD include:

- Ambulatory pH monitoring to measure the frequency and duration of reflux episodes: performed by placing a tube through the nose and into the lower esophagus. The outer tube is connected to a monitor worn on the belt. Acid levels are usually measured for 24 hours.

- Barium swallow to show structural abnormalities and reflux of barium from stomach into esophagus. Performed by using x-rays after client swallows barium.

- Endoscopy (most common test used for diagnosis) to directly visualize tissue erythema, fragility, or erosion and detect esophageal cancer or Barrett's esophagus (precancerous change in the lining of the esophagus). Performed using an endoscope (tube).

- Esophageal manometry to measure pressure of esophageal wave motility and identify LES pressure sufficiency. Performed by inserting water-filled catheter through the nose and into the esophagus. Pressures and peristalsis are measured as the catheter is withdrawn.

Treatment of GERD aims to reduce reflux of gastric juices and abdominal pressure. Dietary management includes:

- Losing weight if obese.

- Eating a low-fat, high-protein diet to reduce acid production.

- Limiting or avoiding chocolate, fatty foods, and mints to ease LES pressure.

- Eating small frequent meals (4 to 6 a day) to help reduce abdominal pressure.

- Avoiding carbonated beverages, which can increase stomach pressure.

- Avoiding meals within 3 hours of going to bed to reduce reflux caused by larger meals.

- Avoiding spicy and high-acid foods, which can irritate the esophageal lining.

- Avoiding alcohol, especially late at night before bedtime.

- Increasing fluid intake to help wash gastric contents out of esophagus.

Other changes include:

- Discontinuing of NSAIDs, as ordered by physician.

- Elevating head of the bed 6 to 12 inches or more to prevent reflux during sleep.

- Stopping smoking to improve pressure on LES.

- Avoiding constrictive clothing (tight clothes increase intra-abdominal pressure).

Drug therapy includes:

- Proton-pump inhibitors—such as omeprazole (Prilosec), lansoprazole (Prevacid), esomeprazole (Nexium), and pantoprazole (Protonix)—to inhibit gastric acid formation. Proton-pump inhibitors are typically the most effective treatment for GERD.

- H_2-receptor blockers—such as nizatidine (Axid), ranitidine (Zantac), and famotidine (Pepcid)—to inhibit gastric acid secretion.

- Antacids—such as aluminum magnesium combinations (Mylanta, Maalox)—to neutralize existing gastric acid.

- Mucosal barrier fortifiers—such as sucralfate (Carafate) to protect the mucosal barrier.

Invasive treatments include:

- Endoscopic intervention to tighten the LES and prevent reflux.

- Surgical intervention to correct LES weakness. May be needed if client does not respond to medical management or problem is complicated by a hiatal hernia. Laparoscopic Nissen fundoplication (LNF) is the most common procedure. Some people choose to undergo surgery to prevent lifelong use of medication to treat GERD.

What can harm my client?

- Long-term untreated GERD causes acidic burning of tissue, leading to esophagitis (erosion and ulceration of epithelium of esophagus).

- Stricture (narrowing of esophagus caused by scar tissue) can lead to swallowing difficulties.

- Barrett's esophagus (a precancerous change in the tissue of the esophagus) can lead to esophageal cancer.

If I were your teacher, I would test you on . . .

- Definition of GERD.

- Causes of GERD and rationales.

- Signs and symptoms of GERD and rationales.

- Pharmacology of drugs for GERD.

- Client education regarding pH and manometry studies.

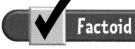

Cimetidine (Tagamet) can inhibit the elimination of other drugs, such as warfarin (Coumadin) and phenytoin (Dilantin), and is used less frequently than the other H_2-receptor blockers.

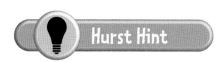

With Nissen, the condition tends to recur in some people so the focus is on identifying risk factors such as smoking, obesity, excessive alcohol intake, poor diet, etc., and making lifestyle changes to eliminate those contributing factors.

- Client education regarding lifestyle changes to improve signs and symptoms.
- Signs and symptoms of more serious problems (bleeding, painful swallowing, weight loss, dysphagia) that require medical attention.

✚ Hiatal hernia

What is it?

A hiatal hernia (Fig. 12-3) occurs when part of the stomach protrudes through the esophageal hiatus (the opening in the diaphragm through which the esophagus passes through). There are two major types of hiatal hernias:

- Sliding: upper segment of the stomach including the esophageal-stomach junction slides through the opening in the diaphragm.
- Paraesophageal: upper segment of the stomach moves into the chest; the esophageal-stomach junction remains in normal position.

▶ Figure 12-3. Hiatal hernia. A hiatal hernia occurs when the upper portion of the stomach slips through the hiatus (the hole between the abdominal cavity and the diaphragm) into the chest cavity.

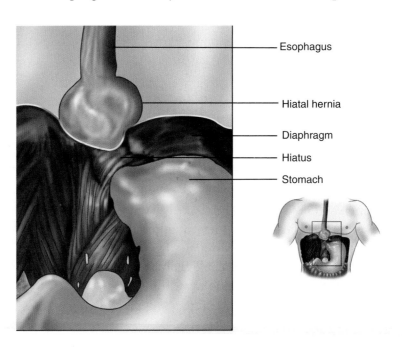

Esophagus

Hiatal hernia

Diaphragm

Hiatus

Stomach

What causes it and why

Table 12-13 shows the causes of hiatal hernias and why these causes occur.

Table 12-13

Causes	Why
Malformation	Larger-than-normal esophageal hiatus that allows a portion of the stomach to enter the thorax
Muscle weakness of the esophageal hiatus	The weakening of this muscle allows a portion of the stomach to move into the thorax
Esophageal shortening	Caused by scarring of the tissue from gastric acids
Obesity	Causes increased pressure variations between thoracic and abdominal cavities, leading to stomach protrusion into the diaphragm

Source: Created by author from References #7 and #8.

Signs and symptoms and why

Small hiatal hernias are usually asymptomatic (without symptoms). Signs and symptoms are usually related to reflux. Table 12-14 shows the signs and symptoms and rationales associated with hiatal hernias.

Table 12-14

Signs and symptoms	Why
Feeling of fullness, smothering, or suffocation after meals	Occurs more with paraesophageal hiatal hernia because part of the stomach is in the thorax. Eating distends the stomach and takes up more room, leading to a decreased ability of the lungs to expand
Anemia	Bleeding of the lining of the hernia may occur with both types of hernias, decreasing the red blood cell count

Source: Created by author from References #5 and #6.

Quickie tests and treatments

Tests for hiatal hernias include:

- Fluoroscopy.

- X-ray studies.

The tests may reveal a hiatal hernia. During the tests, the abdomen may need to be pressed to obtain a definitive diagnosis.

Treatment includes dietary and medical management similar to that for GERD. Remind the client to SIT UP after eating to keep the stomach down.

Surgical repair may be needed if symptoms persist after instituting dietary and medical management:

- Surgery is more common for large paraesophageal hernias.

- The most common technique is the laparoscopic Nissen fundoplication (LNF).

What can harm my client?

- Strangulation (pinching of the hernia, causing it to loose blood supply) can develop. Strangulation leads to a rapid onset of excruciating pain, difficulty swallowing, and radiation of pain into the chest unrelieved by antacids. Immediate surgery is needed.

- Chronic reflux of GERD can lead to esophagitis and esophageal ulceration.

If I were your teacher, I would test you on . . .

- Definition and types of hiatal hernias.

- Causes of hiatal hernia and rationales.

- Signs and symptoms of hiatal hernias and rationales.

- Signs and symptoms and management of hernia strangulation.

- Client education for symptom management.[7]

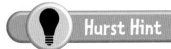

Clients should not take NSAIDs and prednisone at the same time due to ↑ risk of GI irritation.

✚ Peptic ulcer disease (PUD)

What is it?

Peptic ulcer disease (PUD) is an erosion of the lining of the stomach, pylorus, duodenum, or esophagus caused by exposure to hydrochloric acid, pepsin, and *Helicobacter pylori*. *H. pylori* causes damage to the mucosa of the GI tract. Ulcers are named according to the area where they occur. Duodenal ulcers are more common than gastric ulcers. PUD is more common in the elderly and Caucasians. When you hear the term PUD, this is usually referring to either a stomach or duodenal ulcer (Figure 12-4).

▶ Figure 12-4. Peptic ulcers. (From Saladin K. *Anatomy and Physiology: The Unity of Form and Function*. 4th ed. New York: McGraw-Hill; 2007.)

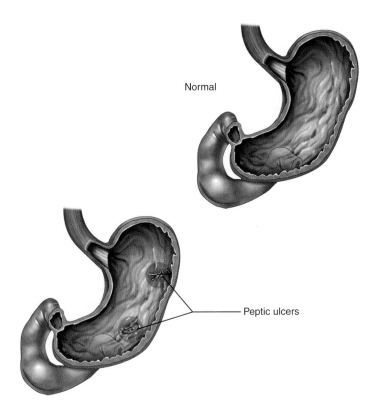

Stress ulcers can be caused by severe illness and trauma (any kind of stress can cause hypersecretion of acid). Many clients in intensive care units are treated to prevent the development of these ulcers.

What causes it and why

Table 12-15 shows the causes of PUD and why these causes occur.

Table 12-15

Causes	Why
Infection (*H. pylori* accounts for 90% of duodenal and 80% of gastric ulcers)	*H. pylori* produces substances that damage the gastric mucosa, leading to irritation and inflammation
Medications: • Aspirin • Nonsteroidal antiinflammatory drugs (NSAIDs) • Theophylline • Caffeine • Prednisone	Aspirin and NSAIDs irritate the lining of the stomach and duodenum and expose it to acid and digestive enzymes, which can injure the epithelium and lead to ulcer formation Theophylline and caffeine stimulate acid production, which can damage the lining of the GI tract and lead to ulceration Prednisone also contributes to gastric irritation just like NSAIDs

(Continued)

Table 12-15. (*Continued*)

Causes	Why
Smoking	Decreases gastric blood flow and delays ulcer healing; nicotine causes vasoconstriction
Stress	Increases acid production that can lead to erosions and ulcerations

Source: Created by author from References #7 to #9.

Signs and symptoms and why

Gastric and duodenal ulcers have differentiating features.

- Gastric ulcers: common in women in labor; clients are malnourished in appearance; pain occurs $1/2$ to 1 hour after meals; food doesn't help but vomiting does; clients tend to vomit blood (hematemesis).

- Duodenal ulcers: common in executive type personalities (type A); clients are well nourished in appearance; pain occurs at night and 2 to 3 hours after meals; food helps; blood appears in stool (melena). Duodenal ulcers are the most common to rupture.

Table 12-16 designates which symptoms go with each type of ulcer. If there is no designation, then the symptom is applicable to both types of ulcer.

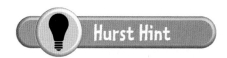

Hurst Hint

Gastric—eating leads to pain.
Duodenal—eating lessens pain.

Table 12-16

Signs and symptoms	Why
Dyspepsia (indigestion) described as gnawing or burning in the left epigastric or upper abdominal area. May be described as sharp, burning, gnawing. Some clients say they feel hungry	Stomach acid and digestive juices erode the lining of the stomach Gastric: pain mainly in the left epigastric area Duodenal: pain mainly in the right epigastric area
Nausea, vomiting after eating, belching, and bloating	GI tract is inflamed. These are other dyspeptic symptoms Ulcers can affect pyloric sphincter which could delay gastric emptying
Weight loss	Gastric ulcers: chronic nausea and vomiting can cause weight loss
Pain 1 to 2 hours after eating	Gastric ulcers: eating promotes motility of stomach and decreases acids and digestive enzymes on eroded areas After eating, an increase in acids and enzymes and a swelling of tissue leading to the small intestine make food passage difficult
Burning or cramping pain in right epigastric or upper abdominal area	Duodenal ulcers: caused by high acid concentrations
Pain 2 to 4 hours after meals or during the night	Duodenal ulcers: eating buffers stomach acids for first 2 hours. Pain returns when stomach is empty
Weight gain	Duodenal ulcers: increased food consumption decreases burning and cramping
Relief from food, milk, antacids	Duodenal ulcers: food, milk, and antacids buffer acids produced in the stomach

Source: Created by author from References #7 to #9.

Quickie tests and treatments

Tests for PUD include:

- Urea breath test or (serum) to detect *H. pylori*. Carbon dioxide excreted in client's breath is measured before and after client drinks carbon-enriched urea solution.

- Serum IgG antibody screening to detect *H. pylori*. Blood test identifies antibodies to *H. pylori*.

- Upper GI endoscopy with tissue biopsy and cytology for microscopic examination. Pyloritek is a biopsy urea test used to detect *H. pylori* per upper GI.

- Upper GI (barium swallow) to visualize changes in GI tract structure and function. (peptic ulcers).

- Esophagogastroduodenoscopy (EGD) to confirm presence of ulcers. Flexible tube (endoscopy) is inserted through the mouth and into the stomach and duodenum. A tissue sample is taken to test for *H. pylori* and gastric cancer.

- Serial stool specimens (stool for occult blood × 3) to detect occult (hidden) blood.

- Gastric secretory studies (gastric acid secretion test and serum gastric level test). These will be elevated in some syndromes such as Zollinger–Ellison syndrome (a condition associated with high levels of gastric acid).

- Complete blood count to detect low hemoglobin level and hematocrit from bleeding.

Treatments:

- Treatment itself decreases pain as mucosa starts to heal.

- A bland diet with no spicy or high-acid foods, which could cause irritation.

- Lifestyle changes includes avoiding irritants such as caffeine, tea, cola, alcohol, and smoking because these substances irritate the lining of the stomach or cause increased release of gastric acid. Coffee stimulates gastrin release and irritates the stomach.

- Meditation.

- Herbs and vitamins to increases healing.

- No bedtime snacks because it increases gastric secretions.

- No NSAIDs or salicylates (such as aspirin). Misoprostol (Cytotec) may be given to reduce the incidence of NSAID-induced ulcers.

- Decrease GI bleeding if applicable (may require surgery to do so).

Drug therapy includes:

- Proton-pump inhibitors—such as omeprazole (Prilosec), lansoprazole (Prevacid), esomeprazole (Nexium), and pantoprazole (Protonix)—to inhibit gastric acid formation.

- H_2-receptor blockers—such as nizatidine (Axid), ranitidine (Zantac), and famotidine (Pepcid)—to inhibit gastric acid secretion.

- Antacids—such as aluminum magnesium combinations (Mylanta, Maalox)—to neutralize existing gastric acid.

- Mucosal barrier fortifiers—such as sucralfate (Carafate) to protect the mucosal barrier.

Infection with *Helicobacter pylori* requires a 2-week course with three drugs. The most common combinations are bismuth subsalicylate (Pepto-Bismol) or a proton-pump inhibitor and metronidazole (Flagyl) and tetracycline (Achromycin) or clarithromycin (Biaxin) and amoxicillin (Amoxil).

What can harm my client?

Bleeding (hemorrhage) may appear as hematemesis (vomiting blood) or melena (blood in stool) and may be treated with:

- Endoscopy to achieve blood-clot formation (cauterizing the vessel, injection of diluted epinephrine, laser therapy, or clipping of bleeding vessel).
- H$_2$-receptor blockers or proton pump inhibitors to help heal the ulcer (for mild bleeding).
- Intravenous (IV) fluids and NPO (nothing by mouth) to allow healing.
- Saline lavage (instilling of saline through an NG tube with repeated withdrawal and insertion until the returns are light pink to clear).
- Surgery (for severe bleeding).

Perforation (ulcers penetrating the wall of the GI tract) causes sudden, excruciating pain in shoulders that becomes more intense with position change or deep breathing, rebound tenderness (pain after the abdomen is pressed and released suddenly; means peritoneal inflammation), and fever. Treatment includes:

- Immediate replacement of fluids and electrolytes via IV route.
- Nasogastric suctioning (use of a tube inserted through the nose into the stomach and connected to low intermittent suction) to remove gastric contents and prevent further spillage.
- Suction turned too high will increase bleeding.
- Emergency surgery and IV antibiotics.

Penetration (ulcer penetrates the stomach or duodenum and continues into adjacent organs), causes continuous pain at the involved site and is treated with:

- Drug therapy.
- Surgery (if drug therapy fails).

Obstruction caused by edema (swelling) or scarring of tissue around an ulcer can decrease the passageway and cause a feeling of fullness, vomiting, regurgitation, and a loss of appetite. Treatment includes:

- Adequate ulcer treatment.
- Nasogastric suctioning (use of a tube inserted through the nose into the stomach and connected to low intermittent suction) until edema subsides.

If I were your teacher, I would test you on . . .

- Definition of PUD.
- Differentiation of 2 types PUD.
- Causes of PUD and rationales.

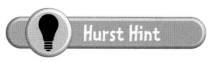

Hurst Hint

Barium studies should not be used if a perforation (tear in the lining) is suspected. Generally, abdominal x-rays are performed to check for free air (a sign of perforation) before these studies.

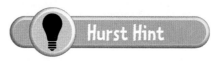

Hurst Hint

Calcium carbonate (Tums) causes rebound acid secretion by triggering gastrin release, and thus is not recommended for ulcer disease.

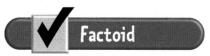

Factoid

Flavored antacids should be avoided because the flavoring increases the emptying time of the stomach.

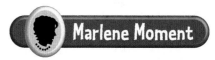

Marlene Moment

You may not have had an ulcer before you started nursing school, but you may get one before it's over!

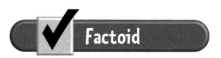

Factoid

As many as 50% of upper GI bleeds result from peptic ulcers.

- Signs and symptoms of PUD and rationales.
- The four types of drugs for stomach disorders.
- Triple-therapy medication options for treating *H. pylori*.
- Differentiating gastritis, gastric ulcer, and duodenal ulcer.
- Complications of PUD.

✚ Achalasia

What is it?

Achalasia is ineffective or absent peristalsis of the distal esophagus that affects movement of food into the stomach. In achalasia, the lower esophageal sphincter (LES) fails to relax or open with swallowing, causing a backup of food material, and the lower esophagus is narrowed above the stomach, leading to a gradual dilation of the esophagus in the upper chest.

What causes it and why

The underlying cause of achalasia is unknown. Table 12-17 shows the current theory on what causes achalasia and why this cause occurs.

Table 12-17

Cause	Why
Denervation of muscle layers of the esophagus	Immune (viral or autoimmune) damage occurs to nerves

Source: Created by author from References #6 to #8.

Signs and symptoms and why

Table 12-18 shows the signs and symptoms of achalasia and associated rationales.

Table 12-18

Signs and symptoms	Why
Difficulty swallowing solids and liquids (main symptom)	Decreased esophageal contractions and tightening of LES
Feeling of food sticking in the lower esophagus	Tightening of LES makes it difficult for food to pass into the stomach
Chest pain	Common when swallowing because of accumulation of food in esophagus
Weight loss	Inability to maintain adequate nutritional intake because of difficulty passing nutrients
Regurgitation of undigested food	Food collects in enlarged esophagus, and as the passage of food becomes more difficult regurgitation can occur
Contents are not acidic because food has not entered the stomach
Typically occurs during sleep
Can lead to aspiration of food into lungs
Halitosis (foul mouth odor)	Regurgitation of undigested food into the throat

Source: Created by author from References #6 to #8.

Hurst Hint

Define Time—Achalasia is a disorder of the esophagus where the rhythmic contractions are significantly decreased and the lower esophageal sphincter fails to relax as it normally does.

Quickie tests and treatments

Tests for achalasia include:

- Barium swallow (x-rays taken after drinking barium) to show an enlarged esophagus that narrows as it reaches the LES and decreased peristalsis.
- Esophagoscopy to visualize enlarged esophagus that is not due to obstruction.
- Biopsy (sample of tissue removed) to rule out cancer.
- Esophageal manometry to measure the pressure of esophageal wave motility. (Achalasia results in increased LES pressure with lack of sphincter relaxation during swallowing.)

Treatment for achalasia includes:

- Having client eat slowly and chew food completely to aid passage through a narrowed LES.
- Having client drink fluids with meals to help prevent a feeling of food sticking to the throat.
- Explaining that warm food and liquids may be swallowed easier than cold ones.
- Elevating the head of the bed 6 to 12 inches to decrease reflux at night.
- Using medications such as nitrates, such as nitroglycerin; or calcium-channel blockers, such as nifedipine (Procardia); to help to relax the sphincter and make food passage easier.
- Using balloon dilation of the narrowed esophagus.
- Using a botulinum toxin (Botox) injection instead of balloon dilation; Botox is injected into the lower esophageal sphincter muscle to provide symptom relief.
- Using surgery (esophagomyotomy), cutting LES muscle fibers to decrease obstruction, if other treatments are unsuccessful.

What can harm my client?

- Weight loss because of an inability to effectively swallow food and liquid.
- Malnutrition from inadequate nutritional intake.
- Esophageal rupture during balloon dilation, which is rare and requires surgical repair.
- Aspiration.

If I were your teacher, I would test you on . . .

- Definition of achalasia.
- Causes of achalasia and rationales.
- Signs and symptoms of achalasia and rationales.
- Education on ways to increase nutritional intake.
- Client preparation for barium swallow[8] (nothing to eat after midnight before the test, removal of jewelry and metal before the test, x-rays taken in various positions after client drinks barium).

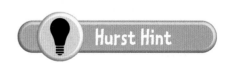

Hurst Hint

Not only will eating before the test cause problems but clients should not smoke before the test either, because this increases gastric secretions and gastric motility.

✚ Malabsorption disorders

What are they?

Malabsorption disorders are disorders in which nutrients are not digested or absorbed properly.

What causes them and why

Table 12-19 shows the causes of malabsorption disorders and why these causes occur.

Table 12-19

Causes	Why
Bile salt deficiencies	If the body is not producing enough bile salts, fats and fat-soluble vitamins are not absorbed adequately
Lactase deficiency (can be genetic or be caused by bacterial overgrowth or viral hepatitis)	Without enough lactase, lactose cannot be broken down for use by the body
Pancreatic enzyme deficiency (can be caused by destruction or obstruction of the pancreas)	Pancreatic enzymes are needed for proper absorption of B_{12}
Infections (viral, bacteria, or parasitic)	Infection injures the intestinal lining and leads to decreased absorption of nutrients
Gastric surgery	Removal of a section of the stomach (the most common cause of malabsorption) prevents adequate mixing of digestive enzymes and acids with food, decreasing digestion of nutrients
Intestinal surgery	Intestinal surgery leads to a loss of surface area for absorption
Lymphatic system blockage from conditions such as lymphoma (cancer of the lymph system) and Crohn's disease	Blockage of lymph flow can lead to a loss of vitamin B_{12}, folic acid, minerals, and lipids
Decreased blood supply	Inadequate blood supply to the GI system reduces the absorption of nutrients
Crohn's disease	The inflammation of Crohn's disease decreases bile salt absorption and leads to fat malabsorption
Ulcerative colitis	The inflammation of ulcerative colitis decreases bile salt absorption and leads to fat malabsorption
Celiac sprue (genetic intolerance to gluten that causes damage to the lining of the small intestine)	Damage to the lining of the small intestine leads to decreased absorption of iron, protein, vitamin B_{12}, and calcium
Tropical sprue (a disease of unknown cause occurring in people who live in tropical areas)	Tropical sprue may be caused by an infectious agent and leads to decreased absorption of vitamin B_2, prothrombin (substance needed for normal blood clotting), folic acid, vitamin B_{12}, and iron

Source: Created by author using References #4 and #8.

Signs and symptoms and why

Table 12-20 shows the signs and symptoms and rationales associated with malabsorption disorders.

Table 12-20

Signs and symptoms	Why
Weight loss	The body is unable to absorb needed nutrients
Steatorrhea (light-colored, bulky, foul-smelling stool)	Fat is inadequately absorbed and eliminated in waste
Diarrhea, flatulence (gas)	Inadequate absorption of nutrients
Increased bruising	Clotting factors such prothrombin are decreased
Edema (swelling)	Results from decreased protein absorption
Anemia	Results from vitamin B_{12}, folic acid, or iron deficiency

Source: Created by author from References #6 to #8.

Quickie tests and treatments

A thorough client history can identify symptoms associated with malabsorption and the onset of problems.

These laboratory findings may indicate malabsorption disorders:

- Decreased mean corpuscular volume (MCV), mean corpuscular hemoglobin (MCH), and mean corpuscular hemoglobin concentration (MCHC) indicate an iron deficiency.
- Elevated MCV may indicate vitamin B_{12} and folic acid deficiency.
- A low iron level may indicate protein malabsorption.
- Low cholesterol levels may result from decreased fat digestion.
- A low calcium level may indicate decreased vitamin D absorption.
- A serum low albumin level indicates protein loss.
- Low levels of vitamin A and carotene may indicate bile salt deficiency.
- A lactose tolerance test with less than a 20% rise in glucose levels above fasting levels indicates lactose intolerance.

Other tests include:

- Biopsy and microscopic examination of small intestine lining to detect abnormalities that may cause malabsorption.
- Stool sample to assess for undigested food, indicating an inability to break down and absorb nutrients.
- Ultrasonography to detect tumors that might be causing malabsorption.
- Barium enema to detect changes in the mucosal lining and determine the underlying cause of malabsorption. Also for tumor identification.

Treatment of the underlying disease improves signs and symptoms of malabsorption.

Dietary management varies according to underlying problem:

- For lactose intolerance, client should avoid dairy products.
- For celiac disease, the client should maintain a gluten-free diet.
- For gallbladder disease and pancreatic insufficiency, the client should maintain a low-fat diet.

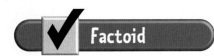

Calcium supplements should be taken to prevent a deficiency of calcium.

- Gastrectomy clients should maintain a high-protein and high-calorie diet and eat small, frequent meals. Should also keep head of bed elevated.
- Clients should take nutritional supplements for their specific deficiencies.
- Clients with tropical sprue or other disorders caused by infection should take prescribed antibiotics.
- Clients with decreased gastric motility should take antidiarrheal agents.

What can harm my client?

Malabsorption of nutrients can lead to long-term complications and death because the body cannot function properly.

If I were your teacher, I would test you on . . .

- Definition of malabsorption disorders.
- Causes of malabsorption disorders and rationales.
- Signs and symptoms of malabsorption disorders and rationales.
- Laboratory findings associated with common malabsorption problems.
- Dietary education of clients with malabsorption syndrome.

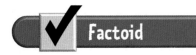

Adenomas are considered precancerous polyps. Generally, the larger the polyp, the greater the chance it is precancerous.

✚ Polyps

What are they?

Polyps are small growths along the lining of the intestinal tract. They are classified according to tissue type (adenomas, hyperplastic, or hamartomatous) and appearance (sessile or pedunculated).

What causes them and why

Most polyps result from hereditary conditions. Table 12-21 shows the causes of polyps and why those causes occur.

Table 12-21

Causes	Why
Familial polyposis	During childhood, polyps develop in the large intestine and rectum and can lead to colorectal cancer
Gardner's syndrome (a rare, inherited disorder characterized by multiple growths—polyps—in the colon)	In addition to precancerous polyps, nonmalignant tumors develop on various parts of the body
Peutz–Jeghers syndrome (characterized by the development of growths called hamartomatous polyps in the gastrointestinal tract—particularly the stomach and intestines)	In utero (before birth), polyps develop in the stomach, small intestine, large intestine or rectum. Typically, they are noncancerous

Source: Created by author from References #5, #8, and #9.

It seems that certain groups of people are more prone to polyps. Clients over age 50, those with a positive family history, those who eat a high fat/low calcium diet, smokers, and those who exercise little/none seem to have a higher frequency of polyps.

Signs and symptoms and why

Most polyps are asymptomatic (without symptoms). Table 12-22 shows the signs and symptoms and rationales associated with polyps.

Table 12-22

Signs and symptoms	Why
Bleeding	Polyp becomes irritated from the passage of intestinal contents, and blood may appear in stool
Abdominal pain and cramping	Large polyps may obstruct the flow of GI contents, causing pain and cramping
Diarrhea or any change in bowel habits	Some polyps can excrete water and salts that lead to excessive watery stools. Some clients may have constipation, increased frequency of bowel movements, or a change in appearance of stool

Source: Created by author from References #5, #8, and #9.

Quickie tests and treatments

Tests for polyps include:

- Digital examination (inserting a gloved finger into the rectum and palpating) to locate a rectal polyp.
- Flexible sigmoidoscopy (examining the lower large intestine through a flexible tube) to detect a polyp.
- Colonoscopy (examining the entire large intestine through a flexible tube) to determine the number of polyps and allow biopsy of one or more.
- Fecal occult blood (blood could be an indicator of cancer).
- Barium may be done to visualize the polyp.

Treatments for polyps include:

- Removal of polyps (polypectomy) because of the risk they will become cancerous. Usually done during colonoscopy. If removal is not possible with colonoscopy, abdominal surgery is performed.
- Removal of a section of the intestine because cancerous polyps may have spread to the area. If familial polyposis is present, the entire large intestine and rectum may be removed.
- Increase calcium intake (studies seem to show calcium can decrease reoccurrence).
- NSAIDs/ASA (seems to decrease reccurrence; can be very irritating to GI tract).
- Exercise, stop smoking, decrease alcohol, eat a low-fat/high-fiber diet.
- Routine colorectal screenings.

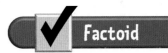

Factoid

Clients needing colonoscopy will receive a liquid substance to drink prior to the test in order to evacuate the bowel of stool contents. This allows for easy visualization of the inside of the colon.

What can harm my client?

- Excessive rectal bleeding.
- Colorectal cancer, the most feared outcome of polyps, especially if tissue type is adenoma.

If I were your teacher, I would test you on . . .

- Definition of polyps.
- Causes of polyps and rationales.
- Signs and symptoms of polyps and rationales.
- Prevention.
- Nursing care for a client after a polypectomy (monitoring for bleeding, fever, and abdominal distention; pain assessment and intervention; signs and symptoms of infection).

✛ Hemorrhoids

What are they?

Hemorrhoids (Fig. 12-5) are varicose (twisted)/distended veins of the anal canal. External hemorrhoids are located below the anorectal junction; internal hemorrhoids form above this junction.

▶ Figure 12-5. Hemorrhoids.

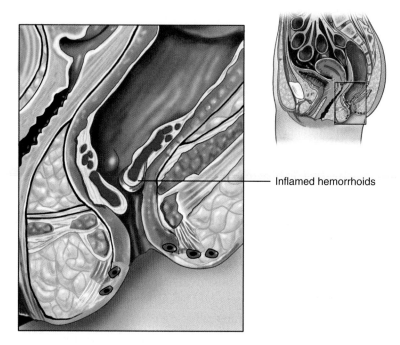

Inflamed hemorrhoids

What causes them and why

Table 12-23 shows the causes of hemorrhoids and why those causes occur.

Table 12-23

Causes	Why
Chronic constipation	Increased intra-abdominal pressure increases pressure in the veins when straining during bowel movements
Pregnancy	Increased circulating fluid volume and increased constipation put more pressure on the veins of the anal canal
Obesity	Can cause increased pressure in the veins of the anorectal area and lead to hemorrhoid development
Heavy lifting, straining, standing for long periods of time	Pressure increases in the venous system with continued heavy lifting or straining

Source: Created by author from References #5 and #6.

Signs and symptoms and why

Table 12-24 shows the signs and symptoms and rationales associated with hemorrhoids.

Table 12-24

Signs and symptoms	Why
Bleeding, usually bright red	Stool passing through the rectum and anus rub the hemorrhoids, causing them to bleed
Itching	Can occur if adequate cleaning of the anal area cannot be performed because of hemorrhoid protrusion
Pain	Results from swelling and irritation of the hemorrhoid

Source: Created by author from References #5 and #6.

Quickie tests and treatments

Tests for hemorrhoids include:

- Digital examination (inserting a gloved finger into the rectum and palpating) to locate hemorrhoids.
- Anoscopy and flexible sigmoidoscopy (examining structures of the rectum and sigmoid colon through a flexible tube) to detect hemorrhoids.

Treatment for hemorrhoids include:

- Sitz bath to relieve symptoms. (Sitz bath is a device that looks like a small basin and is placed between the lids of the toilet. A bag of warm water runs from a bag through a small tube into the basin. The warm water gently sprays and soaks the hemorrhoids.) Some clients prefer to sit in a warm bathtub.
- Nonprescription creams and ointments, such as dibucaine (Nupercainal), anusol to reduce swelling and pain associated with hemorrhoids.

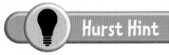

- Compress pads of witch hazel (Tucks) to control symptoms.
- Cleaning anal area by blotting, not wiping, with a moistened wipe. (Sometimes baby wipes are used to reduce abrasion caused by toilet paper.)
- High-fiber diet and increased fluids to manage constipation (client needs to decrease straining with bowel movements). Nuts, coffee, and spicy foods can further irritate hemorrhoids and should be avoided.
- Stool softeners, such as docusate, to help prevent straining during defecation.
- Avoiding long periods of sitting, which can put more pressure on already irritated hemorrhoids.
- Sclerotherapy (injection of material to remove hemorrhoids) to treat bleeding hemorrhoids.
- Band ligation (tying off hemorrhoids with rubber bands) if sclerotherapy is not successful or the hemorrhoids are internal.
- Surgery (hemorrhoidectomy) for hemorrhoids that do not respond to less invasive treatments.

What can harm my client?

- Bleeding after a bowel movement can cause great anxiety. A small amount of blood in the toilet can appear to be a major blood loss. Rarely is the blood loss excessive enough to lead to problems.
- Disruption of daily activities because of pain and swelling. Inability to ride or sit for prolonged periods can affect work and family environment.
- Excessive straining during bowel movements and heavy lifting can exacerbate the symptoms.

If I were your teacher, I would test you on . . .

- Definition of hemorrhoids.
- Causes of hemorrhoids and rationales.
- Signs and symptoms of hemorrhoids and rationales.
- Client education for management (diet, fluids, medications).[7]
- Purpose and use of sitz bath.
- Postoperative care after hemorrhoidectomy.

+ Dumping syndrome

What is it?

Early dumping syndrome is the rapid movement of food from the stomach into the jejunum 30 minutes after a meal.

Late dumping syndrome is the release of an increased amount of insulin, causing hypoglycemia.

What causes it and why

Table 12-25 shows the causes of dumping syndrome and why these causes occur.

Table 12-25

Causes	Why
Gastric surgery: • Gastrectomy (removal of some or all of the stomach). • Gastric bypass surgery (creation of a smaller stomach pouch to decrease intake of food in obese clients) • Gastroenterostomy, gastrojejunostomy (direct connection of stomach to small intestine, bypassing the pylorus) • Fundoplication (surgery to reduce reflux of gastric contents into the esophagus) • Vagotomy (cutting of nerves to stomach to decrease acid production)	These surgeries alter mucosal function and decrease acid, enzyme, and hormone secretions, leading to accelerated gastric emptying. Also, the stomach is structurally altered with surgery (may not have the capacity it once did)
Zollinger–Ellison syndrome (rare disorder involving peptic ulcer disease and gastrin-secreting tumors in the pancreas)	Can lead to damage of the pylorus and changes in the production and release of enzymes, resulting in dumping syndrome

Source: Created by author from References #7 and #8.

Signs and symptoms and why

Table 12-26 shows the signs and symptoms and rationales associated with dumping syndrome.

Table 12-26

Signs and symptoms	Why
Systemic (early dumping syndrome): • Sweating (diaphoresis) • Extreme fatigue and strong desire to lie down • Palpitations • Light-headedness and syncope • Flushing	Early dumping syndrome: these systemic signs and symptoms occur because with rapid gastric emptying, fluid shifts from the intravascular area into the intestinal lumen
Abdominal: • Nausea and vomiting • Abdominal cramping • Bloating and fullness • Diarrhea • Stomach growling (borborygmi)	Early dumping syndrome: abdominal signs and symptoms occur because of distension of the small intestine and increased contractility
Systemic (late dumping syndrome): • Tremors • Inability to concentrate • Sweating (diaphoresis) • Decreased level of consciousness • Hunger • Hypotension (low blood pressure) • Increased heart rate	Late dumping syndrome: these systemic signs and symptoms occur because of a low glucose leve brought on by a pronounced release of insulin

Source: Created by author from References #7 and #8.

Quickie tests and treatments

Use the client history to identify past surgeries that could be causing the dumping and to determine the onset and duration of symptoms. If client has a history of gastric surgery (which they usually do), no further tests are needed as the cause is already known. Dietary management for dumping syndrome:

- Eating 6 small, frequent meals daily.
- Restricting fluid intake during and at least ¹/₂ hour after meals (fluids should be taken inbetween meals).
- Decreasing carbohydrate intake and increasing fat and protein intake (carbs tend to move through the GI tract fast).
- Lying flat (preferably on left side to keep food in stomach longer) after meals to delay gastric emptying and increase venous return.
- Using dietary fiber supplements to delay glucose absorption.

Medical and surgical therapy:

- Remember, the major thing we want to do is DELAY GASTRIC EMPTYING.
- Anticholingeric drugs (dry up secretions in stomach; gastric contents will become less moist and therefore empty more slowly out of stomach).
- Antisecretory agents to delay gastric emptying and inhibit insulin and hormone release.
- Surgery to repair or reconstruct the underlying problem.

What can harm my client?

- Malnutrition and marked weight loss in severe cases.
- Marked anxiety and fear of food (sitophobia).
- Social isolation because of fear of signs and symptoms while in public.

If I were your teacher, I would test you on . . .

- Definition of dumping syndrome.
- Causes of dumping syndrome and rationales.
- Signs and symptoms of dumping syndrome and rationales.
- Client education.
- Medications.

✚ Hernia

What is it?

Hernias are an abnormal protrusion of a loop of bowel through the thin muscular wall of the abdomen.

Hernias can be classified as:

- Reducible hernias: can be placed back into the abdominal cavity with gentle pressure.

- Irreducible (incarcerated) hernias: cannot be placed back into the abdominal cavity.
- Strangulated hernia: blood supply cut off by pressure from the muscle around the hernia.

Table 12-27 describes the four types of hernias.

Table 12-27

Hernia type	Description
Inguinal (Fig. 12-6)	• Protrusion of the spermatic cord (male) or round ligament (female) through the inguinal canal of the abdominal wall • Can be direct (passes through weakness in the wall) or indirect (pushes into the inguinal canal) • Most common type of hernia
Femoral (Fig. 12-7)	• Occurs in the upper part of thigh region, below the groin • More common in females • Femoral canal (area where the femoral artery, vein, and nerve leave the abdominal cavity) enlarges and allows a portion of the intestines to enter
Umbilical (Fig. 12-8)	• Orifice of the umbilicus does not close, allowing protrusion • Most common in infants • Usually closes by age 2 • Can recur later in life because of weakness of the wall at this site
Incisional (ventral)	• Weakness in the abdominal wall, secondary to abdominal surgery

Source: Created by author from References #5, #8, and #9.

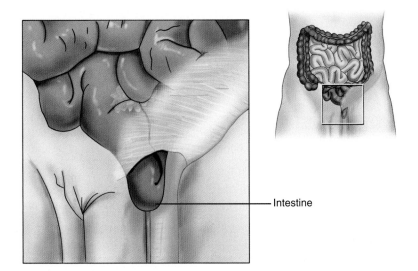

◄ Figure 12-6. Inguinal hernia. The intestine can pass into the scrotal area or into the groin.

Intestine

▶ Figure 12-7. Femoral hernia. The herniated intestine can cause a visible bulge.

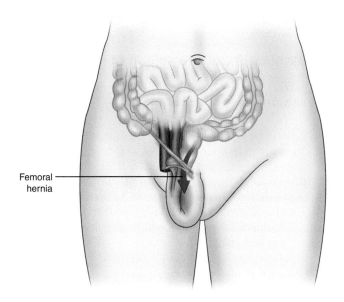

Femoral hernia

▶Figure 12-8. Umbilical hernia.

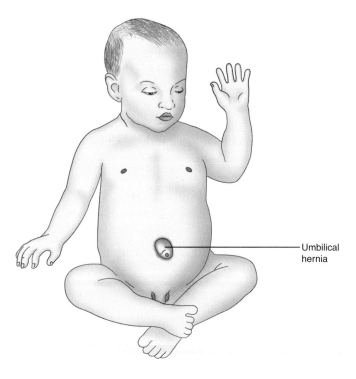

Umbilical hernia

What causes it and why

Table 12-28 shows the causes of hernias and why these causes occur.

Table 12-28

Causes	Why
Congenital	Weakness or incomplete closure of abdominal wall at birth
Increased abdominal pressure	May lead to bulging of contents into the weaker areas of the abdomen
	Conditions that increase this risk are obesity, straining, heavy lifting, prolonged coughing, chronic lung problems, fluid accumulation in the abdomen, and pregnancy
Abdominal surgery	Abdominal surgery leads to weakness in the affected portion of the abdominal wall, which can lead to hernia formation

Source: Created by author from References #5, #8, and #9.

Signs and symptoms and why

Table 12-29 shows the signs and symptoms and rationales associated with hernias.

Table 12-29

Signs and symptoms	Why
Bulging in abdominal cavity	Occurs when intestine and intestinal contents protrude into weakened area of the abdominal wall
	Bulging is worse when standing or lifting, but usually is reduced when lying down
Pain	May precede discovery of bulge. Pain due to pressure created by protrusion

Source: Created by author from References #5, #8, and #9.

Quickie tests and treatments

Use the client history to determine events that may have led to hernia development (weight lifting, bronchitis with extreme coughing, or smoking history leading to chronic coughing) and to obtain a past history of hernias.

A physical examination can help determine the location and size of the hernia and the need for immediate surgery.

If the hernia is strangulated, a complete blood count may be ordered to determine the presence of infection and to prepare for surgical correction.

Client education for hernias includes:

- Explaining why and how to avoid increased abdominal pressure by avoiding lifting any heavy objects, stopping smoking, preventing constipation, and using deep-breathing exercises to decrease chronic cough.

- Explaining the signs and symptoms of strangulation.

- Explaining that the client should use a truss (elastic belt to hold abdominal contents and prevent herniation), which should be applied before getting out of bed.

Surgical interventions include:

- Minimally invasive inguinal hernia repair (MIIHR) or herniorrhaphy, which involves placing a synthetic mesh inside the abdominal wall. A laparoscope (fiber-optic tube to view the herniation) is used, when possible.

- Hernioplasty, which involves placing a mesh patch on the weakened outside wall.

- Traditional surgery, which involves placing the contents of the hernia back into the abdomen and closing the opening.

What can harm my client?

- Incarceration (inability of the contents to return to the abdominal cavity) and strangulation (blood supply cut off to intestines) with potential bowel obstruction and necrosis.

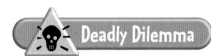

New onset of pain and tenderness at the bulge may signal strangulation (cutting off of blood supply to intestines) and is a surgical emergency.

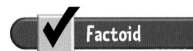

Incarcerated hernias should be reduced before applying a truss.

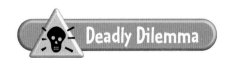

Never forcibly reduce a hernia! It could cause an intestinal rupture.

- Gangrene (death of the intestinal wall) can develop quickly and lead to infection and peritonitis (inflammation of the lining of the abdominal cavity), which if not treated, will result in death!

If I were your teacher, I would test you on . . .

- Definition of hernia.
- Causes of hernias and rationales.
- Signs and symptoms of hernias and rationales.
- Anatomy of inguinal and femoral hernias.[5]
- Client education regarding hernia management.
- Differentiation of signs and symptoms of typical hernia and one that is incarcerated or strangulated.

✚ Intestinal obstruction

What is it?

An intestinal obstruction, which may be mechanical or nonmechanical, is a blockage of the flow of intestinal contents. If not treated, the lining swells with contents and can rupture. A mechanical obstruction is caused by adhesions (bands of fibrous tissue that can connect intestines to intestines, organs, or the abdominal wall), twisting of the intestines, or strangulated hernias creating pressure in the abdominal cavity. A nonmechanical obstruction (paralytic ileus) is caused by impaired peristalsis from abdominal surgery, trauma, and mesenteric ischemia. There is no physical obstruction, just decreased or absent peristalsis.

What causes it and why

Table 12-30 shows the causes of intestinal obstructions and why these causes occur.

Table 12-30

Causes	Why
Birth defects: • Volvulus (twisting of the intestines) • Intussusception (portion of the intestines slides over another area of the intestines)	Mechanical obstruction: birth defects of the GI system can lead to an inability to move contents through the GI tract
Obstruction of small intestine	Mechanical obstruction: may occur from scarring of tissue as a result of ulcers and abdominal surgery Adhesions (tissue of one area sticks to another area) can lead to a collapse of a portion of the intestines
Obstruction of large intestine	Mechanical obstruction: can result from stool impaction, inflammatory bowel disease (IBD), diverticulitis (from scar tissue or adhesions)
Cancer	Mechanical obstruction: the growth of malignant cells can block the intestinal tract
Worms	Mechanical obstruction: a large number of parasitic worms in the GI tract can form an obstruction
Surgery	Nonmechanical obstruction: handling of the intestines leads to temporary loss of function

(Continued)

Table 12-30. (*Continued*)

Causes	Why
Electrolyte imbalance	Nonmechanical obstruction: hypokalemia can increase the risk of paralytic ileus
Peritonitis (inflammation of the abdominal wall)	Nonmechanical obstruction: irritation from contents leaking into abdominal cavity can lead to inflammation with decreased or absent peristalsis
Decreased blood flow to the bowel	Nonmechanical obstruction: can lead to ischemia and decreased or absent peristalsis

Source: Created by author from References #6 and #9.

Signs and symptoms and why

Table 12-31 shows the signs and symptoms and rationales associated with intestinal obstruction.

Table 12-31

Signs and symptoms	Why
Abdominal cramping and pain	Passageway through the GI system can be partially or completely blocked. Pain may be intermittent with periods of relief
Abdominal distention with peristaltic waves	Results from an inability of food, gas, or digestive enzymes to pass through the obstruction. Peristaltic wave is when you can actually see the abdomen moving up and down. This is the intestine trying to move bowel contents past the obstruction
Bowel changes	Obstipation (absence of stool) occurs with complete blockage because contents cannot pass through the GI system Diarrhea (ribbon-like stools) may occur with a partial obstruction because liquids can pass but solid contents cannot
Bowel sound changes	Bowel sounds are high-pitched proximal to the obstruction (called borborygmi) and absent distal to obstruction; as obstruction worsens, bowel sounds will become absent
Vomiting and anorexia (lack of interest in eating)	Occurs because of accumulation of contents The farther up the GI tract the obstruction is, the quicker vomiting occurs. The further down the GI tract the obstruction is, the more food, gas, and fluids can accumulate before the body begins to rid itself of them
Fluid and electrolyte imbalances	Can occur because of the body's inability to absorb nutrients to maintain balance. Vomiting and diarrhea can also lead to imbalances
Fever	If an obstruction leads to a rupture, infection can quickly develop in the abdominal cavity (bacterial peritonitis). Fever occurs as the body tries to fight the infection and is usually low grade
Hiccups	Seen in all types of obstructions may be due to stimulation of the phrenic nerve

Source: Created by author from References #6 and #9.

Quickie tests and treatment

Tests for intestinal obstruction include:

- Abdominal computed tomography (CT) scan to show the location and cause of the obstruction and air in the abdomen (an indication of rupture).

- Abdominal x-ray (flat and upright x-ray) to show distention above obstruction and free air below the diaphragm, indicating perforation of the intestines.

- Complete blood count (CBC) to detect bleeding (low hemoglobin and hematocrit) and infection (elevated white blood cell count).
- Chemistry studies to assess for fluid imbalances (elevated creatinine and blood urea nitrogen levels) and electrolyte imbalances (decreased sodium, chloride, and potassium levels).
- Endoscopy or barium enema to determine the cause of lower bowel obstruction.
- Arterial blood gases to determine acid base imbalance.

Treatment may include NPO (nothing by mouth) status for the client and nasogastric tube placement (tube inserted into the nose and passed into the stomach) and suctioning to remove materials blocked by the obstruction. Care of a nasogastric tube involves:

1. Confirming proper tube placement with x-rays.
2. Ensuring that the nares are cleaned and monitoring for skin breakdown at tube-insertion site.
3. Ensuring the tube is secured to nares, using tape or foam patch.
4. Checking potency of tube at least every 4 hours (may be flushed with 30 mL of saline if GI contents are thick and plug tube).
5. Monitoring contents being suctioned (documenting color, consistency, and amount).
6. Assessing suction equipment to ensure correct settings (Levin tubes require low intermittent suction, and Salem pump tubes are set on low continuous suction).

Other treatment may include:

- Fluid and electrolyte replacement administered by intravenous (IV) route to replace fluid and electrolytes lost due to vomiting and nasogastric suctioning.
- Pain management including assessment of character, intensity, and location. Analgesics may be withheld until it is known if the client has a perforation or peritonitis.
- Antibiotics if perforation has occurred.
- Antiemetics to prevent further vomiting.
- Exploratory surgery to find and correct mechanical obstruction. Sometimes, obstruction can be removed using barium enemas or passing an endoscope into the lower colon.
- Temporary colostomy, a procedure that brings the intestine through the abdomen with an opening (stoma) made in the abdomen.
- Correction of acid–base imbalance.

What can harm my client?

- Strangulation of an intestinal segment can lead to necrosis, perforation, and peritonitis.
- Severe electrolyte imbalances, especially a potassium imbalance, can lead to arrhythmias (abnormal changes in the heart rate and rhythm).

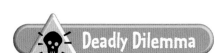

Deadly Dilemma

Barium enemas are not used if perforation of the intestinal wall is suspected. This test can cause further distention and push contents into the abdominal cavity!

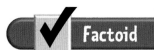

Factoid

Analgesics such as morphine can further slow GI motility and lead to increased nausea and vomiting or gastroparesis.

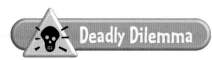

Deadly Dilemma

Changes in pain description from intermittent to constant or an increase in intensity should alert you to the possibility of perforation. Report these changes to the physician immediately!

- Acid-base imbalances: metabolic alkalosis can occur if blockage is high in small intestine (if there is an obstruction in the upper part of the small intestine, then the client will primarily begin to vomit hydrochloric acid from the stomach because the secretions cannot go forward. If the obstruction is lower in the GI tract, then the client will vomit the HCl acid first, then intestinal secretions that are alkalotic. Since the client has lost a lot of base this leaves them in metabolic acidosis).

- Shock and/or death related to perforation.

- Pulmonary complications due to decreased lung expansion related to abdominal bloating and pressure pressing on diaphragm.

If I were your teacher, I would test you on . . .

- Definition and differentiation of types of obstructions.
- Causes of intestinal obstructions and rationales.
- Factors that contribute to the development of obstructions.
- Signs and symptoms of intestinal obstructions and rationales.
- Signs of strangulation or rupture of intestines.
- Bowel sound assessment findings.
- Nursing care for nasogastric tubes.[5]
- Postsurgical management.
- Management of colostomy.

✦ Appendicitis

What is it?

Appendicitis is an acute inflammation of the appendix (Fig. 12-9). The appendix is a little sac on the intestine that can get filled with bowel contents, become inflamed, and possibly rupture. Surgery for appendicitis is one of the most common abdominal surgeries.

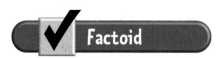

Factoid

The appendix is not an essential organ in the digestive process.

◄ Figure 12-9. Appendicitis.

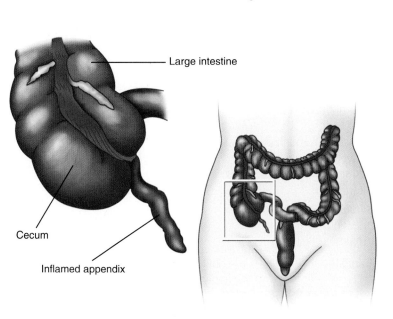

Large intestine

Cecum

Inflamed appendix

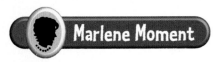

The appendix has no known function in adults, so why do I have to have it? If I'm ever your surgical patient, please make sure they go ahead and take this thing out before I have a problem. Okay?

What causes it and why

Table 12-32 shows the cause of appendicitis and why this cause occurs.

Table 12-32

Cause	Why
Obstruction	When the opening of the appendix becomes obstructed, inflammation and infection can occur. Obstruction can be a result of fecal mass, tumor, stricture, worms, and viral infections

Source: Created by author from References #7 and #9.

Signs and symptoms and why

Table 12-33 shows the signs and symptoms and rationales associated with appendicitis.

Table 12-33

Signs and symptoms	Why
Pain: • Usually around the umbilical area, getting increasingly worse, becoming more constant and severe • In a few hours, pain progresses to an area in the right lower quadrant, known as McBurney's point (1/3 of the distance from the anterior superior iliac spine to the umbilicus), where the base of the appendix typically lies. Remember, the appendix can be in different anatomical locations for different people, resulting in a variation of clinical presentations (i.e., rectal and low back pain for retroperitoneal appendicitis) Rebound tenderness (pain after the abdomen is pressed and released suddenly) occurs at this location • Pain increases with cough or sudden movement, which could be suggestive of peritoneal irritation • Fetal position can help alleviate symptoms, which is a strong clue for appendicitis	Pain results from swelling caused by inflammation. Rupture of appendix can lead to increased pain
Abdominal rigidity	Could be related to abdominal guarding or appendix perforation with peritonitis

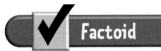

Abdominal guarding is when the client is literally "guarding" the area to prevent further pain. They may hold an arm over it or muscles may be tight because they are so tense.

(Continued)

Table 12-33. (*Continued*)

Signs and symptoms	Why
Nausea and vomiting	May result from the onset of pain or the inflammatory process in the GI tract. Nausea and vomiting are most likely during the onset of umbilical pain
Increased white blood cell (WBC) count and fever	As bacteria lodge in the appendix, inflammation and infection develop. Temp may start as low grade but if it elevates above 101°F, we think peritonitis
Loss of appetite	Caused by pain, nausea, and vomiting

Source: Created by author from References #7 and #9.

Quickie tests and treatments

A client history and physical examination can reveal when symptoms began and if the client has pain at McBurney's point.

Tests for appendicitis may include:

- Complete blood count (CBC) to determine if the white blood cell (WBC) count is greater than 10,000/mL, which indicates an infection.
- Computed tomography (CT) scan to determine if the appendix is inflamed.
- Urinalysis to rule out a urinary tract infection, which can have similar symptoms.

Treatment for appendicitis may include:

- NPO (nothing by mouth) order on admission to acute care facility.
- Intravenous (IV) fluids to prevent dehydration and electrolyte disturbances.
- Opioid analgesics to reduce pain before surgery.
- Immediate surgery for removal of appendix (appendectomy).
- Antibiotics are given after surgery for prophylactic reasons even if the appendix didn't rupture.

What can harm my client?

- Rupture of the appendix, causing a leakage of pus into abdominal cavity (peritonitis). A rupture can occur within 24 to 48 hours of the onset of symptoms, so immediate surgical removal is a priority.

If I were your teacher, I would test you on . . .

- Definition of appendicitis.
- Causes of appendicitis and rationales.
- Signs and symptoms of appendicitis and rationales (focus on onset of pain, location, duration).
- Appropriate comfort measures and client care measures.[5–8]
- Laboratory findings.

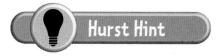

Hurst Hint

Pain that increases with movement and is relieved by flexion of the knees may indicate rupture of the appendix.

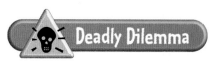

Deadly Dilemma

If rupture of the appendix occurs, mass infection can spread rapidly throughout the body. This is a medical emergency!

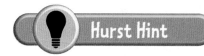

Hurst Hint

Avoid using heat for pain management, because heat will increase blood flow to the appendix and increase inflammation.

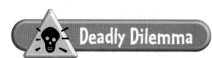

Deadly Dilemma

Do not give laxatives or enemas to a client with appendicitis! This can cause perforation of the appendix! If perforation is suspected, elevate the HOB to keep bowel contents down in one area; client will be going to surgery shortly.

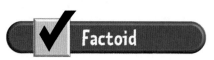

Factoid

Before the advent of modern medicine, death related to appendicitis was usually related to peritonitis. The use of antibiotics and early surgical intervention has really improved the outcomes of people who develop appendicitis. Hooray for modern medicine!!!

- Signs of perforation.
- Preoperative nursing interventions.

✚ Peritonitis

What is it?

Peritonitis is an acute inflammatory disorder of the peritoneum (lining of the abdominal cavity).

What causes it and why

Table 12-34 shows the causes of peritonitis and why these causes occur.

Table 12-34

Causes	Why
Rupture (perforation) of organs. This is the most common cause	Rupture of the appendix, intestines, stomach, or gallbladder allows bacteria to enter the peritoneal cavity
Infection	Inflammation of other organs (pancreas) or other inflammatory processes (pelvic inflammatory disease) can irritate the cavity and lead to peritonitis. Also, fluid accumulation (ascites) from liver disease, and complications of surgery, could lead to infection of the peritoneum
Wound	Penetrating wounds can allow foreign material to enter the abdominal cavity

Source: Created by the author from References #7 to #9.

Signs and symptoms and why

Table 12-35 shows the signs and symptoms and rationales associated with peritonitis.

Table 12-35

Signs and symptoms	Why
Pain: • Generalized pain progressing to more localized pain is common • Rebound tenderness (pain after the abdomen is pressed and released suddenly) is common and occurs as quick movement of peritoneal fluid occurs when pressure is released	From the inflammation of the lining of the peritoneal cavity
Abdominal rigidity aggravated by movement (board-like abdomen); abdomen distention	Caused by widespread inflammation and increased fluid in the abdominal cavity

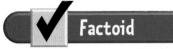

Factoid

People undergoing peritoneal dialysis (procedure used when kidneys are unable to filter waste products of the body) are at risk of having bacteria enter the abdominal cavity through drains used during the procedure.

(Continued)

Table 12-35. (*Continued*)

Signs and symptoms	Why
Decreased peristalsis leading to decreased bowel sounds	Results from absence of normal movement of contents through the GI tract
Increased pulse	Occurs as fluid leaves the GI tract and moves into the peritoneal cavity (hypovolemia)
Decreased urinary output	Kidneys begin to retain fluid because of decreased fluid in the vascular system
Elevated white blood cell (WBC) count and fever (heart rate goes up as fever increases especially in the pediatric population)	Results from bacterial infection development
Nausea and vomiting	Inflammation, infection, and irritation of GI tract. Remember, the peritoneum covers the entire abdominal cavity
Fluid and electrolyte imbalances	Dehydration due to vomiting or leakage of GI contents into the abdominal cavity
Hiccups	Results from irritation to the diaphragm

Source: Created by author from References #7 to #9.

Quickie tests and treatments

A client history and an assessment of the abdomen can reveal the signs and symptoms of peritonitis.

Tests:

- Abdominal x-rays (to identify perforated bowel).

- Fluid biopsy to determine the type of infection and determine best treatment option.

- Complete blood count (CBC) to determine if the white blood cell (WBC) count is elevated which indicates an infection.

- Chemistry profile to determine fluid and electrolyte imbalances.

- Blood cultures to identify invading pathogen.

- ABGs need to be monitored. Remember, abdominal problems can lead to pulmonary complications, which can alter the ABGs.

- Peritoneal lavage to assess for bleeding and presence of infection by Gram stain (RBCs and WBCs will be present in fluid). See Factoid.

Treatments may include:

- NPO order to ensure no further leakage of contents into the peritoneal cavity (applicable only if bowel perforation is the cause).

- Fluid and electrolyte replacement via the IV route to replace the fluids lost in the peritoneum.

- Antibiotics to treat infection.

- Nasogastric tube insertion to decompress stomach and intestine (See "Intestinal obstruction" earlier in the chapter for care of a nasogastric tube).

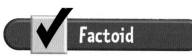
Factoid

Peritoneal lavage or "tap" is a procedure performed for a quick assessment to see if there is abdominal bleeding. Saline is drained through a small opening into the abdomen and then allowed to drain back out. If it is red, you have blood!

- Pain management with IV medications. A patient-controlled analgesia (PCA) pump may be used to administer continuous low doses of analgesics and for the client to initiate bolus doses according to regulated settings.
- Surgical excision, repair, or resection of perforated section or organ and drainage of abscess. If peritonitis is due to an inflammation such as pelvic inflammatory disease or acute pancreatitis, surgery is usually withheld, and the underlying problem is treated. Wound care (site care) may be needed after surgery. Surgery doesn't fix peritonitis. It only fixes the cause!
- Temporary colostomy, a procedure that brings the intestine through the abdomen with an opening (stoma) made in the abdomen (applicable only if perforated intestine is the cause).
- Oxygen, if needed, depending on respiratory status.
- Semi-Fowler's position to promote drainage of peritoneal contents downward and localized in one area. Also facilitates adequate respiratory function because abdominal contents could be pressing on diaphragm which could impede respirations.

What can harm my client?

Peritonitis is a potentially fatal condition!!!

- Renal failure can develop as circulating volume decreases (related to hemorrhage), leading to decreased perfusion of the kidneys.
- If treatment is not started quickly, septicemia (bacterial invasion of the blood) can occur, leading to multiorgan failure.
- Shock can develop from hypovolemia caused by fluid leaking into the abdominal cavity (hemorrhage).
- Respiratory distress can occur as increasing pressure is placed on the diaphragm.

If I were your teacher, I would test you on . . .

- Definition of peritonitis.
- Causes of peritonitis and rationales.
- Signs and symptoms of peritonitis and rationales.
- Fluid and electrolyte assessment and administration.[10]
- Care of nasogastric tube.
- Pain management.
- Complications of peritonitis.
- Positioning.

✛ Crohn's disease

What is it?

Crohn's disease is a type of chronic inflammatory bowel disease (IBD) that can affect the entire alimentary system but typically involves a portion of the small intestine (ileum; Fig. 12-10). In the affected area, the intestine thickens, narrowing the lumen. All layers of the intestinal wall are affected. Onset is between ages 15 and 30, and the condition affects

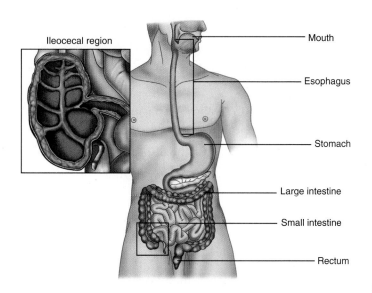

Ileocecal region

Mouth
Esophagus
Stomach
Large intestine
Small intestine
Rectum

◄ Figure 12-10. Crohn's disease is usually found in the ileocecal region, which is the last few inches of the ileum (small intestine) and the beginning of the cecum (large intestine).

more women than men. Crohn's disease is characterized by remissions and exacerbations.

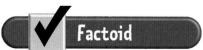

Factoid

Crohn's disease involves all layers of the small intestine and is characterized by regional segments of involvement. It's also referred to as regional enteritis.

What causes it and why

The etiology of Crohn's disease is unknown, but it is thought to be an autoimmune response. Table 12-36 shows possible causes of Crohn's disease and why these causes occur.

Table 12-36

Causes	Why
Smoking	Has been proposed as a risk factor in developing the disease. May also facilitate exacerbations
A familial or genetic predisposition such as immunoregulation of inflammation in the intestinal tract	The disease affects Caucasians, Jews, and upper middle class, urban populations. Family members tend to develop the disease with similar patterns and age of onset

Source: Created by author from References #5 to #7.

Signs and symptoms and why

Table 12-37 shows the signs and symptoms and rationales associated with peritonitis.

Table 12-37

Signs and symptoms	Why
Pain: • Crampy abdominal pain most often in the right lower quadrant (ileum is the typical area of involvement) • Periumbilical pain before and after bowel movements	Pain results from inflammatory process
Weight loss and malnutrition	From lack of eating, malabsorption, and chronic inflammatory process
Chronic diarrhea	Associated with inflammatory process
Elevated temperature	From severe inflammatory process
Fluid and electrolyte imbalances	From malabsorption of food and fluid

Source: Created by author from References #5 to #7.

Quickie tests and treatments

The client history may reveal a family history of the disorder or the client's ongoing bouts of diarrhea associated with abdominal cramping. Tests may include:

- Upper GI barium swallow or barium enema to detect areas with cobblestone appearance.
- Colonoscopy to diagnose the disorder if barium swallow does not.

Treatments for Crohn's disease may include:

- Bowel rest (NPO).
- Dietary supplements and total parenteral nutrition (food solutions given through the IV route) during severe exacerbations. Fish oil may help maintain remission.
- Low-residue diet when acute episode is over. Includes decreasing intake of foods that can irritate GI tract (spicy foods, caffeinated beverages, and alcohol) and taking nutritional supplements to provide needed nutrients. Low-fiber, low-fat diet high in calories, protein, and carbohydrates with vitamin and mineral supplements.
- Corticosteroids to decrease inflammation, pain, and diarrhea. Corticosteroids can also increase appetite.
- Immunosuppressants (other than corticosteroids) to suppress response to antigens.
- Antidiarrheal to decrease diarrhea and control fluid and electrolyte loss.
- Sulfasalazine to reduce inflammation.
- Antibiotics to treat abscess (accumulation of pus from infection) and fistula (abnormal passageway between organs or vessels) and to help induce remission.
- Opioid analgesics or antispasmodics to control pain and decrease diarrhea.
- Surgery if obstruction or perforation occurs.
- Intake/output (I&O).
- Daily weight.

What can harm my client?

- All layers of the small intestine are affected and can develop fissures, ulcerations, and abscesses leading to severe dehydration with electrolyte imbalances, malnutrition (leading to anorexia), and possibly even peritonitis leading to sepsis.
- Inflammation and scarring can lead to obstruction caused by strictures.
- Hemorrhage, bowel perforation.

If I were your teacher, I would test you on . . .

- Definition of Crohn's disease.
- Causes of Crohn's disease and rationales.
- Signs and symptoms of Crohn's disease and rationales.

⚠ Deadly Dilemma

Barium studies should be withheld if risk of perforation is high. The increased pressure in the GI tract can increase the risk of perforation.

✔ Factoid

Fistulas are common in acute episodes of Crohn's disease. Adequate nutrition and maintenance of fluid and electrolyte balance are imperative because severe diarrhea and malabsorption of nutrients vital to human life can occur. To promote fistula healing, the client may need 3000 or more calories per day. Strict intake and output are imperative!

- Education of client regarding dietary management and medication therapy.
- Pharmacology of medications.
- Symptoms requiring immediate attention.
- Differentiating Crohn's disease from ulcerative colitis.
- Complications.

✚ Ulcerative colitis

What is it?

Ulcerative colitis is a chronic inflammatory bowel disease that affects the mucosal layer of the large intestine and rectum. Inflammation leads to eroded lesions (Lieberkühn's crypts) along the lining of the large intestine. The disease most often begins in the rectum and moves toward the cecum. Sometimes only the rectum is involved, which is called ulcerative proctitis. Onset typically occurs between ages 15 and 40.

What causes it and why

The etiology is not fully understood. Table 12-38 shows possible causes of ulcerative colitis and why these causes occur.

Table 12-38

Causes	Why
Infection, allergy or overactive immune response (autoimmunity)	Environmental factors such as viral or bacterial infections, dietary insults, immunologic problems
Familial (genetic) predisposition	Predisposition for illness is increased among nuclear family members. It is most common in whites of Jewish descent

Source: Created by author from References #6 to #8.

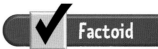

Factoid

A person has a 10 times greater risk of developing this disorder if she has a first-degree relative who has it.

Signs and symptoms and why

Table 12-39 shows the signs and symptoms and rationales associated with ulcerative colitis. These signs and symptoms are intermittent; flare-ups can occur gradually or quickly.

Table 12-39

Signs and symptoms	Why
Left-quadrant abdominal pain (may be crampy)	Multiple ulcerations, diffuse inflammation with continuous involvement of large intestine Pain increases with severity of illness

(Continued)

Table 12-39. (*Continued*)

Signs and symptoms	Why
Fecal urgency and/or diarrhea Painful straining (tenesmus) Frequent, painful bowel movement (up to 20 liquid bloody stools daily with pus and mucus) Rectal bleeding Increased bowel sounds	Ulceration in the colon and rectum
Anorexia (lack of desire to eat)	May occur because of the pain associated with consumption of food and fear of diarrhea
Weight loss	From frequent diarrhea and anorexia Can lead to fluid and electrolyte imbalances as flare-ups become more frequent and severe

Source: Created by author from References #5 to #7.

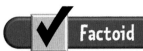

Ulcerative colitis usually involves only the mucosal layer of the large intestine, with ulceration and inflammation in a continuous segment.

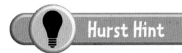

Bloody diarrhea mixed with mucus and often pus is a cardinal sign of ulcerative colitis!

Quickie tests and treatments

Tests for ulcerative colitis may include:

- Sigmoidoscopy or colonoscopy (use of a flexible tube to view colon) to detect the presence and extent of ulcerations.

- Barium enema to differentiate Crohn's disease from ulcerative colitis.

- Stool sample to rule out infectious agent and detect blood.

- Complete blood count (CBC) to determine if the white blood cell (WBC) count is elevated, which indicates an infection. Hemoglobin and hematocrit may be low due to bleeding.

- Chemistry profile to detect decreased sodium, chloride, and potassium levels resulting from chronic diarrhea.

- Serum albumin measurement to detect decreased level.

- Erythrocyte sedimentation rate (ESR) to detect an increase in response to inflammation.

- Rectal biopsy to differentiate ulcerative colitis from other diseases such as cancer.

Treatments may include:

- NPO or clear liquids to allow the bowel to rest.

- Total parenteral nutrition (TPN) may be given to restore nitrogen balance in cases of severe diarrhea with dehydration.

- Dietary modifications to decrease or eliminate high-bulk foods (raw fruits and vegetables) and use a low-residue diet. Foods such as milk products, alcohol, and caffeinated beverages may further aggravate the disorder.

- Bed rest.

- Use of antiinflammatory medications, such as sulfasalazine.

- Corticosteroids to decrease inflammation and frequency of flare-ups.
- Sulfasalazine given PO is the drug of choice for acute and maintenance therapy.
- Immunosuppressant to maintain remission of symptoms.
- Antidiarrheals to control frequency and consistency of stools.
- Treatment of anemia with iron supplements or transfusions for excessive bleeding.

Surgery may be indicated if other treatments are unsuccessful. Removal of large intestine and rectum will cure the disorder. This can be accomplished in three ways:

1. Removing the colon, rectum, and anus and placing an ileostomy (bringing the terminal end of the ileum through an opening in the abdominal wall, called a stoma). A pouch system is attached to the abdomen for drainage of GI contents.

2. Removing the colon, rectum, and anus and forming a pouch from the terminal ileum. Stool is stored in this reservoir until it is drained with a catheter. The reservoir is connected to a stoma flush with the skin with a nipple-like valve that prevents the use of an external pouch and decreases skin irritation caused by the external pouch.

3. Removing the colon and rectum, suturing the ileum to the anal canal, creating an ileoanal reservoir, and preserving the rectal sphincter. A temporary ileostomy is performed to allow healing to the surgical site.

What can harm my client?

- Increased risk for colon cancer.
- Liver disease.
- Malnutrition and anemia.
- Perforation.
- Hemorrhage.
- Electrolyte imbalances.
- Growth retardation in children.
- Possibility of infertility in females.
- Toxic megacolon (a condition in which the large intestine enlarges and, if not treated, can rupture).
- Toxic colitis (damage to the intestinal wall that leads to an absence of contractions to move contents through the GI tract).

If I were your teacher, I would test you on . . .

- Definition of ulcerative colitis.
- Causes of ulcerative colitis.
- Signs and symptoms of ulcerative colitis and rationales.
- Pharmacology of prescribed medications.
- Client education regarding dietary restrictions.

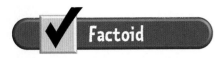

Factoid

IBS is not an inflammatory condition, and anatomic abnormalities are not present. It does not lead to inflammatory bowel disease and is not a life-threatening disorder

- Surgical interventions and postoperative nursing care.
- Differentiating ulcerative colitis from Crohn's disease.
- Complications.

✛ Irritable bowel syndrome (IBS)

What is it?

Irritable bowel syndrome (IBS) is a chronic intestinal disorder characterized by altered intestinal motility and an increase in visceral sensations.

What causes it and why

Table 12-40 shows possible causes of IBS and why these causes occur.

Table 12-40

Causes	Why
Emotions	The digestive system is controlled by the brain, and emotions such as stress and fear can lead to abnormal contractions of the GI tract
Food	Certain foods (coffee, tea, raw fruits and vegetables, dairy products, and fatty foods) can trigger an abnormality of the contraction–relaxation cycle of the GI system Eating too quickly can trigger IBS
Hormones	Changes in hormonal levels during menstruation can trigger IBS IBS affects women three times more frequently than men

Source: Created by author from References #4 and #9.

Signs and symptoms and why

The primary manifestation of irritable bowel syndrome can be either diarrhea, constipation, or both (see Table 12-41).

Table 12-41

Signs and symptoms	Why
Left lower quadrant abdominal pain	The pain of IBS generally begins after eating and is relieved with defecation. It occurs with abnormal contractions (spasms) of the colon
Bloating, flatulence(gas), constipation	Abnormal contraction and relaxation of the digestive tract traps gas and stool Constipation leads to a feeling of fullness, and abdominal distention may occur
Diarrhea (possibly with mucus in the stool and possibly alternating with constipation)	Eating triggers dumping of contents into the large intestine; diarrhea typically starts within a few minutes of eating. Mucus in the stool results from mucosal irritation Pain and cramping may occur with onset of diarrhea and resolve after a bout of diarrhea
Anxiety, depression	Related to fears of a loss of bowel control and an IBS episode in public Viscous circle begins as these emotions further increase episodes of IBS

Source: Created by author from References #4 and #9.

Quickie tests and treatments

The client history reveals the onset of symptoms, precipitating factors, and frequency of episodes. The physical exam is typically normal, although the lower abdomen may be tender.

Tests for IBS include:

- Sigmoidoscopy to rule out inflammatory bowel disorders, such as Crohn's disease and ulcerative colitis. Findings for IBS are normal because it does not affect the anatomy of the digestive tract.

- Stool examination to rule out other disorders.

- Upper GI barium swallow or barium enema to rule out other disorders with similar symptoms. The onset of colon spasm during the test supports the diagnosis of IBS.

- Lactose intolerance testing to determine if IBS is related to milk ingestion.

Treatment for IBS varies, depending on precipitating factors and the type of IBS (predominantly constipation, predominantly diarrhea, or a combination of the two).

Dietary management includes:

- Increasing the intake of high-fiber foods (30 to 40 g/day) and osmotic laxatives if constipation is the primary clinical manifestation.

- Increasing fluids to 8 to 10 cups/day.

- Antidiarrheals improve stool consistency in those whose primary clinical manifestation is diarrhea.

- Avoiding caffeine, alcohol, fructose, and foods that can trigger an IBS episode.

- Avoiding dairy foods, if lactose intolerance is the problem.

- Consuming smaller meals to help decrease episodes of IBS.

Other treatment includes:

- Antidepressants, anticholinergics, analgesics such as Tylenol or Ultram to manage pain.

- Stress management (relaxation strategies and antianxiety drugs).

- Antidiarrheals, such as loperamide (Imodium) for diarrhea-predominant IBS.

- Bulk-forming laxatives, such as psyllium (Metamucil) for constipation-predominant IBS.

- Anticholinergics or antispasmodics, such as dicyclomine (Bentyl), to treat cramping.

What can harm my client?

- Depression from this chronic condition.
- Sexual dysfunction.
- Interference with work and sleep.
- Decreased quality of life.
- Sometimes leads to unnecessary surgery related to misdiagnosis such as cholecystectomies, appendectomies, or partial colectomies.

If I were your teacher, I would test you on . . .

- Definition of IBS.
- Causes of IBS and rationales.

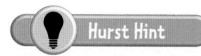

IBS symptoms can manifest as predominantly diarrhea, predominantly constipation, or a combination of the two. It is marked by periods of remission followed by exacerbation when exposed to causative factors.

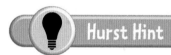

Because IBS doesn't change the appearance of the bowel mucosa, GI testing is done to rule out other disorders. Generally, these test results are normal with IBS, though colon spasms may occur during testing.

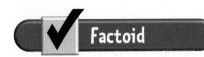

Factoid

Diverticula are pouch-like herniations that can occur anywhere along the intestinal tract. They tend to occur at weakened areas of the intestinal wall and most commonly appear in the sigmoid colon.

- Signs and symptoms of IBS and rationales.
- Differentiation of IBS from inflammatory bowel disease.
- Psychological impact of chronic conditions.[5,7,10]
- Management of IBS.

✛ Diverticulitis

What is it?

Diverticulitis is an acute inflammatory bowel disease characterized by inflammation or infection of blind pouches (diverticula) in the bowel mucosa.

What causes it and why

Table 12-42 shows possible causes of diverticulitis and why these causes occur.

Table 12-42

Causes	Why
Low-fiber diet	A low-fiber diet often leads to constipation, which increases the pressure on the colon wall and traps bacteria-rich stool in the diverticula
Decreased colon motility	Decreased colon motility slows the passage of GI contents and increases the risk of food and bacteria being trapped in diverticula

Source: Created by author from References #7 to #9.

Signs and symptoms and why

Table 12-43 shows the signs and symptoms and rationales associated with diverticulitis.

Table 12-43

Signs and symptoms	Why
Pain in the left lower abdominal quadrant that may be intermittent at first but becomes progressively steady	Pain occurs from irritation and inflammation of the diverticulum
Fever	From bacterial infection in the diverticula, which can even lead to abscess formation
Weakness and fatigue	From the inflammatory process and frequent episodes of diarrhea
Changes in bowel elimination, alternating between constipation and diarrhea	An unexplained problem that occurs frequently with this disorder
Anemia	May occur with rupture of the diverticula
Rectal bleeding	May occur with rupture of the diverticula

Source: Created by author from References #7 to #9.

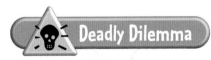

Deadly Dilemma

Pain over the entire abdominal area with rebound tenderness (pain after the abdomen is pressed and released suddenly) may indicate peritonitis.

Quickie tests and treatments

Tests for diverticulitis include:

- CT scan or ultrasound to detect abscesses or thickening of the bowel from diverticulitis.
- Abdominal x-rays to detect the presence of free air or fluid, which indicates perforation.
- CBC (complete blood count) to detect an increased white blood cell (WBC) count caused by inflammation and infection, and to detect low hemoglobin and hematocrit, which would indicate bleeding due to perforation.
- Colonoscopy to diagnose diverticulitis and determine the extent of the disease.
- Barium enema to detect diverticula.

Treatments may include:

- An initial liquid diet.
- Progression to a soft diet in 2 to 3 days.
- Low-fiber diet and stool softeners for several weeks after acute episode.
- After healing, a high-fiber diet and increased fluid intake to prevent constipation.
- Avoidance of laxatives, which increase the motility of intestines, and enemas, which increase pressure in the intestines.
- IV (intravenous) antibiotics to treat severe infections.
- Oral antibiotics to treat mild diverticulitis.
- Pain control, including rest and analgesics (pain medications).
- Surgery (colon resection with removal of involved area), if symptoms persist after typical treatment.

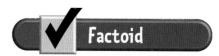

Factoid

Colonoscopy and barium enema are not performed during acute inflammation because of the risk of perforation of sensitive diverticula.

What can harm my client?

An abscess can lead to rupture and peritonitis, requiring immediate medical attention.

- Hemorrhage.
- Bowel obstruction.
- Fistula formation.
- Septicemia.

If I were your teacher, I would test you on . . .

- Definition of diverticulitis.
- Causes of diverticulitis and rationales.
- Signs and symptoms of diverticulitis and rationales.
- Acute management.
- Client education regarding diet and symptom control after an acute episode.
- Complications.

+ Cirrhosis

What is it?

Cirrhosis is severe, potentially fatal scarring and fibrosis of liver tissue.

What causes it and why

Table 12-44 shows possible causes of cirrhosis and why these causes occur.

Table 12-44

Causes	Why
Chronic alcoholism	The products produced when alcohol is broken down act as a toxin, leading to inflammation. With prolonged use, scar tissue develops and the liver is unable to function properly
Viral or autoimmune hepatitis	Immune and inflammatory responses are stimulated, leading to hepatocyte damage and eventually scarring of the liver tissues
Inherited or genetic disorders (hemochromatosis and alpha$_1$-antitrypsin)	In hemochromatosis, excess iron builds up in the body, is stored in organs such as the liver, and eventually destroys the liver cells Alpha$_1$-antitrypsin is a genetic defect that results in deficient liver protein, leading to liver cell destruction
Bile duct obstruction	Bile builds up
Right-sided heart failure (the inability of the heart muscle to pump efficiently to meet the body's needs)	The liver becomes engorged with venous blood as the heart's ability to pump weakens. This congestion prevents nutrient-rich blood from entering the liver, leading to hepatic cell death and fibrosis
Drugs and toxins	Exposure of the liver to some drugs and environmental toxins can lead to hepatic cell damage

Source: Created by author from References #5, #6, and #9.

Signs and symptoms and why

In the early or mild stage of cirrhosis, a person may be asymptomatic (without any symptoms). Late-stage symptoms result from the overall deterioration of liver function. Table 12-45 shows the signs and symptoms and rationales associated with cirrhosis. It is important for you to review and understand NORMAL liver functions. Knowing what is normal will help the signs and symptoms make sense as well as increase your test grade!

Table 12-45

Signs and symptoms	Why
Jaundice	Normally, bilirubin (a product of the breakdown of unusable red blood cells) is carried in bile to the small intestine and removed. If the liver cannot excrete bilirubin into bile or if bile flow is obstructed, bilirubin accumulates in the blood and is deposited in the skin. This leads to the yellow discoloration of the skin and sclera of jaundice (seen in sclera first) Skin deposits may cause itching Urine becomes dark because the kidneys are excreting larger amounts of bilirubin
Fluid in the abdomen (ascites)	One of the major functions of the liver is to synthesize albumin. If liver is sick, then albumin cannot be made so serum albumin level goes down. As a result, fluid leaves the vascular space and can move into the peritoneum (ascites). See Factoid
Hepatomegaly (enlarged liver)	Caused by inflammation and interstitial swelling
Nausea, anorexia, and abdominal discomfort	Anytime liver is not functioning properly, toxins cannot be metabolized. Toxins accumulate and make the client feel really bad. Also, the liver will probably be enlarged. When the liver enlarges, the capsule surrounding it stretches. This capsule is filled with nerves and causes the client discomfort/pain. This same capsular stretching occurs in the pancreas (i.e., pancreatitis)
Malnutrition	Decreased production and release of bile impairs the absorption of fat and fat-soluble vitamins
Spider angiomas (lesions with red centers radiating outward into branches), ecchymosis (bruising), and petechiae (pinpoint, red-purple rash)	Skin changes result from decreased absorption of vitamin K. The lack of vitamin K prevents sufficient production of clotting factors, leading to increased risk of bleeding and bruising
Increased medication sensitivity	Because the liver is unable to metabolize medications
Splenomegaly (enlarged spleen)	Bloodflow to the liver may become obstructed by fibrosis and scarring, leading to portal hypertension (high pressure in portal vein). This leads to a diversion of blood flow to the spleen. Blood is stored in the spleen and taken from the general circulation resulting in: • Anemia (decreased red blood cells) • Thrombocytopenia (decreased platelets) • Leukopenia (decreased white blood cells)
Esophageal varices (dilated veins in the esophagus) just like a hemorrhoid	Results from portal hypertension (high blood pressure in portal vein/liver). This causes back pressures through the esophagus, which causes vessels to distend
Neurologic effects: • Confusion, mood changes, behavioral changes, and agitation • Hepatic encephalopathy • Asterixis (rapid back and forth movement of the wrist), sometimes called a flapping tremor	When the liver is unable to remove toxins from the blood, they accumulate, leading to deterioration of brain processes and neurological symptoms. The major toxin that accumulates in the blood with liver problems is ammonia. Ammonia can affect neurological status of the client in many ways
Shortness of breath	Increased fluid in the abdomen places more pressure on the thoracic cavity, leading to decreased lung expansion

Source: Created by author from References #5, #6, and #9.

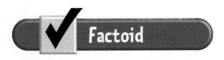

Factoid

Albumin is a very large protein that is responsible for holding fluid in the vascular space. If albumin is deficient then the fluid will shift.

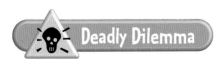

Deadly Dilemma

Esophageal varices may abruptly begin to bleed, leading to hemorrhage and death. This is a medical emergency!!!

Quickie tests and treatments

Tests for cirrhosis include:

- Ultrasound or CT scan to show shrinkage or an abnormal appearance of liver. If radioactive isotopes are used, the scan can show functioning versus nonfunctioning areas of the liver.
- Laboratory studies—bilirubin, albumin, alanine transaminase (ALT), aspartate transaminase (AST), prothrombin time, and serum ammonia—to check for elevated values, which indicate hepatic cell destruction. These are the common lab values elevated with almost any type of liver disease.
- Liver biopsy to confirm the diagnosis microscopically.
- Esophagoscopy to determine the presence of esophageal varices.
- Paracentesis for examination of ascetic fluid for cell, protein, and bacterial count.

No known medical cure is available. The goal of treatment is to prevent the progression of the disease by treating causes and complications. The client can:

- Immediately stop alcohol consumption to slow the progression of cirrhosis.
- Take vitamins (thiamin, folate) and nutritional supplements for malnutrition to correct nutritional deficiencies.
- Decrease sodium intake (less than 2 g/day) to control fluid accumulation/ascites (sodium causes fluid retention).
- Restrict fluid intake to 1000 to 1500 mL daily, if serum sodium levels are decreased. Water intake causes the blood to become dilute. Dilution decreases the serum sodium.
- Use frequent rest periods or periods of bed rest to help conserve energy depleted from decreased nutritional intake. Bed rest also helps to induce diuresis (the supine position causes an increase in kidney perfusion; more urine is produced).
- Diuretics to help with excess fluid.
- Paracentesis for relief of ascites.
- Albumin administration to help maintain osmotic pressure (albumin to help hold fluid in the vascular space).
- Pain management if indicated.
- Liver transplant (possible, depending upon the cause).

The client's nurse should:

- Monitor medications that are usually metabolized in the liver.
- Give diuretics to rid the body of excess fluid. If diuretics are nonpotassium sparing, the client may need potassium supplements.
- Elevate the head of the bed at least 30 degrees to decrease shortness of breath.
- Implement bleeding precautions.

Depending on the client's condition, the following may be required:

- Paracentesis (using a needle to drain fluid from peritoneal cavity) to manage ascites.

- Esophagogastric intubation (balloon placed into the esophagus and inflated to put pressure on bleeding sites) or endoscopic sclerotherapy (placing a flexible tube into the esophagus and using an agent that causes sclerosing of the bleeding area) for bleeding esophageal varices. If sclerotherapy is unsuccessful, endoscopic banding may be performed. This technique involves banding of the varices causing strangulation and eventually fibrosis of the area.

- Blood transfusions for significant bleeding, resulting in low hemoglobin and hematocrit levels (anytime the liver is sick, bleeding can occur; must take bleeding precautions).

- Hepatitis A vaccine (HAV) and hepatitis B vaccine (HBV), because the client is more susceptible to hepatitis, which would further destroy liver function.

What can harm my client?

- Bleeding esophageal varices that may lead to hemorrhage and death, if treatment is not readily available!
- Coagulopathies.
- Peritonitis.
- Liver failure may progress to a need for a liver transplant. If a transplant is not available, the result is death!!
- Progression to liver cancer (hepatoma).
- Susceptibility to contracting hepatitis A or B.
- Hepatic encephalopathy.

If I were your teacher, I would test you on . . .

- Definition of cirrhosis.
- Causes of cirrhosis and rationales.
- Signs and symptoms of cirrhosis and rationales.
- Complications.
- Liver function tests that indicate liver damage.
- Dietary and medication considerations.
- Community resource education (Alcoholics Anonymous).
- Client education regarding the HAV and HBV.[7]
- Management of client with esophageal varices:
  1. Assessment of bleeding (onset and volume).
  2. Assessment of blood pressure, pulse, and respirations.
  3. Insertion of IV line for fluid infusion (blood loss leads to decreased circulating volume and decrease in blood pressure). Fluid replacement is critical for organ function.

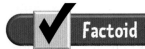

Factoid

Cholecystitis is more common among women and Mexican-American clients.

Hurst Hint

In nursing school (many years ago), we were taught to be alert for high-risk clients who might present to the hospital with a new onset of pain. The 3 F's (fair, fat, female) were introduced as a way to remember the most commonly diagnosed population. We could actually add a fourth F and include family history. So remember when you are assessing a client with an acute onset of pain, if the 4 F's apply, you may very well be dealing with cholecystitis.

4. Management of the airway (head of bed elevated if blood pressure is adequate, position client on side to prevent aspiration, suction oral cavity to help remove blood from mouth).

5. Insertion of nasogastric tube to remove gastric contents before endoscopy. (See "Intestinal obstruction" earlier in the chapter for care of a nasogastric tube).

6. Preparation for esophagogastric intubation, endoscopic sclerotherapy, or endoscopic banding, as ordered by physician.

7. Procedure for blood administration.

- Management of a client undergoing paracentesis:

1. Obtaining consent for the procedure.

2. Positioning the client (supine or semi-Fowler's position; or sitting up, if tolerated).

3. Educating client regarding purpose of procedure, use of numbing agent, needle insertion into the abdomen, and postprocedure problems to report.

4. Monitoring and reporting complications (increased temperature; excessive bleeding or drainage of insertion site; blood in urine; increased or new onset of severe abdominal pain; increased warmth, redness, or tenderness of abdomen).

5. Vital signs prior to procedure and frequent vital signs thereafter.

✚ Cholecystitis

What is it?

Cholecystitis is an inflammation of the gallbladder. About 90% of cases result from gallstones (accumulation of solid crystals) obstructing the cystic duct. If cholecystitis occurs without gallstones, it is usually after a major illness or injury (acalculous cholecystitis). Cholecystitis affects about 1 million new clients annually. It can be acute (sudden onset of inflammation) or chronic (long-term inflammation with repeated gallbladder attacks of pain).

What causes it and why

Table 12-46 shows possible causes of cholecystitis and why these causes occur.

Table 12-46

Causes	Why
Acute cholecystitis: edema, inflammation, and impaction of gallstones in cystic duct	Responses to obstruction of bile duct; buildup of bile in gallbladder causes irrigation and pressure
Chronic cholecystitis: fibrotic thickening of gallbladder wall and incomplete emptying	Responses to repeated acute attacks or chronic irritation of gallstones

Source: Created by author from Reference #3, #7, and #8.

Signs and symptoms and why

Table 12-47 shows the signs and symptoms and rationales associated with cholecystitis.

Table 12-47

Signs and symptoms	Why
Severe acute right upper quadrant (RUQ) and epigastric pain (4 to 6 hours after eating a fatty meal) radiating to shoulder and right scapula and aggravated by breathing movement. Pain usually lasts more than 12 hours, and abdominal muscles become rigid within a few hours of the onset of pain	Pain occurs from the obstruction of the cystic duct of the gallbladder or a spasm as the stone moves through the duct
Nausea and vomiting	Due to severity of pain occurring during the attack
Fever	An elevated temperature may occur in response to inflammation
Indigestion (dyspepsia), gas (flatulence), and belching (eructation)	A lack of bile decreases the ability of the GI tract to break down meals that are high in fat, disrupting the normal digestion process
Steatorrhea (fatty stools)	A lack of bile leads to decreased absorption of fats and steatorrhea

Source: Created by author from References #3, #6, and #8.

Quickie tests and treatments

Tests for cholecystitis may include:

- Complete blood count (CBC) to detect an elevated white blood cell count (WBC), which indicates inflammation and infection.
- Serum amylase levels to detect an elevation, which occurs with common bile duct stone or pancreas involvement.
- Ultrasound to check for gallstones in the gallbladder and thickening of the gallbladder wall (from chronic inflammation).
- X-ray to identify gallstones as calcium versus cholesterol.
- ERCP (endoscopic retrograde cholangiopancreatography) to visualize the pancreatic and bile ducts for presence of stones.

Treatments may include:

- NPO (nothing by mouth) order and administration of intravenous (IV) fluids and electrolytes; being NPO allows the GI tract time to rest.
- Progression to a low-fat diet after acute symptoms subside.
- Pain control (opioids and comfort measures to reduce the intensity of pain).
- Antispasmodics or anticholinergics to reduce biliary colic.
- Antibiotics to prevent infection.
- Laparoscopic cholecystectomy (removal of gallbladder through tubes inserted through the abdomen).

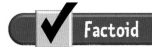

Acute or chronic cholecystitis gallbladder attacks begin with pain.

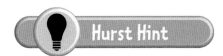

Morphine typically is not ordered because it can cause biliary spasms.

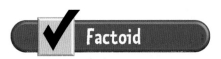

Elderly clients can experience confusion and even seizures when given meperidine (Demerol) for pain control!

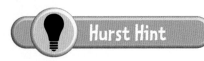

Long-term symptoms of infection (elevated temperature, increased white blood cell count, malaise, chills) warrants further investigation.

What can harm my client?

If a gallbladder attack continues for more than a few days, one of these complications may be the reason:

- Perforation of gallbladder.
- Gangrene (death of tissue).
- Abscess (pocket of infection).
- Ileus (cessation of normal movement of intestines).
- Pancreatitis (inflammation of the pancreas), if gallstones have obstructed the pancreatic duct.

If I were your teacher, I would test you on . . .

- Definition of cholecystitis.
- Causes of cholecystitis and rationales.
- Signs and symptoms of cholecystitis and rationales.
- Nursing interventions for a client admitted with cholecystitis.
  1. Maintaining NPO status and administering IV fluids and electrolytes.
  2. Pain assessment and interventions (remember to assess and document pain scale, type of pain, description of pain, location of pain, precipitating factors that increase pain). Provide pain medications as needed, but don't forget things like rest and relaxation techniques, which may be used with medications to control pain. Pain follow-up within 30 to 45 minutes with documentation of effectiveness.
  3. Preparation for surgery (signed consent, education on procedure) and assessment after procedure (vital signs monitoring, incision assessment).
- Client education on dietary recommendations, if gallbladder is not removed. (Fatty foods may be reduced between episodes.)
- Pharmacology of medical management.[7,8]
- Complications.

✚ Pancreatitis

What is it?

Pancreatitis is an acute or chronic inflammation of the pancreas (Fig. 12-11). Acute pancreatitis results when pancreatic enzymes are activated while still in the pancreas (they are not supposed to activate until they get to the small intestine). Since the purpose of a digestive enzyme is to digest, the pancreatic enzyme that is trapped in the pancreas begins to eat the pancreas. This leads to a cascade effect of inflamed cells releasing additional enzymes. The process of the pancreas eating itself is called autodigestion (auto means self). Chronic pancreatitis results when progressive, recurring episodes of acute pancreatitis cause structural changes, and functional capabilities of the pancreas become damaged.

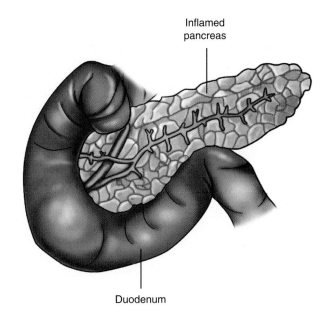

Inflamed pancreas

Duodenum

◄ Figure 12-11. Pancreatitis.

What causes it and why

Table 12-48 shows possible causes of pancreatitis and why these causes occur.

Table 12-48

Causes	Why
Toxic metabolic processes (alcoholism, medications)	Alcohol causes scar tissue to form throughout the GI tract. This causes blockages (due to scar tissue) in the pancreas resulting in trapped pancreatic enzymes. These trapped enzymes start eating the pancreas. Various medications, such as furosemide, can cause an irritation of the pancreas
Biliary obstruction (gallstones, stenosis of sphincter of Oddi)	A gallstone can fall and block the pancreatic duct leading to autodigestion
Trauma	Blunt trauma or penetrating wounds can damage the pancreas Endoscopic and surgical procedures can also cause damage
Viral infections	Some viral infections, such as mumps, can lead to an inflammation of the pancreas
Cancer	Pancreatic cancer can lead to an inability of the pancreas to function normally, resulting in inflammation
Unknown origin	Chronic pancreatitis can occur from unknown etiology; tropical countries have an increased incidence

Source: Created by author from References #7 to #9.

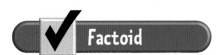

Factoid

Alcohol use accounts for 80% of chronic pancreatitis; however, do not automatically assume that someone who has pancreatitis is an alcoholic.

Signs and symptoms and why

Table 12-49 shows the signs and symptoms and rationales associated with pancreatitis. Remember, the GI tract is one system. When one organ gets sick, another organ in the system can be affected as well. For example, a sick pancreas can lead to a sick liver, and vice versa. A sick liver can lead to a sick esophagus (esophageal varices). You will better understand as you continue to learn.

Table 12-49

Signs and symptoms	Why
Pain	Severe left upper abdominal pain that may radiate to the back or epigastrium radiating to the left shoulder or back. Occurs because of the inflammatory process in the pancreas
	Movement and coughing may intensify the pain as well as lying supine
	Abdomen may become rigid because client may be guarding, have peritonitis or may be hemorrhaging
Nausea and persistent vomiting	GI tract is upset
Decreased or absent bowel sounds	From decreased motility of intestines and possible ileus. Anytime the GI system gets sick, it can shut down. Electrolyte imbalances can cause a paralytic ileus
Respiratory distress (increased respiratory rate, shallow breathing, pulse rate greater than 100, decreased oxygenation) Atelectasis (collapse of tissues in lungs)	Atelectasis, effusion, and pneumonia can result due to escaping pancreatic enzymes from the peritoneum to the pleural cavity
Fluctuation in blood pressure (typically low)	In pancreatitis, vasodilation frequently occurs due to chemicals that are released. Also, proteins are leaking into the peritoneal space related to tissue destruction which leads to an ultimate circulating loss of protein in the vascular space. Volume in vascular space goes down as does the blood pressure
Fever	Inflammatory process
Malaise and decreased level of consciousness	Accumulation of toxins released during pancreatic digestion; decreased oxygenation; shock; if liver is involved ammonia level could go up leading to LOC
Steatorrhea (fatty, frothy, foul-smelling stools)	Decreased pancreatic enzymes
Cullen's sign (bluish discoloration around navel)	Bleeding
Turner's sign (grayish-blue discoloration of flank area)	Hemorrhaged blood settles to flank area when supine. Pancreatic enzymes are leaking
Ascites (possibly)	Pancreatic duct can rupture causing fluid to leak into the peritoneum; pancreas is digesting itself, so fluid could leak out of the pancreas

Source: Created by author from References #7 to #9.

Quickie tests and treatments

Tests for pancreatitis may include:

- Increased serum amylase and lipase (enzymes produced in the pancreas). Amylase may be normal in chronic pancreatitis. Lipase usually elevates after amylase and is considered a more specific indicator of acute pancreatitis than amylase.

* Increased AST/ALT if liver is involved.

* Electrolyte disturbances related to dehydration.

* Elevated white blood cell (WBC) count (leukocytosis) related to inflammation or possible infection.

* Decreased serum albumin related to sick liver.

* Elevated glucose levels (may or may not be elevated) because the pancreas is unable to produce and release insulin. Remember, think glucose problems with pancreas problems.

* Urine amylase may be elevated.

* Increased bilirubin if liver is involved.

* Elevated alkaline phosphatase when anything is going on in the gut.

* Elevated calcium may be seen in 25% of clients; however, many clients have hypocalcemia (pancreas loses calcium into the peritoneal space when it digests itself). Now we have to worry about seizures.

* Abdominal ultrasound to identify gallstones, mass, or pseudocyst.

* Endoscopic ultrasonography can detect pancreatic changes related to chronic pancreatitis.

* Abdominal x-rays to detect ileus. May show pancreatic calcifications or gallstones. This could suggest alcohol or liver problems as the cause.

* Chest x-rays to detect pulmonary complications such as pleural effusion and atelectasis. Pleural effusions are most commonly seen on the left but may be bilateral.

* CT scan to detect structural changes and size of pancreas (may be enlarged) and calcification of ducts; will show perfusion deficits in areas of necrosis.

* ERCP (endoscopic retrograde cholangiopancreatography) to locate obstructions and ductal leaks. Can help to diagnose chronic pancreatitis. Will also differentiate inflammation and fibrosis from carcinoma.

* Percutaneous fine-needle aspiration biopsy to differentiate chronic pancreatitis from cancer of the pancreas by examining cells.

Treatments may include:

* Dietary management:

  1. NPO (nothing by mouth) to decrease gastric secretions; when secretions go into the stomach, the pancreas thinks its time to make more enzymes which increases pain.

  2. Administration of IV fluids and electrolytes to prevent or treat dehydration, electrolyte imbalances, and shock from decreased circulating volume.

  3. Nutritional support using total parenteral nutrition (TPN). This involves placement of an access device in a large vein to administer lipids and other nutritional components.

* Prophylactic antibiotic therapy to avoid infection or treat existing infection.

- Nasogastric placement and suctioning (using a tube inserted through the nose into the gastric area to remove air and gastric contents. (See "Intestinal obstruction" earlier in the chapter for care of a nasogastric tube). This relieves gastric stasis, distention, and is helpful if ileus is present. It is very important to keep the stomach empty and dry.
- Oxygen administration using nasal cannula or, in severe cases, a ventilator (machine that supplies oxygen and maintains respirations). Oxygen deprivation may be present due to pain, anxiety, acidosis, abdominal pressure, or pleural effusions.
- Pain management, typically including narcotics such as meperidine (Demerol); as well as proper positioning (fetal positioning); PCA pump may be used.
- Anticholinergic drugs to dry up secretions.
- Replacement of pancreatic enzymes for chronic pancreatitis. These are typically taken orally with meals.
- Antacids, H_2-receptor blockers, or proton pump inhibitors to decrease gastric acid content or prevent gastric enzyme production. Prevents stress ulcer formation which is a common complication related to acute illnesses.
- Sodium bicarbonate to reverse metabolic acidosis.
- Insulin to treat hyperglycemia if present.
- Prevention of complications (i.e., pulmonary)–cough and deep breathing to improve respiratory function.
- Vital signs including temp as well as skin color.
- I&O and daily weights.
- Daily abdominal girth if pancreatic ascites is suspected.
- Oral hygiene daily.
- Surgical intervention to treat the underlying cause, such as surgical repair of trauma or incision and drainage of a pseudocyst (a collection of tissue and fluid that can enlarge and become infected or rupture); debridement or pancreatectomy to remove pancreatic necrotic tissue; cholecystectomy for pancreatic related to gallstones.
- ERCP (endoscopic retrograde cholangiopancreatography) to remove gallstones.
- Once acute pancreatitis is resolved, gradually resume low-fat, low-caffeine diet as tolerated.
- Rest with gradual increase in activity.
- Minimize stress to prevent recurrent acute attacks which could lead to chronic pancreatitis.
- Teach alcohol avoidance.
- Recommend AA.

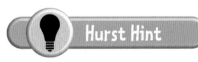

Hurst Hint

Morphine is generally avoided because it may cause spasms of the sphincter of Oddi.

What can harm my client?

- Seizures related to hypocalcemia.
- Arrhythmias related to electrolyte imbalances.

- Pancreatic ascites which accentuates shock due to decreased volume in the vascular space.
- Pancreatic abscess.
- Pancreatic pseudocyst which can rupture.
- Pulmonary infiltrates, pleural effusion, ARDS (acute respiratory distress syndrome).
- Peritonitis (inflammation of the abdominal wall).
- Ileus (cessation of movement of the contents of the stomach and intestines).
- ARDS (acute respiratory distress syndrome) from atelectasis and damage to lungs.
- Shock from blood and pancreatic fluid moving into the abdominal cavity and decreasing the volume of circulating blood.
- Infection of the pancreas, requiring antibiotics may require surgical removal of infected tissue. Infection is the most common cause of death may be related to sepsis with multiorgan dysfunction or failure.
- Hemorrhage with hypovolemic shock.
- Acute renal failure.
- Increased severity of pain can indicate worsening OR inadequate pain management.

If I were your teacher, I would test you on . . .

- Definition of pancreatitis.
- Causes of pancreatitis and rationales.
- Signs and symptoms of pancreatitis and rationales.
- Lab values related to pancreatitis (normal vs. abnormal).
- Nursing management: diet, oxygen, IV site observation, care, pain management, total parenteral nutrition (TPN) care.
- Potential complications.
- NG tube placement and maintenance (NG care).

SUMMARY

The GI system consists of the main organs of digestion—oral cavity, esophagus, stomach, small intestine, and large intestine—and is aided by the liver, gallbladder, and pancreas in converting the nutrients of food into energy and breaking the nondigestible material into waste for excretion. Diseases and disorders of the GI system can be acute or chronic and can result in malabsorption, malnutrition, fluid and electrolyte imbalances, and compromised organ function. Many conditions compromise the quality of daily living and thus have accompanying psychosocial implications. Some conditions, when untreated, can be life threatening. The nurse's knowledge of GI diseases and expertise in client care, treatment, and education are critical for the client's optimal outcomes.

PRACTICE QUESTIONS

1. Which of the following statements about GERD is correct?

1. Heartburn and regurgitation are the most common symptoms of GERD.

2. Without the presence of heartburn, GERD is most likely not the diagnosis.

3. The length of time the client has had symptoms has no long-term implications.

4. GERD assessment is done with the client history only.

Correct answer: 1. Heartburn and regurgitation are the most common symptoms; however, their absence does not rule out GERD. Complaints of frequent throat clearing, hoarseness upon waking, and a sensation of having food stuck in the throat are also symptoms. Long-term effects of untreated GERD can lead to esophagitis and esophageal cancer.

2. Clients with hiatal hernia should be educated to manage the symptoms of heartburn and regurgitation by:

1. Eating a snack immediately before going to bed.

2. Allowing an hour to recline after a meal.

3. Sleeping lying flat without using a pillow.

4. Eating more frequent, smaller meals.

Correct answer: 4. Eating a snack immediately before going to bed, allowing an hour to recline after a meal, and sleeping lying flat without using a pillow would aggravate heartburn and regurgitation. The client with hiatal hernia should remain upright after eating; reclining after meals is recommended for clients with dumping syndrome.

3. Irritable bowel syndrome (IBS) and inflammatory bowel disease (IBD) are two:

1. Names for the same disease.

2. Degrees of severity of the same disease.

3. Distinct types of disease, affecting different segments of the colon but with the same tissue pathology.

4. Distinct types of disease, affecting different segments of the colon with different tissue pathology.

Correct answer: 4. IBS and IBD are distinct diseases. With IBS, the intestinal tissue does not change. With IBD, all layers of the small intestine (Crohn's disease) and the mucosal layer of the large intestine (ulcerative colitis) are affected.

4. Appropriate treatment when assessing and preparing a client with acute appendicitis for surgery would include:

1. Administering a laxative or enema for surgical bowel prep.

2. Applying an ice pack to the right lower quadrant, placing the client in Fowler's position, and maintaining an NPO (nothing by mouth) order.

3. Applying a heat pad to the area of abdominal pain.

4. Having the client walk to avoid postoperative complications.

Correct answer: 2. Applying an ice pack to the right lower quadrant and keeping the client as comfortable as possible are appropriate treatments. The NPO status is necessary for anesthesia and surgery. A heat pack and laxative or enema may cause rupturing of the appendix. The client cannot tolerate ambulation.

5. Crohn's disease and ulcerative colitis are inflammatory bowel diseases that:

1. Have similar symptoms and etiology, affect the same intestinal areas and layers, and have the same long-term risks.

2. Have similar symptoms and etiology, affect different intestinal areas and layers, and have the same long-term risks.

3. Have different symptoms and etiology, affect different intestinal areas and layers, and have different long-term risks.

4. Have similar symptoms and etiology, affect different intestinal areas and layers, and have different long-term risks.

Correct answer: 4. Crohn's disease and ulcerative colitis have similar symptoms and are thought to have the same etiology. However, Crohn's disease affects mostly the small intestine and all layers of the wall; ulcerative colitis involves the large intestine and rectum and only the mucosal layer. Crohn's disease clients are at risk for fistulas and perforations. Ulcerative colitis clients are at risk for colon cancer.

6. Hepatitis A, B, C, D, and E have:

1. Similar symptoms but different modes of transmission, clinical course, and prognoses.

2. Different symptoms but the same mode of transmission, clinical course, and prognoses.

3. Different symptoms, modes of transmission, clinical course, and prognoses.

4. Similar symptoms, modes of transmission, clinical course and prognoses.

Correct answer: 1. The symptoms are similar in the five different types of hepatitis, but the modes of transmission, the clinical courses, and prognoses are different.

7. The treatment of GI diseases is based on:

1. The client learning to live with the disease because there are no known cures.

2. Stress management techniques because stress is the primary cause of most GI diseases.

3. Multiple modalities for managing inflammation, controlling pain, preventing infection, improving diet and nutrition, and making lifestyle changes to avoid triggering factors.

4. Managing one symptom at a time to ensure complete effectiveness.

Correct answer: 3. No cure exists for many GI diseases and disorders, but treatment and management include such steps as taking prescribed medications, improving diet and nutrition, and making lifestyle changes to avoid factors that trigger or exacerbate symptoms. Stress management is a key element of client education, but stress is no longer considered the primary cause.

8. Proton-pump inhibitors are prescribed to:

1. Potentiate the transport of hydrogen ions.

2. Inhibit gastric acid formation.

3. Increase gastric acid section.

4. Form a protective barrier on the mucosa.

Correct answer: 2. Proton-pump inhibitors bind to enzymes to prevent hydrogen ions transport and inhibit gastric acid formation. H_2-receptor blockers inhibit gastric acid secretion, and sucralfate agents enhance the mucosa barrier.

9. The three medications prescribed for gastritis and peptic ulcer disease associated with *H. pylori* are:

1. Two antibiotics and one H_2-receptor blocker or proton-pump inhibitor taken sequentially over several months.

2. Three different antibiotics in three separate courses to ensure full eradication of *H. pylori.*

3. Two antibiotics and one H_2-receptor blocker, antacid, or proton-pump inhibitor for a 14-day course.

4. One antibiotic, one H_2-receptor blocker or proton-pump inhibitor, and one antacid.

Correct answer: 3. The triple therapy for gastritis and peptic ulcer disease associated with *H. pylori* consists of two antibiotics and one H_2-receptor blocker, antacid, or proton-pump inhibitor taken for 14 days. The drugs are taken together. The 14-day course of the antibiotic is more effective than a 10-day regimen.

10. Which of the following are true of GI diseases and disorders? Select all that apply.

1. Anxiety and stress can exacerbate some GI diseases and disorders.

2. GI diseases and disorders result from viral or bacterial infection, the immune response, or compromised integrity of the structure or function of the affected organs.

3. Psychological influences are the primary cause of GI diseases and disorders.

4. GI diseases and disorders primarily affect the elderly population.

Correct answers: 1 & 2. Psychological influences are not the primary cause of GI diseases and disorders. However, anxiety and stress can exacerbate some of them. The pathophysiology is caused by viral or bacterial infection, the immune response, or compromised integrity of the structure or function of the affected organs. GI diseases and disorders affect people of all ages.

References

1. Dawson SG. Gastrointestinal system function, assessment, and therapeutic measures. In: Williams LS, Hopper PD, eds. *Understanding Medical Surgical Nursing.* 2nd ed. Philadelphia: Davis; 2003:473–504.

2. Oliver MV, Zaloum R, Burkel WE. Digestive system. In: Oliver MV, Burkel WE, eds. *Rapid Review Anatomy Reference Guide.* Skokie, IL: Anatomical Chart Company; 1996:21–22.

3. Kennedy EB, Scanlon V. Liver, gallbladder, and pancreas functions and assessment. In: Williams LS, Hopper PD, eds. *Understanding Medical Surgical Nursing.* 2nd ed. Philadelphia: Davis; 2003:506–543.

4. Minocha A, Adamec C. *The Encyclopedia of the Digestive System and Digestive Disorders.* New York: Facts on File; 2004.

5. Smelzer SC, Bare BG, eds. *Brunner and Suddarth's Textbook of Medical-Surgical Nursing.* 10th ed. Philadelphia: Lippincott Williams & Wilkins; 2004.

6. Beers M, Fletcher A, Porter R, et al. *Merck Manual of Medical Information.* 2nd home ed. New York: Merck; 2003.

7. Corwin E. *Handbook of Pathophysiology.* 3rd ed. Philadelphia: Lippincott Williams & Wilkins; 2008.

8. Antczak S, Berger N, Tagan W, et al. *Just the Facts: Pathophysiology.* Ambler, Pa: Lippincott Williams & Wilkins; 2005.

9. Ignatavicius D, Workman L. *Medical-Surgical Nursing.* 5th ed. St. Louis: Elsevier Saunders; 2006.

Bibliography

Hurst Review Services. www.hurstreview.com.

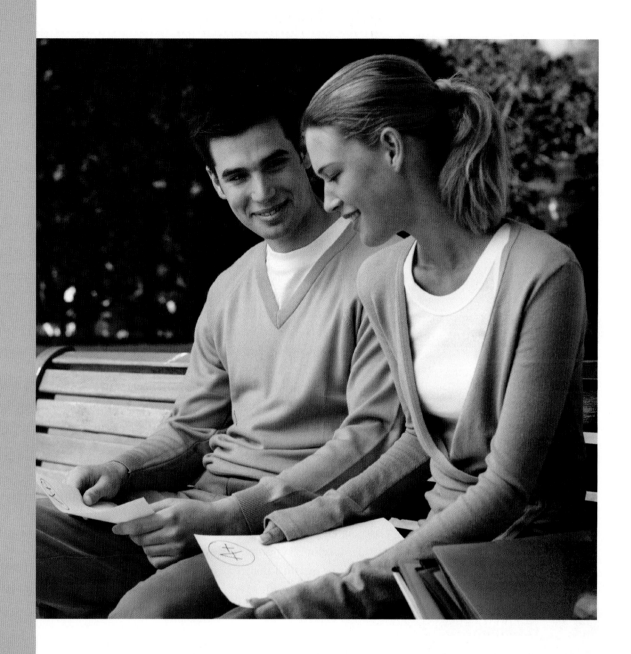

13 Nutritional Abnormalities

OBJECTIVES

In this chapter, you'll review:

- The causes and signs and symptoms of malnutrition.
- The key psychosocial and physiological manifestations of anorexia nervosa.
- The major differences between anorexia nervosa and bulimia nervosa.

LET'S GET THE NORMAL STUFF STRAIGHT FIRST

Adequate nutrition is essential for all our body functions. Proper intake of food substances breaks down to chemicals that provide energy, support growth, and maintain and repair our body tissues. Calories provide energy that is used to support every function of the body. Energy is expended in activity and rest. Malnutrition is a condition where a person does not receive, or is unable to use, an adequate amount of calories and nutrients to maintain body functions. This chapter explores the most common nutritional abnormalities in order to improve your nursing care of clients with these illnesses.

✚ Protein–energy malnutrition

Nutritional deficiency—or protein–energy malnutrition (PEM)—occurs due to deprivation of protein, calories (energy), or both. PEM is mainly associated with a deficit in nutrition and energy in young children of underdeveloped countries. However, PEM is also evident in industrialized nations in institutionalized children and those with complex diseases, such as cancer. In these types of diseases, nutrition is a constant battle and requires nursing attention.

What is it?

Nutritional deficiencies, malnutrition, and PEM basically are the same thing: lack of adequate energy needed to maintain homeostasis of the body.

What causes it and why

PEM is caused by a decreased intake in nutrients or the body's inability to effectively process nutrients to be used as energy. In response to this, the body begins breaking itself down to provide energy. Additionally, the metabolism begins to slow in order to conserve energy.

Signs and symptoms and why

Table 13-1 details the signs and symptoms and why these signs and symptoms occur in general malnutrition.

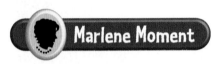

Marlene Moment

I knew I was burning calories as I watched that lady on the television exercise!

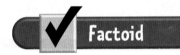

Factoid

A 4-year-old child with protein–energy malnutrition will look the age and size of a typical 2-year-old.

Table 13-1

Signs and symptoms	Why
Decreased adipose tissue	Body breaks down fat for energy in the absence of adequate calories
Protruding bones	Loss of adipose tissue and muscle
Thin, dry skin	Lack of nutrients
Alopecia	Lack of nutrients
Cachexia—muscle wasting muscle atrophy	Body breaks down muscle for energy in the absence of nutrients
Cognitive deficits	Lack of blood flow to the brain
Immunosuppression	Body's lack of energy and nutrients to fight infection
Diarrhea	Decreased acid production in the stomach can't fight bacteria
Heart atrophy	Lack of nutrients to support heart size
Heart failure	Red blood cell (RBC) count is low due to malnutrition; heart pumps harder and faster to provide what few oxygenated RBCs are left; finally heart wears out
Respiratory failure	Respiratory muscles—diaphragm—waste away due to starvation
Apathy and irritability	Low blood flow to the brain
Amenorrhea	Body tries to conserve energy; decreased levels of estrogen, luteinizing hormone, follicle stimulating hormone, and thyroid hormone
Low body temperature	Metabolism decreases
Decreased activity tolerance	Low energy
Edema	Serum protein (albumin) drops, causing fluid to leak out of the vascular space. Fluid begins to leak out of the vascular space into the interstitial space, abdomen, and other areas
Dull hair and dry, brittle nails	Fats are needed to keep hair and nails healthy

Source: Table created by author from Reference #1.

Quickie tests and treatments

Tests to detect malnutrition include bloodwork to evaluate albumin levels, electrolytes, total protein, and renal function. An electrocardiogram (EKG) is useful in measuring cardiac function. Treatment includes treating the underlying disorder with nutritional, hydration, and electrolyte therapy.

What can harm my client?

Malnutrition causes many complications. With altered acid production by the digestive system, frequent, fatal diarrhea—dysentery—occurs. Enzymes are in short supply because of the deteriorating gastrointestinal (GI) tract. Due to this deteriorating GI tract, food that is consumed can't be digested and absorbed. The cardiovascular system pumps a reduced amount of

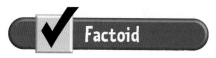

Factoid

Loss of body fat is first noticed in the face.

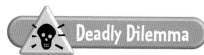

Deadly Dilemma

After 8 to 12 weeks of no nutrient intake, death will occur, if not sooner.

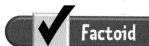

Factoid

Albumin, a protein in our body, acts like a sponge to hold fluid in the vascular spaces.

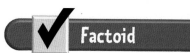

Factoid

The body burns up protein sources first in the presence of a calorie deficit.

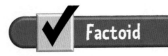

Factoid

Protein (albumin) holds on to fluid in the vascular space. When the albumin level is low, fluid starts to leak out into the tissue (interstitial space), and the client develops total body edema—anasarca.

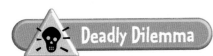

Deadly Dilemma

If the protein (albumin) is not replenished in the vascular space, then ALL of the fluid could leak out and cause vascular collapse.

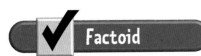

Factoid

Anemia causes the heart to beat faster, which circulates RBCs to provide oxygen to the body. If the heart beats quickly, with excessive force, and for an extended period of time, heart failure can occur.

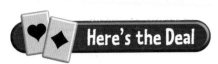

Here's the Deal

Anorexia nervosa is not an appetite problem. Deep-seated problems related to identity and autonomy are the root of the disorder.

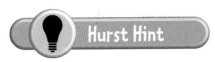

Hurst Hint

Clients may have bulimia nervosa in addition to anorexia nervosa.

blood, causing decreased heart rate and low blood pressure. Heart failure occurs due to the heart wearing out. It beats fast and hard to pump what little vascular volume is left. It will then wear out. Fluid accumulates in the arms, legs, and abdomen due to the decrease in protein—or osmotic pressure. The respiratory system slows due to reduced lung capacity, resulting in failure. The blood becomes low in iron, affecting its ability to carry oxygen. Anemia often leads to heart failure and occasionally sudden death. The immune system cannot fight infections or repair wounds, which can lead to death.

If I were your teacher, I would test you on . . .

Guaranteed that you'll see information related to the items in this list come test time!

- What is the cause of PEM?
- What are the signs and symptoms associated with malnutrition?
- Which diagnostic tests are used to detect malnutrition?
- What treatments are associated with malnutrition?

✚ Anorexia nervosa

Anorexia nervosa is an illness that results in malnutrition. Anorexia occurs mainly in industrialized societies. Let's look at this eating disorder more closely.

What is it?

Anorexia nervosa is an eating disorder of self-induced starvation. People with anorexia nervosa:

- Refuse to maintain a minimal normal body weight—15 % less than normal for age and height.
- Have a fear of weight gain.
- Have a distorted view of their body.

These patients view themselves as overweight, when actually they are underweight. Anorexia nervosa occurs mainly in young women, but is increasing in males. An interest in weight reduction and excessive physical exercise develops. Many patients with anorexia nervosa weigh less than 70 pounds and develop amenorrhea (lack of menstrual cycle).

Anorexia also means loss of appetite. In many medical conditions, patients experience anorexia due to disease states or side effects of medications. In anorexia nervosa, the patient feels hunger but refuses to eat. Anorexia nervosa is not loss of appetite in this case, but the denial of food with the purpose of self-starvation due to the fear of becoming overweight.

What causes it and why

Anorexia nervosa is a psychological disorder, not a physical one, although it does have physiologic effects. Some of the factors contributing to the development of anorexia nervosa are:

- Societal pressures to be thin.
- Family dynamics.

- Developmental stress.
- Personality characteristics.
- Triggers, such as abuse.

Anorexics do not perceive themselves as having an illness. This is the most difficult part of the disease. Until anorexics admit they have a disorder, they cannot be helped. One cause of anorexia nervosa is the client's feeling of lack of control. Since they feel they cannot control their life, they choose to control their eating habits in order to gain full control of their body. Controlling or domineering parents are also a causative factor. Some clients are so unhappy that they starve themselves in an attempt to literally vanish. Self-punishment for poor life choices and heredity also play a role.

Signs and symptoms and why

Table 13-2 demonstrates the key psychological signs and symptoms associated with anorexia nervosa and the cause of their occurrence.

Table 13-2

Psychological signs and symptoms	Why
Meticulous, compulsive, intelligent, high achiever, low self-concept; always been the perfect child	Personality of client who develops this disorder
Unusual and excessive concerns over weight and diet, as client is already thin	Etiology unknown
Constantly thinking about diet and weight, which increases as client becomes thinner	Etiology unknown
Complains of being fat when the client is emaciated	Etiology unknown
Denies being too thin and denies any problem exists	Etiology unknown
Resists treatment	Denies that a problem exists; fears weight gain
Hides and wastes food; denies this behavior	Etiology unknown
Constant thoughts of food in the presence of hunger, but will not eat	Etiology unknown
Cooks elaborate meals and collects recipes	Etiology unknown
Binges and purges by vomiting and using laxatives, diuretics, enemas; denies this behavior	Compulsion to lose weight
Places severe food restrictions on self	Compulsion to lose weight
Depression	Cause is different for each patient
Excessive exercise	Compulsion to lose weight

Source: Table created by author from Reference #3.

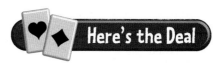

Here's the Deal

Since family problems may be an underlying cause of anorexia nervosa, family therapy is an important part of treatment.

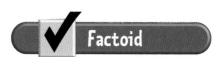

Factoid

Anorexia nervosa mainly affects middle- to high-income families.

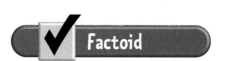

Factoid

Clients with eating disorders may be hyperactive, fidget, and chew gum constantly to burn more calories.

Table 13-3 describes the physical signs and symptoms of anorexia nervosa and why these signs and symptoms occur.

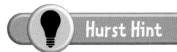

Anorexics may develop calluses on their knuckles from inserting their fingers into the oropharynx to induce vomiting. The knuckles scrape against the top teeth, causing calluses.

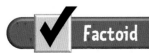

The esophagus may erode and ulcerate due to excessive vomiting.

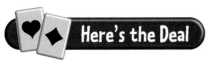

One criterion for diagnosing anorexia nervosa according to the *Diagnostic and Statistical Manual of Mental Disorders* (DSM) is the absence of 3 consecutive menstrual cycles.

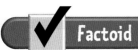

In male anorexics, the testosterone levels fluctuate, leading to erectile dysfunction and low sperm counts.

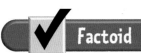

Some clients may experience metabolic acidosis as the body burns fat for energy. When fat is burned, ketones are produced. Ketones are acids, which make the blood acidic.

Table 13-3

Physical signs and symptoms	Why
Excessive weight loss of 15% of body weight or more	Malnutrition
Amenorrhea	Body tries to conserve energy; decreased levels of estrogen, luteinizing hormone, follicle-stimulating hormone, and thyroid hormone
Breast atrophy	Starvation; body uses fat for energy
Decreased libido	Low energy; decreases in estrogen, luteinizing hormone, follicle-stimulating hormone, and thyroid hormone
Decreased vital signs	Metabolic processes slow down to conserve energy; blood pressure drops due to decreased volume (less volume, less pressure); norepinephrine decreases—adrenal glands aren't working due to malnutrition; decreased norepinephrine contributes to a decreased heart rate
Hypothermia	Poor body insulation due to decreased adipose tissue; metabolism purposefully decreases to conserve energy and calories
Cold hands and feet	Decreased blood flow
Edema	Decreased protein in diet (protein holds on to fluid in the vascular space causing edema)
Lanugo—fine hair on the face and body	The body produces fine hair to insulate the body
Fluid and electrolyte imbalances	Poor intake; vomiting; use of diuretics, enemas, and laxatives
Arrhythmias	Electrolyte imbalances
Congestive heart failure (CHF)	Heart pumps hard and fast to supply what little fluid is present; it finally wears out
Dehydration	Decreased fluid intake
Fainting	Decreased blood flow to the brain
Gum disease; teeth enamel erosion	Excessive vomiting
Metabolic alkalosis	Acid loss due to vomiting creates alkalosis
Muscle atrophy; adipose loss	Starvation
Postural hypotension	Decreased fluid volume

(Continued)

Table 13-3. (*Continued*)

Physical signs and symptoms	Why
Anemia	Decreased red blood cell production due to starvation
Immunosuppression	Malnutrition
Fractures	Brittle bones due to malnutrition
Leg cramps	Hypokalemia due to decreased intake
Decreased gastric emptying	Gastrointestinal system slows to absorb as many nutrients as possible
Parotid gland enlargement and soreness	Excessive vomiting resulting in increased salivation

Source: Table created by author from References #2, #3, and #4.

Quickie tests and treatments

Tests to aid in the diagnosis of anorexia nervosa are an electrocardiogram (EKG), laboratory tests (elevated urea nitrogen and electrolyte imbalances), and an Eating Attitude Test. Treatments include therapy, nutritional counseling, anxiolytics, and antidepressants.

What can harm my client?

The following complications of anorexia nervosa can harm your client:

- Electrolyte imbalances leading to arrhythmias.
- Renal failure.
- Congestive heart failure (CHF).
- Suicide.
- Decreased immune system.

It is important to provide a thorough nursing assessment and interventions to prevent these complications and ensure a positive outcome for your clients.

If I were your teacher, I would test you on . . .

- The signs and symptoms and causes of anorexia nervosa and why they occur.
- Treatment and specific nursing interventions for anorexia nervosa.
- How malnutrition affects the body.
- Signs and symptoms of heart failure.
- Monitoring renal function in the anorexic patient.
- Recognition of life-threatening electrolyte imbalances.
- Nursing interventions to correct electrolyte imbalances.
- Emotional support of the client with anorexia nervosa.

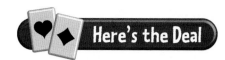

Here's the Deal

The client with anorexia nervosa may have lanugo, but she loses scalp hair due to malnutrition.

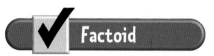

Factoid

The dentist may be the first to identify anorexia nervosa due to enamel erosion of the client's teeth.

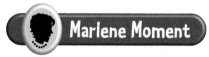

Marlene Moment

You must weigh your client first thing in the morning after voiding on a daily basis. Only a hospital gown is to be worn . . . the client wears the gown, not you!

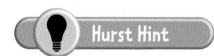

Hurst Hint

Make sure the client does not try to sneak a drink of water prior to weighing.

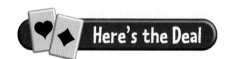

Here's the Deal

When food is being reintroduced during treatment, the nurse must monitor the client during meals and for at least 1 hour after meals to make sure the client does not vomit.

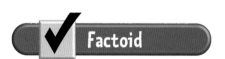

Factoid

Many clients have only one episode of anorexia nervosa. With a full recovery, relapse is uncommon.

✚ Bulimia nervosa

Bulimia nervosa is a behavioral disorder that affects young Caucasian women in Western society. Let's take a closer look . . .

What is it?

Bulimia nervosa is an eating disorder that is characterized by binge eating and purging. The client eats an enormous amount of food, and then induces vomiting. These patients are also known to use diuretics and laxatives as a way of getting rid of extra fluid and food. The bulimic is like the anorexic in that she fears weight gain. Binge–purge episodes can be precipitated by hunger, boredom, anger, anxiety, and depression. Bulimics spend much of their day in a starved state and suffer from malnutrition. Binge episodes generally occur every day or more often. Purging then occurs in an attempt to regain a sense of control and to eliminate the calories ingested. Purging may occur as many as 20 times a day. Bulimics do not generally have the dangerously low weight levels like anorexic patients. They will be in their normal weight range but at the lowest weight (in that range).

What causes it and why

The social pressures to be thin are a major contributing factor to the development of bulimia nervosa. The appetite regulation center in the hypothalamus is thought to be involved. There is dysregulation of neurotransmitters such as serotonin and other hormones. Bulimic patients tend to have depression, suicidal ideation, and impulsive behavior. Bulimics are more likely than anorexics to have been victims of sexual abuse.

Signs and symptoms and why

The signs and symptoms of bulimia nervosa are the same as anorexia nervosa with the addition of esophageal strictures due to excessive self-induced vomiting—acid erodes the lining of the esophagus, forming strictures from the scar tissue development.

Quickie tests and treatments

Tests used to diagnose bulimia nervosa are the Beck Depression Inventory, Eating Attitude Test, and laboratory tests to detect metabolic acidosis and metabolic alkalosis. Treatment includes cognitive and family therapy and selective serotonin reuptake inhibitors (SSRIs) such as paroxetine (Paxil) and fluoxetine (Prozac).

What can harm my client?

As with anorexia nervosa, complications due to electrolyte imbalances are a major concern. Other possible complications are:

- Complications listed under the discussion of anorexia nervosa earlier in the chapter.

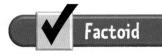

Factoid

After bulimics complete a binging episode—which they do find enjoyable—they experience intense self-criticism and depression.

- Ruptured stomach (leading to hemorrhage) from excessive vomiting.
- If syrup of ipecac is used to induce vomiting, cardio toxicity can occur.
- Excessive vomiting causes the esophageal sphincter to relax, which may result in aspiration pneumonia.
- Unrecognized signs of depression and suicide attempt.

If I were your teacher, I would test you on . . .

- What is bulimia nervosa?
- What factors contribute to bulimia nervosa?
- What does a patient with bulimia nervosa look like?
- What physical conditions may result from bulimia nervosa and why?
- Recognition of life-threatening electrolyte imbalances.
- Nursing interventions to correct electrolyte imbalances.
- Psychological support and referrals for clients with bulimia nervosa.

✚ Anorexia nervosa and bulimia nervosa at a glance

Table 13-4 outlines the differences between anorexia nervosa and bulimia nervosa.

Table 13-4

Anorexia nervosa	Bulimia nervosa
Possible binging	Frequent binging on high-calorie foods
Emaciated appearance	Thin; may be within normal weight range
Amenorrhea	Amenorrhea uncommon
Starvation	Binge and purge
Denies problem exists	Realizes problem exists
Possible hospitalization	Hospitalization uncommon
Substance abuse uncommon	Substance abuse common
Prefers healthy food when eating	Prefers sweet, high-calorie foods
Psychological disorder	Behavioral disorder

Source: Table created by author from Reference #2.

SUMMARY

Caring for clients with nutritional abnormalities requires compassion and sound knowledge of the complications associated with malnutrition. For those clients who have an eating disorder, strict attention to psychological disturbances such as depression and possible suicide are of the utmost importance.

PRACTICE QUESTIONS

1. When providing nutritional teaching to a client, the nurse knows the most important nutrient for body function is:

   1. Protein.

   2. Water.

   3. Carbohydrates.

   4. Lipids.

   Correct answer: 2. It's a fact . . . water is the MOST important nutrient found in the body, because every cell requires it to function properly.

2. A 7-month-old client is admitted to the emergency department (ED) for dehydration. While assessing the client's general appearance, the nurse notes the client is very small for its age and appears to have very little muscle or fat. The nurse suspects the client has:

   1. Protein-energy malnutrition (PEM).

   2. Anorexia nervosa.

   3. Bulimia nervosa.

   4. Leukemia.

   Correct answer: 1. These are typical symptoms of PEM—lack of energy to maintain homeostasis of the body. Anorexia nervosa and bulimia nervosa are not seen in a 7-month-old. These are not signs of leukemia.

3. A 15-year-old client presents to the ED after collapsing in class. Upon examination, the nurse finds the client has tooth erosion, an irregular heart rate, and is 10 lbs underweight. The nurse suspects:

   1. Anorexia nervosa.

   2. Bulimia nervosa.

   3. Hyperkalemia.

   4. Gastroenteritis.

   Correct answer: 2. Tooth erosion is very prevalent with bulimia due to excessive self-induced vomiting. Tooth erosion may exist with anorexia nervosa, but is not seen as frequently as with bulimia nervosa. The client would be hypokalemic from vomiting, not hyperkalemic. Tooth erosion is not associated with gastroenteritis.

4. The body burns which nutrient first in the presence of a calorie deficit?

   1. Fat.

   2. Carbohydrate.

   3. Vitamins.

   4. Protein.

Correct answer: 4. The body burns up protein sources first in the presence of a calorie deficit.

5. How does anorexia nervosa lead to metabolic acidosis?

1. The body burns fat for energy.

2. Acid loss is created due to vomiting.

3. Metabolic process slowing excessively.

4. The adrenal glands function slows down due to malnutrition.

Correct answer: 1. When fats are broken down for energy, ketones are produced. Ketones are acids. This leads to metabolic acidosis.

6. A 36-year-old client expresses a loss of appetite and is not eating. An appropriate nursing intervention is:

1. Administer an antiemetic.

2. Provide foods the client likes.

3. Insert a nasogastric (NG) tube for feedings.

4. Provide the client with privacy.

Correct answer: 2. Antiemetics are given for nausea and vomiting. Inserting an NG tube at this point is a premature intervention. How does privacy increase appetite? It doesn't! The correct answer is to give the client foods she likes, please!

7. A major energy source for the body is which nutrient?

1. Proteins.

2. Minerals.

3. Carbohydrates.

4. Water.

Correct answer: 3. Carbohydrates are the major energy nutrient.

8. When assessing a client's nutritional status, which is indicative of malnutrition?

1. Dull hair.

2. A body mass index (BMI) of 24.

3. Moist mucous membranes.

4. Soft abdomen.

Correct answer: 1. A body mass index of 24 is normal, as are moist mucous membranes and a soft abdomen. Dull hair and dry, brittle nails indicate malnutrition.

9. Why do most clients with anorexia nervosa resist treatment?

1. Lack of insurance.

2. Fear of purging in front of others.

3. Fear of weight gain.

4. Lack of self-confidence.

Correct answer: **3.** Most anorexics resist treatment because they fear weight gain and they often deny that they have a problem. The other answer choices are inappropriate.

10. Bulimics are at risk for which complication?

1. Ruptured spleen.

2. Aspiration pneumonia.

3. Constipation.

4. Congestive heart failure (CHF).

Correct answer: **2.** Bulimics are at risk for a ruptured stomach (leads to hemorrhage) from excessive vomiting; cardio toxicity if syrup of ipecac is used to induce vomiting; aspiration pneumonia from relaxation of the esophageal sphincter due to excessive vomiting; and depression and suicide attempt.

References

1. Whitney E, Rolfes SR. *Understanding Nutrition.* 10th ed. Belmont, CA: Thompson Wadsworth; 2005.

2. Ignatavicius DD, Workman ML, Mishler MA. *Medical-Surgical Nursing Across the Health Care Continuum.* 3rd ed. Philadelphia: Saunders; 1999.

3. Huether SE, McCance KL. *Understanding Pathophysiology.* 3rd ed. St. Louis: Mosby; 2004.

4. Porth CM. *Essentials of Pathophysiology.* 2nd ed. Philadelphia: Lippincott Williams & Wilkins; 2007.

Bibliography

Hurst Review Services. www.hurstreview.com.

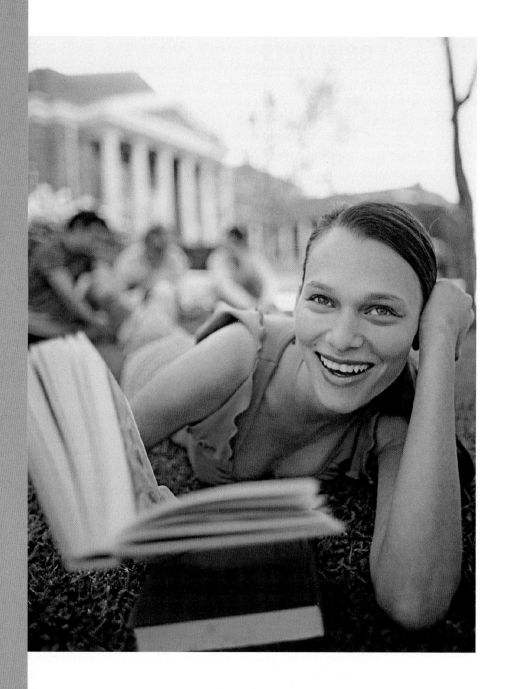

CHAPTER

14 Endocrine System

OBJECTIVES

In this chapter, you'll review:

- The normal function of the endocrine system.
- The relationship between abnormal endocrine hormonal levels and resulting endocrine disorders.
- Need-to-know information regarding common endocrine disorders, causes, signs and symptoms, treatment, and important patient education tidbits.

LET'S GET THE NORMAL STUFF STRAIGHT FIRST

Along with the nervous system and the immune system, the endocrine system plays a crucial role in the communication and regulation of body systems. The endocrine system consists of glands and other glandular tissues that produce, store, and secrete hormones (chemical substances). Most hormones are released into the blood circulation from a **single** gland (adrenals, pituitary, thyroid gland) and transported to specific target cells in another area of the body. The hormones act as change agents for important functions in the body. Testosterone is the exception to this rule. Testosterone is secreted by two glands, the adrenal glands and the testes. There are sites throughout the body that constantly monitor the levels of hormones in the blood. The hypothalamus is the main gland that keeps track of all the hormone levels.

Hormones are part of either a positive or a negative feedback loop. Most hormones work through a negative feedback loop. When the hypothalamus senses high levels of a certain hormone, it sends out a signal that says, "Don't make any more for a while!" This allows the hormone level to come back down into normal range. When a certain hormone level gets too low, the hypothalamus says, "Hey! You need to start producing and secreting some more." The endocrine system has a role in reproduction, growth and development, and energy metabolism and regulation.

✚ Which glands belong to the endocrine system?

The following glands help the endocrine system function properly (Fig. 14-1):

- Hypothalamus.
- Pituitary.
- Thyroid.
- Parathyroids.
- Adrenals.
- Pancreas.

- Ovaries.
- Testes.
- Pineal glands.
- Thymus.

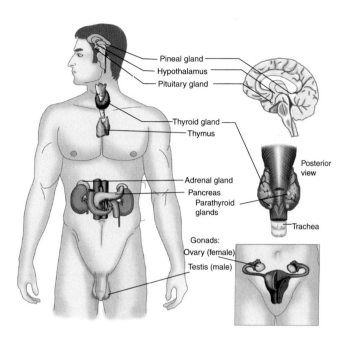

◀ Figure 14-1. The major organs in the endocrine system. (From Saladin K. *Anatomy and Physiology: The Unity of Form and Function.* 4th ed. New York: McGraw-Hill; 2007.)

✚ More on hormones

The word hormone in Greek means "to stir up." Think about the effects that happen in the body when you are terrified—you get a surge of adrenaline—or during sexual activity—sex hormones are all stirred up! Hormones are either made of protein molecules or steroid molecules. Endocrinology is the study of hormones.

Table 14-1 lists the hormones associated with each gland.

Table 14-1

Gland	Hormone
Hypothalamus	Corticotropin-releasing hormone (CRH)
	Thyrotropin-releasing hormone (TRH)
	Gonadotropin-releasing hormone (GnRH)
	Growth hormone inhibitory hormone (AKA somatostatin)
	Growth hormone releasing hormone (GHRH)
	Prolactin-inhibiting hormone (PIH)
	Melanocyte-stimulating hormone (MSH)
Anterior pituitary	Thyroid-stimulating hormone (TSH)
	Adrenocorticotropic hormone (ACTH, corticotropin)
	Luteinizing hormone (LH)
	Follicle-stimulating hormone (FSH)

(Continued)

Table 14-1. (*Continued*)

Gland	Hormone
	Prolactin (PRL)
	Growth hormone (GH or somatotropin)
	Melanocyte-stimulating hormone (MSH)
Posterior pituitary	Vasopressin (antidiuretic hormone [ADH])
	Oxytocin
Thyroid	T3
	T4
	Calcitonin
Parathyroid	Parathyroid hormone
Adrenal cortex	Glucocorticoids (aka cortisol)
	Mineralocorticoids (aldosterone)
Adrenal medulla	Epinephrine
	Norepinephrine
Ovary	Estrogen
	Progesterone
Testes	Testosterone
Pancreas	Insulin
	Glucagon
	Somatostatin

Source: Created by author from References #1 to #3.

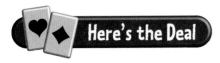

Endocrine glands secrete chemical substances directly into the circulation to be transported to their target cells. Exocrine glands secrete substances into ducts to be released into a body cavity or on to a body surface.

✚ How do endocrine hormones work?

The endocrine hormones are chemical messengers that are secreted by the endocrine organs. These hormones are transported through the blood to target cells where they bind to specific receptor sites and exert their action on the cell. The receptors then recognize the specific hormone and a cellular response follows. Hormones do not cause reactions; instead they regulate tissue responses. Some hormones require a protein carrier to regulate tissue responses. Hormone levels are controlled by the pituitary gland and by a series of feedback systems, both negative and positive. In other words, sensors in the endocrine system detect changing levels of hormones and then take action to correct the problem and facilitate the return to homeostasis. Hormones are released by three different mechanisms:

1. Hormonal mechanism: for example, the hypothalamus secretes hormones that stimulate the anterior pituitary gland to secrete hormones that stimulate other endocrine glands to secrete hormones . . . that's a lot of secreting of hormones!

2. Humoral mechanism: for example, capillary blood contains a low concentration of calcium that stimulates secretion of parathyroid hormone. Parathyroid hormone makes serum calcium go up.

3. Neural mechanism: preganglionic SNS fiber stimulates the adrenal medulla cells to secrete catecholamines.

Hormones affect all body tissues and organs, making it difficult sometimes to assess for dysfunction of the endocrine system. I know this sounds very difficult, but I'm going to make it a lot easier for you by explaining how the key endocrine glands function and how this relates to endocrine illnesses! Read on!

✚ Thyroid gland

The thyroid gland lies under the larynx and takes iodine from the blood to make thyroid hormones (Fig. 14-2). When thyroid hormone levels get low, the hypothalamus is triggered to release thyroid-releasing hormone (TRH):

→ TRH triggers the anterior pituitary to release thyroid-stimulating hormone (TSH).

→ TSH stimulates the thyroid gland to produce thyroid hormone that is released into the blood.

→ Metabolism increases and energy levels increase (Fig. 14-3).

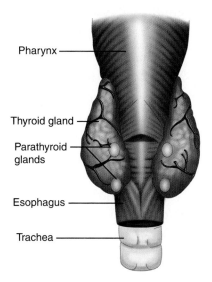

◀ Figure 14-2. Thyroid gland (posterior view).

Pharynx

Thyroid gland

Parathyroid glands

Esophagus

Trachea

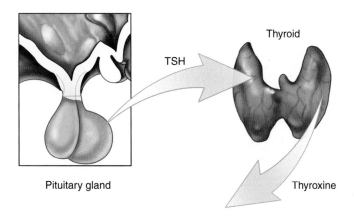

◀ Figure 14-3. The pituitary gland secretes TSH, and this will result in the thyroid releasing T4. (From Saladin K. *Anatomy and Physiology: The Unity of Form and Function.* 4th ed. New York: McGraw-Hill; 2007.)

TSH

Thyroid

Pituitary gland

Thyroxine

Following are some facts you should know about the thyroid gland:

- A drop in body temperature, stress of any kind, and low levels of T4 trigger the process outlined earlier. For example, decreased body temperature results in production of thyroid hormone in order to increase body temperature. This is a normal compensatory mechanism.

- For the body to produce adequate amounts of thyroid hormone, adequate amounts of protein and iodine (which is definitely not a problem with my diet) must be taken in.

- The thyroid produces 3 hormones: T3, T4, and calcitonin.

Let's focus on T3 and T4 first:

- Thyroid hormone is located in the body in 2 forms: T3 and T4.

- Fancy word for T3 = triiodothyronine.

- Fancy word for T4 = thyroxine.

- Since these words are not easy to remember or say, we just say T3 and T4.

- Both T3 and T4 increase metabolic rate of cells and tissues.

- T4 is the precursor to T3.

- T3 regulates the metabolic rate of all cells and all processes of cell growth and tissue differentiation.

- T3 and T4 indirectly increase blood glucose levels.

- When thinking about thyroid hormones think energy and metabolism! You either have too much or not enough.

- When you hear the term "thyroid hormone," this means T3 and T4 in combination. They differ in structure (their looks), but their function is the same.

- T4 and T3 are just out there in the body floating around having a great time. At some point in time T4 moves into the cell and is converted to T3 (which is the **most active** form of thyroid hormone). This is just a normal process that occurs in the body.

- Being cold *increases* the conversion of T4 to T3.

- Things such as stress, starvation, certain dyes, and certain drugs like steroids, beta-blockers, PTU (propylthiouracil), and amiodarone *decrease* the conversion of T4 to T3.

How does thyroid hormone affect the body?

Thyroid hormone:

1. Increases the metabolism of protein, fat, and glucose.

2. Increases body temperature in response to an elevated metabolism, which produces body heat.

3. Increases the use of oxygen as metabolism increases.

4. Aids in the development of the neural and skeletal systems in fetuses.

5. Helps regulate secretion of growth hormone.

6. Aids in production of red blood cells.

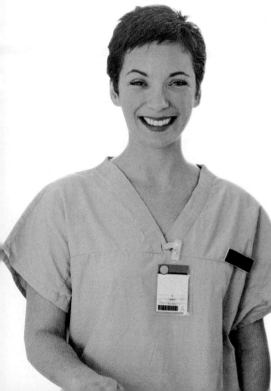

7. Affects respiratory rate: too much thyroid hormone increases respiratory rate, and too little decreases respiratory rate.

8. Aids in normal growth and development.

Which illnesses are associated with thyroid hormone problems?

Too much thyroid hormone = hyperthyroidism.

Too little thyroid hormone = hypothyroidism.

If hypothyroidism occurs in the very young, it is called cretinism.
    Let's look at another hormone produced by the thyroid: calcitonin.

How does calcitonin affect the body?

Calcitonin:

- Targets the bones, kidneys, and epithelial cells of the intestines.

- Lowers serum calcium by sending a signal to the thyroid that says, "stop secreting calcitonin; calcium is too low; we need calcium from the bones." Therefore, calcitonin secretion decreases, calcium is released from the bone, and serum calcium goes up.

- Decreases blood/serum calcium in three ways:

    1. Decreases intestines' ability to absorb calcium (so calcium is lost).

    2. Decreases osteoclast activity in the bones. Osteoclasts break down bone and release calcium from the broken-down bone into the blood/serum. If osteoclasts are not active, this process does not occur and serum calcium goes down.

    3. Decreases calcium resorption from the kidney tubules. If calcium is not being reabsorbed by the tubules, it is being excreted out of the body.

Which illnesses are associated with calcitonin problems?

You've never heard of the disease hypercalcitoninemia because it doesn't exist! Calcitonin problems manifest themselves as signs and symptoms rather than a disease. With calcitonin problems, think bone problems. If the calcitonin level is too high, then the serum calcium is going to be low as calcium is being driven back into the bone. If the calcitonin level is too low, then the serum calcium level will be too high as calcium is being released from the bone and into the blood, causing weak and brittle bones. Therefore, you must have a strong understanding of hypercalcemia (same as hypophosphatemia) and hypocalcemia (same as hyperphosphatemia). Remember, the electrolytes; phosphate and calcium; have an inverse relationship.

    Increased levels of calcitonin in the blood (low serum calcium) are associated with:

- Thyroid cancer: medullary carcinoma of the thyroid, which occurs with something called multiple endocrine neoplasia syndrome; this syndrome is a very rare genetic cancer disorder.

- Cancer of the lung, breast, small cell (oat cell) carcinoma, and pancreatic cancers.

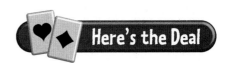

If thyroid hormone levels are high, TSH release is decreased. If thyroid hormone levels are low, TSH release is increased.

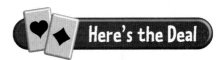

Bone resorption is always a confusing concept. Bone resorption occurs when osteoclasts break down bone and release calcium from the bone into the blood. This causes the serum calcium to go up. The word "resorption" makes it confusing because it sounds like the bone is ABSORBING the calcium. Not happening!

- Chronic renal failure.
- Zollinger–Ellison syndrome.
- Pernicious anemia.
- Liver disease.
- Complications with pregnancy at term.

Decreased levels of calcitonin in the blood (low serum calcium) may lead to:

- Kidney stones.
- Osteoporosis.

LET'S GET DOWN TO SPECIFICS

Let's get down to the specific illnesses that can occur when the endocrine system is not in homeostasis. When the endocrine system is out of balance, it affects your clients in predictable ways. We will explore what happens, what the experience is like for the client, and how it can be managed.

✚ Hyperthyroidism

What is it?

Hyperthyroidism is due to an overactive thyroid that leads to increased levels of thyroid hormone. As a result, the body's metabolism is significantly increased. Let's get something straight right now! Hyperthyroidism is hyperthyroidism. Yes, there are many different causes of it and the names of the hyperthyroid disease may vary depending upon the cause. However, all of the different diseases have the same end result—too much thyroid hormone.

   Many times people will say hyperthyroidism is the same thing as Graves' disease, and they will use the terms interchangeably. Graves' disease is an autoimmune disorder that **causes** hyperthyroidism. If you come across a test question on Graves' disease, think hyperthyroidism!

What causes it and why

Table 14-2 shows the causes and why associated with hyperthyroidism.

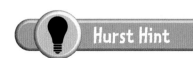

Hyperthyroidism is mainly seen in females and is most common after childbirth or during menopause.

Table 14-2

Causes	Why
Graves' disease	These clients have a gene that causes antibodies to stimulate the thyroid to produce and secrete excess thyroid hormones in the blood
Hashimoto's thyroiditis: most common thyroid disorder in the U.S.	Overactive thyroid due to an autoimmune attack of the thyroid; 50% of clients develop hypothyroidism

(Continued)

Table 14-2. (*Continued*)

Causes	Why
Infected thyroid: viral or bacterial thyroiditis	Virus or bacteria invade the thyroid, causing more thyroid hormone to be released
Thyroiditis: acute, inflammatory problem; thyroid does return to normal with treatment	Inflammation of the thyroid gland causes stored thyroid hormone to be released
Toxic nodules (adenoma), tumors, thyroid cancer	Tumors and nodules can produce too much thyroid hormone
Overactive pituitary: very rare cause	Produces too much TSH, which triggers thyroid gland to release thyroid hormone
Any severe illness	Body's natural response is to produce more hormones for energy
Toxic substances and radiation exposure	Causes inflammation that releases stored thyroid hormone

Source: Created by author from References #1, #2, and #4.

Did you notice that no matter the illness, the client's primary problem was the same?

Too much thyroid hormone!

Signs and symptoms and why

Table 14-3 shows the signs and symptoms and rationales associated with hyperthyroidism.

Remember this: thyroid hormones give you energy and increase metabolism!

Table 14-3

Signs and symptoms	Why
Goiter	Overstimulated and overworked thyroid; hypertrophy of thyroid
Thyroid may be palpable; may auscultate a bruit	Enlarged thyroid; circulation to area increases, causing bruit
Nervousness, jitteriness, tremor	Too much energy; stimulation of sympathetic nervous system; muscles react more vigorously due to an increased effect on neural synapses
Heat intolerance, sweating	Increased metabolism
Weight loss in the presence of increased appetite	Increased metabolism
Increased bowel movements; hyperactive bowel sounds	Hyperactive GI system
Exophthalmos (protrusion of eyeball): only seen with Graves' disease	Fluid accumulates behind the eye, which pushes the eye forward; increased fat deposits around the eye

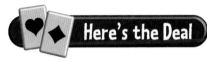

Here's the Deal

Hashimoto's thyroiditis can cause hyperthyroidism or hypothyroidism. The client's symptoms depend on which phase of the disease she is in.

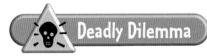

Deadly Dilemma

Excessive palpation of a goiter can cause a release of thyroid hormone that could throw the client into thyroid storm.

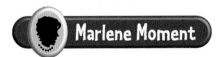

Marlene Moment

Hmmm . . . losing weight while still eating? Might be OK for a month or so!

(*Continued*)

Table 14-3. (*Continued*)

Signs and symptoms	Why
Decreased concentration, mood swings	Hyperstimulated central nervous system
Clumsiness	Increased spinal cord activity
Moist, smooth, flushed warm skin	Increased metabolism causing sweating and warmth; vasodilation helps body heat escape
Fine, soft hair; premature graying; hair loss; weak nails	Dermal layer of skin is affected; increased circulation causes increased growth and brittleness of hair and nails
Normal blood pressure; increased pulse (90 to 160 beats/minute at rest); bounding pulse; arrhythmia; palpitation (atrial fibrillation in clients over age 50)	Increased cardiac output; systemic vasodilation effect to help rid the body of heat. The two counteract each other, keeping the BP in a close to normal range. BP will go up if the client begins to go into thyroid storm; arrhythmias and palpitations due to stimulation of nervous system
Increased cardiac output	Heart is working hard and is pumping more blood out to the systemic circulation; however, if the heart continues to work this hard over a period of time, then heart failure (left ventricular hypertrophy) can begin, which would result in a decreased cardiac output; depends on how long your client has had untreated hyperthyroidism
Increased respiratory rate	Body is using more oxygen since it is in a hypermetabolic state; client breathes faster to get more oxygen in
Dyspnea on exertion	Body is in a hypermetabolic state and uses more oxygen. If the heart is failing due to stress, cardiac output decreases, preventing blood from moving forward into the systemic circulation. If the blood is not being pumped out to the body, then it is going to start to go backward into the lungs. No wonder the client is short of breath!
Menstrual problems (amenorrhea); fertility problems	Thyroid hormone controls FSH and LH, which are very important in regulation of ovulation and menses; too much thyroid hormone will alter these normal mechanisms
Decreased libido	Thyroid gland influences all hormones
Gynecomastia in men (rare)	Thyroid gland influences all hormones; may cause an increase in estrogen

Source: Created by author from References #4 and #5.

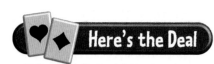

Here's the Deal

Hyperthyroidism may be confused with pheochromocytoma, sepsis, sympathomimetic ingestion, and psychosis/mania.

WILL SOMEBODY PLEASE EXPLAIN WHAT A GOITER IS?   Okay, I will
(Fig. 14-4). A goiter is an enlarged thyroid. Normally, the thyroid cannot
be seen when looking at someone. However, you can feel it, especially
when the client swallows. A goiter is usually easy to spot. The neck may
be enlarged all the way around or just in one spot. You've probably seen
pictures of this in your med-surg books.

Goiter can accompany hyperthyroidism and hypothyroidism. How?
In hyperthyroidism, the thyroid is working overtime making more
hormones and pumping them into the blood. Anytime an organ is
working hard it hypertrophies—just like the biceps muscle when
biceps curls are done on a regular basis. In hyperthyroidism, the thyroid
enlarges because it is working very hard to make thyroid hormones, thus
causing a goiter.

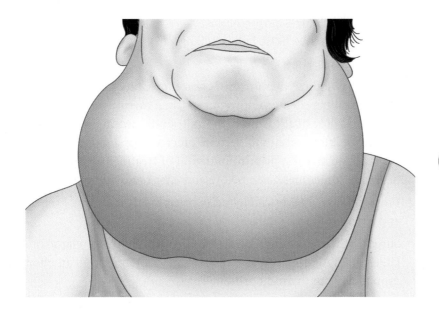

◀ Figure 14-4. Goiter. (From Saladin K.
*Anatomy and Physiology: The Unity of
Form and Function.* 4th ed. New York:
McGraw-Hill; 2007.)

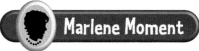

This is either a goiter or this
patient could have swallowed a
football. Note: This picture is an
extreme example; most goiters are
not this drastic!

Quickie tests and treatments

Tests:

- Thyroid-stimulating hormone (TSH): low or undetectable.

- T3 and T4: increased.

- Radioactive iodine uptake test (scan): increased.

- Pregnancy test: hyperthyroidism can occur during the first 4 months
  of pregnancy when hCG levels are high; pregnancy can cause
  hyperthyroidism.

- CT or MRI of the eye orbit if client has exophthalmos, especially if it
  is unilateral: monitor for pressure on the optic nerve or orbital
  contents.

- Antinuclear antibody (ANA): presence of autoimmune marker
  because Graves' disease is an autoimmune disease affecting the thyroid
  gland.

- Fine-needle biopsy: etiology of nodular lesions. This is the preferred
  approach to clients with thyroid masses.

Treatment:

- Depends on the severity of the disease and is client specific.
- Monitor for arrhythmias; maintain pulse at 80 beats/minute.
- Propylthiouracil (Propyl-Thyracil) and methimazole (Tapazole): inhibits thyroid hormone synthesis.
- Potassium iodide (Pima), Lugol's solution, sodium iodide (Iodotope): block hormone release.
- Propylthiouracil (Propyl-Thyracil) and dexamethasone (Decadron): prevent conversion of T4 to T3.
- Beta-blockers (atenolol [Tenormin]): decrease effects of thyroid hormone; decrease tachycardia and nervousness.
- Acetaminophen: decreases fever; aspirin is contraindicated because it displaces thyroid hormone from thyroglobulin, causing thyroid hormone levels to increase.
- Manage congestive heart failure (CHF).
- Manage dehydration.
- Radioactive iodine: treatment of choice for Graves' disease; given slowly until the client is euthyroid (normal thyroid function). Only a single oral dose of I^{131} is needed. Contraindicated in pregnancy and clients are informed not to become pregnant for 3 months after treatment. Pregnancy test prior to initiation of treatment. Antithyroid drugs are sometimes given before and after radioiodine treatment.
- Propylthiouracil (Propyl-Thyracil): preferred drug during pregnancy and breast-feeding.
- Surgery (thyroidectomy): when the client continues to relapse or has a large goiter. All or part of the thyroid may be removed in an effort to drop the serum thyroid hormone levels.

  Monitor for hypocalcemia postop: parathyroids may be removed during surgery.

  Iodine compounds such as potassium iodide (Pima), Lugol's solution, and SSKI may be given preoperatively. They decrease vascularity in order to prevent bleeding postop. They must be given with milk or juice with straw, because they stain the teeth.
- Thyroid storm treatment: antithyroid drugs prevent the conversion of T4 to T3; beta-blockers to decrease sympathetic effects such as increased blood pressure and tachycardia; corticosteroids to decrease conversion of T4 to T3; increase fluids and caloric intake to hydrate and maintain strength; monitor for CHF and stroke; administer oxygen; decrease body temperature; sedate for comfort.
- Ophthalmologic treatment: eye lubricants such as artificial tears, petrolatum, and lacrilube; sunglasses for the sun. At night, elevation of the bed (to decrease fluid retention behind eyes) and eye protectors during sleep can be helpful to protect the protruding eye.
- Client may require referral to specialist for high doses of prednisone, orbital irradiation, or decompression of the orbit by surgery in order to save vision.

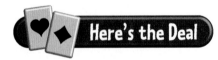

Here's the Deal

Agranulocytosis (white blood cell count drops very low) can develop as a side effect of the antithyroid drugs. Signs of this include sore mouth, sore throat, rash, and fever. A white blood cell count should be checked prior to initiating therapy.

What can harm my client?

- Extreme tachycardia.
- Extreme hyperpyrexia.
- Arrhythmias.
- If respiratory rate increased significantly, may induce respiratory alkalosis.
- Hypocalcemia, which could occur postthyroidectomy.
- Thyroid storm—hyperthyroidism multiplied by 100, in my opinion. This is a medical emergency manifested by high fever, tachycardia, CHF, angina, agitation, restlessness, and delirium. Mortality rate is high.
- When the thyroid is destroyed by radioactive iodine, thyroid hormone levels will drop. This is expected. However, that little piece of thyroid that is left is sitting there looking at the blood saying, "Where did all the hormones go?!" So the small piece of functioning thyroid that is left goes crazy and overproduces hormones. This is called a rebound effect. It is rare, but can be life threatening.

If I were your teacher, I would test you on . . .

- Causes and why.
- Signs and symptoms and why.
- Nursing care associated with tests and treatments.
- Importance of monitoring for arrhythmias, CHF.
- Promotion of client comfort (decreasing activities, maintaining a cool room, wearing less clothing, elevating the head of the bed (HOB) for dyspnea, promoting a calm atmosphere).
- Importance of nutrition and hydration.
- Treatment of hypothermia.
- Eye care (eye drops for exophthalmos).
- Effects of prolonged hypertension.
- Side effects of medications and related client teaching.
- Counseling on body image (goiter, gynecomastia).
- Counseling on sexual problems.
- Fluid imbalances (sweating a lot, diarrhea, increased metabolism).
- Electrolyte imbalances (especially postthyroidectomy, postradioactive iodine).
- Safety precautions (clumsiness).
- Thyroid storm recognition and treatment.
- How radioactive iodine works.
- Complication to watch for: postradioactive iodine (hypothyroidism, rebound thyroid storm).
- Care of the client postthyroidectomy.
- Care of client receiving I^{131}.

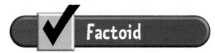

There are two types of iodine: dietary iodine and medicinal iodine. They each have totally different actions.

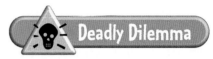

Asthmatics and diabetics should not be given beta-blockers. Beta-blockers can cause bronchospasm and mask the signs of hypoglycemia.

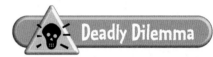

Postradioactive iodine. The client should stay away from babies, not kiss anyone, and cover the mouth and nose when coughing and sneezing for 24 hours after treatment as the iodine can be shed in saliva.

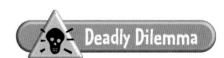

Be sure to watch for hypocalcemia postop thyroidectomy, as this electrolyte imbalance can affect the airway, the heart, and cause seizures!

✚ Hypothyroidism

What is it?

Hypothyroidism is characterized by underactivity of the thyroid gland. As a result, the thyroid does not produce enough thyroid hormone, which slows all body functions and metabolism.

- Low levels of thyroid hormone lead to a decreased metabolic rate (everything slows down).

- An insufficient amount of thyroid hormone causes abnormal lipid metabolism, with increased cholesterol and triglyceride levels. These two things increase the presence of atherosclerosis and cardiac disease. The etiology of this particular aspect of hypothyroidism is not well understood.

- The terms "myxedema" and "hypothyroidism" are frequently used interchangeably (especially in test questions). Different sources explain myxedema different ways. Some sources say myxedema is actually a condition (basically edema) that results from prolonged hypothyroidism. Other sources say that when hypothyroidism becomes severe, it is then called myxedema. The fluid associated with myxedema is made of mucins that trap water in the interstitial space. Pleural, cardiac, and abdominal effusions are a result of this process. Mucinous edema = myxedema.

- Myxedema coma is a rare presentation of untreated hypothyroidism. It is usually seen in elderly women with chronic hypothyroidism. It is an end-stage manifestation of hypothyroidism.

  Major symptoms include cardiovascular collapse, hypoventilation, hyponatremia, hypoglycemia, and lactic acidosis. The death rate for myxedema coma is extremely high, so it is a life-threatening emergency. Severe hypothyroid clients are at risk for myxedema coma when exposed to the following conditions: acute illness, anesthesia, surgery, hypothermia, chemotherapy, sedatives, rapid withdrawal of thyroid medications, and untreated or under-treated hypothyroidism.

- Cretinism is when hypothyroidism is present at birth. This is very dangerous if not detected early, because it can lead to slowed mental and physical development. A baby's thyroid level is checked in the hospital prior to discharge. If the baby does not develop appropriately, does sleep a lot, or does gain an unusual amount of weight, a thyroid panel may be repeated. Once detected, treatment is immediate.

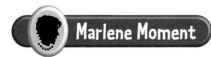

Here's the Deal

Myxedema is the worst-case scenario of hypothyroidism. If a test question says "myxedema," think hypothyroidism.

Marlene Moment

If your new baby is the "best baby in the whole world" because she does not wake up during the night, she never cries or fusses, and she is still gaining weight, you in turn feel great (because you've been sleeping so well) and have started a new step aerobics class, then you MAY want to have the baby's thyroid hormone levels checked. This scenario is just too good to be true!

What causes it and why

There are three classifications of hypothyroidism:

1. Primary: the problem is located within the gland itself.

2. Secondary: the problem is located in the pituitary.

3. Tertiary: the problem is in the hypothalamus.

The most common type of hypothyroidism is primary hypothyroidism. Table 14-4 shows the causes and why of primary hypothyroidism.

Table 14-4

Causes	Why
Hashimoto's thyroiditis (most common cause of hypothyroidism)	The thyroid is gradually destroyed and produces decreased amounts of thyroid hormone
Congenital defects	Poor or absent thyroid development in utero
Thyroidectomy (surgically induced hypothyroidism)	If you do not have a thyroid, you cannot make thyroid hormone
Radiation therapy used in treatment for cancers of the head and neck	Loss of thyroid tissue decreases hormone output
Antithyroid medications (drug induced)	Decreased thyroid hormone production
Thyroiditis	Bacterial or viral infection causes decreased thyroid hormone
Pituitary failure (very rare)	Cannot produce TSH, so thyroid hormone levels drop
Pregnancy	Immune system response where antibodies attack the thyroid, thus decreasing output of thyroid hormones
Iodine deficiency	Dietary iodine is necessary for thyroid hormone production; this is only seen in certain parts of the world (in the United States, dietary iodine is added to table salt)
Medications (aka drug goitrogen) Lithium carbonate (Eskalith) Iodide Propylthiouracil (Propyl-Thyracil) Methimazole (Tapazole) Sulfonamides Amiodarone (Cordarone) Inteferon alpha (Alferon N) Interleukin 2 (Proleukin)	Can cause a decreased output of thyroid hormones

Source: Created by author from References #1 and #2.

Notice something? No matter what the cause of hypothyroidism, the end result was the same:

→ low thyroid hormone levels!

Signs and symptoms and why

Picture yourself being so tired and sluggish, gaining weight, and not having energy or enthusiasm. Hmmmmm. Sounds like nursing school!

Table 14-5 shows the signs and symptoms and associated causes of hypothyroidism.

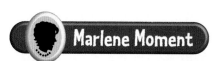

Udder stuff . . . in the United States, it is rare to have a dietary iodine deficiency, as we use plenty of iodized salt. Our dairy farmers have been on top of iodine deficiency for a long time as they use iodine to sterilize the milk cow's udders, so now we have plenty of iodine in our dairy products as well! Thank you, dairy farmers!

Table 14-5

Signs and symptoms	Why
Slowed thinking, decreased attention span, clumsiness, slowed movements, slurred speech	Low energy
Decreased heart rate leading to low cardiac output; decreased temp	All body processes are slowed; metabolism is slowed leading to a decreased temp
Fluid volume excess	If cardiac output is decreased (from low heart rate), then renal perfusion is compromised, leading to decreased fluid excretion. If fluid is not excreted, it remains in the body and builds up causing volume excess
Fatigue	Low energy
Puffy hands, feet, and eyes	Fluid retention
Intolerance to cold temperatures; cold hands and feet	Decreased metabolic rate and decreased heat production; client is already cold and can't tolerate being colder
Increased weight	Slowed metabolism; weight gain is not because the client is eating more but because metabolism is slowed
Decreased caloric requirements	When metabolism is slowed, fewer calories are needed
Constipation (can lead to megacolon)	Slowed GI tract related to low energy
Change in reproductive function (no ovulation—also called anovulation)	When the thyroid is sick, the reproductive system is usually affected; the thyroid has an effect on FSH, LH, and prolactin levels
Dry, flaky skin; thinning hair; may lose outer third of eyebrows; brittle fingernails	Lack of nutrients to cells
Prolonged deep tendon reflex (especially ankle jerk); ataxia, nystagmus	TH affects neural control of muscle tone; a decrease in TH causes muscles to react slowly

Source: Created by author from References #1 and #2.

Quickie tests and treatments

Tests:

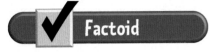

Hypothyroidism may be confused with depression, heart failure or hypoalbuminemia (due to edema).

- Newborn screening is performed in all states after delivery and prior to leaving the hospital. Remember that the infants can still develop hypothyroidism several weeks later even though they had a normal TSH while hospitalized.

- TSH: elevated. Thyroid says to the brain, "We need stimulation in order to produce thyroid hormone. Send MORE, send MORE!" This occurs in primary hypothyroidism. No matter how much TSH is sent, the thyroid hormone levels stay the same. In pituitary insufficiency, the TSH may be decreased or normal. If the pituitary is the main problem, then it may have difficulty secreting TSH.

- Serum T3 and T4: decreased, especially T4.
- Blood tests for antibodies: because Hashimoto's thyroiditis is an autoimmune problem.
- Thyroid scan or sonogram: detects structural abnormalities.
- CT and MRI: detects pituitary or hypothalamic lesions causing secondary hypothyroidism.
- Cholesterol: elevated due to abnormal lipid metabolism.
- EKG: shows varying degrees of bradycardia.

Treatments:

- Levothyroxine (Synthroid) is the treatment of choice even in pregnant women. Watch for cardiac problems, especially in the elderly (heart rate and workload of heart are going to go up). Remember, too, most hypothyroid clients have high cholesterol and triglycerides.
- Women who take estrogen may require higher doses of thyroid supplement.
- Levothyroxine must be continued for life and may need to be adjusted periodically throughout the client's life by testing TSH levels and monitoring clinical status.
- IV levothyroxine is given for myxedema in the hospital. These clients will need warm blankets due to hypothermia. Sometimes, intubation is needed for assisted mechanical ventilation.

What can harm my client?

- Sedating a hypothyroid client could kill him as his body is depressed already.
- Myxedema coma: includes stupor, hypoventilation, hypoglycemia, hyponatremia, hypotension, and hypothermia.
- Chest pain and myocardial infarction from coronary artery disease may occur. Remember, I said that hypothyroid patients have abnormal lipid metabolism.
- Heart failure.
- Megacolon.
- Replacement therapy should be started slowly because it will speed up heart rate and increase blood pressure and all other body processes. Thyroid hormone replacement therapy could cause BIG problems in people with known cardiovascular complications. Remember, thyroid hormone replacement speeds up everything, which increases workload on the heart.
- In children with cretinism, slowed mental and physical development is the main result of untreated or under-treated hypothyroidism.
- Infertility.

If I were your teacher, I would test you on . . .

- Nutritional requirements including importance of high-fiber diet.
- Treatment for constipation.
- Monitor for signs of hyperthyroidism when treatment begins.

- Importance of teaching client to report chest pain and tachycardia, especially when treatment begins.
- Safety precautions because of the general slowing of all intellectual functions. Assessment of cardiac output and sign of cardiac failure.
- Teach client importance of reporting infections.
- Correction of hypothermia.
- Importance of avoiding sedation.
- Skin care.
- Assessment of respiratory function.
- Monitoring client response to thyroid replacement therapy especially in clients with cardiovascular problems.
- Sign and symptoms of hypothyroidism.
- Counseling on sexual problems including infertility.
- Need for life-long thyroid replacement therapy.
- Recognizing myxedema coma.

PARATHYROID GLANDS

The parathyroid glands are attached to the bottom of and behind the thyroid. We have four parathyroids, each about the size of a pea. The parathyroid glands regulate calcium in the blood. The parathyroid glands secrete parathyroid hormone (PTH) which **makes the serum calcium level go up.** PTH works by pulling calcium from the bone, then placing it in the blood. It decreases calcium excretion from the kidneys and stimulates calcium resorption through the gastrointestinal tract.

- As with any hormone in the body you can have too much or too little of that hormone.

  Too much PTH = hyperparathyroidism = hypercalcemia, hypophosphatemia, bone damage, and renal damage.

  Too little PTH = hypoparathyroidism, hypocalcemia, hyperphosphatemia, hyperreflexia, and cognitive changes (altered sensorium).

- What causes an increase in the secretion of PTH? Low blood calcium. When blood calcium is low, PTH secretion increases, which causes calcium to be pulled from the bone. This causes bone breakdown and the serum calcium to go up.

- What causes a decrease in PTH secretion? High serum calcium or high serum magnesium. Magnesium is chemically similar to calcium. If serum calcium is high, then PTH is not released. PTH is only released when more calcium is needed in the blood.

✚ Hyperparathyroidism

Hyperparathyroidism is a major parathyroid problem.

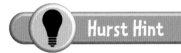

Factoid

PTH makes the serum calcium increase.

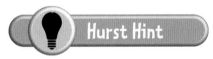

Hurst Hint

The parathyroids have nothing to do with the thyroid. The thyroid is all about energy. The parathyroids are all about calcium.

Hurst Hint

Remember, calcium and phosphorus have an inverse relationship. When one is elevated, the other is decreased.

What is it?

Hyperparathyroidism is overactivity of the parathyroid glands, resulting in excess production of PTH, consequently leading to increased serum calcium (hypercalcemia). Remember, when PTH is secreted, it pulls calcium from the bone and places it in the blood. Therefore, serum calcium goes up.

What causes it and why

Table 14-6 shows the causes and associated explanations for hyperparathyroidism.

Table 14-6

Causes	Why
Dysfunction of the parathyroid gland (example: adenoma of one of the four parathyroid glands), which is considered a primary dysfunction	Adenoma is a benign tumor. These adenomas secrete PTH and are responsible for hypercalcemia
Renal failure: example of secondary cause of hyperparathyroidism	Certain medical conditions can cause the parathyroids to produce too much PTH in response to chronically low levels of serum calcium. In renal failure, phosphorus is not excreted, causing hyperphosphatemia, and therefore causing hypocalcemia (due to inverse relationship). This circumstance (hypocalcemia) stimulates the parathyroids to produce more PTH
Vitamin D deficiency	Without vitamin D, calcium isn't absorbed well. As a result, the parathyroids produce PTH to get the serum calcium back up
Pregnancy and lactation	Hormones stimulate the parathyroid glands. This is why it is more common in women than in men and children

Source: Created by author from References #1, #3, and #4.

Signs and symptoms and why

To understand the symptoms seen with hyperparathyroidism you must remember this: CALCIUM ACTS LIKE A SEDATIVE. Most sources say "calcium acts like a central nervous system depressant." That's okay too, but "sedative" is easier to remember. When you have too much calcium in the body, everything is sedated. When you do not have enough calcium in the body, everything is hyperactive, making the muscles tight and twitchy. Don't forget this: When you think about the parathyroid glands, the first thing you should think of is CALCIUM. You've either got too much or not enough in the blood/serum (calcium, that is).

Many times the signs and symptoms of hyperparathyroidism go unnoticed. The client may have a fracture, kidney stones, or muscle weakness that, considering the circumstances, may provide a red flag that hyperparathyroidism may be the cause.

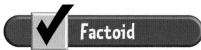

Factoid

Twice as many women as men develop primary hyperparathyroidism.

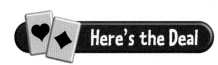

Here's the Deal

Hyperparathyroidism is most commonly caused by a tumor.

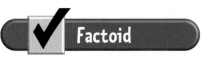

Factoid

There are four parathyroid glands. However, just for your information, it is not uncommon for some people to have five parathyroid glands, or more. This does not mean these people will experience hyperparathyroidism. It just means they have a lot of parathyroids!

Table 14-7 shows the signs and symptoms and associated reasons for hyperparathyroidism.

Table 14-7

Signs and symptoms	Why
Neurological: depression, confusion, lethargy, decreased level of consciousness (LOC)	Too much calcium has a sedative effect
Arrhythmias	Calcium is essential in the function of muscles. Any and all muscles can be affected by calcium problems, and your heart is definitely a muscle
Gastrointestinal: nausea, vomiting, weight loss, constipation. These are the most common symptoms seen in mild cases of hyperparathyroidism	Sedative action of calcium causes everything to be slowed down. If everything is slowed, the small intestine (smooth muscle) is slowed, decreasing peristalsis. Calcium is essential in nerve function
Kidney stones (renal calculi): extreme tendency for renal calculi	Most kidney stones are made from calcium; hyperparathyroidism is caused by too much calcium in the blood
Muscular: atrophy of muscles with weakness and fatigue, decreased deep tendon reflexes (DTRs), fractures, and kyphosis (curvature) of the spine.	Calcium is essential to muscle function and affects muscle tone. Too much calcium causes sedation of the muscles
Osteoporosis puts the client at risk for fractures	Calcium is pulled from the bone into the blood serum

Source: Created by author from References #1, #3, and #4.

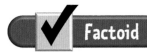

Factoid

Hypercalcemia often will cause no signs and symptoms, but those who are symptomatic often complain of problems with "bones, stones, abdominal groans, psychic moans, with fatigue overtones!" (Source CMDT 2005, McGraw Hill, Tierney, McPhee, and Papadakis)

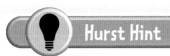

Hurst Hint

Remember: calcium acts like a sedative. When answering test questions about calcium, think muscles first. Don't forget the smooth muscles of the body such as found in the airway or intestines.

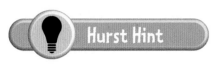

Hurst Hint

PTH makes serum calcium increase.

Quickie tests and treatments

Tests:

- PTH hormone: elevated.

- Serum calcium: elevated (hypercalcemia)—serum calcium above 10.5 mg/dL or ionized calcium greater than 5.4 mg/dL.

- Serum phosphate: low, less than 2.5 mg/dL (hypophosphatemia). Why? When PTH is increased, calcium is pulled from the bone, as is phosphate. However, PTH stimulates renal excretion of phosphate.

- Urinalysis: elevated phosphate due to excessive loss of phosphate in the urine.

- 24-hour urine collection: tests kidney function and measures the amount of calcium excreted in the urine.

- If hyperparathyroidism is due to renal failure, the serum phosphate increases because the kidneys can't excrete phosphorus.

- Alkaline phosphatase: increase because so much calcium is being pulled from the bone. Anytime the bone is significantly disturbed, alkaline phosphatase goes up (bone cancer, multiple myeloma, etc.) Why? When osteoblasts are active, they secrete large quantities of alkaline phosphatase.

- Bone mineral density test or x-ray: determines degree of osteoporosis.
- Imaging studies: detect the presence of a tumor or abnormal parathyroid gland and identify location prior to surgery; identify possible kidney stones.

Treatments:

- Parathyroidectomy: calcium, phosphorus, and magnesium levels must be monitored closely and treated promptly; serum calcium will drop during the first 5 days postop.
- Treat severe hypercalcemia with hospitalization and intense hydration with IV saline to flush out the calcium (monitor for secondary congestive heart failure).
- Bisphosphonates for hypercalcemia: some are given PO to elevate the phosphorus level in the blood and therefore decrease the serum calcium.
- Drugs to inhibit bone resorption: calcitonin (SQ Calcimar); calcitonin drives calcium into bone.
- Glucocorticoids: decrease calcium absorption in the intestines and increase renal excretion of calcium as well.
- Limit foods high in calcium.
- Dialysis: removes excess calcium; also used in clients who are in renal failure.
- If client is on digoxin (Lanoxin), be very cautious as toxicity to digoxin is likely.
- Avoid thiazide diuretics: thiazides have a tendency to cause calcium retention.
- Avoid calcium-containing antacids or supplements.
- Strain urine for stones.
- Turn client gently: high risk for pathological fractures.
- When giving rapid fluid replacement to flush out calcium, check lung sounds frequently to prevent fluid volume excess and pulmonary edema.
- Watch for development of peptic ulcer: high serum calcium causes stomach to produce excessive acid.
- Watch for arrhythmias.
- Provide an acidifying diet (helps ↓ formation of stones).
- Acidic drugs are frequently used for treatment of renal stones.

What can harm my client?

- Kidney stones.
- Renal failure.
- Osteoporosis leading to fractures.
- Hypoparathyroidism postop.
- Cardiac problems due to calcium imbalances.
- Ulceration of upper GI tract (peptic ulcer disease), which could possibly cause hemorrhage perforation (when serum calcium is high, the stomach produces too much acid, which irritates tissues).
- Fluid volume overload with rapid saline administration.

If I were your teacher, I would test you on . . .

- Causes and why.
- Signs and symptoms and why.
- How the parathyroids work.
- Nursing care associated with care and treatments (e.g., 24-hour urine collection).
- Ways to prevent kidney stones (drink lots of fluids).
- Ways to build bone mass (exercise, weight bearing).
- Importance of taking vitamin D to enhance calcium absorption.
- Importance of stopping smoking (smoking increases bone loss).
- Food sources high in calcium should be avoided.
- How to monitor for hypocalcemia postop.
- How to administer calcitonin (Cibacalcin) at home.
- Importance of reporting signs and symptoms of tetany (numbness and tingling around the mouth or extremities).
- Postop care of the client who has had a parathyroidectomy (importance of keeping calcium gluconate at the bedside).
- Drug therapy used in treatment.
- How electrolytes are affected by hyperparathyroidism and why.

✚ Hypoparathyroidism

What is it?

Hypoparathyroidism is underactivity of the parathyroid gland leading to inadequate production of PTH. As a result, the serum calcium goes down and the serum phosphorus goes up because PTH normally stimulates renal excretion of phosphate. In hypoparathyroidism, the bones remain intact.

What causes it and why

Table 14-8 shows the causes and why of hypoparathyroidism.

Table 14-8

Causes	Why
Damage to or accidental removal of the parathyroid glands during a thyroidectomy or surgery for throat or neck cancer; most common cause of hypoparathyroidism	Decreased amounts of PTH causes serum calcium levels to drop
Autoimmune destruction of the parathyroid gland	Decreased amounts of PTH causes serum calcium levels to drop
Radiation treatments of face and neck	Parathyroids are destroyed leading to decreased PTH secretion
Hypomagnesemia: as seen in alcoholism due to poor nutrition and increased excretion by kidneys	Must have adequate magnesium levels for the parathyroid to secrete PTH

Source: Created by author from References #1 and #2.

Signs and symptoms and why

Remember, with hypoparathyroidism there is not enough calcium so the client is not sedated. Instead, everything tightens! Table 14-9 shows the signs and symptoms and associated reasons for hypoparathyroidism.

Table 14-9

Signs and symptoms	Why
Neurological: hyperactive reflexes, irritability, seizure activity, anxiety, stridor, laryngospasm	Calcium is essential to muscle function. In the case of hypoparathyroidism, the client's calcium is low, thus <u>preventing</u> a sedative effect on the body
Arrhythmias	Heart is made of muscle and calcium is essential for muscle function
Musculoskeletal: tetany, positive Chvostek's and Trousseau's signs, increased deep tendon reflexes (DTRs). Bones remain intact	Low calcium. Calcium acts like a sedative and with hypoparathyroidism there is not enough calcium. No sedative = hyperactivity, excitability. In regard to the calcification of bones, this occurs because the calcium moves from the serum and blood <u>into</u> the bones
Carpal pedal spasm	Lack of calcium, which is necessary for proper neuromuscular function (not enough sedative)
Tingling of the mouth or extremities	Lack of calcium, which is necessary for proper neuromuscular function (not enough sedative)
Integumentary: skin is dry, nails are brittle, alopecia (thinning of the hair), and malformation of the teeth	Hair loss and skin changes can occur, as calcium has a role in nutrition. Adequate nutrition is crucial for hair growth and quality as well as skin cell development. Low calcium can also cause a defect in cellular immunity, which can affect hair and skin cell development. If a client is hypocalcemic, then the client is also hyperphosphatemic. Phosphorus plays a role in cell division; therefore, too much phosphorus can affect the cells of the skin and hair. Either of these symptoms is usually seen with prolonged calcium deficiency

Source: Created by author from References #1 and #2.

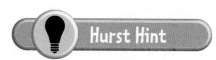

Hurst Hint

Chvostek's sign is unilateral contraction of facial muscles when the cheek is tapped. Trousseau's sign is a hand tremor in response to the pumping up of a blood pressure cuff on the same arm.

Quickie tests and treatments

Tests:

- Serum calcium: low.
- Serum phosphate: high.
- PTH: decreased.
- Urine calcium: decreased.

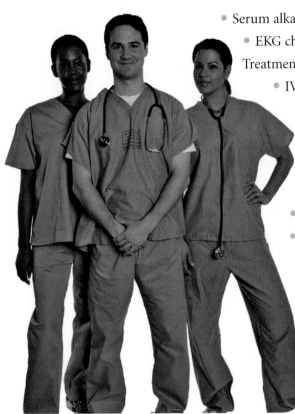

- Serum alkaline phosphatase: normal.
  - EKG changes associated with hypocalcemia.
- Treatments:
  - IV calcium.
    - Calcium acetate given with meals to bind phosphate: lowers the serum phosphorus and increases serum calcium.
    - Medications to decrease seizures and relax muscles: used until calcium level normalizes.
    - Increased dietary intake of calcium.
  - PO calcium.
    - Estrogen replacement in postmenopausal women: helps with calcium regulation.
    - Avoid digitalis preparations in the presence of calcium imbalances, which could cause toxicity.
    - Vitamin D added to the diet to enhance calcium absorption.
    - Thiazide diuretics to enhance calcium retention.
    - Monitor for and treat arrhythmias.
    - Phosphorus-binding drugs (Maalox, Mylanta, Amphojel): lower serum phosphorus which increases serum calcium.
- Avoid carbonated soft drinks: contain phosphorus.
- PTH is given only occasionally due to the extreme expense and it is has not been shown to be very effective.

What can harm my client?

- Arrhythmias.
- Laryngospasm.
- Seizures.
- Rapid administration of calcium. (Heart could stop)

If I were your teacher, I would test you on . . .

- Caring for clients with anxiety, confusion, or decreased level of consciousness.
- Signs and symptoms and why.
- Causes and why.
- Assessing Chvostek's and Trousseau's signs.
- Assessing tolerance of heart rhythm changes and need for heart (telemetry) monitoring.
- Pertinent assessment after parathyroidectomy.
- Safety precautions (including seizure precautions) with hypocalcemia.
- Importance of monitoring airway closely due to potential for laryngeal spasm.
- Nursing care associated with administration of IV calcium.

- Dangers associated with administration of IV calcium.
- Assessment of neuromuscular status.
- Identification of high calcium foods.
- Importance of administering digoxin with caution (toxicity).
- Drug therapy for hypoparathyroidism.

ADRENAL GLANDS

There are two adrenal glands. They live in the penthouse of the kidney (the top floor, that is) and have an inner layer and an outer layer. The inner layer is called the adrenal medulla, which is functionally related to the sympathetic nervous system, which secretes epinephrine and nor-epinephrine in response to sympathetic stimulation. The outer layer is called the adrenal cortex, which produces hormones called corticosteroids.

There are 2 distinct parts of the adrenal glands, which secrete entirely different sets of hormones:

1. Adrenal cortex produces glucocorticoids, mineralocorticoids, and sex hormones.

2. Adrenal medulla produces epinephrine and norepinephrine.

Let's talk about the adrenal cortex first.

✚ Adrenal cortex

The hormones the adrenal cortex produces are frequently called steroids. We (not me!) have been able to isolate over 30 steroids from the adrenal cortex, but only two are of major significance to the normal endocrine function of the human body. The first is aldosterone, which is the principle mineralocorticoid. The second is cortisol, which is the principle glucocorticoid.

Different books will tell you different things about the hormones of the adrenal cortex. This may totally confuse you. Here is a safe way to remember this information:

- Adrenocorticotropin hormones (ACTH): the pituitary secretes ACTH, which then stimulates the adrenal cortex to release hormones. The major hormones the adrenal cortex secretes are corticosteroids. Corticosteroid is the term used when referring to any secretion of the adrenal cortex. They include glucocorticoids, mineralocorticoids, and sex hormones (androgens). **However, 99% of the time, when the term "corticosteroid" is used, it means glucocorticoid.** There are different types of glucocorticoids, and they are generally referred to as steroids. The most important and most potent glucocorticoid is cortisol. Remember, steroids are produced naturally in the body, but there are also synthetic steroids we administer as drugs (cortisone, prednisone, solumedrol, solucortef, hydrocortisone, etc.). In many texts, the terms ACTH, cortisol, steroids, and glucocorticoids are used interchangeably, probably because the majority of steroids that are administered are glucocorticoids. This is okay as long as you know how things are really classified.

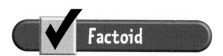

Factoid

Kidney stones may occur with either hypo- or hyperparathyroidism, but most commonly in hyperparathyroidism. In hyperparathyroidism, the serum calcium is high, so there is plenty of calcium available to form kidney stones due to calcium levels being proportionate in the urine and blood. In hypoparathyroidism, calcium is excreted through the kidneys, so stone formation is possible.

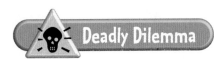

Deadly Dilemma

Many heart attacks occur during the early morning hours when people are coming out of REM sleep, as this is a very stressful time for the body.

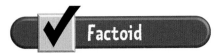

Factoid

Most exogenous forms of cortisol (prednisone, dexamethasone, hydrocortisone) are usually ordered by the physician to be given early in the morning in an effort to mimic our own body's (endogenous) cortisol secretion.

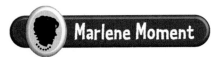

Marlene Moment

The steroids produced by the adrenal cortex (cortical steroids) are made from cholesterol. See! Cholesterol is good for you!

- Cortisol: the majority of cortisol is secreted early in the morning, especially when coming out of REM sleep. Coming out of REM sleep is very stressful on the body and cortisol helps fight stress. This is why our body was made to secrete the majority of our "steroids" during this time (to help fight the stress of waking up).
- A few examples of <u>adrenal</u> steroids include cortisol, corticosterone, and aldosterone. A few examples of <u>synthetic</u> steroids include cortisone, prednisolone, methylprednisone, and dexamethasone.

✚ Functions of glucocorticoids

Let's look at <u>some</u> important functions of glucocorticoids. You must understand these or you'll be lost later. Glucocorticoids:

1. Stimulate gluconeogenesis (the formation of carbohydrates from proteins and other substances by the liver).
2. Provide amino acids and glucose during times of stress.
3. Suppress the immune system due to powerful immunosuppressive and antiinflammatory properties.
4. Stimulate fat breakdown. Fatty acids are released and used for energy production. Glucocorticoids are considered to be catabolic steroids as they break down the body's stored resources during times of need. They are not the same as anabolic steroids athletes sometimes take to build up their muscles—and cause "roid rage." (haha!)

What causes an increase in corticosteroid secretion?

All of the examples listed below are times when the body is stressed and needs more cortisol. Glucocorticoids help mobilize fuels needed during stress (amino acids, glucose, fatty acids).

- Physical trauma.
- Cold.
- Burns.
- Heavy exercise.
- Infection.
- Shock.
- Decreased oxygen.
- Sleep deprivation.
- Pain.
- Fear.
- Emotional upset and anxiety.

Chronic stress causes fat to be deposited in the midsection (abdomen). Why? The cause is really unknown but may mean the body is preparing a place to pull potentially needed fuel from. Watch those waistlines in nursing school!

What causes a decrease in corticosteroid secretion? Taking exogenous forms of steroids and diseases such as Addison's disease cause a decrease in corticosteroid secretion.

Administering steroids

Think about this: when administering a steroid, you better look it up to see what type of action it has so you will know what kind of effects to look for in your client.

For example:

1. Prednisone is the most commonly used glucocorticoid due to its high glucocorticoid activity.

2. Dexamethasone has a high glucocorticoid effect, but has a small amount of mineralocorticoid activity, too. So now you have to worry about fluid retention in addition to the effects of glucocorticoids.

3. Hydrocortisone has more mineralocorticoid activity than prednisone, but primarily has glucocorticoid activity.

✚ Mineralocorticoids

Let's look at the mineralocorticoids

There is one major mineralocorticoid—aldosterone. Aldosterone causes sodium and water retention in the vascular space and potassium excretion from the body. Therefore, aldosterone plays a major role in body fluid regulation.

What causes an increase in aldosterone secretion?

Low blood levels of sodium trigger the renin–angiotensin system. If the sodium level is low, the kidneys retain it in order to build the blood level back up. The renin–angiotensin system kicks in, resulting in retention of sodium and water in the vascular space. Remember, anytime sodium is retained, potassium is excreted (due to their inverse relationship).

An increase in aldosterone secretion is also caused by:

• Low fluid volume levels in the vascular space as in shock or hypovolemia (same mechanism as listed above).

• High blood levels of potassium: when potassium levels are high in the blood, this means the sodium levels are low, as sodium and potassium have an inverse relationship. Therefore, aldosterone is secreted, which causes sodium and water retention in the vascular space and causes potassium excretion out of the body. This helps bring the serum potassium back into the normal range.

What causes a decrease in aldosterone secretion?

Under normal circumstances, aldosterone secretion decreases if fluid volume is elevated in the vascular space. This is a normal compensatory mechanism. There is also a disease, called hypoaldosteronism, where there is not enough aldosterone being produced.

Which illnesses are associated with aldosterone?

The illnesses associated with aldosterone are:

1. Hyperaldosteronism (one type is Conn's syndrome): obviously from the name, TOO MUCH aldosterone is produced in hyperaldosteronism. As a result, sodium and water are retained and the vascular volume is increased to the point of fluid volume excess (hypervolemia). So, when

studying hyperaldosteronism be sure to review hypervolemia. In addition, you must not forget that potassium is EXCRETED in this disease. You better review hypokalemia as well when studying this disease.

2. Hypoaldosteronism: obviously from the name, NOT ENOUGH aldosterone is being produced in hypoaldosteronism. As a result, sodium and water are lost from the vascular space to the point of fluid volume deficit (shock, hypovolemia). Be sure to review hypovolemia when studying this disease. In addition, since sodium and water are excreted from the body, potassium is retained. You should review hyperkalemia when studying this disease.

✚ Sex hormones

Sex hormones are actually made by the adrenal cortex and the gonads, which include the ovaries and testes.

Gonadocorticoids is one name for sex hormones. Another name is androgens—think masculine characteristics.

Sex hormones are usually broken down into three categories:

1. Androgens, testosterone being the main one.

2. Estrogens, estradiol being the main one.

3. Progestagens, progesterone being the main one.

The majority of testosterone in males is produced during puberty; therefore, this is when we see secondary sexual characteristics begin to form.

MAJOR ADRENAL CORTEX DISEASES (ADDISON'S AND CUSHING'S)

Which diseases are associated with adrenal cortex problems?

1. Cushing's disease—too many steroids.

2. Addison's—not enough steroids.

Let's talk about Addison's disease first.

✚ Addison's disease

Addison's disease is the same as adrenal hypofuntion or adrenal insufficiency.

What is it?

In Addison's disease, the adrenal cortex does not produce enough steroids—also known as adrenal hypofunction. Remember, the term "steroid" includes glucocorticoids, mineralocorticoids, and androgens (sex hormones). If you want to get picky, there are two types of Addison's disease:

1. Primary, due to the adrenal gland itself.

2. Secondary, due to problems outside of the adrenal gland.

We are just going to study plain ole Addison's disease. Be aware there are different and more complex forms of every disease, but the most common adrenal hypofunction disease studied in nursing school is Addison's disease.

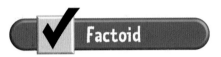

Factoid

Synthetic androgens (sex hormones) are referred to as anabolic steroids.

Factoid

DHEA is an androgen we are hearing a lot about in the news for treating depression, chronic fatigue, cardiovascular disease, and many other problems. It has also been promoted as a natural supplement with antiaging qualities—builds muscle strength and improves memory.

HERE'S WHAT HAPPENS IN ADDISON'S DISEASE In Addison's disease (adrenocortical insufficiency):

- The client does not have enough glucocorticoids, mineralocorticoids, and sex hormones. However, the focus—to get more questions right on your test—is on aldosterone, the major mineralocorticoid.

- Normally, aldosterone makes us retain sodium and water (in the vascular space) and lose potassium. For example, if volume in the vascular space gets low, aldosterone is produced and sodium and water are retained, which makes the vascular volume go up. Potassium is excreted too, because sodium and potassium always do the opposite of each other (inverse relationship). Sodium and water retention is a good thing if your volume is low. This is a great compensatory mechanism of the body.

- If there is **not enough** aldosterone, as with Addison's disease, the body cannot hold on to sodium and water anymore so, the body begins to lose (excrete) sodium and water. As a result, the vascular volume drops. So, now you have to go back and review all the signs and symptoms of hypovolemia!

- If sodium and water are excreted, then potassium is saved in the vascular space. The client becomes hyperkalemic. Now you have to review the signs and symptoms of hyperkalemia!

- Based on the above information, there are three key points I want you to remember regarding Addison's disease:

Not enough steroids.

Shock.

Hyperkalemia.

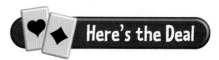

Exogenous refers to something that comes from outside the body. Endogenous refers to something that comes from inside the body. For instance, we produce steroids inside our body (endogenous). You can also take steroids (exogenous).

What causes it and why

Table 14-10 shows the causes of Addison's disease and why these causes occur.

Table 14-10

Causes	Why
Immune problem: known as a primary cause, if you want to get picky	Antibodies kill the adrenal tissue, decreasing steroid secretion
Bilateral adrenalectomy: known as a primary cause, if you want to get picky	Lack of adrenal glands makes it impossible to produce adrenal hormones (also called steroid hormones)
Hypopituitarism: known as a secondary cause, if you want to get picky	If the pituitary is not functioning, then the adrenals can't be triggered to secrete steroids
Sudden withdrawal of steroid medication: known as a secondary cause, if you want to get picky	Sudden decrease in circulating corticosteroids because adrenals are suppressed during steroid therapy. This is why you have to wean off steroids to allow sufficient time for the adrenals to kick back in

Source: Created by author from References #2 and #4.

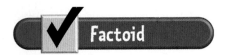

Factoid

The most common cause of Addison's disease is an autoimmune response. The adrenal cortex loses about 90% of its function before any clinical manifestations appear.

CASE IN POINT   Imagine you have a client who is taking steroids—let's say prednisone (Deltasone)—as ordered by a physician. Since prednisone is an exogenous form of steroid, the client's adrenal glands shut down and stop making all steroids: glucocorticoids, mineralocorticoids, and androgens. The adrenal glands see no need to work since the body is getting steroids from somewhere else. If the client STOPS taking the exogenous form of steroid (the prednisone pill), then all of a sudden there is NO steroid in the body (endogenous or exogenous). When the onset of Addison's disease is this sudden, it is called an addisonian crisis.

Signs and symptoms and why

The signs of decreased aldosterone predominate when studying Addison's disease. However, since Addison's disease is a decrease in **all of the steroids** of the cortex, you will see signs and symptoms of glucocorticoid insufficiency as well. The client usually does not have any signs of sex hormone insufficiency, but anything is possible! The signs and symptoms of Addison's disease can come about slowly or abruptly (addisonian crisis).

Table 14-11 shows the signs and symptoms and why of Addison's disease.

Table 14-11

Signs and symptoms	Why
Asthenia (weakness)	The cardinal symptom due to fluid and electrolyte imbalances
Fluid volume deficit including dehydration, weakness and fatigue as early symptoms	Sodium and water are excreted. You better review the signs and symptoms of hypovolemia (shock)!
Salt cravings	Sodium loss
Orthostatic hypotension is common; vertigo, syncope	Sodium and water (volume) are lost from vascular space due to lack of aldosterone. Hypotension is also due to decreased ability for vessels to constrict and a decreased total peripheral resistance
Hyperkalemia: begins with muscle twitching, then proceeds to weakness and then flaccid paralysis (don't forget about potential arrhythmias)	Since sodium and water are lost, potassium is retained in the vascular space
Sodium imbalances	If water is lost (blood is concentrated), then the client will be hypernatremic; if sodium is lost (blood is dilute), the client will be hyponatremic; if sodium and water are lost equally, there will be no change in serum sodium. So who knows!
Decreased bowel sounds; GI upset	Hyperkalemia

(Continued)

Table 14-11. (*Continued*)

Signs and symptoms	Why
Muscle weakness, fatigue, muscle wasting, muscle ache	Decreased glucocorticoids causes decreased ability to maintain contractions and avoid fatigue; cortisol deficit (glucocorticoid deficit) causes problems with fat, protein, and carbohydrate metabolism
Hyperpigmentation: especially in the creases of the skin, elbows, nipples, and pressure points; bronze skin. The gums and mucous membranes become bluish-black	Increased levels of ACTH; ACTH is very similar to melanocyte-stimulating hormone
Increased risk of infection	Anytime your steroids are messed up, you are at risk for infection. Infection is a stressor. The body can't handle stress because there are no steroids! Remember cortisol?
Hypoglycemia: be sure to review the signs and symptoms of hypoglycemia	Steroids are responsible for gluconeogenesis, which causes a rise in blood glucose. Steroids are decreased, so blood sugar drops due to inability to carry out gluconeogenesis
Very little axillary and pubic hair (mainly in women)	Decreased sex hormones
Inability to handle emotional or physical stress	Decreased glucocorticoids, which help the body deal with stress

Source: Created by author from References #1 and #2.

Quickie tests and treatments

Tests:

- Serum cortisol levels: less than 10 µg/dL in the morning.
- Urine tests: show decreased corticosteroid concentrations.
- Serum sodium: decreased due to excretion.
- Serum potassium: increased due to retention.
- Blood glucose: decreased because not enough steroids cause blood glucose to go down.
- Serum ACTH: increased because the pituitary secretes ACTH when adrenocortical secretions are low.
- CT and MRI of head: to detect pituitary tumors.
- EKG: detects rhythm changes due to hypovolemia and hyperkalemia.
- CBC: neutropenia (low white blood cell count); anytime steroids are not in balance, the immune system is altered.
- Hematocrit and eosinophils: elevated because blood is hemoconcentrated due to fluid loss.
- CT: may show adrenal atrophy. If the adrenals aren't working, "SHRINKAGE!" as George Castanza on *Seinfeld* would say.

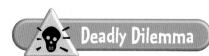

In Addison's disease, if sodium and water loss is severe, the client can go into shock and cardiovascular collapse.

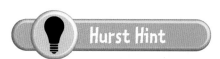

The client should avoid precipitating factors such as infection, trauma, and temperature extremes that could trigger an addisonian crisis.

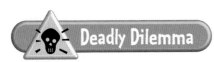

For clients who take steroids, teach them to never stop taking the steroid suddenly, as this could result in an addisonian crisis, shock, and death.

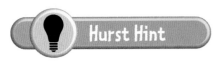

When treated promptly, adrenal crisis subsides quickly, with blood chemistry and vital signs returning to normal.

Treatments:

- IV fluids (IVFs): for clients in shock due to fluid losses.
- Monitor for arrhythmias due to retention of potassium.
- Correct hyperkalemia.
- Replacement therapy including glucocorticoids and mineralocorticoids: may be given IV until client stabilizes. In mild cases, hydrocortisone alone may be adequate. Hydrocortisone is the drug of choice to replace glucocorticoid and fludrocortisone (Florinef) is given to replace minearalcorticoid. Lifetime steroid replacement is usually necessary.
- Fludrocortisone acetate (Florinef) has a potent sodium-retaining effect. Be sure to monitor for this.
- DHEA (androgen) given to some women with adrenal insufficiency: replacement of sex hormone.
- Immediate and aggressive treatment of all infection with an increased dosage of hydrocortisone: infection can trigger an addisonian crisis.
- Increase hydrocortisone in the case of trauma, surgery, or other forms of stress.
- Addisonian crisis: IV bolus of hydrocortisone and administered continuously until the client is stabilized. Don't forget to give IV fluids.

What can harm my client?

- Acute adrenal (addisonian) crisis: severe sudden drop in blood pressure, nausea and vomiting, very high temperature, cyanosis.
- Life-threatening arrhythmia due to hyperkalemia.
- Hypovolemia and shock if severe fluid loss occurs.
- Infection: immune system is impaired anytime steroids are out of balance.
- Adverse effects of steroid therapy.
- Hypoglycemia.

If I were your teacher, I would test you on . . .

- Causes and why.
- Signs and symptoms and why.
- Nursing care associated with tests and treatments.
- Nursing interventions related to stress (adjusting medications in times of stress).
- Identification of and emergency treatment of addisonian crisis: hypotension, shock, coma; treatment includes rapid fluid replacement and steroid replacement.
- Important teaching points for the client in regard to steroid replacement therapy: take with food; take as directed; never stop taking steroids abruptly; watch for weight gain daily; increase medication dosage in times of stress; anticoagulants and insulin decrease effectiveness of steroids; if client is diabetic, monitor blood glucose carefully.

- The diet recommendations for clients with Addison's disease are tricky. A high-sodium and low-potassium diet is needed. Dietary sodium replaces the sodium that is excreted, and dietary potassium is limited due to the existing potassium excess. HOWEVER, if the client is undergoing steroid replacement therapy, remember that steroids generally cause sodium and water retention and potassium excretion. In this case, the client would need a low-sodium diet with increased potassium.

- Proper room assignment for someone on steroids. (Can't be around anyone with infection or communicable disease)

- Signs and symptoms of infection and how steroid use affects infection.

- Infection control and prevention in the client.

- Monitoring daily weights and intake and output.

- Forcing fluids until mineralocorticoid takes effect.

- Monitoring for Cushing's effects in clients taking steroids: (for example: fluid retention in the eyes and face.)

- Promoting client sleep: steroids can cause insomnia, especially if given after lunch, as they stimulate the CNS.

- Monitoring for hypoglycemia.

- Teach client how to avoid an adrenal crisis.

- Teach client to wear a medical alert bracelet.

- Teach client to keep a hydrocortisone injection on hand during times of stress.

- Teach client signs and symptoms of PUD. (Peptic ulcer disease)

- Teach client to identify and avoid stressors.

✛ Cushing's syndrome and Cushing's disease

Cushing's disease is also called hypercortisolism.

What is it?

Let's differentiate between Cushing's syndrome and Cushing's disease first. Many times the terms are used interchangeably, but this is incorrect. Let me re-emphasize, when someone is receiving steroids as a drug, this is referred to as "exogenous" steroids. In other words, the steroids came from **outside** of the body. At some time, you may see the statement, "The client is producing too much glucocorticoid **endogenously.**" This means the client is producing too much glucocorticoid from within her own body. Remember, the adrenal cortex is responsible for producing steroids.

Basically, with each type of Cushing's you have too many steroids. The client either has an ACTH excess (coming from the pituitary) or a cortisol excess. As a result of the ACTH excess, the adrenal cortex is hyperstimulated and produces too many steroids. The client whose by the pituitary problem started with the adrenal gland itself will overproduce steroids too. Some clients are GIVEN steroids as a drug and the steroid builds up in their blood. Other clients make too many of their own steroids. With all these conditions, the client has TOO MANY STEROIDS!

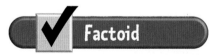

Factoid

ACTH is produced by the anterior pituitary to stimulate the adrenal cortex to produce adrenocortical hormones.

WHAT'S THE DIFFERENCE BETWEEN CUSHING'S SYNDROME AND CUSHING'S DISEASE? Here's the difference between Cushing's syndrome and Cushing's disease:

1. Cushing's syndrome is any condition where there is a high level of glucocorticoids (Fig. 14-5). This may be seen in a client who is receiving steroids as a medication (exogenous form of steroid) for problems such as asthma, COPD, autoimmune disorders, organ transplants, cancer (used with chemotherapy), or allergic responses. Cushing's syndrome is more common than Cushing's disease.

2. Cushing's disease is a condition where the **body** produces excess ACTH. Lots of diseases may cause this, such as any malfunction of the pituitary like a pituitary tumor, bilateral adrenal hyperplasia, malignancies, and adrenal adenoma or carcinoma.

▶ Figure 14-5. Cushing's syndrome. **A.** Client prior to syndrome. **B.** Client 4 months after diagnosis of syndrome. (From Saladin K. *Anatomy and Physiology: The Unity of Form and Function.* 4th ed. New York: McGraw-Hill; 2007.)

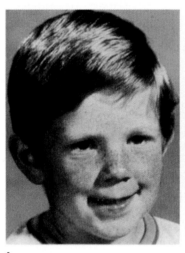
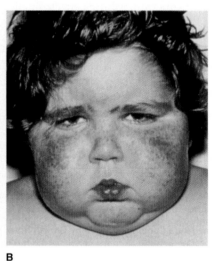

A   **B**

Even though we differentiated between the terms Cushing's syndrome and Cushing's disease, we will just be using the term "Cushing's" from now on.

In general, think of Cushing's as a disease where there are too many steroids present. The major steroids the body produces are glucocorticoids, mineralocorticoids, and sex hormones (also called androgens). The major steroid that the client with Cushing's has too much of are glucocorticoids, but you can have too much aldosterone and sex hormones as well.

Signs and symptoms and why

The signs and symptoms of Cushing's depend on how long and how much steroid the patient has been exposed to, if there is androgen excess or not, and if there are tumors secreting cortisol (steroids). As always, every patient is different. Some patients will have all the symptoms listed below and some could have a few of the symptoms listed below.

Now let's get specific and look at how each steroid affects the body when there is an excess.

Glucocorticoids have four major effects:

1. Influence mood.

2. Alter defense mechanisms.

3. Cause protein breakdown, altered fat metabolism, and altered distribution of fat.

4. Inhibit insulin.

When you think of Cushing's, you probably think of the client having a moon face due to fluid retention and fat deposition, buffalo hump, skinny arms and legs, and a large abdomen.

Table 14-12 shows the signs and symptoms and reasons behind them for Cushing's.

Table 14-12

Signs and symptoms	Why
Glucocorticoids	
Mood changes: depression, euphoria, irritability, and excess energy that can lead to insomnia	Steroids play a part in neurotransmission, which can lead to mental changes; steroids give you energy
Skinny arms and legs	Muscle wasting and protein breakdown; muscles are mainly made of protein
Thin skin	Fibroblasts are inhibited, which leads to a loss of collagen and connective tissue; this leads to thin skin and poor wound healing; little or no scar formation results
Muscle weakness	Protein breakdown
Poor wound healing	Lack of protein slows wound healing; protein is needed to help wounds heal
Bruising	Capillary weakness due to protein loss (capillaries have a lot of protein), which leads to bleeding and ecchymosis; when capillaries are weak they leak fluid out into the tissue, which produces ankle edema
Ketonuria	When the body breaks down fat, something called a KETONE is produced; ketones are acids and cause the body to be more acidic, which naturally puts the client at risk for metabolic acidosis
Buffalo hump: excess deposition of fat across the top of the back and shoulders	Altered fat metabolism and improper distribution of fat
Truncal obesity: deposition of fat in the trunk	Altered fat metabolism and improper distribution of fat
Pink/purple stretch marks on the breasts, abdomen, thighs	Protein collagen fibers in subcutaneous tissue are diminished due to protein breakdown, resulting in development of striae where they have been torn apart
Risk for infection	Excess steroids in the blood decrease the body's ability to make as many lymphocytes and antibodies as needed to fight infection. This also affects the body's ability to show signs and symptoms of inflammation
Hyperglycemia	Glucocorticoids inhibit insulin. If insulin is inhibited, glucose won't move into the cell, and the client becomes hyperglycemic. This is *why* you must perform frequent blood sugar checks on clients who receive steroids as part of their medical care
	Also, glucocorticoids promote hepatic gluconeogenesis
Glycosuria	Kidneys lower excess blood sugar by excreting it through the urine

(Continued)

Table 14-12. (*Continued*)

Signs and symptoms	Why
Osteoporosis	Steroids cause calcium excretion through the GI tract. The body works to replace the **blood** calcium (which has been lost through the GI tract) by pulling extra calcium from the bone into the blood. Why does this happen? Because your body wants your serum (blood) calcium to remain normal. When the body starts pulling the calcium from the bone to put it in the blood then brittle bones result. Yes, the calcium level in the blood went up, but we have a client who IS STILL MAKING too many steroids. This process just repeats itself, which makes the bones more and more brittle and weak
Peptic ulcer	Steroids cause increased gastric secretions, which eat away at the gastric mucosa
Mineralocorticoids	
Fluid volume excess	Fluid retention of sodium and water
Hypertension	Fluid retention of sodium and water
Hypokalemia	Sodium retention and potassium excretion
Sodium imbalances	Retention of sodium and water; retention of more sodium than water can cause **hypernatremia;** or, retention of sodium and water can be equal causing a normal level of sodium. When answering test questions, think hypernatremia first with cushing's
Muscle weakness	Hypokalemia
Androgens (sex hormones)	
Voice deepening (female)	Adrenal androgen stimulation
Beard growth (hirsutism) (female)	Adrenal androgen stimulation
Menstrual irregularities (female)	Hormones are out of balance
Thinning hair (female)	Adrenal androgen stimulation
Ruddy complexion (same as facial plethora) (female)	Adrenal androgen stimulation
Decreased libido (female and male); impotency (male only)	Decreased testosterone production; yes, females have testosterone, too

Source: Created by author from References #1 to #3.

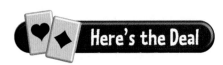

Here's the Deal

A client who receives heavy-duty steroid therapy in the hospital may develop steroid psychosis. Conversely, a client who receives a steroid injection at the doctor's office may just simply develop insomnia and irritability.

Quickie tests and treatments

Tests:

- Serum cortisol level: in Cushing's, there are more steroids present in the blood in the morning and lesser amounts in the afternoon.
- Serum ACTH: determines the origin of the problem (pituitary or adrenal gland).
- Dexamethasone suppression test: determines the etiology of the problem.
- Midnight serum cortisol level: increased.
- 24-hour urine collection: increased levels of steroids.
- Serum sodium: increased (mineralocorticoids cause sodium retention).

- Serum potassium: decreased (mineralocorticoids cause potassium excretion).
- Serum glucose: elevated (steroids make blood glucose go up).

Treatments:

- Treatment varies depending on the cause. For example, did the problem start in the pituitary gland or the adrenal gland?
- Transphenoidal resection of the pituitary adenoma: This tumor causes increased production of steroids; the rest of the pituitary usually returns to normal function; this is also called transphenoidal hypophysectomy.
- Craniotomy: depends on the size of the pituitary tumor.
- Bilateral laparoscopic adrenalectomy: if there is an adrenal cortex tumor, may take one or both adrenals; if both are removed, client will require lifelong steroid replacement.
- Gamma knife surgery: normalizes urine free cortisol within 12 months.
- Radiation: suppresses ACTH producing tumor or destroys the pituitary.
- Ketoconazole (Nizoral) 200 milligrams every 6 hours with monitoring of liver enzymes: ketoconazole and metyrapone (Metopirone) can help suppress hypercortisolism in inoperable adrenal carcinoma.
- Surgical resection of adrenal neoplasms.
- Adrenal carcinoma treated with mitotane (Lysodren): toxic to the cortex; known as a medical adrenalectomy or drug induced adrenalectomy.
- Monitoring daily weights, intake and output, and vital signs. Watch for signs of hypervolemia; restrict fluids as ordered; prevent fractures; implement fall precautions; and monitor for and prevent infections. Be sure to select a roommate who doesn't have an infection for the Cushing's client in semiprivate room.
- Monitor blood glucose; care for wounds due to delayed healing, if applicable; implement dietary measures; help client cope with body image disturbances.

What can harm my client?

- Profound immunosuppression: client may acquire *Pneumocystis carinii*, as this is a common source of pneumonia in this population.
- Hypervolemia leading to CHF and pulmonary edema.
- Suicide due to severe body image changes; adolescence is the age group that is usually preoccupied with body image.
- Fractures from osteoporosis.
- Addisonian crisis from steroid levels dropping too low (acute deficit of cortisol) as a result of treatment. In Cushing's there are too many steroids, so when we start treatment, steroid levels should drop. There is a chance that the steroid levels could drop too low, which could cause an addisonian crisis.

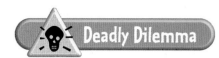

Excess steroids can cause immuno-suppression and infection. Things that do not make most people sick can make clients who take steroid therapy very, very ill!

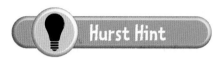

Both males and females may have a decreased sex drive (libido). When there are high levels of adrenal steroids, this interferes with the ability of the pituitary gland to secrete LH and FSH and for the testes to make testosterone, resulting in testicular atrophy and feminization such as gynecomastia.

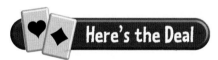

In pediatric clients, suspect Cushing's if increased obesity in the presence of delayed height on the growth chart exists.

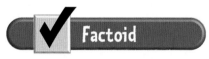

There are many treatments that may require the client to take lifelong glucocorticoids, mineralocorticoids, and possibly sex hormones. Two examples are bilateral adrenalectomy or a hypophysectomy.

If I were your teacher, I would test you on . . .

- Causes and why.
- Signs and symptoms and why.
- Nursing care associated with treatments.
- Care of clients who are depressed, angry, confused (e.g., using therapeutic communication).
- Importance of administering steroids in the morning.
- Maintaining safe blood glucose levels.
- Care of a slow-healing wound.
- Typical vital signs found in a Cushing's client.
- Signs and symptoms of hypokalemia.
- Administration of potassium supplements.
- Recognition and management of CHF and pulmonary edema.
- Care of an immunosuppressed client.
- Care of a hypervolemic client.
- Management of gastric ulcers.
- Diet high in calcium to prevent osteoporosis.
- Care of the client undergoing a craniotomy.
- Care of the client undergoing a transphenoidal hypophysectomy.
- Care of the client undergoing an adrenalectomy.
- Fall and fracture prevention.
- Care of the client undergoing body image changes.

✚ Adrenal medulla

The adrenal medulla is a sympathetic nerve ganglion that has secretory cells. The hormones secreted by the adrenal medulla are called the "fight or flight" hormones. These hormones are under the control of the sympathetic nervous system. The adrenal medulla hormones are:

1. Epinephrine (also known as adrenaline).

2. Norepinephrine (also known as noradrenaline).

Epinephrine and norepinephrine together are referred to as catecholamines. Catecholamines are a crucial part of the body's response to stress. The different actions of catecholamines are to:

- Increase heart rate.
- Cause peripheral blood vessels to constrict so blood pressure goes up.
- Increase sweating.
- Cause glycogen to convert to glucose (increases energy).
- Cause bronchial tubes to dilate (to breathe more air in).
- Decrease digestion (blood is sent to more important places like your heart).
- Lower urine output (to conserve fluid).
- Increase alertness.

Without the adrenal glands, stress is not tolerated. Remember, the last near miss you had in a car accident? That rush of panic, increased heart rate, and sheer terror—that is how epinephrine (epi) and norepinephrine (norepi) make you feel.

✚ Pheochromocytoma

The major adrenal medulla problem we will discuss is pheochromocytoma.

What is it?

Pheochromocytoma is a benign catecholamine-secreting tumor of the adrenal medulla. In 85% of the cases, the tumor is in the adrenal medulla. The tumor may present in other sympathetic nervous system (SNS) tissues in the body such as the urinary bladder, carotids, vertebral tissue, neck, thorax, abdomen, and pelvis, but mainly this tumor is in the adrenal medulla. The term pheochromocytoma got its name due to the pheochromocyte, which is a chromaffin cell in the adrenal medulla. A tumor in the chromaffin cells of the adrenal medulla that secretes catecholamines (epinephrine and norepinephrine) is called a pheochromocytoma. It secretes way too much epi and norepi IN BOLUSES. This increase in epi and norepi puts the client at risk for cerebral hemorrhage, cardiac failure, and death if left untreated. Secondary hypertension can be caused by pheochromocytoma.

What causes it and why

The cause of pheochromocytoma is unknown. Some cases of pheochromocytoma can occur with certain disorders such as multiple endocrine neoplasia syndrome.

Signs and symptoms and why

Table 14-13 shows the signs and symptoms and rationales associated with pheochromocytoma. Remember, the signs and symptoms are seen as "episodes." The client may say, "I have these spells where my heart beats out of my chest, my head pounds, and my blood pressure gets real high." These episodes may last from minutes to hours.

Table 14-13

Sign and symptoms	Why
Hypertension: intermittent, fluctuating, occurs rapidly and stops abruptly; hypertension is THE major sign that alerts the physician to a possibility of pheochromocytoma	Vasoconstrictive properties of epi and norepi secreted in boluses
Apprehension, sense of impending doom	The sympathetic nervous system (SNS) is stimulated because epi and norepi are being released

(Continued)

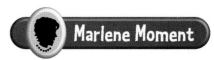

Marlene Moment

Catecholamines are what you get a surge of when you are about to take a big test!

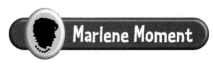

Marlene Moment

When you get a surge of catecholamines, your pupils get big and your alertness increases, so you can better see who is about to beat you up!

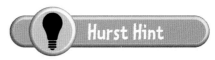

Hurst Hint

The client with pheochromocytoma has a tumor that secretes epi and norepi in boluses. The tumor does not secrete these chemicals constantly, or the client would die.

Table 14-13. (*Continued*)

Sign and symptoms	Why
Pupillary changes	In "fight or flight" situations, the eyes dilate in order to see the source of the fear and to react as needed
Severe headache	Increase in blood pressure (hypertension) in the small vessels of the brain
Nervousness, tremors	Stimulation of SNS by epi and norepi
Tachycardia, chest pain	Increased heart rate due to vasoconstrictive properties of epi and norepi. The heart attempts to push against the increased pressure that occurs as a result of vasoconstriction or in an effort to move blood forward and out to the vital organs
Palpitations	SNS is stimulated
Hyperglycemia (hypoglycemia could occur at some point as body is in hypermetabolic state and is using up glucose stores)	Glycogenolysis (conversion of glycogen to glucose in the liver and muscles) and suppression of insulin caused by catecholamine stimulation
Cold extremities	Vasoconstriction caused by epi and norepi. Blood is shunted away from the extremities (peripheral circulation) to the vital organs
Excessive perspiration	Stimulation of SNS; epi and norepi increase metabolism
Flushing	Increased blood pressure and delivery of more blood to central part of body as a result of peripheral vasoconstriction

Source: Created by author from References #3 and #5.

Quickie tests and treatments

Tests:

- Vanillylmandelic acid (VMA) test: 24-hour urine specimen to detect urinary catecholamines and metanephrines (inactive metabolite of epinephrine); these values are elevated in 90% or more of the cases of pheochromocytoma. A 24-hour urine test is necessary because the client secretes **boluses** of epi and norepi, not a continuous secretion. When you think about the VMA, think about "vanilla"—any food with vanilla alters the test.

- Blood test for serum epinephrine and norepinephrine can be drawn during or following an attack. The client should remain quiet during collection because any stress or activity can cause epi/norepi secretion. Serum catecholamines are elevated and are best tested during an "attack."

- CT or MRI of the abdomen: identifies tumor. These should not replace biochemical testing and are less reliable when used alone for the detection of pheochromocytoma.
- Nuclear imaging for visualizing pheochromocytomas: allows crisper image that can be viewed in three dimensions.
- Chest x-ray: assesses the lungs for pulmonary edema; high blood pressure can cause CHF.

Treatments:

- Monitor blood pressure closely preop: use the same arm every time for consistency.
- Alpha-adrenergic blockers (beta-blockers) to control blood pressure: phentolamine (Regitine); nitroprusside (Nitropress) for uncontrolled hypertension; labetalol (Normodyne); esmolol (Brevibloc).
- Calcium-channel blockers to control blood pressure.
- Fluid replacement: as vasoconstriction is relieved with medications, blood pressure drops. This is when fluid replacement begins to prevent hypotension.
- Metyrosine (Demser): decreases formation of epi/norepi.
- No caffeine: caffeine increases blood pressure.
- No sudden position changes, as this can cause a surge of epi and norepi.
- Decrease stress: stress can cause a surge of epi/norepi.
- Surgery to remove the tumor is the treatment of choice. One or both adrenal glands may be removed depending if the tumor is unilateral or bilateral. Postop care includes meticulous blood pressure monitoring, because it could take up to 3 weeks to stabilize the blood pressure. Monitor for **hypotension** postop. If the client is unable to have surgery due to pre-existing conditions, the condition will be managed with medications.
- Decrease activity: keeps blood pressure down; decreases workload on heart.
- Dark room: decreases anxiety.
- EKG: monitors for possible arrhythmias.
- Neurological checks: monitor for possible intracranial bleed.

What can harm my client?

- Cerebral hemorrhage: high blood pressure can cause vessels in brain to rupture and bleeding into brain or skull, resulting in increased intracranial pressure.
- Heart failure: high blood pressure stresses the heart.
- Myocardial infarction: hypertension stresses the heart and could cause ischemia.
- Renal failure: severely high blood pressure can damage the kidneys.
- Arrhythmias.
- Severe hypertension.
- Palpation of abdomen: can cause surge of epi and norepi.

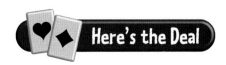

Pheochromocytoma can be confused with drug use of amphetamines, crack, and cocaine.

If I were your teacher, I would test you on . . .

- What is it?
- What causes it and why.
- Signs and symptoms and why.
- Assessment of vital signs, urinary output, and neurological status.
- Identifying stressors that cause hypertensive crisis and client strategies to avoid them.
- Minimizing stressors and keeping the environment calm.
- Teaching clients to avoid stimulants such as smoking and caffeine and to change positions slowly to avoid surges of epi and norepi.
- Teach clients to regularly monitor blood pressure.
- Never palpate the abdomen due to increased risk for stimulating more secretions from the tumors.
- Diet indications including increasing calories and vitamins and minerals, and decreasing sugar.
- How to deal with multiple signs and symptoms until treatment occurs.
- Monitoring for heart failure, cerebrovascular accident, myocardial infarction, shock, and renal failure.
- Administration of IV antihypertensive medications for hypertensive crisis.
- Procedure for collecting a 24-hour urine specimen.
- Foods to teach client to avoid during collection of 24-hour urine specimen for pheochromocytoma.
- Care of the client undergoing an adrenalectomy.

PANCREAS

The pancreas produces the hormone insulin. The function of insulin is to carry glucose from the vascular space (bloodstream) into the cell. When this mechanism is working properly, the blood sugar stays within a normal range. When the glucose can get into the cell, it can be used for energy. You must have insulin to carry glucose into the cell because glucose can't magically go into the cell without insulin. If the glucose cannot get into the cell, the glucose will stay in the vascular space (bloodstream) and build up to dangerously high levels depending on the degree of pancreatic dysfunction.

✚ Insulin

The pancreas lies under the stomach. Pancreatic tissue consists of 1 to 2 million islets of Langerhans. Beta, alpha, and delta cells make up the islets of Langerhans. The beta cells make up about 60% of the islet cells and are responsible for secreting insulin. The alpha cells make up about 25% and are responsible for secreting glucagon. The delta cells secrete somatostatin.

What triggers the release of insulin?

High blood glucose levels trigger the release of insulin from beta cells. Insulin binds with cell receptors, causing cellular uptake of glucose across the cell membrane and out of the blood.

What does the pancreas secrete?

The pancrease secretes:

1. Glucagon—produced by the alpha cells.
   - Mobilizes glucose, fatty acids, and amino acids into the blood.
   - Promotes conversion of glycogen (stored glucose in liver) to glucose through glycogenolysis, gluconeogenesis, and ketogenesis. Glucose is then secreted into the circulation, increasing the blood sugar.
2. Somatostatin—produced by the gamma cells; also known as growth-inhibiting hormone.
3. Insulin.
   - Promotes storage of glucose, fatty acids, and amino acids.
   - Accelerates movement of glucose out of blood and into cells (lowers blood sugar).
   - Inhibits release of glucose by liver (keeps blood sugar down).

> ✔ **Factoid**
>
> Normal blood glucose ranges between 70 and 120 mg/dL. When the blood glucose is too high, the client is hyperglycemic.

✚ Diabetes mellitus

Diabetes is a Greek word that means to siphon or to pass thru. Mellitus is Latin and refers to something sweet or honey. Sometimes I'd like to know where they get these names for diseases.

What is it?

Diabetes mellitus (DM) occurs when there is not enough insulin to carry the glucose out of the vascular space and into the cells. Our pancreas is supposed to produce and secrete insulin. Insulin is required to move glucose out of the vascular space and into the cell. If glucose is not pulled from the vascular space, it will build up in the blood. The cells need the glucose (sugar) for energy. Without insulin, the body enters a state of catabolism. Catabolism means to tear down and anabolism means to build up. The cells need energy, so they begin to break down fats and proteins. FAT breakdown (not protein breakdown) leads to ketone formation. Ketones are acids. This increase in ketones in the blood leads to metabolic acidosis.

There are three types of diabetes mellitus: type I, type II, and gestational diabetes. Let's focus on type I and type II in this chapter. You can worry about gestational diabetes when you take maternity nursing!

WHAT'S THE DIFFERENCE BETWEEN TYPE I AND TYPE II DIABETES?

Type I:

- Begins in childhood or adolescence, usually around the age of 14.
- Also called juvenile diabetes mellitus or insulin-dependent diabetes mellitus.

- The pancreas does not function properly and does not produce insulin at all.
- Even if these clients take a medication to stimulate insulin production, the pancreas still will not produce insulin.
- Oral antidiabetic agents do not work in type I diabetics. Client must take insulin hormone replacement therapy.
- Abrupt onset: the client typically does not even know he has a glucose problem until waking in the emergency department where he recovers from diabetic ketoacidosis. (You'll understand what I'm talking about in one minute!)

Type II:

- Far more common than type I, and accounts for 90% of all diabetes.
- Trend in the United States related to obesity. Childhood diabetes is related to childhood obesity.
- Usually occurs after age 30 and is most commonly seen between the ages of 50 and 60.
- Also known as adult-onset diabetes.
- Nonketotic form of diabetes because there is sufficient insulin production to prevent breakdown of fats leading to ketosis.
- Exact cause is unknown.
- These clients do not have enough insulin, or the insulin they have does not work properly at the cellular level (insulin resistance). The pancreas still works, it's just not working enough or the client is taking in so much glucose (through diet) the pancreas can't keep up.
- Insulin resistance can also be defined as fasting hyperglycemia despite having available endogenous insulin.
- Genetic predisposition to type II diabetes.
- Other risk factors may include obesity, dietary intake, and environmental factors.
- Special diet and an exercise plan are used in an attempt to control the blood glucose.
- Oral agents, and then if these do not do the trick, insulin injections may be used.
- As many as 20% to 30% of clients with type II diabetes require treatment with insulin.
- It is important to understand that type II diabetics may eventually end up with full-blown diabetes mellitus (type I diabetes) due to complete failure of the pancreas to produce insulin. Type II diabetes is a major cardiovascular risk factor.
- The onset for type II diabetes is more subtle and sneaky than type I.
- Type II diabetes is usually found by accident. The client may see the physician for a routine physical exam when type II diabetes is discovered. When a client is treated for a wound that won't heal or for repeated infections (especially vaginal infections) that just won't go away in spite of usual treatments, this will alert the physician to check the blood glucose.

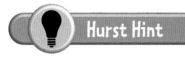

Hurst Hint

Clients with type II diabetes produce just enough insulin so that they do not break down body fat for energy. Therefore, they do not experience diabetic ketoacidosis (DKA).

- Bacteria love a high-glucose environment and will proliferate in this environment. The proliferation of bacteria is one thing that can prolong the healing of a wound.
- When a client has diabetes, the vascular system is compromised, which could impair blood flow to wounds, prolonging wound healing even further.

What causes it and why

Table 14-14 shows the combined causes and explanations for diabetes mellitus types I and II.

Table 14-14

Causes	Why
Beta cells in pancreas are destroyed (can be destroyed by virus); destroyed beta cells do not produce insulin. Insulin produced by the body is referred to as endogenous insulin. The client will need exogenous insulin (not made by the body—e.g., the medication, insulin)	Environmentally triggered autoimmune response where the body attacks itself. The immune system fails to see the pancreatic cells as "self." This autoimmune response may be due to mumps, rubella, cytomegalovirus, a toxin in the body, or an adverse reaction to a drug. Clients with pancreatitis are also at risk for developing diabetes depending on how much of the pancreas is affected
Genetics	Sometimes but not always associated with a family history. There may be a genetic tendency for beta-cell degeneration even in the absence of viral or autoimmune insult. There seems to be a strong genetic factor with type I
Unknown (idiopathic)	That's just the way it is!

Source: Created by author from References #1 to #3.

Signs and symptoms and why

Table 14-15 shows the signs and symptoms and background for type I and II diabetes mellitus.

Table 14-15

Signs and symptoms	Why
Polyuria (large amounts of urine) **Type I**	Blood sugar is high. The kidneys want to help get rid of some of the excess sugar in an effort to bring blood sugar down into normal range. Glucose "spills" into the urine. The kidneys begin excreting sugar particles, but when sugar is excreted, fluid volume goes with it (osmotic diuresis)
Hypovolemia, fluid volume deficit, shock, dehydration **Type I**	Polyuria causes excessive fluid loss from the vascular space

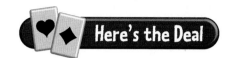

Here's the Deal

Clients with type II diabetes can get their blood glucose under control with diet and exercise, but this is easier said than done. Diet and exercise is hard for everyone, making compliance an issue.

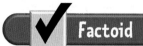

Factoid

Diabetes insipidus (DI) has **nothing** to do with blood sugar. **Diabetes mellitus** (DM) has **everything** to do with blood sugar.

(Continued)

Table 14-15. (*Continued*)

Signs and symptoms	Why
Polydipsia (excessive thirst) **Type I** **Type II (less common)**	Excessive thirst is a result of losing all of the volume from the vascular space
Polyphagia (excessive hunger) **Type I** **Type II (less common)**	The brain is hungry because there is no glucose feeding it! However, if the client eats, he will still be hungry, as the glucose still cannot make it into the cell without insulin
Fatigue and weight loss **Type I**	Lack of glucose in the cells and the breakdown of fat and protein; fluid losses
Glycosuria (glucose in the urine) **Type I and II**	Excessive amounts (greater than 200 mg/dL) of glucose in the bloodstream that spills over into the urine
Ketonuria **Type I**	The body breaks down fat for energy. When fat is broken down, ketones are produced. Ketones are acids. This acid is excreted through the kidneys into the urine
Metabolic acidosis **Type I**	Ketone production causes the blood to become more acidotic
Kussmaul respirations (an increase in rate and depth of respiration) **Type I**	In metabolic acidosis, the lungs will try to compensate by blowing off carbon dioxide (which is acid) in an effort to bring the pH back into normal range
Fruity breath **Most common in type I**	Fat breakdown causes breath changes, causes an acetone smell
Hyperkalemia followed by hypokalemia **Type I and II**	In the presence of acidosis, potassium "leaks" out of cell and hydrogen is "hidden" in the cell
	Administering insulin and fluids will correct the pH by preventing ketone formation. With the administration of insulin and fluids to correct DKA, potassium will move quickly back into the cell. Now, the client is at risk for hypokalemia. Anytime a client is hypokalemic, you should "worry" about arrhythmias
Decreased level of consciousness, coma, death **Type I**	Acidosis; brain does not like it when the pH is out of balance, so neuro changes occur

Source: Created by author from References #1 to #3.

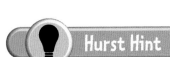

Hurst Hint

Glucose "spills" into the urine once the blood glucose level reaches approximately 200 mg/dL. However, it does vary from person to person.

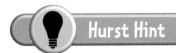

Hurst Hint

You must know all the signs and symptoms of fluid volume deficit, as they are very applicable here! We studied these symptoms in Chapter 1.

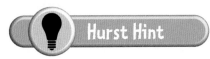

Hurst Hint

You better know all of the signs and symptoms of metabolic acidosis and why the signs occur! We studied these in Chapter 2. These signs and symptoms are very applicable!

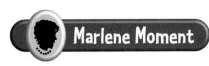

Marlene Moment

I know you love to assess someone's breath! Did you know breath changes are significant indicators of systemic disease?

Quickie tests and treatments

Tests (types I and II combined):

- Urinalysis: glucosuria (sugar in the urine) and ketonuria (ketones) may be present.

- A fasting blood sugar of 126 mg/dL on more than one occasion is diagnostic. Therefore, further evaluation with a glucose challenge is unnecessary.

- If diabetes is suspected but fasting blood sugar is less than 126 mg/dL, a standardized oral glucose tolerance test may be initiated (generally done in clinic setting).

- Must be free from acute illness for glucose tolerance test. Medications that impair glucose tolerance include diuretics, oral contraceptives, glucocorticoids, niacin, and phenytoin (Dilantin).

- The glucose tolerance test has largely been replaced by documentation of fasting hyperglycemia due to the lack of standards.

- HbAIC (glycosylated hemoglobin): is produced by a reaction between protein and glucose. The level is obtained at the time of diagnosis and obtained every 3 months. American Diabetes Association recommends HbAIC to be less than 7%. If consistently 8%, then therapy should be re-evaluated.

- Blood and urine for renal function tests to detect presence of kidney damage.

- Monitor arterial blood gases (ketoacidosis) and vital signs.

Treatment (types I and II combined):

Table 14-16 compares the different types of insulin used in treatment.

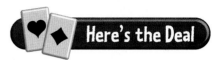

Here's the Deal

The severity of the signs and symptoms in diabetes mellitus vary depending on the client. Some clients may have only the three Ps—polyuria, polydipsia, and polyphagia—but some may have every sign and symptom to the point of coma.

Table 14-16

Generic name	Brand name	Onset (hours)	Peak (hours)	Duration (hours)
Insulin aspart	Novolog	0.25	1–3	3–5
Insulin lispro	Humalog	0.25	0.5–1.5	3–4
Regular human insulin	Humulin R	0.5	2–4	6–8
	Novolin R	0.5	2.5–5	8
Human insulin isophane suspension	NPH	1.5	4–12	24
Human insulin zinc suspension	Lente	2.5	7–15	22
Human insulin extended zinc suspension	Ultralente	4–6	8–20	28
Insulin glargine	Lantus	2–4	None	24
70% insulin aspart protamine suspension/30% insulin aspart	NovoLog Mix 70/30	0.25	1–4	24
75% insulin lispro protamine suspension/30% insulin lispro	Humalog Mix 75/25	0.25	1–2	24
70% human insulin isophane suspension (NPH)/30% regular insulin	Humulin 70/30	0.5	2–12	24
	Novolin 70/30	0.5	2–12	24
50% Human insulin isophane suspension (NPH)/50% regular insulin	Humulin 50/50	0.5	3–5	24

Source: Created by author from References #4 and #5.

- Diabetic diet (usually based on exchanges) recommended by the American Diabetic Association (ADA) with emphasis on timing of meals and appropriate snacks.
- Exchange lists can be obtained from the ADA.
- High soluble fiber content in diet such as beans, oatmeal, apple skin, etc., because soluble fiber slows glucose absorption from the intestine, therefore offering a favorable effect on blood sugar.
  - Weight loss if overweight.
  - Some clients are taught to administer regular insulin or insulin lispro for each 10 or 15 g of carbohydrates eaten at meals.
  - Exercise as prescribed by the physician.
  - Artificial sweeteners are OK in the diabetic diet.
  - Self-monitoring of blood glucose using a glucometer.
  - Scrupulous foot care.
  - Maintain IV access.
  - IV fluids.
  - Potassium as prescribed.
  - Consult MD if signs or symptoms persist or worsen.
  - Instruct insulin self-administration.
  - Oral hypoglycemics for type II diabetes.
  - Drugs for neuropathy.
  - Regular eye exams.
  - Urine test for microalbuminuria to detect early kidney damage.
  - Type II may require oral hypoglycemics and insulin.
  - Strict control of lipids with cholesterol medication, as these clients are at risk for cardiovascular disease.
  - Foot care.
- Hemoglobin AIC every 3 to 6 months. This helps determine average blood glucose over a period of several months. Remember, there may be fluctuations not detected by accuchecks. These fluctuations cause tissue damage; therefore, the AIC is a useful diagnostic tool in maintaining strict control of blood glucose.

THINK ABOUT THIS   A diagnosis of impaired glucose tolerance (IGT) means that the client has prediabetes. This stage of development is between normal glucose metabolism and a diagnosis of diabetes. This occurs when the fasting plasma glucose is between 100 and 126 mg/dL. When endogenous insulin is not working well at the cellular level (insulin resistance) and is accompanied by hypertension, lipid abnormalities, and central obesity, the client has features of metabolic syndrome (syndrome X).

What can harm my client?

- Diabetic ketoacidosis.
- Coma.
- Myocardial infarction.

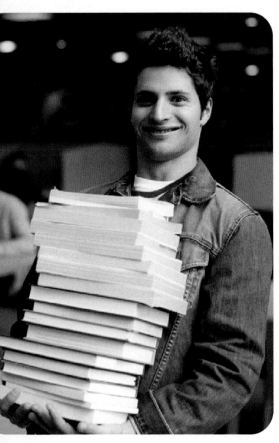

- Retinopathy (vision problems and blindness).
- Amputations related to complications from infected and poor healing wounds.
- Kidney failure.
- Smoking (causes more vasoconstriction, leading to compromised tissue perfusion to heart, kidneys, legs, feet, etc.).

If I were your teacher, I would test you on . . .

- Type I specifics.
- Type II specifics.
- Causes and why.
- Signs and symptoms and why.
- Complications of each type of diabetes: diabetic ketoacidosis, kidney failure, MI, retinopathy, amputations, etc.

✛ Diabetic ketoacidosis (DKA)

DKA is an acute complication of diabetes.

What is it?

DKA occurs in 2% to 5% of type I diabetics. Infection is most often the cause. The 3 Ps—polyuria, polydipsia, and polyphagia—usually precede full-blown DKA.

Pathway to DKA:

1. Lack of insulin.
2. Glucose cannot enter cells.
3. Cells are starved.
4. Body breaks down fat for energy.
5. Fat = ketones.
6. Ketones = acids.
7. Metabolic acidosis = DKA.

What causes it and why

Table 14-17 shows the causes and explanations for DKA.

Table 14-17

Causes	Why
Uncontrolled diabetes	If blood glucose is not monitored closely, the sugar level in the blood will increase
Insufficient insulin dose OR Unknown new-onset type I diabetes	Not enough insulin medication is taken to bring blood glucose down into normal range

(Continued)

Table 14-17. (*Continued*)

Causes	Why
Skipping routine insulin dose	Seen frequently in adolescents and elderly; forget to take insulin, which causes blood glucose to go up
Stress	Any form of stress increases blood glucose (this is normal); however, a diabetic needs to monitor blood glucose during times of stress to adjust insulin dose accordingly to keep blood glucose in the normal range
Taking medications that interfere with insulin secretion	Cause blood glucose to go up; affect the normal action of insulin (which is to bring the blood glucose down)

Source: Created by author from References #3 and #4.

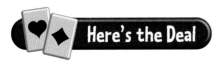

Here's the Deal

When a diabetic gets sick, she should monitor her blood glucose even more closely and adjust the insulin dose accordingly. If she does not, she can develop DKA and wind up in the ED.

Signs and symptoms and why

The signs and symptoms of DKA are the same as seen with diabetes mellitus (see Table 14-15). Let me emphasize some of the most severe symptoms, but you better know the other symptoms, too!

1. Decreased level of consciousness due to metabolic acidosis and shock.

2. Severe hypovolemia due to shock.

3. Electrolyte imbalances, especially potassium problems.

In addition, the client will have polyuria initially to excrete excess sugar particles. When the sugar is excreted by the kidneys, fluid is excreted along with it. As a result, the client becomes hypovolemic. When hypovolemia occurs, polyuria progresses to oliguria and, maybe, anuria—the kidneys are either trying to hold on to what little fluid the body has left, or they might not be adequately perfused. Remember, you must monitor intake and output closely to prevent as much kidney damage as possible.

Quickie tests and treatments

Tests:

- Urinalysis: glycosuria, ketonuria.
- Blood gases: low pH indicating ketoacidosis (metabolic acidosis).
- Blood chemistry: high serum potassium.
- Blood test for kidney function BUN and creatinine.

Treatments:

- First and foremost is prevention, which involves teaching the client to recognize early signs and symptoms.
- In severe ketoacidosis, the client is hospitalized, possibly in the ICU.

- Vitals signs are monitored constantly while fluids (0.9% normal saline to replenish vascular volume) are replaced intravenously in order to correct electrolyte imbalances and shock.

- Potassium may be added to the IV solution at some point if the serum potassium falls. **NOTE:** insulin will also drive potassium back into the cell, causing decreased serum potassium (hypokalemia).

- Indwelling catheter in comatose clients in order to closely observe intake and output.

- Nasogastric tube to prevent vomiting and aspiration.

- The client should not receive sedatives or narcotics, as he already has a decreased level of consciousness.

- Insulin replacement (IV piggyback or PUSH) to correct insulin deficiency and correct acidosis.

- Treatment of associated infections that may be potential culprits.

The major things that can harm the client in DKA are shock, renal failure (from hypovolemia and poor perfusion), metabolic acidosis; remember, everything you learned with type I diabetes is applicable here!

> **Hurst Hint**
>
> The only kind of insulin that can be given to treat DKA is IV insulin.

✚ Hyperglycemic hyperosmolar nonketotic (HHNK) syndrome

This complication presents in a similar way as DKA but without acidosis and usually with higher blood sugar levels. Again, the body is making just enough insulin to prevent breakdown of body fat. If there is no breakdown of body fat, then no ketones are formed. No ketones = no acidosis. This client will not experience Kussmaul respirations because they are not acidotic.

You must understand the content presented earlier in the chapter under "Diabetes mellitus" for a complete understanding of HHNK syndrome as it is all interrelated.

Quickie tests and treatments

Tests:

- Serum glucose: severe elevation of glucose, ranging from 600 to 2400 mg/dL.

- Serum blood chemistry: hyponatremia related to mild dehydration. Serum sodium can increase as dehydration progresses. Ketosis and acidosis are usually absent or mild.

Treatments:

- Fluid replacement to correct hypovolemia (also will help hyperglycemia).

- Insulin replacement.

- Potassium replacement if needed. Remember, potassium may drop as it is driven along with glucose back into the cell.

- Phosphate replacement, if needed, due to hypophosphatemia, which develops during insulin therapy.

✚ Hypoglycemia

What is it?

Hypoglycemia occurs when the blood sugar is too low, less than 70 mg/dL. It is uncommon in those who do not have diabetes. The brain is very sensitive to low levels of blood glucose, so hypoglycemia must be dealt with quickly. If blood sugar falls below normal range, the brain triggers the adrenal glands to release epinephrine. Other responses of the body include glucagon release by the pancreas and growth hormone release from the pituitary gland. All of theses responses contribute to the release of sugar into the blood by the liver.

What causes it and why

Table 14-18 shows the causes and explanations for hypoglycemia.

Table 14-18

Causes	Why
Too much endogenous or exogenous insulin; oral antidiabetic agents	Decreases blood sugar
Decreased food intake	Decreases blood sugar; is worsened if client takes oral antihyperglycemics or insulin
Increased activity	Increases cellular metabolism

Source: Created by author from References #3 and #5.

Signs and symptoms and why

Table 14-19 shows the signs and symptoms and the background for hypoglycemia.

Table 14-19

Signs and symptoms	Why
Sweating, increased pulse, nervousness, irritability, tremors—early symptoms	Stimulation of SNS; release of epinephrine
Dizziness, headache, slurred speech, decreased coordination, confusion—late symptoms	CNS becomes depressed due to lack of glucose

Source: Created by author from References #3 and #5.

Quickie tests and treatments

Tests:

- Low capillary glucose via finger-stick is usually followed by serum glucose to confirm the decreased glucose value.

Treatments:

- Administer a simple sugar such as soda, orange juice, apple juice, or hard candy in nonsevere cases and conscious clients. Give 4 oz, which is half a cup, or 4 sugar cubes.

- After the blood sugar increases, add a complex carbohydrate and protein: half of a peanut butter sandwich, milk, and cheese crackers, or a diabetic nutrition bar.

- In unconscious clients, D50W per large-bore IV/angiocath or injectable glucagon (IM) when there is no IV access (glucagon converts liver glycogen to glucose). After glucose stabilizes and the client wakes up or regains consciousness, give snack or small meal, because the effects of D50W or glucagon are temporary. In other words, the client's blood sugar will bottom out again.

- If the client is at home and is unconscious, place jelly or honey under the tongue for rapid absorption. There are products available for purchase at drug stores that can be used to increase the blood sugar rapidly under these same circumstances. The question often arises regarding what to do in the event that you do not know whether the client is passed out on the floor because of hypo- or hyperglycemia. Treat as if hypoglycemia is the cause. Then call 911!

- Prevent aspiration in nonalert clients because glucagon can cause vomiting. Nausea frequently accompanies hypoglycemia.

- Focus on prevention, which includes client teaching regarding eating and taking insulin regularly with appropriate snacks. The client should always keep a snack or hard candy with her at all times.

- Clients should wear an ID bracelet or carry an ID card in order to assist others in providing prompt treatment.

- Evaluate the result of treatment by monitoring blood glucose levels for several hours, as this is a more reliable indicator of hypoglycemia than signs and symptoms during this phase.

What can harm my client?

- Brain damage due to prolonged hypoglycemia.
- Permanent organ damage.
- Death.

If I were your teacher, I would test you on . . .

- Definition of hypoglycemia.
- Causes and why.
- Signs and symptoms and why.
- Treatment (difference between hypo- and hyperglycemia).
- Importance of following simple sugar with protein.
- Effects of hypoglycemia on the body.
- Peak times and duration of insulin.

✔ **Factoid**

Milk is very good for getting the blood sugar up rapidly (approximately one cup is adequate). Milk not only has sugar but also has protein, which keeps the blood sugar up for a longer period of time.

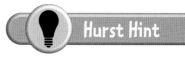 **Hurst Hint**

You need to know when the client's antidiabetic agents (insulin or oral) are peaking, because this is when your client needs to be eating a snack to prevent hypoglycemia. Refer to the insulin chart under treatment for type I diabetes.

PHENOMENA ASSOCIATED WITH DIABETES

Table 14-20 shows the phenomena associated with diabetes.

Table 14-20

Phenomena	Factors
Somogyi phenomenon	Rebound phenomenon that occurs with type I diabetes. Characterized by normal or increased blood glucose levels at bedtime, but blood glucose drops in early morning hours (2 to 3 A.M.) usually because nighttime insulin dose is too high. The client's body attempts to compensate by producing counterregulatory hormones (stimulating gluconeogenesis and inhibiting peripheral glucose absorption) to increase blood glucose, resulting in hyperglycemia on awakening
Dawn phenomenon	Decrease in the tissue sensitivity to insulin that occurs between 5 and 8 A.M. (prebreakfast hyperglycemia) thought to be caused by a release of nocturnal growth hormone causing decreased cellular glucose uptake. Occurs in type I and II diabetes

Source: Created by author from References #2 and #3.

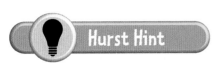

Hurst Hint

Remember . . . High insulin dose in the evening causes low blood sugar around 2–3 A.M. with rebound blood sugar elevation on awakening. Somogyi phenomenon.

CHRONIC COMPLICATIONS OF DIABETES

Chronic complications of diabetes are characterized as macrovascular (large vessel) or microvascular (small vessel).

Macrovascular:

- Coronary artery disease, peripheral vascular disease, and cerebrovascular disease are common in poorly managed diabetics and increase mortality (death) rates for this population.
- Related to associated problems like hypertension, sedentary lifestyle, lipid abnormalities, and smoking as well as hyperglycemia.
- Remember, a large majority (80% or greater) of clients with type II diabetes are obese.

Microvascular:

- Nephropathy (kidney damage), neuropathy (an example is erectile dysfunction or burning of the feet), and retinopathy (damage to the retina) occur in patients with diabetes.
- Evidence supports the theory that these microvascular complications occur less when glucose is better controlled.
- Hyperglycemia = microvascular complications.
- Hyperglycemia not only damages vessels but nerves as well.
- Neuropathies are nerve dysfunctions related to progressive deterioration of nerves leading to decreased nerve function.
- Damage to sensory nerve fibers lead to pain and loss of sensation. The etiology is not completely understood.
- Increased levels of sorbitol and fructose in the nerves act as "poisons," causing damage to cells, resulting in pain, paresthesias, or numbness.
- Paresthesia refers to burning, prickling, or stinging sensation. Sugar kills nerves.

Whether macrovascular or microvascular, these complications are a result of changes to the vessel lining due to hyperglycemia. These vessels thicken and narrow, decreasing blood flow to the area, resulting in ischemia and/or necrosis. Smaller blood vessels leak or are destroyed, thereby decreasing the delivery of nutrients and oxygen to tissues.

Table 14-21 compares the different chronic complications of diabetes.

Table 14-21

Complication	Why
Cataracts	Due to accumulation of protein on the lens of the eye and chronic dehydration of lens
Blindness	Associated with retinopathy
Foot and leg problems	Peripheral vascular disease
Neurogenic bladder (without tone)	Nerve damage (neuropathy)
Gastroparesis	Slowed motility secondary to hyperkalemia. Remember, hyperkalemia starts with muscle twitching, then muscle weakness, and can progress to paralysis; can also be due to nerve damage
Repeated infections (vaginal)	Bacteria thrive in a high-glucose environment
Delayed wound healing	Macrovascular changes leading to poor circulation

Source: Created by author from References #4 and #5.

Quickie tests and treatments

Tests and treatments depend on the cause of the diabetic complication.

What can harm my client?

- Chronic hyperglycemia leads to complications.
- Unresolved infection.
- DKA.
- HHNK syndrome.
- Coma and death.
- Amputation.

If I were your teacher, I would test you on . . .

- Managing a client's blood sugar and avoiding complications.
- Caring for the hypovolemic client.
- Signs and symptoms of diabetes.
- Signs and symptoms of DKA.
- Key client education points (including DKA and HHNK prevention).
- Explain why a client would have polyuria, polydipsia, and polyphagia.

PITUITARY GLAND

The pituitary gland (hypophysis) is often referred to as the master gland even though it is the size of a pea. It is located at the base of the brain (behind the nose) in a little pocket called the sella turcica. The pituitary gland is made up of two parts, the anterior (toward the front of the head) and posterior (toward the back of the head).

The anterior pituitary—also known as anterior hypophysis/ adenohyphosis—secretes the following hormones:

- Growth hormone (GH): controls growth and protein, carbohydrate, and lipid metabolism. Production of growth hormone is controlled by two other hormones:

    1. Somatostatin: inhibits growth hormone.

    2. Somatotropin: stimulates secretion of growth hormone.

The majority of growth hormone is secreted during sleep. Other factors that increase secretion of growth hormone are exercise, stress, hypoglycemia, starvation, and hypothyroidism.

- TSH: stimulates the thyroid gland to produce thyroid hormones T3, T4, and calcitonin.

- ACTH (adrenocorticotropic hormone): stimulates adrenal cortex to release corticosteroid hormones including glucocorticoids, mineralo-corticoids, and the androgens (sex hormones).

- Gonadotropic hormones:

    1. Prolactin: stimulates breast growth and production of milk.

    2. FSH: stimulates development of egg and sperm and secretion of sex hormones.

    3. LH: stimulates the production of progesterone and regulates ovulation in women, and regulates testicular growth, testosterone production, and androgen production in men.

    4. To stimulate the release of these gonadotropic hormones, gonadotropin-releasing hormone (GnRH) must be present. GnRH is released from the hypothalamus.

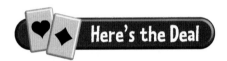

Here's the Deal

You may have the greatest pituitary in the world, but if you do not have adequate hypothalamic stimulation, GH will not be released.

✚ Let's break it down

Here's another way to look at it:

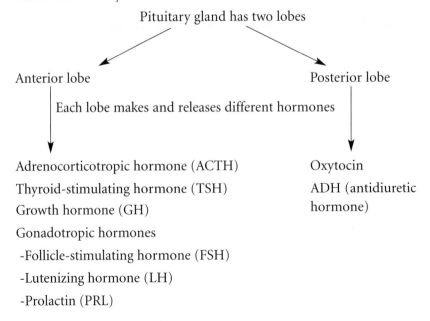

The posterior pituitary—also known as neurohyphosis—secretes:

- Oxytocin: important for cervical dilatation prior to birth, and helps the uterus to contract during labor and delivery, especially during the second and third stages. In breast-feeding (lactating) mothers, oxytocin causes milk to be "let down" into area of breast where baby can suckle and receive milk.

  Which diseases are seen with oxytocin problems? There really aren't any diseases or disorders associated with endogenous (made by the body) oxytocin. However, oxytocin can be given as a drug in the exogenous form called Pitocin. Pitocin is used frequently to induce labor and is associated with serious side effects such as uterine rupture due to overcontraction.

- Vasopressin—also known as antidiuretic hormone (ADH): when ADH is secreted, **WATER** is retained in the vascular space.

ANTIDIURETIC HORMONE (ADH)

The normal action of antidiuretic hormone (ADH) is to retain WATER in an effort to increase vascular volume. When water is retained, urine output drops. The urine that is excreted is now more concentrated because there is not as much water in the urine. An important point to understand is sodium is not being retained.

Don't get ADH and aldosterone confused. When you think of ADH, think WATER! When you think of aldosterone, think sodium AND water.

What diseases are seen with ADH problems?

1. Not enough ADH = diabetes insipidus (DI).
2. Too much ADH = syndrome of inappropriate ADH secretion (SIADH).

✚ What causes an increase in ADH secretion?

Anytime vascular volume is low (as in hemorrhage), ADH is secreted in an effort to replenish the vascular volume by retaining more water.

- Increased blood (serum) osmolarity: osmolarity tells us how much water and particles are in a solution. Osmolarity goes up when there are more particles than water in a solution (hemoconcentration). In an effort to get the particle-to-water ratio back in balance, ADH is secreted and water is retained. This decreases the concentration of the blood (because it is being diluted), and therefore decreases the osmolarity.

- Hypernatremia: the serum sodium can go up for two reasons. The water level in the blood may be too low, or the sodium level can be too high. With either circumstance, the particle-to-water ratio is out of balance. Hypernatremia is the same as dehydration—not enough water in the blood. ADH is secreted and water is retained in the vascular space—notice I did NOT say "sodium and water." The blood becomes more dilute and the serum sodium comes down.

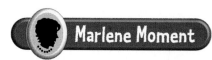

Marlene Moment

If you are a breast-feeding mom, hearing your baby cry, thinking about your baby, or smelling your baby can cause the letdown reflex to occur. However, beware. This reflex can kick in at Pizza Hut too, when you hear someone else's baby cry or smell another baby; even sitting in the chair where you frequently feed your baby can cause letdown.

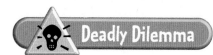

Deadly Dilemma

Any form of nipple stimulation can cause oxytocin to be released and therefore cause uterine contractions. If someone is in premature labor, nipple stimulation is a contraindication, as it could cause premature birth.

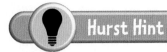

The only electrolyte that is affected by the amount of water in the vascular space is sodium. If the water level in the blood is too high (making it dilute), the sodium level will go down. If the water level in the blood is too low (making it concentrated), the sodium level will go up.

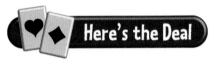

Anytime the body is low on volume (shock), the body compensates by holding on to fluid any way it can. One chemical that helps fight shock and replenish volume is ADH.

✚ What causes a decrease in ADH secretion?

Anytime vascular volume is high (hypervolemia), ADH secretion decreases. If ADH is not secreted, the kidneys cannot hold on to water. The kidneys will excrete water, making vascular volume decrease. This is a normal compensatory mechanism.

- Decreased blood (serum) osmolarity: serum osmolarity goes down when there is more water as opposed to particles in a solution (diluted blood). One cause of decreased blood osmolarity is when there is too much water in the vascular space. Excess water in the blood causes it to become too dilute. When there is water excess, ADH secretion is decreased so the kidneys won't hold on to water, and the body excretes water so the blood becomes less dilute. This brings the particle-to-water ratio back into normal range again.

- Hyponatremia: another cause of decreased ADH secretion is a decreased serum sodium level. There **really** may be a deficit of sodium or there may be so much water in the blood that it is diluting the number of sodium particles present. ADH secretion decreases and the kidneys excrete water. This makes the blood less dilute, which brings the serum sodium level back up.

THINK ABOUT THIS "Concentrated" makes the numbers go up, and "dilute" makes the numbers go down. The specific numbers I am talking about are sodium, osmolarity, specific gravity, and hematocrit. These four things can be measured in any fluid except for hematocrit—you need blood for this. For example, if I am dehydrated, this means my blood plasma is concentrated because there is not enough water and too many particles in the plasma. In this case, the serum sodium, serum osmolarity, specific gravity of blood, and hematocrit will go up— concentrated makes numbers go up. Also, in this circumstance, the urine output is decreased because the body is trying to hold on to what little fluid is left. The kidneys, if functioning properly because they are still being perfused, will still try to put out at least 20 to 30 mL/hr to get rid of toxins and electrolytes as they normally would. This little bit of urine that is being put out is very concentrated. Remember, the kidneys are holding on to water when dehydrated if they are working properly. Therefore, the urine sodium, urine osmolarity, and specific gravity of urine are increased as well.

✚ Diabetes insipidus (DI)

What is it?

Diabetes insipidus occurs when the posterior pituitary does not secrete enough ADH. Therefore, the kidneys start excreting more water. The vascular volume decreases to the point of shock and the blood becomes concentrated. The urine output continues to increase in spite of the shock, resulting in very dilute urine. This is weird because normally when somebody is in shock, the urine output will decrease, because the

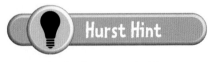

In DI the body cannot hold on to water because there is not enough ADH.

kidneys either are not being perfused or the body is holding on to what little fluid it has left.

Let's talk about another concept. Do you agree that **NORMALLY** blood and urine like to do the same thing? They like to mirror each other, don't they? Yes, they do! Think about it. When someone drinks a lot of water, the blood is dilute and the urine is dilute because they mirror each other. In dehydration, the blood is concentrated and the urine is concentrated. In hyperglycemia, there is a lot of glucose in the vascular space, so the blood has a lot of glucose in it and the urine has glucose in it as well (glucosuria). See? They like to do the same thing!

Well, GUESS WHAT? Blood and urine DO **NOT** mirror each other when someone has diabetes insipidus. In DI, there is not enough ADH, so water is **not** being retained in the vascular space. The urine output increases, and the urine that is being put out is dilute due to the high volume-to-particle ratio. The volume is depleted and the blood becomes concentrated because **water** is being lost out of the vascular space. Normally when the blood becomes depleted and concentrated, urine output decreases to help save volume. In DI, there is no ADH to help hold water in. Large amounts of dilute urine are being put out even though the client is going into shock. In DI, the blood is concentrated and the urine is dilute. The blood and urine are opposite of each other.

There are four types of diabetes insipidus:

1. Primary DI (neurogenic): due to disorder in the pituitary or hypothalamus.

2. Secondary DI (neurogenic): due to craniotomy, trauma, or surgery (the pituitary/hypothalamus are altered).

3. Nephrogenic DI: occurs when kidney tubules are insensitive to ADH (inherited). Abnormality resides in the kidney.

4. Drug induced DI: the name says it all!

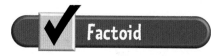

Factoid

Neurogenic DI refers to DI that originates as a consequence of a problem in the brain.

What causes it and why

Table 14-22 shows the causes and explanations for DI.

Table 14-22

Causes	Why
Decrease in production or release of ADH	May be due to a tumor in the pituitary or a defect in the hypothalamus
Inability of the kidney to respond to ADH (nephrogenic)	The renal tubules and the collecting tubes are not able to respond to the ADH. It is not because there is not enough ADH; there is little to no water resorption
Tumor in the pituitary or hypothamus glands (neurogenic)	The pituitary is extremely sensitive to any kind of foreign stimulation

(Continued)

Table 14-22. (*Continued*)

Causes	Why
Skull trauma, injury, CVA, brain infections	Anytime the pituitary is upset, DI or SIADH can occur (you never know which one)
Surgery	If the pituitary is removed, not enough ADH is being produced, is it? NO! If the pituitary is even touched during brain surgery, DI or SIADH could occur
Drug induced—lithium (Eskalith), alcohol, general anethestics	These drugs interfere with the kidney's response to ADH
Rare causes: brain disease, brain hemorrhage, or cerebral aneurysm	Anything going on in the brain can upset the pituitary (pressure on it, etc.)
Psychogenic polydipsia	Psychiatric disorder where the client drinks excessive amounts of water. This suppresses ADH secretion

Source: Created by author from References #1 to #3.

Signs and symptoms and why

Table 14-23 shows the signs and symptoms and associated background for DI.

Table 14-23

Signs and symptoms	Why
Thirst and polyuria (sudden onset)	Not enough ADH; water is excreted by the kidneys in large amounts; thirst is your body's way of saying "drink fluids, you've lost too much"
Dehydration (you better review all the signs and symptoms of dehydration, because they are very applicable here)	Excessive loss of water from the vascular space
Polydipsia (excessive thirst)	Polyuria causes dehydration; the osmoreceptors relay the message (dehydration) to the brain, so that it will trigger the sensation of thirst (client needs increased water intake)
Hypotension	Excessive loss of water from the vascular space (less volume = less pressure) and decreased peripheral resistance
Tachycardia	The heart rate increases; the heart is trying to pump the decreased volume to perfuse vital organs

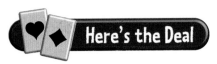

Here's the Deal

Let the "D" in diabetes insipidus help you to remember "diuresis." Now you will get more questions right on your test!

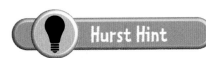

Hurst Hint

Anytime something is going on in the head (craniotomy, sinus surgery, stroke, whatever!), worry about the pituitary. The least little thing can upset the pituitary and trigger DI or SIADH when you least expect it.

(*Continued*)

Table 14-23. (*Continued*)

Signs and symptoms	Why
Decreased central venous pressure (CVP)	If the vascular volume is decreased, then the volume inside the heart chambers is decreased, so CVP goes down (less volume = less pressure)
Irritability	Brain changes associated with dehydration and sodium imbalances; your brain doesn't like it when volume is too low or when sodium is out of balance
Changes in LOC: lethargy to possible coma	Hypernatremia since so much water has been lost. The brain doesn't like it when sodium is too high or too low. Neuro changes begin as a result
Vision changes	If a tumor is causing DI, the tumor might be pressing on the optic nerve
Weight loss	When water is lost, weight is lost
Headache	Cellular dehydration of brain

Source: Created by author from References #1 to #3.

Quickie tests and treatments

Tests:

- Serum osmolarity increased and urine osmolarity decreased (same with specific gravity).
- Serum sodium up (dehydrated); urine sodium down (dilute urine).
- Specific gravity of blood up; urine specific gravity down.
- Urine output must be greater than 4 L in 24 hours.
- Fluid deprivation test—also known as dehydration test: this test can be very dangerous, as fluids are being withheld in a client who is putting out large amounts of dilute urine. We are trying to see if the urine output decreases when fluid is withheld, as it normally would. If the client keeps putting out large amounts of dilute urine, then DI is suspected.
- Hypertonic saline test: hypertonic saline is administered IV. This solution contains a large number of sodium particles. As a result, the sodium level in the blood will increase. Normally, a high sodium level in the blood triggers ADH to be released, so water will be retained (the blood needs more water for dilution; dilution will bring the serum sodium down into normal range). This release of ADH causes the urine output to drop. If the urine output does not drop as it normally would, DI is suspected.
- Hematocrit: increased; blood is hemoconcentrated due to water loss (blood gets thicker too).
- BUN: increased; anytime the blood is concentrated, the BUN goes up.
- Serum vasopressin: low.

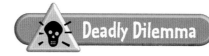

In diabetes insipidus, the amount of urine output can be anywhere from 4 to 30 liters a day! Get fluid replacement started quickly!

If DI occurs as a result of some type of brain injury, the symptoms usually appear 3 to 6 days postinjury and can last for up to 10 days. So be very watchful of the vital signs and urine output during this time.

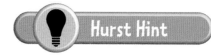

1000 milliliters = 2.5 pounds.

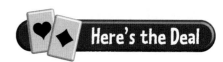

Diabetes insipidus has NOTHING to do with your blood sugar. So don't pick Accu-checks Q4 hours on a test!

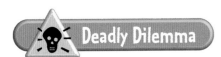

- Vasopressin challenge test: desmopressin acetate is given intranasally or IV with a subsequent monitoring of urine volume 12 hours pre- and postchallenge.
- MRI of the pituitary and hypothalamus.

Treatments:

- Medications: Diabinese (chlorpropamide) or Novo-Propamide (avo-chlorpropamide) to produce ADH. These drugs also help the ADH that is already being produced work better. ADH is given to keep the water level in balance. Desmopressin acetate (DDAVP), synthetic ADH, is given intranasally. Lypressin (Diapid) is the same type of drug, but it is short acting. Aqueous vasopressin (Pitressin) may be given.
- Maintain fluid volume, monitor intake and output, assess vital signs, check lab work often, encourage fluids.

What can harm my client?

- Shock due to hypovolemia.
- Hypernatremia.
- Treatment using DDAVP can cause increased water retention (fluid volume excess and high blood pressure) if not taken properly.

If I were your teacher, I would test you on . . .

- Clinical manifestations of diabetes insipidus.
- Differentiation of diabetes mellitus and diabetes insipidus.
- Treatment and care of clients with diabetes insipidus.
- Monitoring of fluid balance.
- Signs and symptoms of hypovolemic shock.
- When client is discharged, teach signs that client needs a dose of ADH (DDAVP); the signs are polyuria and polydypsia.
- The importance of teaching the client about daily weights.
- The importance of teaching the client when to call the physician.
- Drug therapy associated with diabetes insipidus.

✚ Syndrome of inappropriate antidiuretic hormone (SIADH)

What is it?

SIADH is when too much antidiuretic hormone (ADH) is produced. When this happens, the client goes into fluid volume excess or hypervolemia. The fluid in the vascular space becomes very dilute due to WATER retention. This dilute fluid decreases the serum sodium and the client becomes hyponatremic. Normally, when someone is hypervolemic, urine output increases in an effort to get rid of the excess fluid. Not here! Since there is so much ADH being produced, the kidneys hold on to water, so urine output goes down. This makes everything worse!

What causes it and why

Table 14-24 explores the causes and why of SIADH.

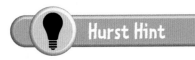

Table 14-24

Causes	Why
Drugs such as NSAIDs, morphine, metaclopramide (Reglan), and antidepressants	Increases the action or the production of ADH
Tumors in the lungs, pancreas, prostate, and brain	Tumors can secrete ADH or a vasopressin-like substance that increases the amount of water retained in the body
Infections: meningitis, encephalitis	Infection in the brain can affect the pituitary gland
Head injury	Pituitary is extremely sensitive to any foreign stimulation
Cancer of the kidney	Decreases response to the ADH

Source: Created by the author from References #2, #4, and #5.

Signs and symptoms and why

Table 14-25 shows the signs and symptoms and why of SIADH.

Table 14-25

Signs and symptoms	Why
Decreased urinary output	Too much ADH causes water retention, not excretion
Hyponatremia	Water retention dilutes the serum sodium
Hypertension	Fluid retention causes volume to go up. Remember, MORE VOLUME = MORE PRESSURE!
Tachycardia	The heart only wants volume to go in one direction, and that direction is forward; if the fluid doesn't go forward, it's going to go backward into the lungs
Increased central venous pressure (CVP). CVP is determined by the amount of blood returning to the right side of the heart. The greater the amount, the greater the pressure. CVP is measured in the right atrium	Water retention causes fluid volume excess. Hypervolemia leads to more blood return to the right side of the heart. More volume = more pressure
Decreased hematocrit, serum sodium, specific gravity, BUN, and osmolarity	Blood is diluted, which makes these numbers decrease (hemodilution)
Edema	Water retention; when the vascular space is overloaded with fluid, it will leak out into the interstitial space
Change in level of consciousness (LOC)	Hyponatremia is present. The brain does not like it when sodium is out of balance
Vision changes	If a tumor is the cause of the SIADH, then the tumor could be pressing on the optic nerve
Weight gain	When water is retained, weight is gained

Source: Created by author from References #1 and #2.

RECAP   Now let's think about a few of the signs and symptoms we have read.

Let's talk about the normal first. The body is always trying to compensate. The body wants to fix any problems before they get out of hand.

A client with SIADH experiences fluid volume excess. Water is retained in the vascular space. When a client experiences fluid volume excess, what happens to the urine output? Normally, the urine output goes UP because the body knows that it is not supposed to have that much volume in the vascular space. The kidneys try to rid of the fluid by causing diuresis.

In SIADH, what happens to the client's urine output? It is going DOWN! That is weird! That is not supposed to happen because the client is in vascular overload! Well, the client with SIADH goes into fluid volume excess, and the urine output goes down because of too much ADH. Water is retained in the vascular space. The more fluid retained, the worse the client becomes.

Again, do you agree that NORMALLY blood and urine like to do the same thing? They like to mirror each other? YES! Well, guess what? Blood and urine DO NOT mirror each other in SIADH. The urine is very concentrated, because water is retained in the vascular space due to TOO MUCH ADH. The blood is dilute due to fluid retention (specifically water) in the vascular space. Understanding this will help you get more test questions right!

Here's a quick visual aid to help you remember the difference between DI and SIADH.

Meet S$\bar{\text{i}}$ (pronounced sigh) and D$\bar{\text{i}}$ (pronounced die)

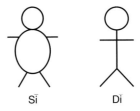

Notice S$\bar{\text{i}}$ has retained way too much fluid and D$\bar{\text{i}}$ has lost way too much!

Quickie tests and treatments

Tests:

- Serum sodium: decreased.
- Urine sodium: increased.
- Serum osmolarity: decreased.
- Urine osmolarity: increased.
- Specific gravity of blood: decreased.
- Specific gravity of urine: increased.
- BUN: decreased due to hemodilution.
- Urine output: decreased.
- Serum ADH: increased.

Treatments:

- Treat the cause.
- Diuretics: pulls fluid out of the body; watch serum sodium closely as the diuretic could make hyponatremia worse.
- Hypertonic saline IV: builds the sodium level back up. Monitor the client as excess sodium could pull fluid into the vascular space and throw the client into CHF and pulmonary edema quickly. Also, anytime sodium is being manipulated, the brain could become unhappy.

- Lithium (Eskalith): monitor client because lithium + sodium imbalance = toxicity.
- Demeclocycline (Declomycin): commonly used medication.
- Fluid restriction; keep mucous membranes moist by allowing the client to rinse; do not let him swallow.
- Do not use water in tube feedings, use saline instead.
- Use saline with nasogastric tube irrigations: client doesn't need any more plain water.
- Monitor intake and output.
- Monitor daily weights: a gain of 1 kilogram equals a gain of 1000 milliliters of fluid.

What can harm my client?

- Seizures.
- Cerebral edema.
- Confusion.
- Coma.
- Water intoxication.

If I were your teacher, I would test you on . . .

- Causes and why.
- Signs and symptoms and why.
- Effects on osmolarity, specific gravity, sodium, and BUN.
- Dangers associated with administration of hypertonic saline.
- Drugs used for treatment.
- Importance of limiting water intake.
- Difference between DI and SIADH.

SUMMARY

The endocrine system affects many organs and life processes. This review of the endocrine system provides you with a better understanding of a complicated body system to allow you to care for your clients safely and teach them the information needed to improve their quality of life.

PRACTICE QUESTIONS

1. A client displays the following symptoms: laboratory results indicating hyponatremia and hyperkalemia, heavy pigmentation of the skin in sun-exposed areas, muscle weakness, and poor appetite. Based on these symptoms, the client is most likely exhibiting which illness?

   1. Diabetes insipidus.

   2. Myxedema.

   3. Cushing's syndrome.

   4. Addison's disease.

Correct answer: 4. The clinical presentation of Addison's disease includes low sodium, high potassium, hyperpigmentation of the skin, anorexia, and muscle weakness.

2. A client presents to the physician's office with severe headache, palpitations, and profuse sweating. The nurse suspects the client is experiencing:

   1. Hypothyroidism.

   2. Pheochromocytoma.

   3. Cushing's syndrome.

   4. SIADH.

   Correct answer: 2. Pounding headache, sweating, and palpitations are classic signs of pheochromocytoma.

3. A client admits to frequent urination, thirst, and weight loss. The client is diagnosed with diabetic ketoacidosis (DKA). The nurse knows DKA is caused by:

   1. Severe lack of insulin.

   2. Too much insulin.

   3. High-calorie diet.

   4. Excessive exercise.

   Correct answer: 1. Clients with type I diabetes can develop DKA when there is not enough insulin present, usually because the client forgets to take his or her prescribed insulin. Type I diabetics require insulin in their system 24 hours a day.

4. In diabetes insipidus, one of the hallmark causes is:

   1. Increased production of ADH.

   2. Increased response of the kidney to ADH.

   3. Decreased production of ADH.

   4. Dehydration.

   Correct answer: 3. The primary cause of diabetes insipidus is lack of ADH. The body loses water at a fast rate, putting the client at risk for hypovolemia.

5. Which of the following symptoms is the most diagnostic sign of hypoparathyroidism?

   1. Exophthalmos.

   2. Dyspnea.

   3. Numbness and tingling of hands and feet.

   4. Tetany.

   Correct answer: 4. In hypoparathyroidism, low calcium levels can cause tetany, one of the chief signs of this disease.

6. Another name for hypothyroidism is:

1. Addison's disease.

2. Graves' disease.

3. Cushing's disease.

4. Diabetes mellitus.

Correct answer: 2. Hyperthyroidism is also known as Graves' disease.

7. When discharging a client who is diagnosed with hyperaldosteronism, the nurse would assure that the client understands (select all that apply):

1. The importance of maintaining health care appointments to monitor blood pressure and electrolytes.

2. If taking spironolactone (Aldactone), the possibility of side effects of gynecomastia, impotence, or menstrual disorders may exist.

3. Glucose intolerance may develop.

4. To eat only a high-sodium diet

Correct answers: 1, 2, & 3. It is important to monitor blood pressure and electrolytes, especially potassium, in clients diagnosed with hyperaldosteronism. Clients should also be aware of the side effects of spironolactone therapy, chance of developing glucose intolerance, and importance of maintaining a low-sodium diet.

8. The adrenal medulla secretes which of the following groups of hormones?

1. Glucocorticoids, mineralocorticoids, and androgens.

2. Insulin, glucagon, and somatostatin.

3. Epinephrine and norepinephrine.

4. T3, T4, and calcitonin.

Correct answer: 3. The medulla of the adrenal gland causes the release of epinephrine and noreinephrine.

9. When discharging a client who is diagnosed with hypothyroidism, the nurse knows that the client needs further education when the client states:

1. "I will make sure I take my levothyroxine sodium (Synthroid) until I feel better."

2. "I know that I will probably be taking hormone replacement therapy for the rest of my life."

3. "I should report any chest pain, nervousness, or weight loss to my doctor."

4. "I will try to stay on my low-calorie diet as recommended."

Correct answer: 1. Clients diagnosed with hypothyroidism should understand that taking hormone replacement therapy (levothyroxine sodium [Synthroid]) is likely a lifelong process and that therapeutic doses are determined based on lab findings and the client's response.

10. A client asks a nurse to explain the difference between type I and type II diabetes. The nurse's best response would be:

   1. "There is no a difference between the two types once the client with diabetes starts taking insulin."

   2. "In type I diabetes, the client can eat what and when he wants."

   3. "In type I diabetes, the client does not produce any insulin, and in type II diabetes there is an insufficiency of insulin along with insulin resistance."

   4. "Though both types of diabetes can require insulin, oral diabetic medications can also help to decrease blood glucose."

Correct answer: 3. Type II diabetes may eventually require insulin to aid in blood glucose management. Type II diabetes is usually managed with oral agents, diet, and exercise. Type I diabetes produces no insulin and does not respond to oral agents.

References

1. Anderson KN, Anderson LE. *Mosby's Pocket Dictionary of Medicine: Nursing & Allied Health*. 3rd ed. St. Louis: Mosby; 1998.

2. Christensen BL, Kockrow EO. *Adult Health Nursing*. 5th ed. St. Louis: Mosby; 2006:516–564.

3. Lemone P, Burke K. *Medical-Surgical Nursing*. 3rd ed. Upper Saddle River, NJ: Pearson Education; 2004:438–471.

4. Lewis SL, Heitkemper MM, Dirksem SR, et al. *Medical-Surgical Nursing*. 7th ed. St. Louis: Mosby; 2007:1234–1322.

5. Porth CM. *Pathophysiology: Concepts of Altered Health States*. 6th ed. Philadelphia: Lippincott Williams & Wilkins; 2002:891–923.

6. Hypoaldosteronism: Aldosterone deficiency syndromes. *Scientific American Medicine 2000*. Available at http://enotes.tripod.com/hyperaldosteronism.htm. Accessed August 25, 2007.

7. *Current Medical Diagnosis & Treatment*. Lange edited by Tierney, McPhee, and Papadakis 44th ed. McGraw Hill; 2005.

Bibliography

Hurst Review Services. www.hurstreview.com.

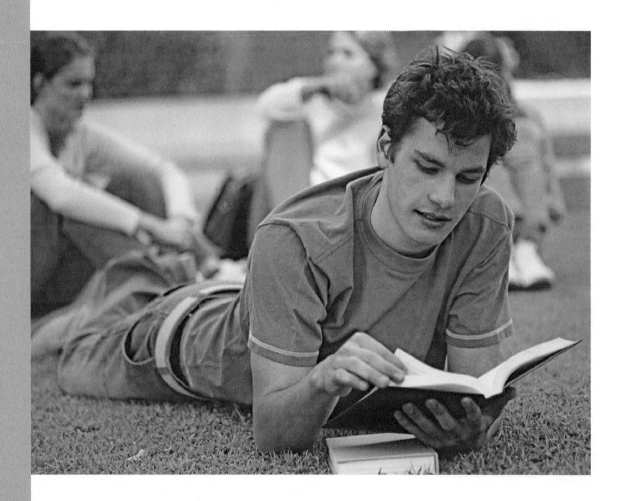

CHAPTER

15 Renal System

OBJECTIVES

In this chapter, you'll review:

- The function of the renal system.
- The causes, signs and symptoms, and the treatments for renal system disorders.
- The complications associated with renal system disorders.

LET'S GET THE NORMAL STUFF STRAIGHT FIRST

The kidneys are the main excretory organs. While working along with other body systems, the kidneys help to maintain homeostasis, fluid and electrolyte balance, and acid–base balance. Some of their functions include:

- Reception of one-fifth of the circulatory blood from cardiac output.
- Production of erythropoietin, which stimulates red blood cell production and maturation.
- Activation of vitamin D: kidneys convert vitamin D to its active form so calcium can be absorbed in the GI tract. Other names for the active form of vitamin D are calcitriol and 1,25-dihydroxycholecalciferol.
- Secretion of renin—a hormone that has an effect on blood pressure and electrolytes.
- The juxtaglomerular (JG) cells of the renal afferent arteriole recognize a decreasing vascular volume. Here's what happens: JG cells release renin → something called renin substrate is converted to angiotensin I (A-I) → a converting enzyme then converts A-I to angiotensin II → A-II tells the adrenal cortex to secrete aldosterone → sodium and water are retained in the vascular space → vascular volume goes up, increasing blood pressure (more volume equals more pressure).

Remember, when sodium and water are retained, potassium is excreted. Therefore, renin may cause the serum potassium to decrease.

✚ Which kidney structure does what?

Table 15-1 shows the different structures of the kidney and their related functions.

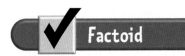

Here's the Deal

Anytime someone's kidneys are sick, look for anemia due to a decrease in erythropoietin.

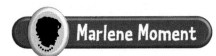

Factoid

Angiotensinogen has a new name . . . renin substrate.

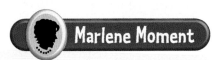

Marlene Moment

Did you know you have one million nephrons per kidney? That's a lot of nephrons!

Marlene Moment

When you think of a glomerulus, think of a roller coaster with many "loops." The glomerulus is made of lots of loops!

Table 15-1

Kidney structure	Function
Nephron (the nephron consists of many different structures, shown in Figure 15-1)	This is where urine is formed regulating water and soluble substances by filtering the blood, reabsorbing what substances are needed, and excreting the rest as urine. When we do not take in much fluid, the nephron makes our urine more concentrated (still gets rid of the bad stuff, but keeps the fluid)
Glomerulus	Capillary tuft that receives its blood supply from an afferent arteriole of the renal circulation; filters out water and **tiny** particles in the blood
Glomerular capsule or Bowman's capsule	Filters blood

(Continued)

Table 15-1. (*Continued*)

Kidney structure	Function
Proximal convoluted tubule (PCT)	The only tunnel between the Bowman's capsule and the loop of Henle; moves water and solutes from place to place. The PCT has a role in fluid absorption, sodium resorption and pH regulation
Loop of the nephron or loop of Henle	Street that connects the PCT to the distal convoluted tubule; reabsorbs water and certain ions from urine
Distal convoluted tubule (DCT)	The tunnel between the loop of Henle and the collecting duct system; transports ions and is regulated by the endocrine system; has a role in regulating pH, potassium (K), sodium (Na), and calcium (Ca) levels
Collecting ducts	Consists of many ducts and tubules that connect the nephron to the ureter. The collecting duct is normally impermeable to water; however, it becomes permeable (lets water come through) in the presence of antidiuretic hormone (ADH). As much as three-fourths of the water from urine can be reabsorbed as it leaves the collecting duct by osmosis. Levels of ADH determine whether urine will be concentrated or dilute. Dehydration results in an increase in ADH (causes water retention) secretion, causing a concentrated urine; while water sufficiency (adequate water levels in the body) results in low ADH secretion, causing water excretion and dilute urine

Source: Created by author from Reference #1.

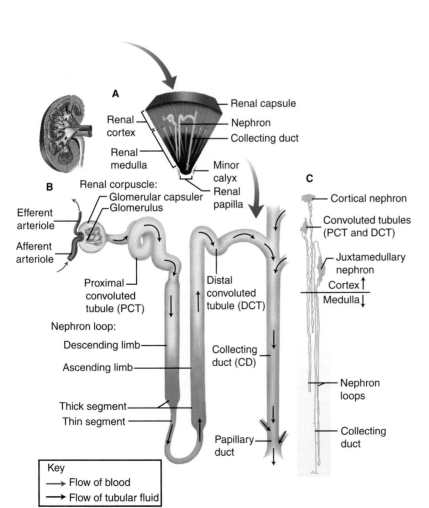

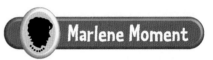

Marlene Moment

Did you know the Bowman's capsule was named after Sir William Bowman in the 1800s? He was a British surgeon and anatomy dude. Now don't ask me how the proximal convoluted tubule got its name!

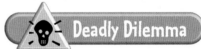

Deadly Dilemma

There are cells in the PCT called proximal tubular epithelial cells. Acute tubular necrosis (which can lead to rapid kidney failure) occurs if these cells are damaged from antibiotics (especially "mycins") or bacteria.

◄ Figure 15-1. Microscopic anatomy of the nephron. **A.** Location of a nephron in one lobe of the kidney. **B.** Structure of a nephron. **C.** Three nephrons. (From Saladin K. *Anatomy and Physiology: The Unity of Form and Function.* 4th ed. New York: McGraw-Hill; 2007.)

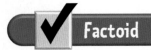

Factoid

The majority of diuretics act specifically on some part of the nephron. For example, thiazides act on the DCT and therefore do not allow Na or Cl to be reabsorbed.

Hurst Hint

If the body secretes a lot of ADH, water is retained in the vascular space, which concentrates urine. If the body does not secrete ADH, then water is excreted, which dilutes the urine.

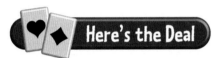

Here's the Deal

The collecting duct system is the kidney's last chance to manipulate fluid and electrolyte balance.

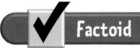

Factoid

Normally, everyone has two kidneys. However, humans can live a normal life with just one kidney.

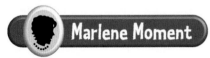

Marlene Moment

Did you see the lady on *Oprah* who found her true love online and it just so happened he needed a kidney? He gave her the ring, got her kidney, and dumped her. Please be careful who you give your kidney to.

Good stuff to know

The following is basic information that is important to know about the renal system.

1. Normal glomerular filtration rate (GFR) is approximately 125 mL/min.

2. The kidneys have the ability to manipulate their own internal blood pressure (BP). This enables the kidney to keep the GFR somewhat constant. However, if systolic BP drops below 70 mm Hg, the kidney can no longer maintain its own BP and the GFR will either drop significantly or cease altogether. This is BAD!

3. Normal urine output is approximately 1 to 3 L/day.

4. Albumin (a type of protein) and globulin (another type of protein) are very large particles. They are so large they cannot fit through the openings in the glomerulus. So, as a rule, these two proteins are not normally found in the urine, and should be a red flag to you if they are present. There are disease processes that can damage the glomerulus and cause protein to leak into the urine.

5. The kidneys reabsorb some glucose from the blood, but there is a limit as to how much they can reabsorb. This "limit" is called the renal threshold. As long as the blood glucose does not go over 220 mg/dL, ALL the blood glucose is reabsorbed and goes back to the blood. As a result, there is no glucose in the urine. However, if the blood glucose goes over 220 mg/dL, then the excess is excreted from the body through the urine. This is your kidneys' way of helping you maintain a normal blood glucose level.

LET'S GET DOWN TO SPECIFICS

Let's look at the causes, signs and symptoms, and treatments for the most common renal illnesses.

✚ Glomerulonephritis

What is it?

Glomerulonephritis is an acute inflammation of the glomerulus that can lead to chronic disease. In glomerulonephritis, the glomeruli capillaries become inflamed and impair the kidney's ability to filter urine. Glomerulonephritis is typically preceded by a group A beta-hemolytic streptococcal infection of the throat. Other illnesses that precede glomerulonephritis are impetigo, upper respiratory tract infections, mumps, varicella zoster virus, Epstein–Barr virus, hepatitis B, and HIV. The antigen–antibodies deposit in the glomerulus in the presence of these infections. This causes thickening and scarring of the glomerular filtration membrane, which leads to decreased GFR. Medications such as gold used in the treatment of rheumatoid arthritis, may also cause glomerulonephritis due to antigen–antibody complexes deposited in the glomeruli. When the glomerulus is damaged, protein and blood cells can leak out into the urine. The bottom line is this: if your glomerulus is not working properly, then everything having to do with kidney function is messed up!

OTHER IMPORTANT THINGS TO KNOW   Glomerulonephritis is:

1. Mainly seen in boys ages 3 to 7, but can be seen at any age.
2. Treatable with full recovery in 60% of adults. However, there is a great chance of permanent renal damage, which can progress to chronic renal failure, especially in the elderly population.
3. A severe illness, which can vary from client to client depending on how much of the glomerulus is damaged.

What causes it and why?

Table 15-2 describes the causes and explanations for glomerulonephritis.

Table 15-2

Causes	Why
Streptococcal infection (post-streptococcal glomerulonephritis); this is the BIGGIE! Poststrep glomerulonephritis usually occurs 7 to 12 days after the initial infection	Antibodies lodge in the glomerulus due to strep infection of the throat or skin and cause scarring; antibodies attach to an antigen forming an antigen–antibody complex, which can damage kidneys
Immune mediated response which is a noninfectious cause	Inflammation of blood vessels in the kidney called vasculitis; due to various autoimmune disorders or related to antigen–antibody complexes
Viruses and parasites	Antigen–antibody mediated

Source: Created by author from References #3, #4, and #6.

Signs and symptoms and why

Signs and symptoms usually subside in 10 to 14 days. Table 15-3 describes the signs and symptoms and background for glomerulonephritis.

Table 15-3

Signs and symptoms	Why
Asymptomatic	Latent symptoms due to slow progression of disease
Hematuria, proteinuria (proteinuria may persist for months)	When the glomerular membrane is damaged (inflammation, thickening, scarring), the openings in the glomerulus enlarge, allowing protein and blood to leak out. Glomerular bleeding can occur and make the urine acidic (blood is slightly acidic)
Edema found mainly in hands and face	When glomerulus is damaged and inflamed, the GFR decreases (not as much blood passing through glomerulus), so sodium and water are retained. Anytime the kidneys are sick, odds are fluid retention will occur as they are unable to excrete properly

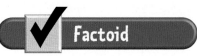

Factoid

Goodpasture's syndrome is a rare type of glomerulonephritis seen mainly in males aged 20 to 30 years.

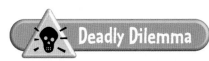

Deadly Dilemma

Glomerulonephritis is the major cause of chronic renal failure.

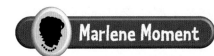

Marlene Moment

Adults and children with sore throats and fever should be tested for strep throat and treated promptly with antibiotics if they test positive for the bacteria to avoid poststrep glomerulonephritis!

(Continued)

Table 15-3. (*Continued*)

Signs and symptoms	Why
Malaise, headache, nausea and vomiting	Retention of toxins; kidneys are unable to filter and excrete bad substances properly; toxins make you feel bad
Elevated blood pressure and fluid volume overload with weight gain	Related to decreased urine output with subsequent fluid volume excess
Dark urine that contains blood (smoky, coffee-colored appearance that looks like a cola-colored soft drink or tea); possible first sign of glomerulonephritis	Red blood cells and protein that are not normally allowed through the kidney now pass through due to damage
Anemia	Kidney produces erythropoietin under healthy conditions, which is responsible for red blood cell production. With renal failure, erythropoietin production is impaired, which interferes with red blood cell production; blood is excreted in the urine
Dyspnea, engorged neck veins, cardiomegaly, pulmonary edema, periorbital edema	Circulatory overload
Hypertension (with possible headache)	Circulatory overload
Confusion, somnolence, seizures	Circulatory overload; sodium imbalances can also affect the level of consciousness and cause seizures
Oliguria (one of the first symptoms)	Kidneys are unable to excrete properly; worsens as GFR decreases

Source: Created by author from References #3, #4, and #6.

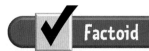

When doctors suspect glomerulo-nephritis, a needle biopsy of the kidney is usually performed to confirm the diagnosis and to determine the amount of scarring.

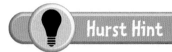

Chronic glomerulonephritis may progress to kidney failure which can cause nausea, vomiting, difficulty breathing, itching, and fatigue.

Quickie tests and treatments

Tests:

- Serum electrolytes: elevated due to decreased excretion.

- Serum protein and albumin: decreased because these substances leak from the blood supply into the urine; albumin can also be decreased as fluid is retained, causing a dilution effect on the blood, which makes albumin even lower.

- Urinalysis: positive for blood, protein, white blood cells.

- 24-hour urine specimen for creatinine clearance and for total protein assay: client may lose up to 3 grams of protein every 24 hours.

- Serum BUN and creatinine: elevated due to decreased excretion.

- Renal ultrasound or x-ray of kidneys, ureter, and bladder (KUB): may show kidney enlargement.

- Renal biopsy: monitor health of kidney tissue.

- GFR: decreased due to inflammation (may be less than 50 mL/min); the older the client, the more decreased the GFR. GFR is measured through a creatinine clearance test.

- Antistreptolysin-O titer: elevated in presence of glomerular damage due to strep.

- Other immune tests may be performed as glomerulonephritis can be due to an immune system problem such as antinuclear antibodies, decreased C3 complement, and IgG present in serum (also known as cryoglobulins).

- Throat culture: positive if glomerular damage is due to strep.

Treatments:

- If BUN is increased and oliguria is present, then dietary protein should be limited or restricted. Under normal circumstances, protein breaks down into urea and is excreted by the kidneys. However, if the kidneys are not working correctly, then urea is not excreted and BUN will go up. Limited or restricted intake of dietary protein keeps BUN from increasing.
- Low-sodium diet until kidney function normalizes: sodium causes fluid retention.
- Monitor fluid intake closely due to edema and fluid retention.
- Diuretics help kidneys get rid of excess sodium and water.
- Phosphate-binding drugs (Amphojel): decrease phosphorus in the blood and increase serum calcium.
- H$_2$-blockers and proton pump inhibitors treat stress ulcers.
- Steroids depending on the cause (autoimmune disease): decrease inflammation in the glomerulus so membranes can heal.
- Treat infection (strep) with antibiotics.
- Monitor intake and output.
- Measure weight daily at the same time each day.
- Bed rest: decreases metabolic demands on the body, but also induces diuresis, which is good; supine position perfuses the kidneys → increased urine production.
- Increase carbohydrate intakes to improve energy and to prevent body from breaking down protein for energy.
- Dialysis or kidney transplant: treatment for chronic glomerulonephritis.
- Plasmapheresis: removes antibodies.
- Diuretics and blood pressure medications: decrease extra fluid volume.

THINK ABOUT THIS   Creatinine is formed from creatine phosphate, which is stored in the muscle and is normally excreted by the kidneys. It is produced constantly and is directly related to muscle mass. Serum creatinine and GFR are inversely related. A rise in serum creatinine suggests renal disease, because the kidneys are unable to excrete it. If creatinine rises by 50% in the blood, then GFR has gone down by 50%—in other words, 50% decrease in kidney function. When the GFR is decreased, the glomerulus is not filtering as it should because it is sick. Therefore, you see a rise in the serum creatinine. GRF cannot be measured directly. It has to be calculated. GFR is an estimate of renal function and is calculated by a formula using urine and plasma creatinine (don't worry; the physician will do the calculating). Since urine creatinine is needed to figure GFR,

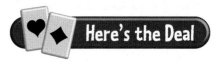

BUN is not as reliable a test as serum creatinine because BUN is affected by several things such as protein intake and fluid volume status. Creatinine is produced constantly and does not fluctuate as readily as BUN.

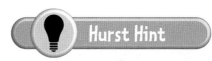

Most sources say that a high-protein diet does not have any bad effect on the kidneys unless kidney damage already exists. This is why you will see different amounts of dietary protein limited or restricted for varying kidney diseases.[1]

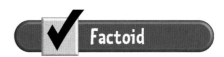

ACE inhibitors have been shown to decrease the decline in kidney function and may be prescribed for different types of kidney disease, especially if the kidney disease progresses to the chronic phase.

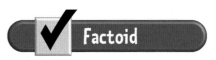

When collecting a sample to determine creatinine clearance, you must take a 24-hour urine specimen and one blood sample.

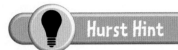

Creatinine clearance is the most sensitive indicator of renal function and is used to document and follow the progression of renal disease.

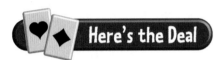

Hypertensive encephalopathy is a medical emergency and requires immediate treatment to reduce the blood pressure.

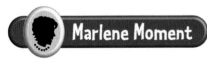

Take the time to understand the structure of the kidney and how it works. This knowledge will help you to think through test questions related to fluid volume deficit and excess, or fluid and electrolyte imbalances.

how do we get this value? A creatinine clearance value from the 24-hour urine specimen is used.

Creatinine clearance is the amount of creatinine excreted from the kidneys in 24 hours. This is one reason to obtain a 24-hour urine specimen. Creatinine clearance is used to determine the rate of glomerular filtration. There is no way to determine exactly what the GFR is, but creatinine clearance is used to help determine an estimate of GFR. Specifically, the creatinine clearance measures the amount of blood that is cleared of creatinine in 1 minute. This value is plugged into a formula to determine GFR.

What can harm my client?

- Too much protein in the diet.
- Renal failure, resulting in dialysis.
- Hypertension.
- Congestive heart failure.
- Hypertrophy of the heart.
- Hypertensive encephalopathy (medical emergency), seizures.
- Pulmonary edema.
- Urinary tract infections.
- Fluid and electrolyte imbalances.
- Sepsis.

If I were your teacher, I would test you on . . .

- Definition of glomerulonephritis.
- Signs and symptoms of glomerulonephritis and why.
- Causes of glomerulonephritis and the impact on fluids and electrolytes.
- Complications and related treatment.
- Nursing interventions such as monitoring intake and output and daily weights.
- Diet modifications.
- Function of albumin and related kidney function tests.
- How age affects GFR.
- Medication side effects; the use of steroids and how this affects client roommate selection (client may be immunosuppressed).

✚ Nephrotic syndrome

What is it?

Nephrotic syndrome produces inflammation of the glomerulus just as in glomerulonephritis but the damage is more severe with severe loss of protein, which causes hypoalbuminemia (low protein in the blood). Albumin is responsible for maintaining or "holding on to" fluid in the vascular space. Without albumin, fluid leaves the vascular space and enters the interstitial tissue, causing edema. The fluid collects in the tissues, decreasing the circulating vascular volume. The kidneys act as they normally do in the case of decreased vascular volume by initiating the renin–angiotensin system. Aldosterone is produced causing retention of sodium and water, but there is not enough albumin in the vascular space to hold on to the sodium and water. Subsequently, they collect in the interstitial space, causing total body edema.

What causes it and why

Table 15-4 explores the causes and background associated with nephrotic syndrome.

Table 15-4

Causes	Why
Diabetes: most common cause; diabetic nephropathy	Soon after the onset of diabetes, the kidney's filtration system becomes stressed, which causes proteins to leak into the urine. This causes the pressure in the blood vessels of the kidneys to increase. Hyperglycemia contributes to the deterioration of blood vessels in the kidneys, thickening of the glomerular basement, and sclerosis of the glomerulus. Remember that sugar damages vessels and the kidneys are very vascular organs with many vessels. Microalbuminuria (albumin in the urine) occurs in the early stages of kidney disease with progression to end-stage renal disease
Autoimmune diseases	Infiltration of inflammatory cells into the glomerulus causing intrarenal vasoconstriction, which results in loss of protein through the kidney. Thought to be antigen–antibody mediated (antibody attaches itself to antigen, forming an antigen–antibody complex that can sometimes damage the kidneys)
Viral infections	Same as with autoimmune diseases
Drugs	Some drugs are toxic to the kidneys: NSAIDs, amino-glycosides, "mycin" antibiotics, amphotericin B, some chemotherapeutic drugs, lithium, IV contrast dye
Immune mediated response (allergic reaction) to insect bites such as pollens, poison ivy, and poison oak	Antigen–antibody complexes deposit in the kidney

Source: Created by author from References #5 and #7.

Many causes of nephrotic syndrome are unknown but can be related to many other diseases such as Hodgkin's disease, syphilis, hepatitis, HIV, allergic reactions, diabetes, and lupus. These diseases damage the glomerular capillary membrane, resulting in small holes in the capillaries and leakage of protein into the urine.

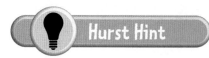

Hurst Hint

The three major things to remember about nephrotic syndrome are proteinuria, hypoalbuminemia, and hyperlipidemia.

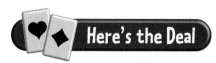

Here's the Deal

Normally, a person loses less than 150 milligrams of protein in the urine in a 24-hour period. In nephrotic syndrome, urination of more than 3.5 grams of protein during a 24-hour period—or 25 times the normal amount—is seen.

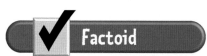

Factoid

Total body edema is called anasarca.

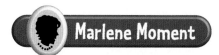

Marlene Moment

Pay attention to the kidney function of diabetic patients! Diabetes is the most common cause of nephrotic syndrome.

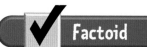

Factoid

Nephrotic syndrome may develop gradually or suddenly and can occur at any age. Small amounts of albumin may leak into the urine undetected for years.

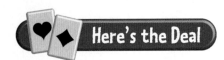

Here's the Deal

Nephrotic syndrome results in excess protein in the urine which may cause foam to form in the toilet water.

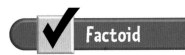

Factoid

Nephrotic syndrome affects men more often than women.

Signs and symptoms and why

Table 15-5 shows the signs and symptoms and rationales of nephrotic syndrome.

Table 15-5

Signs and symptoms	Why
Pitting edema, periorbital edema, ascites, weight gain	Fluid from the vascular space leaks into the tissue as there is no protein or albumin to hold on to the fluid; early morning periorbital edema can be one of the earliest signs (fluid accumulates around the eyes when the client lies down)
Muscle atrophy and/or extreme wasting (cachexia)	Nutrients—especially protein—are lost in the urine
Abdominal ascites and tissue edema	Excess retention of sodium and water with collection of fluid in the peritoneal cavity
Loss of appetite (anorexia), fatigue, malaise, headache, and diarrhea	Edema and accumulation of toxins
Dyspnea	Pulmonary effusion; pulmonary edema; pressure on the diaphragm related to ascites and edema
Oliguria, anuria	Severe decline in renal function leads to inability to excrete urine
Infection of the abdominal cavity and peritoneum	Antibodies that fight infection are lost in the urine or not produced in normal amounts
Anemia (depends on degree of kidney damage)	When kidneys are sick, erythropoietin production is compromised
Pale skin	Severe edema disrupts the normal appearance of skin
Hypotension	Fluid moves from the vascular space into the tissue, decreasing blood pressure

Source: Created by author from References #1, #2, and #5.

Quickie tests and treatments

Tests:

- Urinalysis: 24-hour urine determines the degree of protein loss (usually very high level of protein in urine); presence of high levels of sodium and low levels of potassium; urine lipid levels are high; urine appears foamy due to excess protein in the urine.

- Creatinine clearance: decreased.

- Blood tests: low level of serum albumin, decreased total protein; high lipid concentration; decreased hemoglobin and hematocrit; increased or decreased blood clotting proteins.

- Increased lipid levels include high triglycerides and low-density lipids (LDL) [bad lipids]: lipoproteins and albumin increase in an attempt to compensate for albumin loss; elevated lipid levels lead to atherosclerosis in the client with nephrotic syndrome.

- Renal ultrasound: determines extent of kidney damage.
- Serum and urinary electrophoresis: differentiates between normal renal function, glomerular proteinuria, and tubular proteinuria.
- Glycemic tests: determine glycemic control.
- Kidney biopsy: determines cause and extent of kidney tissue damage; also helps confirm diagnosis.

Treatments:

- Prevention or vigorous treatment of urinary tract infections.
- Angiotensin-converting enzyme inhibitors (ACE): decrease proteinuria and lipid levels. Don't forget that these drugs can increase serum potassium in those who have renal disease.
- Low-sodium diet: sodium causes fluid retention.
- Diet low in saturated fat: client is already hyperlipidemic due to nephrotic syndrome.
- Avoidance of nephrotoxic substances: prevents further damage to the kidneys.
- Hemodialysis or peritoneal dialysis in severe disease.
- Adjustment of medications as renal function changes: the sicker the kidney, the lower the dose of medication required.
- Renal transplant: depends on how much kidney damage is present.
- Small, frequent meals: more tolerable when stomach capacity is reduced due to abdominal ascites.
- Diuretics: help decrease fluid accumulation, but may increase the risk for blood clots, because diuretics can cause hemoconcentration of blood.
- Anticoagulants: reduce risk of blood clots.
- Allergy shots: can reverse nephrotic syndrome caused by allergens.
- Reduction or restriction of dietary protein: protein restriction of 0.6 g/kg/day in clients with GFR less than 25 mL/min prior to the start of dialysis. After starting dialysis, the amount of dietary protein may be altered depending on the client's needs.
- Steroids: decrease inflammation and prevent leakage of protein from the glomerulus.
- Albumin infusion: albumin pulls fluid back into the vascular space, but this presents a risk for circulatory overload; the physician may add furosemide (Lasix) to the infusion to prevent heart failure and pulmonary edema.

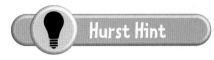

Hurst Hint

The treatment of nephrotic syndrome always involves treating the underlying medical condition causing this problem.

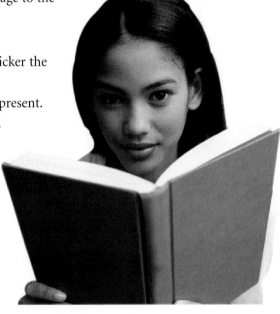

What can harm my client?

- Recurrent infections due to a loss of immunoglobulins (proteins) that are responsible for helping fight infection (kind of like antibodies).
- Loss of binding proteins, which could lead to low levels of ions (iron, copper, and zinc) and hormones such as thyroid and sex hormones.

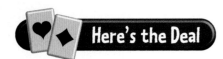

Here's the Deal

Patient education is really important when treating nephrotic syndrome. Patients should be advised to limit their salt intake, take vitamin D supplements, and try to reduce their cholesterol and triglyceride (fats in the blood) levels.

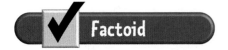

Factoid

Renal failure is a decrease in the glomerular filtration rate (GFR) detected by an elevated serum creatinine.

- Drug overdose, because many drugs have to bind to a protein for transport. With insufficient binding proteins, the drugs remain unbound or free (active).
- Retinopathy.
- Untreated hypertension.
- Thrombotic complications—pulmonary embolism, deep vein thrombosis, renal vein thrombosis—due to an impaired coagulation system (related to loss of coagulation factors).

If I were your teacher, I would test you on . . .

- Causes of nephrotic syndrome and why.
- Signs and symptoms and why.
- Complications associated with protein loss.
- Medication administration and possible side effects.
- Patient education regarding infection control, blood pressure and glycemic control, and low-sodium, low-protein diet.

✚ Renal failure
What is it?

Acute renal failure occurs over days to weeks and decreases the kidneys' ability to filter metabolic waste products from the blood. Chronic kidney failure is a decrease in the kidneys' ability to filter metabolic waste products from the blood, which occurs over months to years. Renal failure develops when the glomerular filtration rate is less than 20% to 25% of normal.

Renal failure can be categorized into three categories: prerenal, intrarenal, and postrenal. Prerenal failure results from decreased blood flow to the kidney. Intrarenal failure occurs from disorders that disrupt the structural integrity of the kidney. Postrenal failure occurs from problems that interfere with urine leaving the kidney.

Examples (Fig. 15-2):

- Prerenal failure: not enough blood reaches the kidneys.

  Hypovolemia due to hemorrhage, dehydration, excessive loss of GI fluids, excessive fluid loss related to burn injuries.

  Decreased vascular filling.

  Anaphylactic shock, septic shock.

  Heart failure and cardiogenic shock.

  Decreased renal perfusion related to drugs.

- Intrarenal failure: damage to the inside of the kidney.

  Acute tubular necrosis due to prolonged renal ischemia, nephrotoxic drugs, heavy metals, hemoglobinuria, myoglobinuria, acute glomerulonephritis, and pyelonephritis.

- Postrenal failure: urine is not able to leave the kidney.

  Bilateral ureteral obstruction.

  Bladder outlet obstruction.

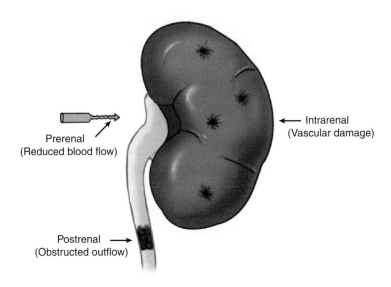

◀ Figure 15-2. Pre-, intra-, and postrenal failure.

What causes it and why

Table 15-6 describes the causes and explanations for acute and chronic renal failure.

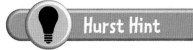

Anything that decreases cardiac output can cause renal failure because not enough blood reaches the kidneys.

Table 15-6

Acute renal failure	Causes and why
Renal failure develops when glomerular filtration rate is less than 20% to 25% of normal.	• Anything causing hypotension, decreased heart rate, or decreased cardiac output such as myocardial infarction or heart failure, shock related to hemorrhage, sepsis, or anaphylaxis. All of these are examples of situations which can impair renal blood flow, causing hypoperfusion of the kidney and drop in glomerular filtration rate
	• Infection, nephrotoxic agents, and severe transfusion reactions can all lead to renal toxicity, necrosis, ischemia, and loss of renal function
	• Dehydration: not enough fluid reaches the kidneys
	• Medications: antibiotics, NSAIDs, ACE inhibitors, and vasodilators can precipitate acute renal failure and should be used with extreme caution
	• Rhabdomyolysis: necrosis of skeletal muscle that causes an accumulation of myoglobin (protein) in the glomerulus
	• Herbal remedies: cause nephrotoxicity
	• Obstruction (e.g., kidney stone, enlarged prostate): increases pressure in kidney tubules, leading to decreased GFR
	• Glomerulonephritis and pyelonephritis

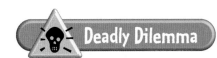

Rhabdomyolysis is a serious, life-threatening condition which may be caused by trauma to the body, viral infections, or a toxic reaction to medication. Up to 85% of patients with significant traumatic injuries may experience rhabdomyolysis a cause of acute renal failure.

(Continued)

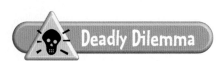

Deadly Dilemma

End-stage renal disease occurs when serum creatinine rises above 2 mg/dL or creatinine clearance drops below 60 mL.

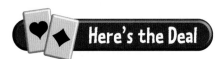

Here's the Deal

ACE inhibitors are used to slow the decline of renal function. However, clients who are in chronic renal failure have kidneys that are already dead.

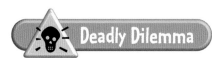

Deadly Dilemma

Renal failure prohibits the excretion of potassium, which causes serum potassium to increase. This is why we do not put clients diagnosed with renal failure on ACE inhibitors as these drugs cause potassium retention, which can worsen the hyperkalemia that causes killer arrhythmias!

Table 15-6. (*Continued*)

Chronic renal failure	Causes and why
Also called end-stage renal disease (ESRD); clients can live with it for many years; the same illnesses that cause acute renal failure can cause chronic renal failure. ESRD develops when the glomerular filtration rate is less than 5% of normal. This is the final stage of renal failure, and the client will require dialysis or a transplant. This stage is also referred to as uremia—urine in the blood—where everything the kidneys used to excrete is now staying in the blood. There are a reduced number of renal capillaries and there is scarring of the glomeruli. The tubules are atrophied and fibrotic and the entire mass of the kidney is reduced	• Systemic diseases: diabetes mellitus, hypertension; chronic glomerulonephritis; pyelonephritis; obstruction of urinary tract; polycystic kidney disease; vascular disorders; infections; medications; and toxic agents that damage the kidneys' small blood vessels causing metabolic products to build up in the body • Systemic lupus erythematosus (SLE): antibodies damage the glomeruli (tiny blood vessels) and tubules (tiny tubes) of the kidneys • Environmental/occupational agents such as lead, cadimum, mercury, and chromium: toxins build up in the blood and damaged kidneys cannot remove them • Renal failure can also be idiopathic (unknown cause)

Source: Created by author using References #1 to #3.

PHASES OF ACUTE RENAL FAILURE   We are going to discuss acute and chronic renal failure signs and symptoms as one. There are some obvious signs and symptoms that you need to know when studying renal failure. There are four phases of ACUTE renal failure that we need to review first.

1. Onset: when the initial problem begins (obstruction, MI, glomerulonephritis). It is very important to identify and treat the initiating cause, as this can influence the extent of kidney damage that occurs. We want rapid identification and treatment of the cause to save the kidneys. This phase continues until oliguria begins. Waste products such as creatinine and urea begin to build up in the blood. This phase can last hours to days.

2. Oliguric phase: this phase lasts 8 to 14 days. As you can tell from the name of the phase, urine output drops (less than 400 mL/24 hrs) or ceases (urine output less than 50 mL/24 hrs). The kidneys do not respond to fluid challenge tests or diuretics. Waste products (creatinine and urea) continue to increase in the blood. Electrolyte imbalances begin.

3. Diuretic phase (also called high output phase): begins 2 to 6 weeks from the onset of the oliguric phase and lasts about 10 days. The kidneys improve and begin to produce urine rapidly. The amount of urine output can be up to 10 liters per day. Electrolytes such as serum potassium begin to drop. BUN falls late in this phase.

4. Recovery phase: can last up to 6 months. The client may resume activities of daily living but will not have as much energy as before. The client is susceptible to further kidney damage during this time.

Signs and symptoms and why

The initial symptoms of renal failure depend on the type of renal failure. For example, if the initiating cause is a heart problem (prerenal failure), the following could occur: arrhythmia such as bradycardia is present → cardiac output drops → client experiences decreased level of consciousness, hypotension, decreased peripheral pulses, decreased urine output → if the bradycardia is not resolved, the kidneys are not getting adequate blood flow, which can precipitate kidney failure.

Prior to the client exhibiting signs and symptoms of renal failure, the client will exhibit symptoms specific to the initiating cause.

In chronic renal failure, the client may exhibit additional symptoms that may not resolve until dialysis or a renal transplant are performed.

Table 15-7 shows the signs and symptoms and associated rationales of acute and chronic renal failure.

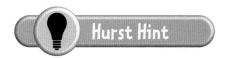

Remember, when the kidneys fail serum potassium goes up, serum phosphorus goes up, serum magnesium goes up, and serum calcium goes down.

Table 15-7

Signs and symptoms	Why
Acute renal failure	
Edema of feet, ankles, hands, face	Retention of fluid due to poor kidney perfusion and excretion
Cola-colored urine	Concentrated urine due to decreased output less than 1 pint/day; oliguria is decreased urine output; anuria is no urine output
Fatigue, decreased concentration, irritability, anorexia, nausea, pruritus, unpleasant taste in mouth	Buildup of toxins; toxins make you feel bad!
Circulatory overload: increased edema, wet lung sounds, shortness of breath, hypertension, headache, weight gain	Decreased excretion of fluid; fluid volume builds up in the body
Electrolyte imbalances	Sodium may be normal, increased, or elevated; If client is retaining excess water, dilutional hyponatremia can occur; serum sodium depends on the amount of water in the vascular space. The kidneys normally excrete potassium, so if kidneys are not working, then serum potassium goes up. Serum phosphorus increases because the kidneys cannot excrete it from the body, and serum calcium will decrease due to the inverse relationship of phosphorus and calcium. Serum magnesium increases
BUN: increased	Urea is not being excreted by kidneys so it builds up in blood
Creatinine clearance: decreased	Poor GFR
Changes in arterial blood gases (ABGs)	Since the kidneys are sick, they retain hydrogen (H+) while excreting bicarbonate. This causes metabolic acidosis to occur. The normal secretion of bicarbonate is also impaired
Hemoglobin and hematocrit: decreased	Erythropoietin production is decreased
Specific gravity: normal or fixed	Specific gravity is the particle to water ratio in a fluid. A high concentration of particles in a fluid makes specific gravity go up; a low concentration of particles in a fluid makes specific gravity go down

(Continued)

Table 15-7. (*Continued*)

Signs and symptoms	Why
Chronic renal failure	
Mental status changes: confusion, encephalopathy, seizures	Increased waste products in the blood cause changes in the brain
Bruising and bleeding	Accumulation of waste products and toxins cause damage to the blood vessels
Hypertension	Diseased kidneys produce hormones that increase blood pressure and cause circulatory overload
Muscle twitches, muscle weakness, cramps, neuropathy, pain	Metabolic wastes damage the muscles and nerves
Pericarditis, angina	Accumulation of metabolic wastes affect the heart muscle
Yellow-brown skin, uremic crystals on skin, pruritis	Metabolic wastes are excreted through the skin since they aren't excreted in the urine
Uremic fetor: fishy odor of the breath	Metabolic wastes cause breath odor
Bone pain, increased risk of fractures	Impaired formation and maintenance of bone tissue (renal osteodystrophy)

Source: Created by author using References #1 to #3.

WHAT IS "FIXED" SPECIFIC GRAVITY?   One of the most important functions of the kidneys is to concentrate and dilute urine according to how much fluid we take in. If you drink a lot of water, urine is diluted. If you become dehydrated, urine is concentrated. When renal failure exists, the kidneys lose the ability to concentrate or dilute urine. When renal failure is suspected, a fluid challenge test is performed. The client is given a bolus of saline. Normally, when a bolus IV of saline is given, urine output increases and the urine becomes more dilute. In the presence of renal failure, the specific gravity of urine will not change no matter how much fluid is given or withheld. Hence, the specific gravity is fixed.

Quickie tests and treatment

Tests:

* Blood tests for electrolytes, BUN, creatinine, urea, arterial blood gasses, triglycerides, parathyroid hormone, vitamin D, complete blood count: determine presence and extent of renal failure.
* Parathyroid hormone (increased); calcitriol (decreased); calcium absorption (impaired); phosphate (increased): impaired formation and maintenance of bone tissue (renal osteodystrophy).
* Urinalysis: determines specific gravity and presence of protein.
* Ultrasound: detects enlarged bladder; hydronephrosis.
* Computed tomography (CT): detects size of kidneys.
* Angiography: detects obstruction.
* Kidney biopsy: determines extent of renal damage.

Treatments:

* Hemodialysis or peritoneal dialysis (if necessary): removes toxins.
* High-calorie, low-protein, low-sodium, low-potassium, low-phosphorus, and low-magnesium diet: controls hypertension, uremia, acidosis,

hyperlipidemia, edema, circulatory overload, and accumulation of toxins.

- Fluid restriction: controls circulatory overload and hypertension.
- Diuretics: reduce circulatory overload and hypertension.
- Antibiotics: treat infections.
- Removal of urinary obstructions: prevents further damage to the urinary system.
- Controlling hyperglycemia with medication, diet, and exercise: slows deterioration of kidney function.
- Angiotensin-converting enzyme (ACE) inhibitors: slows progression of disease.
- Erythropoietin: improves anemia.
- Blood transfusion: improves severe anemia.
- Kidney transplant: improves kidney function.

THINGS YOU NEED TO KNOW   Before we go any further, let's look at three treatments for renal failure: hemodialysis (Fig. 15-3), peritoneal dialysis, and continuous renal replacement therapy (CRRT).

1. Hemodialysis.
    - The dialysis machine acts as the glomerulus in the kidney by filtering toxins from the blood.
    - Blood leaves the client's body through an arteriovenous (AV) shunt inserted in the artery, flows through the machine, and re-enters the body via a vein.
    - Heparin is used to prevent clotting, but if the client is allergic to heparin, alteplase (Cathflo Activase) or sodium citrate is administered 3 to 4 times a week.
    - Clients must follow a strict diet that limits potassium, phosphorus, magnesium, and sodium while receiving dialysis treatment.
    - Electolytes and blood pressure are continuously monitored, especially in those clients with an unstable cardiovascular system.
    - The client has a graft, fistula, AV shunt, or temporary catheter (Asch catheter), which is utilized for short-term access while the permanent access matures. The temporary catheter is typically used for 90 days or less.
    - Clients who receive dialysis are at high risk for suicide. They may even purposefully alter their diet to achieve death.
    - Do not draw blood, start an IV, or give medications through the access device. Do not obtain blood pressures or stick the client's arm where there is an alternate circulatory access! No pressure or constriction should be applied to the affected arm; not even a watch should be worn.
    - Palpate the alternate circulatory access site for a thrill—a cat purring sensation that pulsates. Auscultate the device for a bruit. Remember to palpate the thrill and listen for the bruit to ensure the device is patent.

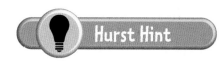

Acute renal failure is usually reversible with medical treatment. If it goes untreated, acute renal failure can progress to end-stage renal disease, uremia, and death.

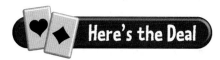

Renal failure can be treated in three ways:
1. Hemodialysis can be used to filter toxins from the blood
2. Peritoneal dialysis can be used to draw toxins into fluid placed into, and drained from the body cavity
3. Continuous renal replacement therapy can be used to slowly detoxify 80 mL of blood at a time (as opposed to 300 mL with hemodialysis)

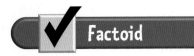

Factoid

Hemodialysis is the "gold standard" in the treatment of renal failure in the absence of a transplanted kidney.

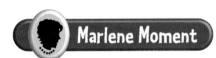

Marlene Moment

Patients who have continuous ambulatory peritoneal dialysis (CAPD) must make this their "full-time job" by having dialysis four times per day seven days a week!

2. Peritoneal dialysis.

- Dialysate is warmed to prevent vasoconstriction and is infused into the peritoneal cavity by gravity through a catheter. The amount of dialysate administered is 2000 to 2500 mL at the time.

- The solution remains in the peritoneal cavity for the period of time as ordered by the physician. Then, the bag is lowered and the fluid and accumulated toxins are drained. The drained fluid is clear to straw-colored. If the fluid is cloudy, assume an infection is present.

- There are two types of peritoneal dialysis: continuous ambulatory peritoneal dialysis (CAPD) and continuous cycle peritoneal dialysis (CCPD). CCPD occurs at night while the client is sleeping, allowing for more freedom for the client.

- Clients who receive CAPD must be able and willing to undergo dialysis 4 times per day 7 days per week. These clients usually complain of back pain due to the weight of the fluid in the peritoneal cavity.

- Clients with a colostomy cannot participate in CAPD due to risk of peritonitis (infection), which includes symptoms of abdominal pain and cloudy fluid.

- Clients undergoing peritoneal dialysis experience a constant sweet taste in the mouth due to the high glucose content of the solution. This may affect their appetite.

- Other complications of peritoneal dialysis are hernia, altered body image, constipation due to decreased peristalsis, and low protein due to loss of protein through the peritoneum during dialyzing.

3. Continuous renal replacement therapy (CRRT).

- CRRT is performed in the ICU in clients who have fragile cardio-vascular status and those who are sensitive to drastic fluid shifts.

- Hemodialysis is more aggressive than CRRT, because at any given time there are approximately 300 mL of blood being filtered through the dialysis machine. With CRRT, there are only 80 mL of blood running through the machine.

▶ Figure 15-3. Hemodialysis. Blood is pumped to a dialysis chamber, where it flows through a membrane surrounded by dialysis fluid. Blood leaving the chamber passes through a bubble trap to remove air before it is returned to the patient's body. (From Saladin K. *Anatomy and Physiology: The Unity of Form and Function.* 4th ed. New York: McGraw-Hill; 2007.)

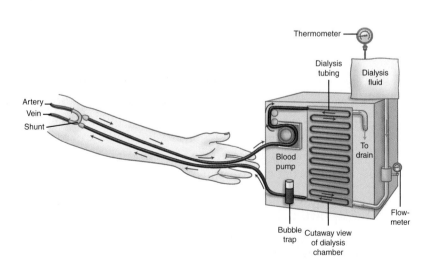

What can harm my client?

- Infection.
- Pulmonary edema.
- Sepsis.
- Shock.
- Depression related to chronic illness.
- Refer back to the clinical manifestations or signs and symptoms. There could be a great number of things.

If I were your teacher, I would test you on . . .

- Causes and why of renal failure.
- Signs and symptoms and why of renal failure.
- Medication administration and possible side effects.
- Client education regarding diet, fluid restriction, and lifestyle changes.
- Importance of monitoring intake and output, urine characteristics, and daily weights.

✦ Pyelonephritis

What is it?

Pyelonephritis is a bacterial infection of one or both kidneys.

What causes it and why

Chronic pyelonephritis is an inflammatory and/or infectious process. The most common cause is reflux of urine into one or both kidneys. Urethrovesical reflux is the reflux of urine from the urethra into the bladder. Vesiculoureteral reflux is the backup of urine into the ureters from the bladder. Ascending bacteria of the renal system can lead to scarring and atrophy of the kidneys. Chronic pyelonephritis is a major cause of renal failure and end-stage renal disease.

Table 15-8 shows the causes and associated rationales for pyelonephritis.

Table 15-8

Causes	Why
Infections of the bladder; urinary tract infections (UTI)	Bacteria travel through the urethra to the bladder, up the ureters, and into the kidneys
Repeated catheterizations	Introduce bacteria into the urinary tract
• Structural abnormality, obstruction (kidney stone, enlarged prostate, bladder tumors)	• These conditions cause an obstruction to the flow of urine; urine is not able to wash bacteria from the body
• Reflux of urine from the bladder into the ureters	• Urine flows backward into ureters
• Trauma	• If the urinary tract is damaged, urine is not excreted, causing stasis of urine and bacterial overgrowth

(Continued)

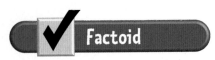

Factoid

The majority of cases of pyelonephritis are caused by *Escherichia coli* (and we all know where this comes from!). You can never teach "front to back" wiping enough! Other gram-negative bacteria such as *Proteus*, *Klebsiella*, *Enterobacter*, and *Pseudomonas* are common causative agents as well.

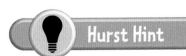

Hurst Hint

Acute pyelonephritis is considered a soft-tissue infection, but cystitis is considered a mucosal infection.

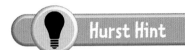

Hurst Hint

The client with chronic pyelonephritis is usually asymptomatic except in the presence of an acute exacerbation.

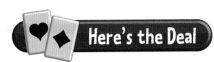

Here's the Deal

Elderly clients may not show the typical signs of pyelonephritis such as fever. The symptoms may be vague, and a family member may report that the client isn't acting in a usual manner.

Table 15-8. (*Continued*)

Causes	Why
Diabetes (a risk factor rather than a cause)	Hyperglycemia increases bacteria production in the urine; bacteria can proliferate in a high-glucose environment
Pregnancy (risk factor)	Enlarged uterus puts pressure on the ureters, which partially obstructs the normal downward flow of urine; pregnancy causes the ureters to dilate and reduces muscle contractions that propel urine down the ureters into the bladder, increasing the likelihood of reflux of urine into the ureters

Source: Created by author from References #1 to #3.

Signs and symptoms and why

Table 15-9 explores the signs and symptoms of pyelonephritis and associated rationales.

Table 15-9

Signs and symptoms	Why
Chills, fever	Infection
Anorexia, nausea, vomiting	Kidneys are unable to excrete toxins; toxins build up in the body
Dysuria, frequency, urgency	Inflammation and infection of kidneys
Pyuria (pus) in the urine	Bacterial growth causes formation of pus, but is not an indicator for pyelonephritis alone because pus in the urine is also present in UTIs
Costovertebral angle tenderness	Infection of kidneys causes tenderness (flank pain)

Source: Created by author from References #1 to #3.

Quickie tests and treatments

Tests:

- Complete blood count (CBC): elevated white blood cell count.
- Urinalysis: pus (white cells and leukocytes in urine), bacteria, and blood.
- Urine culture: identifies causative microorganism.
- Ultrasound for complicated pyelonephritis: determines cause when fever does not respond to treatment after 72 hours (most likely cause is obstruction).
- Blood tests: show elevated white blood cells or bacteria in the blood if sepsis is suspected.
- Intravenous urography: determines obstruction.

Treatments:

- Antibiotics: type and dosage depend on causative organism and location of infection; some clients can be treated on an outpatient basis as long as they are not dehydrated and are able to take medications by mouth. Sulfamethoxazole and trimethoprim (Bactrim), Septra, or fluoroquinolone (Ciprofloxacin) for 10 to 14 days is the usual treatment If the client is hospitalized, intravenous penicillin or an aminoglycoside is started to combat gram-negative bacteria.

- Antipyretics: control fever and inflammation.

- Urinary analgesics: relieve discomfort.

- Surgery: removal of kidney stone, obstruction, or structural abnormality if indicated.

- Monitor fluid intake and output.

- Fluids to dilute the urine (unless contraindicated) as with UTIs: increases flow of urine.

- Hospital admission only in severe cases; mild cases can be treated and followed outpatient. In the inpatient setting, IV ampicillin (Omnipen) and an aminoglycoside are administered prior to culture results. Antibiotics are adjusted accordingly after sensitivity results have been obtained.

- If the client is having significant flank pain, administer analgesics as ordered and encourage client to reposition themselves as needed.

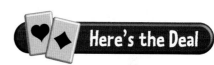

Intravenous pyelogram (IVP; Fig. 15-4) is not indicated during acute pyelonephritis, because findings are normal in up to 75% of patients.

◀ Figure 15-4. Intravenous pyelogram. Dye is injected and x-rays are taken.

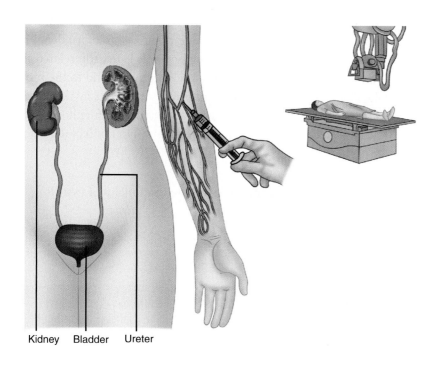

Kidney   Bladder   Ureter

What can harm my client?

- Renal abscess.

- Chronic pyelonephritis that may lead to scarring of the kidney.

- End-stage renal disease (ESRD).

- Sepsis.
- Paralytic ileus.

If I were your teacher, I would test you on . . .

- Definition of pyelonephritis.
- Causes and why of pyelonephritis.
- Signs and symptoms and why of pyelonephritis.
- Diagnostic tests and rationales.
- Importance of monitoring characteristics of urine, pattern of urine, intake and output, and daily weight.
- Complications of pyelonephritis.
- Importance of reporting fever that persists 72 hours after antibiotics are started.
- Teaching regarding antibiotics (take entire prescription).
- Teach client the importance of repeat urine cultures after antibiotics are completed.

✚ Urinary tract infection (UTI)

What is it?

In this section, we will cover the two most common UTIs: cystitis and urethritis. Cystitis is an infection of the urinary bladder, also known as a lower urinary tract infection (UTI). UTI is caused by coliform bacteria (most commonly *E. coli* and enterococci). Urethritis is an infection of the urethra. Sometimes, children can get viral cystitis caused by adenovirus, but this is rarely seen in adults. In men, cystitis is usually related to bacterial invasion of the urethra that spreads upward and to the prostate. Men who have chronic bacterial prostatitis may never actually be completely cleared from the infection because prostatic tissue is difficult to penetrate with antibiotics; therefore, the prostate continues to reinfect the bladder.

What causes it and why

Table 15-10 shows the causes and associated rationales of cystitis.

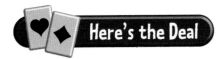

Here's the Deal

Lower urinary tract infection is an umbrella term for infections of the bladder or urethra. Signs and symptoms of both are basically the same; however, the signs and symptoms of cystitis may be more severe.

Table 15-10

Causes	Why
Transmission of microorganisms	*E. coli* and other organisms travel from the urethra to the bladder; bacteria attack and colonize the epithelium of the urinary tract, making urination painful and emptying of the bladder difficult. The urethra is short in women and is located in close proximity to the vagina and anus. Sexual intercourse can introduce bacteria from around the vagina (which is normally colonized) and the anus to the bladder through the urethra. Wiping back to front can also cause transmission of bacteria to the urethra in women. The most frequent cause of UTIs in men is obstruction of the urinary tract due to benign prostatic hyperplasia

(Continued)

Table 15-10. (*Continued*)

Causes	Why
Pregnancy	Cystitis is common in women, especially during reproductive years. Pregnancy can cause incomplete emptying of the bladder due to size and location of the uterus in proximity to the bladder and possibly due to hormonal influence and changes in pH, which can alter normal flora
Stasis of urine flow related to obstruction anywhere in the urinary tract	Kidney stones and/or enlarged prostate can partially obstruct the flow of urine. The urine can't flow leading to proliferation of organisms in stagnant urine
Stasis of urine flow related to structural abnormality (drooping uterus and bladder)	Prevents complete bladder emptying
Stasis of urine flow related to reflux	Reflux occurs when urine moves from the urethra into the bladder (urethrovescical reflux) or from the bladder into the ureters (vesicoureteral). Urethrovesical reflux can occur during normal activities (in women) such as coughing or squatting. Vesicoureteral reflux can occur as a result of congenital defects of the ureters
Impaired immune system	*Candida*, which tends to overgrow in those with impaired immune systems, can attack the bladder
Procedures of the urinary tract (catheterization, cystoscopic procedures)	Organisms are introduced by way of invasive procedures with instruments or other equipment such as catheters
Use of diaphragm	Diaphragms and spermicides (especially used together) can alter the normal flora, allowing other microorganisms to take over
Diabetes	Hyperglycemia encourages bacteria growth in the urinary tract because bacteria love to live in a high-glucose environment
Inadequate voiding	Not taking the time to let the bladder completely empty (bacteria remain in the bladder and multiply causing inflammation and infection)

Source: Created by author from References #1, #2, #5, and #6.

Signs and symptoms and why

Table 15-11 shows the signs and symptoms and why associated with cystitis.

Table 15-11

Signs and symptoms	Why
Pain and burning on urination (dysuria)	Urethra and bladder inflammation; irritation from infection
Frequency, urgency, nocturia, incontinence	Ureter and bladder spasm
Suprapubic or pelvic pain	Inflammation due to infection
Hematuria	Urethra and bladder inflammation and irritation
Back pain	Can be referred pain if uncomplicated lower urinary tract infection, or could be due to more complicated infection and inflammation of upper-level structures
Fever	Infection
Bladder spasms	Inflammation of the bladder

Source: Created by author from References #1 and #2.

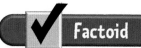

Factoid

The majority of UTIs are caused by bacteria from the intestine or vagina; 86% of UTIs in women are caused by *E. coli.*

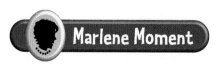

Marlene Moment

I hate it when the uterus droops. Once, a student told me during clinical to come to her female client's room immediately. When I asked why the student said, "My lady has a scrotum!" No, the client had a prolapsed uterus!

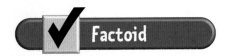

Factoid

Nurses may have an increased incidence of UTIs, as we are unable to take the time to empty our bladders every 2 to 3 hours as recommended.

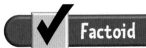

Factoid

Dysuria can also be a sign of vaginitis or an STD infection. This needs to be investigated.

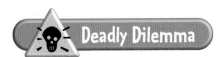

Deadly Dilemma

When assessing your client's signs and symptoms, be sure and look for tenderness of the abdomen with guarding or rebound tenderness, as this could indicate more serious problems than a UTI.

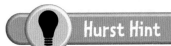

Hurst Hint

In the older adult, the most common signs of UTI are fatigue and change in cognitive status. The elderly person may also present with nausea and vomiting and abdominal pain. The client's caregiver may say that the client isn't acting like herself. THINK UTI!

Quickie tests and treatments

Tests:

- Urinalysis: pus (WBCs), bacteria (bacteriuria), with or without blood (hematuria).
- Urine dipstick: nitrates, which indicate infection.
- Urine culture and sensitivity: determine causative organism to guide treatment.
- Imaging only if pyelonephritis or structural abnormalities, or in the presence of recurrent infections.
- CT scan: detects source and location of obstruction.
- X-ray studies with radiopaque dye: provide images of the bladder, ureters, and kidneys if indicated (if something other than simple cystitis is suspected).
- Cystourethrography: detects reflux of urine from the bladder to the ureters.
- Retrograde urethrography: detects stricture, outpouching, or abnormal fistula of the urethra.
- Bladder cystoscopy: provides further information for cases when cystitis does not improve with treatment.

Treatments:

- Antibiotics: type and dosage depend on causative organism and location of infection; UTIs respond well to antibiotics that are mainly excreted in the urine; the goal is to sterilize the urine quickly. Common antibiotics used are ciprofloxacin (Cipro), nitrofurantoin (Macrodantin), and sulfa drugs such as trimethoprim and sulfamethoxazole (Bactrim or Septra).
- Anticholinergics: relieve bladder spasms that cause sense of urgency.
- Urinary analgesics: relieve urinary burning, urgency, and frequency; phenazopyridine (Pyridium or Urogesic).
- Surgery: removal of kidney stone, obstruction, or structural abnormality.
- Fluids: dilute the urine (unless contraindicated); increasing water intake decreases the concentration of bacteria in the urine.
- Cranberry juice: acidifies the urine, making it more difficult for bacteria to grow; actually has a substance that directly inhibits bacterial growth.

Prevention:

- Cranberry juice.
- Fluids.
- Urinating often; especially after sexual intercourse.
- No spermicides with diaphragm for birth control.
- If chronic, may need to take low-dose antibiotics three times a week or right after intercourse.
- Avoid substances that irritate the bladder such as alcohol, soft drinks, tea, coffee, aspartame.
- Avoid bubble baths, powders, douches, and vaginal deodorants.

What can harm my client?

- Pyelonephritis.
- Recurrent infections can lead to scarring of the urethra and bladder, upper urinary tract infections (UTIs), and kidney damage.
- Sepsis.
- Recurrent infections in children should always be investigated further, because reflux needs to be corrected to prevent renal damage. The procedure is commonly called "deflux."

If I were your teacher, I would test you on . . .

- What is it?
- Causes and why.
- Signs and symptoms and why.
- Diagnostic tests and rationales.
- Educate client regarding all aspects of prevention.
- Explain how taking showers instead of baths can decrease chance of UTI (bacteria from skin sits in bathwater and can re-enter the body).

✚ Hydronephrosis

What is it?

When urine outflow is obstructed, a large fluctuating collection—or mass—of urine forms in the kidney. This mass subsides as retained urine finally passes into the ureters and bladder. Stagnation of urine in the kidneys leads to infection. Hydronephrosis is distension of the kidney with urine that leads to progressive atrophy and eventual destruction of the kidney. The kidney ends up looking like a thin-walled shell filled with fluid. The causative factor, obstruction, has several different types.

What causes it and why

Table 15-12 lists the causes of hydronephrosis and related rationales.

Table 15-12

Causes	Why
Structural abnormalities	Cause backward pressure on the kidney when urine flow is obstructed. Examples: birth defects, BPH, scarring of ureters, cancer, rectal impaction, pregnancy
Kidney or ureter stone	Obstructs the ureters causing urine to backflow into the kidney
Pregnancy	Enlarged uterus puts pressure on the ureters, which partially obstructs the normal downward flow of urine; pregnancy causes the ureters to dilate and reduces muscle contractions that propel urine down the ureters into the bladder, increasing the likelihood of reflux of urine into the ureters

Source: Created by author from Reference #2.

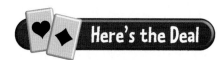

If the urinalysis results are positive for a lot of epithelial cells, this means the specimen is probably contaminated with vaginal secretions. A new specimen must be obtained by using a clean catch midstream approach, or some clients may require catheterization to obtain the sample.

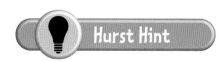

Clients with indwelling catheters may have bacteria in their urine due to colonization but no symptoms of UTI. In this case, treatment is implemented only when symptoms are present.

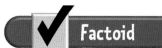

Hydronephrosis is caused by an obstruction of the urinary outflow.

Signs and symptoms and why

Table 15-13 shows the signs and symptoms and explanations associated with hydronephrosis.

Table 15-13

Signs and symptoms	Why
Acute: extreme flank plain on affected side; pain may radiate to groin	Buildup of pressure in the kidney or ureter due to backflow of urine
Chronic: mild discomfort over affected side (sometimes described as dull and aching)	Kidney shifts downward, causing overfilling of the renal pelvis or blockage of the ureters
Anuria, oliguria, hematuria, polyuria	Blockage of the urethra or ureters
Urinary tract infection	Backflow or stasis of the urine encourages bacterial growth
Nausea, vomiting, abdominal pain	Body's immune response
Asymptomatic	If progression of hydronephrosis is slow there may be no symptoms for awhile
Palpable mass over flank area	Seen only in extreme cases; due to enlargement of obstructed area related to the collection of urine

Source: Created by author from Reference #2, #5, and #7.

Hydronephrosis may be acute or chronic. The pain with acute hydronephrosis is severe, whereas the pain with the chronic form is dull and aching. In addition, chronic hydronephrosis can cause a palpable mass in the flank area.

Quickie tests and treatments

Tests:

- Physical exam: distended kidney is palpable.
- Bladder catheterization: detects site of the obstruction.
- Urinalysis: increased white blood cells and presence of red blood cells.
- Ultrasound: detects cause of the obstruction.
- Intravenous urography: detects flow of urine through the kidneys.

Treatments:

- Immediate drainage of urine via needle directly into the kidney through the skin.
- Surgery: remove obstruction.
- Urethral stent: bypasses obstruction (this is used in chronic hydronephrosis).
- Hormone therapy for prostate cancer.
- Prevent and treat infection and/or kidney failure promptly.

What can harm my client?

- End-stage renal failure.
- Infection.
- Improper catheter irrigation technique. For example, using too much force can cause fluid and bacteria to travel back up into the kidney, which can cause hydronephrosis.

If I were your teacher, I would test you on . . .

- What is it?
- What causes it and why.
- Signs and symptoms and why.
- Care of the client undergoing stent placement.
- Care of the client undergoing surgery.
- Patient education regarding side effects of hormone therapy.

✛ Urolithiasis (renal calculi)

What is it?

Urolithiasis is the condition caused by renal calculi (kidney stones), which form in the urinary tract (Fig. 15-5). They are made of crystallized substances (usually calcium oxalate) that the kidney normally excretes. The actual reason for stone formation remains a mystery, but it is believed to be precipitated by many factors. Clients living in the mountains or tropical areas where dehydration is common tend to develop kidney stones. The majority of clients who get kidney stones are males between 20 and 40 years of age. Most stones move down the ureter, causing severe discomfort. Most clients don't know they have a stone unless the stone is moving down the ureter. This movement causes severe pain. The majority of clients (80%) pass the stone spontaneously.

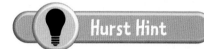

If you have had two kidney stones in your life, you can look forward to having some more, as reccurrences are common.

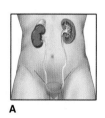

A

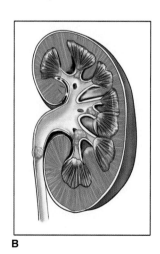

B

◀ Figure 15-5. Kidney stones. **A.** Kidney stones located in the major and minor calyces of the kidney. **B.** Kidney stone located in the ureter.

What causes it and why

In clients with urolithiasis, one of the following exists:

- Increased abundance of substances that promote crystal or stone formation.

- Lack of substances that inhibit crystal formation.
- Excessive excretion of salts in the urine, which results in supersaturation of crystallizing salts that forms calculi.

Table 15-14 shows the causes and related rationales for urolithiasis.

Table 15-14

Causes	Why
Supersaturation of urine with stone-forming substances	Increased concentration of calcium, oxalate, citrate, magnesium, urate, cystine, xanthine, and phosphate lead to calculi formation; different stones are made of different things
Dehydration	Concentrated blood is prone to developing stones
Immobility	When someone is immobile, there is no weight bearing on the bones. If there is no pressure being placed on the bones, then calcium leaves the bone and move into the vascular space (blood), elevating the serum calcium. Also, when immobile, the client is usually more prone to dehydration (the kidneys are perfused more when lying supine, so urine output goes up)
Increased serum and urine calcium	Promotes stone formation
Inflammatory bowel disease; ileostomy; bowel resection	Increased absorption of oxalate
Medications: antacids, acetazolamide (Diamox), vitamin D, laxatives, high doses of aspirin	Urine with a normal pH has a natural way of keeping stones from forming. Certain drugs alter the pH, making the environment for stone formation more conducive
Diseases such as hyperparathyroidism, or multiple myeloma	These diseases cause an increase in the serum calcium level
High purine diet or poor metabolism of purine (like in gout)	Many stones are made of uric acid. If unable to break down purines properly, uric acid accumulates in the blood (hyperuricemia), forms crystals, and promotes stone formation

Source: Created by author from References #1 and #2.

Signs and symptoms and why

Table 15-15 explores the signs and symptoms and why of urolithiasis.

Table 15-15

Signs and symptoms	Why
Severe colicky flank pain that radiates throughout the testicles, groin, and back. Pain commonly originates in back; pain usually stops as soon as the stone has passed	Stone obstructs the ureter, renal pelvis, or drainage tubes
Urinary urgency and frequency with bloody urine (hematuria)	Stone passage down ureter causes spasms
Nausea, vomiting, abdominal discomfort, diarrhea	Nausea and vomiting can be related to the severe pain or the presence of possible infection; the kidneys and intestines share nerves that are stimulated with kidney stones and cause nausea
Fever and chills (if infection is involved)	Immune response to infection; chills and fever are usually associated with stones that are causing obstruction

Source: Created by author from References #1 and #2.

Quickie tests and treatments

Tests:

- Physical exam: flank tenderness; pain in groin area is usually enough to confirm the diagnosis.
- Intravenous urography (IVU) using radiopaque dye: detects stone location and size and if there is any obstruction.
- Urinalysis: detects hematuria and pus; the pH of urine determines if the stone is acid or alkaline.
- Ultrasound and x-rays kidney and upper bladder (KUB): detect some types of stones.
- Computed tomography (CT): used when other tests are inconclusive (used for detecting stone in ureter).
- Basic kidney tests: BUN, creatinine, and electrolytes need to be reviewed to ensure kidneys are working properly.

Treatments:

- Small stones can be treated on an outpatient basis with fluids and pain relief; clients having severe pain, vomiting, fever, or possible obstruction must be hospitalized.
- Hydration therapy (oral or IV): facilitates stone passage through the urinary system; dilutes urine.
- Pain medication: NSAIDs or opioids.
- Extracorporeal shock wave lithotripsy: ultrasound waves break up the stone.
- Percutaneous nephrostolithotomy: stone removal using forceps.
- Stone removal with ureteroscope: removes small stones in lower part of ureter.
- Potassium citrate: dissolves uric acid stones.
- Thiazides reduce renal excretion of calcium; therefore, the calcium content in the urine goes down. The calcium doesn't make it to the kidney but remains in the serum. Thiazides increase serum calcium.
- Surgery is uncommon but is sometimes required.

What can harm my client?

- Residual kidney damage.
- Obstruction.
- Infection.
- Dehydration.
- Hydronephrosis.

If I were your teacher, I would test you on . . .

- The definition of urolithiasis.
- What causes it and why.
- Signs and symptoms and why.

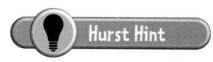

Certain foods may increase the risk of stone formation: spinach, rhubarb, chocolate, peanuts, cocoa, tomato juice, grapefruit juice, apple juice, soda (acidic and contains phosphorus), all types of tea, and berries (contain high levels of oxalate).

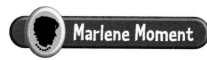

A kidney stone may be as small as a grain of sand or as big as an orange! I hope you're not at work when they pass the orange. You better bring the colander from home to strain out the orange-sized stones! It looks like it is going to be a bad day!

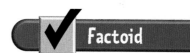

Men and women both get kidney stones, but they are more common in older adults and men. Picture a man having a baby. That is how painful it is but he gets no epidural!

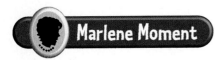

Marlene Moment

It is really important to teach patients to save their kidney stones. The stones can be analyzed to figure out why the stone formed in the first place.

- Importance of straining the urine for 72 hours after the symptoms resolve; clients may use a coffee filter if at home; clients should save the stone for analysis.
- Importance of high-fiber diet to decrease calcium and oxalate absorption.
- Importance of measuring urine output and monitoring basic kidney function tests.
- If urine has clots, the clot must be crushed to assess for stones.
- Importance of ambulation as this helps the stone move out of the body.
- Understanding that blood may stay in the urine for several weeks.
- Specific diets for different types of stones (calcium oxalate, uric acid); uric acid stone diet for calcium oxalate stones.
- Why allopurinol (Alloprim) is given (lowers uric acid when client has uric acid stones).
- Teach client importance of decreasing purines in diet.
- Importance of fluids; how much fluid is recommended and why.

SUMMARY

The renal system works with other systems of the body to maintain homeostasis. As you have seen, when the renal system is compromised, numerous complications can arise. Nurses play an important role in monitoring clients' overall health through proper assessment and care of the renal system.

PRACTICE QUESTIONS

1. One of the major body organs involved with fluid balance and chemical composition is the:

   1. Liver.

   2. Bladder.

   3. Urethra.

   4. Kidney.

   Correct answer: 4. The kidneys and the lungs regulate fluid balance and chemical composition.

2. The main function of the kidneys is to:

   1. Produce calcitriol, erythropoietin, and renin.

   2. Store urine.

   3. Stimulate white blood cell production.

   4. Fight infection.

   Correct answer: 1. The main function of the kidneys is to produce calcitriol, erythropoietin, and renin and to stimulate red blood cell production.

3. What is the cause of frothy urine as found in diabetic nephropathy? Select all that apply.

  1. Hyperglycemia.

  2. Increased white blood cell count.

  3. Bacteria.

  4. Decreased renin.

Correct answers: 1 & 3. Increased sugar and bacteria in the urine cause the frothy consistency of urine as found in diabetic nephropathy.

4. Which of the following diseases is a bacterial infection of one or both kidneys that causes chills, fever, and lower flank pain?

  1. Hydronephrosis.

  2. Acute renal failure.

  3. Pyelonephritis.

  4. Diabetic nephropathy.

Correct answer: 3. Pyelonephritis is a bacterial infection of one or both kidneys that causes chills, fever, and lower flank pain.

5. Which of the following diseases affecting the lower urinary tract causes inflammation of the bladder?

  1. Cystitis.

  2. Chronic renal failure.

  3. Hydronephrosis.

  4. Urolithiasis.

Correct answer: 1. Cystitis—also known as lower urinary tract infection—causes inflammation of the bladder and pain and burning upon urination.

6. In the older adult, what are the most common signs of cystitis? Select all that apply.

  1. Fatigue.

  2. Change in cognitive status.

  3. Burning upon urination.

  4. Nocturia.

Correct answers: 1 & 2. The most common signs of cystitis—or urinary tract infections—in the older adult are fatigue and change in cognitive status.

7. Which medications are used in the treatment of nephrotic syndrome? Select all that apply.

1. Antibiotics.

2. Corticosteroids.

3. Angtiotensin-converting enzyme (ACE) inhibitors.

4. Allergy shots.

Correct answers: 3 & 4. Angiotensin-converting enzyme (ACE) inhibitors prevent proteinuria from worsening and decrease serum lipid concentrations in nephrotic syndrome. Allergy shots are used to reverse nephrotic syndrome caused by allergens, such as poison oak and poison ivy.

8. Which disease causes severe "colicky" flank pain, hematuria, and fever?

1. Cystitis.

2. Diabetic nephropathy.

3. Hydronephrosis.

4. Urolithiasis.

Correct answer: 4. Urolithiasis—or kidney stones—cause colicky flank pain, hematuria, and fever.

9. Which of the following are complications associated with glomerulonephritis? Select all that apply.

1. Hypertensive encephalopathy.

2. Pulmonary edema.

3. Cystitis.

4. Sepsis.

Correct answers: 1, 2, 3, & 4. Hypertensive encephalopathy is a complication of glomerulonephritis and is considered a medical emergency. Pulmonary edema, cystitis, and sepsis are also complications of glomerulonephritis.

10. Which blood test findings are associated with renal failure? Select all that apply.

1. Decreased urea.

2. Increased creatinine.

3. Decreased calcitriol.

4. Anemia.

Correct answers: 2, 3, & 4. The blood test findings associated with renal failure are increased urea, creatinine, BUN, acidosis, potassium, triglycerides, phosphate, and parathyroid hormone; decreased calcium, calcitriol, and sodium; and anemia.

References

1. Steward C, Fallone SM. Renal and urinary tract function. In: Smeltzer SC, Bare BG, eds. *Brunner & Suddarth's Textbook of Medical-Surgical Nursing.* 10th ed. Philadelphia: Lippincott Williams & Wilkins; 2004:1249–1364 .

2. Kidney and urinary tract disorders. In: Beers MH, ed. *Merck Manual of Medical Information.* 2nd home ed. New York: Pocket Books; 2003:819–878.

3. Allen KD, Boucher MA, Cain JE, et al. *Lippincott Manual of Nursing Practice Pocket Guide Medical-Surgical Nursing.* Ambler, PA: Lippincott Williams & Wilkins; 2007.

4. *Glomerulonephritis.* National Kidney Foundation website. Available at: www.kidney.org/ATOZ/atozItem.cfm?id=65. Accessed January 16, 2007.

5. Porth C. *Essentials of Pathophysiology: Concepts of Altered Health States.* 2nd ed. Ambler, PA: Lippincott Williams & Wilkins; 2007.

6. Tierney LM, McPhee J, Papadakis A. *Current Medical Diagnosis and Treatment.* New York: McGraw-Hill; 2005.

Bibliography

Hurst Review Services. www.hurstreview.com.

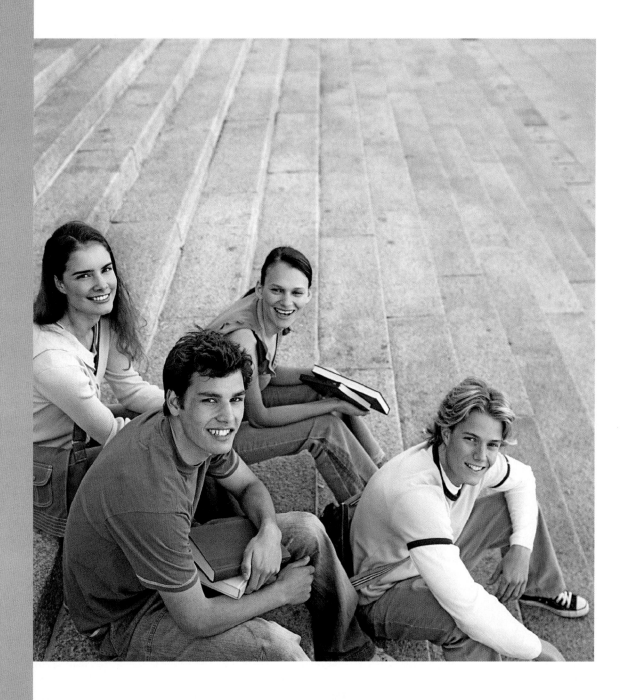

OBJECTIVES

In this chapter, you'll review:

- The key concepts associated with male and female infertility.
- The causes, signs and symptoms, and treatments of selected male and female reproductive disorders including menstrual disorders.
- The complications associated with selected male and female reproductive disorders.

MALE REPRODUCTIVE PATHOPHYSIOLOGY

The male genitourinary system (Fig. 16-1) includes a pair of testes, which secrete male sex hormones (androgens) and produce sperm. Each testicle has hundreds of lobes, with each lobe having one or more long, coiled seminiferous tubules. Estradiol, the primary feminizing hormone, comes from the inside lining of the seminiferous tubules, where it is needed for development and maturation of sperm. The androgens (testosterone, dihydrotestosterone, and androstenedione) normally decrease with aging, creating an imbalance with the existing normal male estrogen (estradiol). The prostate is an accessory gland shaped like a little donut, with the straw-like urethra running right through the center. A function of the prostate gland is to secrete seminal fluid, which bathes and nourishes the sperm. Various seminal ducts lead to the urethra which is the outlet pathway for both semen ejaculation and urine excretion.

▶ Figure 16-1. Male reproductive system. (From Saladin K. *Anatomy and Physiology: The Unity of Form and Function*. 4th ed. New York: McGraw-Hill; 2007.)

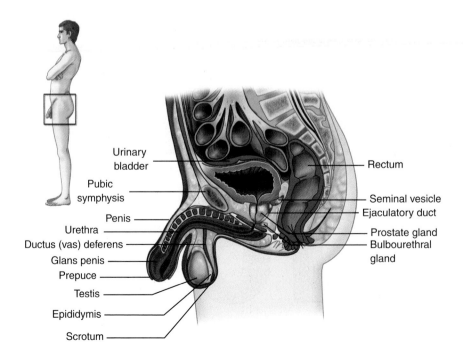

Fertility requires that the male have sufficient sperm, the ability to achieve and maintain an erection and the energy and desire perform sexually. The testes live in the scrotum, which is a thin-skinned sac hanging underneath the penis. The left testicle usually hangs a bit lower than the right in this scrotal sac. The function of the testes is to make sperm and testosterone. The sperm has to have a temperature-controlled environment so a muscle in the wall of the scrotal sac (the cremasteric muscle) swings the testes lower for cooling when temperatures are high, or can pull the testes closer to the body for warmth when it is cold. The epididymis rests posteriorly and laterally on the surface of the testes where sperm is collected and housed. The male reproductive organs are very sensitive to diminished hormone production, blood perfusion, neurological innervation, and psychogenic factors (such as stress, anger, marital discord, or boredom with a partner). Men are naturally concerned with issues such as sexual performance and masculinity that impact self-esteem.

Inflammation is the body's normal response to irritation, trauma, or invading organisms. The signs and symptoms of inflammation are pain, local heat, vasocongestion, redness, swelling, and alteration in normal function. The male reproductive organs become very symptomatic when inflammation occurs. Resultant urinary, gastrointestinal, and sexual dysfunction add to the general misery, which interferes with all aspects of life: activities of daily living, work, recreation, sleep/rest, and sexual relations.

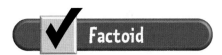

Marlene Moment

I'll never feel the same about doughnuts again.

✔ Factoid

Testosterone is the most abundant and the main testicular hormone.

✚ Benign prostatic hyperplasia (BPH)

What is it?

The most common reproductive disorder in men aged 50 to 80 is benign prostatic hyperplasia (BPH), which occurrs in half of all males aged 50 and older and in 75% of males 80 years and older (Fig. 16-2). This condition is characterized by an abnormal increase in the volume of *normal* prostate cells (hyperplasia), producing enlargement (hypertrophy) of the gland.

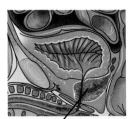

Normal prostate

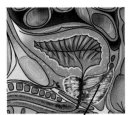

Benign prostatic hypertrophy (BPH)

◀ Figure 16-2. Normal prostate and one with BPH.

Even though the exact cause is unknown, a number of risk factors have been identified:

1. Advancing age.

2. Family history of BPH.

3. Dietary consumption of meat and fat.

4. Race and ethnicity, with the highest incidence in blacks and decreased occurrence in native Japanese.

As the prostate gland grows larger, the urethra, which runs through the center of the gland, becomes compressed. The major problems clients may experience are:

1. Well, obviously, enlargement of the prostate gland.

2. Constriction to the flow of urine (small stream).

3. Stasis of urine and urinary retention.

4. Risk for postrenal failure.

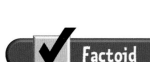

Factoid

Prolonged or severe obstruction somewhere beyond the kidney increases pressure inside of the kidney that may lead to decreased renal function.

What causes it and why

Table 16-1 shows the causes of BPH, and why these causes occur.

Table 16-1

Causes	Why
Hyperplasia of prostate cells	Dihydrotestosterone (DHT)—an androgen—is a metabolite of testosterone. For unknown reasons, it appears this is the primary hormone responsible for stimulating overgrowth of prostate cells. Estrogen also sensitizes the prostate cells to the growth effects of DHT. Even though testosterone levels decrease with aging, the INCREASED estrogen levels might be the ultimate cause of hyperplasia because of their ability to sensitize the cells to the effects of androgens
Hypertrophy of the gland	Overgrowth of prostate cells causes the gland to enlarge or hypertrophy

Source: Created by author from References #1, #3, and #8.

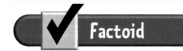

Factoid

A metabolite is any byproduct of metabolism.

Signs and symptoms and why

Table 16-2 shows the symptoms of BPH and why these symptoms occur.

Table 16-2

Signs and symptoms	Why
Urinary hesitancy: difficulty starting the flow of urine due to compression of the urethra by the enlarged prostate gland	The urethra runs through the center of the prostate (the donut), so as it enlarges, it clamps down on the urethra

(Continued)

Table 16-2. (*Continued*)

Signs and symptoms	Why
Small stream of urine	The urethra, which runs through the center of the enlarged gland, is being squeezed, blocking the flow of urine
Frequent urinary tract infections	Stasis and stagnation of urine and urinary retention
Subjective complaint of fullness; feeling that urination is incomplete	Bladder never empties completely due to the urinary obstruction from the enlarged prostate
Frequent awakening at night to void (nocturia)	Our kidneys perfuse more when lying supine. That's why we experience "bedrest diuresis." The combination of incomplete bladder emptying with added nighttime bladder volume due to "bedrest diuresis" causes nighttime urge to void
Dribbling at the end of urination	Diminished force and volume of urinary flow; think of a hose . . . if you turn the water off and there is no forceful stream anymore, the water dribbles or leaks out slowly. It's a mechanical thing
Blood in the urine	Small vessels in the distended bladder stretch and break with frequent straining to void
Fullness and discomfort in the subrapubic/ lower abdominal region	Distention and stretching of the bladder causes uncomfortable sensations of pressure

Source: Created by author from References #1, #3, and #8.

Quickie tests and treatments

Tests:

- Digital exam through the rectum to feel the smooth, nonpainful, enlarged gland.

- Ultrasound to measure the size of the gland and/or the volume of urine remaining in the bladder after voiding.

- A blood test for the carcinogenic prostate specific antigen (PSA) if cancer is suspected.

- A voiding cystourethrogram: x-ray procedure using radiopaque dye, which can detect blockage or constricted stream of urine.

Treatments:

- Conservative, nonsurgical treatments include alpha-adrenergic blockers to relax the smooth muscles of the prostate and neck of the bladder. Examples of alpha-adrenergics are the "o-sins": terazosin (Hytrin) and prazosin (Minipress). Finasteride (Proscar) is a medication that can be used to shrink the prostate.

- Transurethral resection of the prostate (Fig. 16-3): no incision, as the prostate is removed though the urethra. Complications include:

  1. Hemorrhage.

  2. Urinary dribbling, and incontinence afterward.

  3. Since the neck of the bladder is involved (the anatomic location of the prostate is at the neck of the bladder), sperm will flow backward (retrograde ejaculation) into the bladder and mingle with urine, reducing the man's fertility.

- Open surgical resection of the prostate (incision): complications include damaged nerves leading to erectile dysfunction (sexual dysfunction).

▶ Figure 16-3. Transurethral resection of the prostate (TURP). (From Saladin K. *Anatomy and Physiology: The Unity of Form and Function.* 4th ed. New York: McGraw-Hill; 2007.)

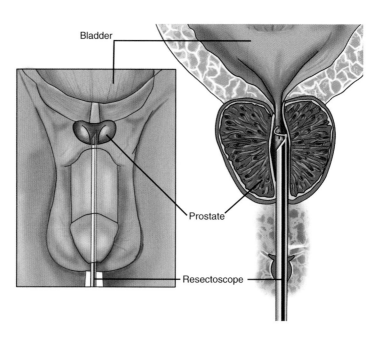

Preventive measures:

- Limit fluid intake after dinner.
- Avoid medications like antidepressants, antiparkinson agents, antipsychotics, antispasmodics, cold preparations (Sudafed), and diuretics.
- Void frequently.
- Urinate, wait a few minutes, then void again.
- Avoid caffeine and alcohol: can cause sudden diuresis.

What can harm my client?

- Acute urinary retention.
- Hydronephrosis leading to postrenal kidney failure.
- Severe hematuria resulting in hemorrhage and anemia.

If I were your teacher, I would test you on . . .

- Causes of BPH and preventive measures.
- Signs and symptoms of BPH and why.

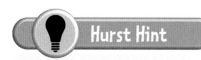

Hydronephrosis is retained urine in the renal pelvis that accumulates and forms a fluctuant cyst.

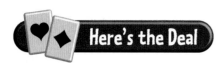

When renal failure occurs, anemia develops due to the lack of erythropoietin production by the kidney. Remember, erythropoietin is the hormone responsible for stimulating red blood cell production.

- Postsurgical precautions.
- Voiding assessment after removal of indwelling catheter (if client had surgery).

✚ Prostatitis

What is it?

Prostatitis is an inflammatory disorder of the prostate. The inflammation is due to bacterium, fungus, virus, or protozoa—also known as acute bacterial infection. An acute bacterial prostatitis may become chronic. Sometimes the prostate is inflamed in the absence of a bacterial infection. The cause of this is unknown. Other times, symptoms exist but no infection or inflammation is present. This type of prostatitis is referred to as noninflammatory prostatitis.

What causes it and why

Table 16-3 explores the causes and related rationales of prostatitis.

Table 16-3

Causes	Why
Acute bacterial prostatitis	Bacteria travel up the urethra to the prostate
Inflammatory prostatitis	Unknown, possibly autoimmune
Noninflammatory prostatitis	Unknown, but may be related to an extra prostatic source (outside of the prostate) such as structural abnormalities of the bladder neck and urethral sphincter
Chronic prostatitis	Progression of acute infection to chronic stage. Possibly related to inadequate treatment or noncompliance with treatment of the initial acute bacterial infection

Source: Created by author from References #2 and #3.

Signs and symptoms and why

Table 16-4 explores the signs and symptoms and why associated with acute bacterial prostatitis, chronic bacterial prostatitis, and inflammatory and noninflammatory prostatitis.

Table 16-4

Signs and symptoms	Why
Acute bacterial prostatitis presents with fever, chills, fatigue	Systemic response to invading microorganisms
Frequent, painful, and urgent need to urinate	Swelling and local inflammatory reaction
Perineal discomfort and low back pain	Local edema compresses nerve fibers and bacterial toxins irritate tissues. Muscle spasm occurs in the bladder, pelvis, and perineum
Blood in the urine (hematuria)	Severe irritation and bacterial toxins damage the lining of the bladder
Chronic bacterial prostatitis presents with frequent, urgent urination, back pain, and perineal discomfort	Severe irritation and bacterial toxins damage the lining of the bladder

(Continued)

Table 16-4. (*Continued*)

Signs and symptoms	Why
Inflammatory prostatitis presents with painful penis and pain in the testicles, scrotum, and rectum. It may also be painful when ejaculation occurs leading to sexual disturbances	Local edema compresses nerve fibers and bacterial toxins irritate tissues. Muscle spasm occurs in the bladder, pelvis, and perineum
Noninflammatory prostatitis	Same as inflammatory prostatitis
Painful defecation	Related to proximity of bowel to prostate

Source: Created by author from References #2 and #3.

Quickie tests and treatments

Tests:

* Digital rectal examination of the prostate: reveals tenderness and swelling of the gland.
* Cultures of the urine and fluid from the penis following prostate massage: identify the causative organism.

Treatments:

* Antibiotics: ofloxacin (Floxin), levofloxacin (Levaquin), ciprofloxacin (Cipro). If antibiotics are not taken for the entire prescribed period, chronic bacterial prostatitis may occur. Long-term treatment with antibiotics is used for chronic prostatitis.
* Frequent ejaculation and periodic prostate massage through the rectum by a physician: promotes evacuation and drainage, relieving pressure and stagnation of seminal fluid.
* Warm sitz baths: relieves symptoms for all types of prostatitis.
* Stool softeners: reduce painful straining.
* Antiinflammatory agents: relieve pain and swelling.
* Analgesics and antipyretics: reduce pain and fever.
* Scrotal support: decreases pain with movement.
* Transurethral prostatectomy (removal of prostate): for complicated cases.
* CT scan or transrectal ultrasound: identifies possible abscess.

What can harm my client?

* Prostatic abscess in those who do not respond to antibiotics.
* Urinary retention leading to kidney infection and kidney failure.
* Prostate stones can be a bothersome complication.
* Epididymis—inflammation and/or infection of epididymis.
* Orchitis: infection of the testis.

If I were your teacher, I would test you on . . .

* What is it?
* Signs and symptoms and why.
* Treatments.

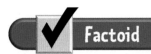

Factoid

The epididymis is a soft structure located on the posterolateral and upper surface of the testis. It stores, matures, and transports sperm.

- Complications.
- Patient education.
- Basic male anatomy.

✚ Epididymis

What is it?

Epididymis is inflammation of the epididymis that may be caused by either a sexually transmitted infection (STI) or from complications of a urinary or prostatic infection. It is usually the result of a bacterial infection, but may be caused by any kind of trauma: surgery, insertion of a urinary catheter, or a kick sustained to the groin. Uncommon causes of epididymis include anatomical abnormalities or side effects of medications such as antiarrhythmics, especially amiodarone hydrochloride (Cordarone). It is important to distinguish epididymis from testicular torsion (Fig. 16-4) or tumor.

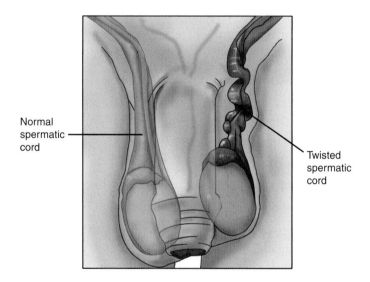

◀ Figure 16-4. Testicular torsion.

Normal spermatic cord

Twisted spermatic cord

What causes it and why

Table 16-5 explores the causes and background related to epididymis.

Table 16-5

Causes	Why
Infection	Travels up the urethra into the epididymis
Trauma	Inflammation to traumatized tissue

Source: Created by author from References #4 and #5.

Signs and symptoms and why

Table 16-6 explores the signs and symptoms and related rationales of epididymis.

Table 16-6

Signs and symptoms	Why
Pain and inflammation with swelling of the affected side including the scrotum, groin, and lower abdomen (almost always appears on one side only)	Infection of epididymis causes tissue inflammation and immune response
Urethral discharge	Infectious pathogens; common organisms that produce epididymis with discharge include gonorrhea, *Chlamydia*, and sometimes gram-negative organisms

Source: Created by author from References #4 and #5.

Quickie tests and treatments

Tests:

- Complete blood count (CBC): elevated white blood cells.
- Urine culture: determines causative organism.
- Ultrasound of scrotum: determines epididymis and rules out torsion.

Treatments:

- Bed rest, scrotal elevation, and support.
- Antibiotics: doxycycline (Vibramycin), rocephin (Ceftriaxone); if client is allergic to doxycycline or rocephin, ofloxacin (Floxin) and levofloxacin (Levaquin) may be used.
- Analgesics: control pain.
- Antipyretics: manage fever.
- Screening of sexual partners: determines if partners require treatment.
- Abstinence of sexual intercourse: until both partners are treated and asymptomatic.

What can harm my client?

- If treatment is delayed, the infection can spread to the testis—known as orchitis—which may result in sterility and/or abscess.

If I were your teacher, I would test you on . . .

- What is it?
- Signs and symptoms and why.
- Treatments and possible complications.
- Medication side effects: amiodarone hydrochloride (Cordarone) can cause self-limited epididymis.
- Protocol for screening and treating sexual partners.

✚ Epididymo-orchitis

What is it?

Epididymo-orchitis is an infection of both the epididymis and testis.

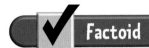
Factoid

Tumors usually present with **painless** swelling.

Factoid

Epididymo-orchitis is an infection of both the epididymis and the testis and is caused by the spread of infection from the epididymis to the testis. Epididymo-orchitis is more common than orchitis because orchitis is usually caused by the mumps virus, which we don't see too much of anymore because of the vaccine.

What causes it and why

Table 16-7 shows the causes and explanations for epididymo-orchitis.

Table 16-7

Causes	Why
Infection of the epididymis	Spreads to the testis from the urethra or bladder via the vas deferens or lymphatics of spermatic cord. If it spreads to the testis, it is called epididymo-orchitis
Infection of the prostate	Spreads to the testis from the prostate
Parotitis (mumps): a viral infection that we do not see much anymore since the advent of the mumps vaccine	This virus attacks the testicles and the parotid glands!

Source: Created by author from References #5, #6, and #9.

Signs and symptoms and why

Table 16-8 shows the signs and symptoms and rationales for epididymo-orchitis.

Table 16-8

Signs and symptoms	Why
Swelling, warmth, redness, and tenderness of affected side with pain	Infection; infectious organism causes inflammation, swelling, and tissue trauma
Fever	Immune response to infection

Source: Created by author from References #5, #6, and #9.

Quickie tests and treatments

Tests:

- Same for epididymis.
- Complete blood count (CBC): elevated white blood cells.
- Urine culture: determines causative organism.
- Ultrasound of scrotum: determines epididymis and rules out torsion.

Treatments:

- Same for epididymis.
- Bed rest, scrotal elevation, and support.
- Antibiotics: doxycycline (Vibramycin), rocephin (Ceftriaxone); if client is allergic to doxycycline or rocephin, ofloxacin (Floxin) and levofloxacin (Levaquin) may be used.
- Analgesics: control pain.
- Antipyretics: manage fever.

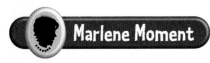

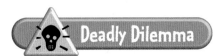

- Screening of sexual partners: determines if partners require treatment.
- Abstinence from sexual intercourse: until both partners are treated and asymptomatic.
- Jock strap: supports testicles against bumps and jarring.

What can harm my client?

- Abscess: may either drain on its own or may need to be surgically drained.
- Delayed treatment: leads to testicular atrophy and sterility.

If I were your teacher, I would test you on . . .

- What is it?
- Current causes of orchitis (i.e., mumps is rarely seen since mumps vaccine was implemented; however, we do still see some cases of it); recognition of epididymo-orchitis.
- Signs and symptoms and why.
- Nursing care to promote comfort and relieve associated symptoms; remember that jock strap.
- Complications or what can harm your client; infertility is the big one here.

✛ Scrotal/testicular torsion

The testicles hang freely in the scrotum from the sperm cord and are enveloped in the tunica vaginalis. The thin-skinned scrotal sac contains the two large olive-shaped glands—the testes. Normally the cremasteric muscle draws the scrotum upward to snuggle the body for maintaining heat and for protection of the testis. Contraction of the cremasteric muscle rotates the left testis counterclockwise and the right testis clockwise. The cremasteric reflex can be stimulated by stroking the inner thigh, which causes retraction of the testis on the same side.

What is it?

Scrotal or testicular torsion is twisting (torsion) of a testis on its spermatic cord. Consequently, the vessels located inside the cord that supply blood to the testis are twisted. The torsion is usually unilateral and can occur because of abnormal development of the spermatic cord or the membrane covering the testis. A scrotal sac which hangs excessively can become twisted. Torsion of the testicles usually happens in young males between puberty and age 25. Torsion can occur spontaneously (even during sleep) or can follow injury or exertion.

What causes it and why

Table 16-9 explores the causes and reasons for scrotal or testicular torsion.

Table 16-9

Causes	Why
Rotation of the testis and twisting of the spermatic cord	• Abnormally positioned testis • Incomplete supporting fascia to the scrotal wall • Loosely attached membranous covering of the testis and sperm cord • Sudden forceful contraction of the cremasteric muscle that elevates testis

Source: Created by author from References #3 and #5.

Signs and symptoms and why

Table 16-10 explores the signs and symptoms and related rationales of scrotal or testicular torsion.

Table 16-10

Signs and symptoms	Why
Excruciating testicular pain unrelieved by rest or scrotal support	Impaired blood flow with twisting and kinking of arteries supplying oxygenated blood to the testicles causes the sudden onset of symptoms. Ischemic pain results anytime blood flow to a body part is interrupted. Anaerobic metabolism leaves the irritating byproduct, lactic acid, in the tissues
Abdominal or pelvic pain	Referred pain from torsion of the testis
Nausea and vomiting	Severe pain stimulates the vomiting center in the brain
Testicular swelling	Compression of vessels and vascular engorgement
Elevated scrotum on the affected side with ecchymosis (bruising)	Secondary to decreased blood flow to the testis from the torsion
Loss of cremasteric reflex on the affected side	Nerves are in close proximity to vessels; nerve compression is present with torsion

Source: Created by author from References #3 and #5.

Quickie tests and treatments

Tests:

• Diagnosis is based on client history and physical assessment.

• Color Doppler ultrasonography: identifies scrotal twisting and vessel compression

• Urinalysis: usually normal.

Treatments:

• Manual reduction: restores some blood flow while awaiting surgery.

• Surgery: ensures complete detorsion.

• Priority treatment: surgery; after 6 to 8 hours from the onset of symptoms it is too late to save the testicles from necrosis.

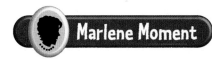

Marlene Moment

If you are working as a school nurse and a 14-year-old student comes to your office complaining of severe testicular pain, do not give him Tylenol and send him back to class. Take the complaint seriously! It's not growing pains!

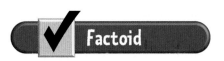

Factoid

Many clients have little or no pain in the testicular area but rather do have pain in the lower abdomen, which can be confused with symptoms of gastroenteritis or appendicitis.

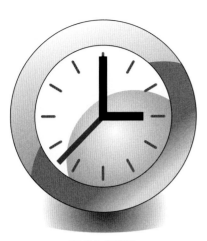

TIME is TISSUE

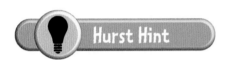

Remember this rule: Time is Tissue! Hurry . . . never delay treatment when torsion is suspected!

What can harm my client?

Scrotal or testicular torsion is a urological emergency that requires immediate surgery! This very painful condition is serious because the blood supply to the testicles can be cut off, resulting in necrosis within 6 to 8 hours if blood flow is not restored. Dead testicles KILL a man's reproductive capability!

If I were your teacher, I would test you on . . .

* Patients at risk for testicular torsion.
* Signs and symptoms and why.
* Why this condition is a medical emergency requiring immediate surgery.
* The role of the school nurse regarding client education and prevention: teenaged boys in sports programs are the focus, but testicular torsion can still occur into early adulthood.

✛ Male sexual dysfunction

What is it?

Male sexual dysfunction is characterized by a male client's inability to attain or maintain an erection—also known as erectile dysfunction (ED). ED causes an inability to achieve orgasm and ejaculate. Ejaculation problems are premature ejaculation (occur too early) or backward ejaculation (retrograde), which causes infertility.

What causes it and why

Male sexual dysfunction may be caused by physical or psychological factors, or a combination of both.

Table 16-11 lists the causes and reasons behind them for male sexual dysfunction.

Table 16-11

Causes	Why
Blood pressure medications	Decrease blood flow into the penis
Antidepressant medications	Decrease sexual desire
Decreased sex drive and performance	Low testosterone levels; trauma to scrotum and penis
Diabetes mellitus, spinal and peripheral nerve disease, pelvic surgery, stroke, alcohol and drugs	Nerve damage to penis
Psychological causes	Work-related stress and anxiety, concern about sexual performance, marital or relationship problems, depression, feelings of guilt, effects of a past sexual trauma

Source: Created by author from References #1 and #5.

Signs and symptoms and why

Table 16-12 addresses the signs and symptoms and rationales of male sexual dysfunction.

Table 16-12

Signs and symptoms	Why
Sexual anxiety, fear of rejection or ridicule, distress related to inability to satisfy sexual partner	Psychological factors
Absence of semen in urine	Inability to ejaculate
Flaccid, soft penis	Side effects of medications; decreased blood flow to the penis

Source: Created by author from References #1 and #5.

Quickie tests and treatments

Tests:

- Urine specimen: detects presence of sperm.
- Sperm count: assesses number and viability of sperm.
- Blood tests: evaluate hormone levels.
- Vascular assessment: evaluation of blood flow to the penis.
- Sensory testing: evaluates the effects of diabetic neuropathy; measures the strength of nerve impulses in reproductive organs.
- Nocturnal penile tumescence and rigidity testing: monitors erections that occur naturally during sleep; determines if a man's erectile problems are due to physical or psychological causes.

Treatments:

- Medications.
    1. For retrograde ejaculation: pseudoephedrine hydrochloride (Sudafed), phenylephrine hydrochloride (Coricidin), or imipramine pamoate (Impril) cause the urinary sphincter to contract and close, preventing backflow of semen; these medications may be harmful to men with hypertension or heart disease.
    2. Antierectile dysfunction agents: sildenafil citrate (Viagra) to achieve and maintain erection.
    3. Testosterone replacement therapy: replaces low levels of testosterone.
- Sexual counseling: explores cause of sexual dysfunction; treats stress, depression, and anxiety.
- Vacuum appliances: pull blood into the cavernous sinuses of the penis; banding at the base of the penis holds the penis erect for penetration. Don't forget to release the band after sex!!
- Limit alcohol intake.
- Smoking cessation.

What can harm my client?

- Side effects of medications, which can lead to hypertensive crisis and increased workload on the heart.
- Use of sildenafil citrate (Viagara) in men concurrently taking nitrates can be dangerous.

If I were your teacher, I would test you on . . .

- Causes and why.
- Signs and symptoms and why.
- Client education regarding sex after heart attack.
- Client coping strategies for sexual dysfunction.
- Patient education regarding sexual dysfunction and management.
- Pathophysiological effects of antihypertensives and alcohol on sexual dysfunction.

✚ Priapism

What is it?

Priapism is a prolonged erection unrelated to sexual stimulation that lasts for hours.

What causes it and why

Sometimes the cause of priapism is unknown.

Table 16-13 explores the causes and reasons behind priapism.

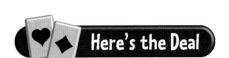

Here's the Deal

Priapism is a urological emergency that does occur in the hospital setting. Nurses need to be able to recognize, assess, and manage priapism.

Table 16-13

Causes	Why
Abnormalities of blood vessels and nerves	Trap blood in erectile tissue
Medications	Certain medications by mouth or those injected into the penis to cause erection
Blood clots, leukemia, sickle cell disease, tumors in the pelvis, or spinal cord injury	Trap blood in erectile tissue

Source: Created by author from References #5, #7, and #8.

Signs and symptoms and why

Table 16-14 shows the signs and symptoms and rationales related to priapism.

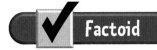

Factoid

One medication responsible for causing priapism is trazodone hydrochloride (Trazorel). Trazodone is commonly prescribed for sleep by some physicians in certain specialties such as chemical dependency units and psychiatric units.

Table 16-14

Signs and symptoms	Why
Painful erection	Trapped blood in erectile tissue causes continued erection

Source: Created by author from References #5, #7, and #8.

Quickie tests and treatments

Tests:

- Client history and physical assessment: determines cause and guides treatment.
- Doppler studies: penile ultrasound confirms diagnosis.
- Computed tomography: determines intrapelvic pathology such as a tumor.

Treatments:

- Analgesics: relieve pain.
- Sedation: decreases anxiety.
- Hydration: improves circulation.
- Catheterization: relieves urinary retention.
- Ice packs: decrease swelling.
- Drugs injected into the corpus cavernosum (erectile tissue): decrease erection.
- Irrigation of the corpus cavernosum (erectile tissue) with saline: decreases swelling and improves blood flow.
- Temporary surgical shunt placement: redirects blood flow.

What can harm my client?

- Ischemia and fibrosis of the erectile tissue, resulting in impotence.

If I were your teacher, I would test you on . . .

- What is it?
- Signs and symptoms and why.
- Causes and why including medication causes.
- Complications.
- Treatment for urologic emergency.

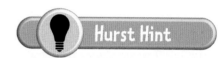

Hurst Hint

If your client complains of a sustained erection, painful or not, and shows it to you, do not assume that he is being inappropriate. Don't dismiss his complaint by storming out of the room because you have been offended! Remember, you are his advocate! Call the doctor immediately!

✛ Testicular cancer

What is it?

Testicular cancer is cancer of the testicle affecting males aged 15 to 35 years.

What causes it and why

Table 16-15 explores the causes and background for testicular cancer.

Table 16-15

Cause	Why
Unknown cause, but may be related to cryptorchidism (undescended testicle), genetic factors, and abnormal testicular development in conditions such as Klinefelter's syndrome	Cause and reasons virtually unknown

Source: Created by author from References #1, #2, and #7.

Signs and symptoms and why

Table 16-16 explores the signs and symptoms and rationales of testicular cancer.

Table 16-16

Signs and symptoms	Why
Enlargement of the testicle with or without discomfort including abdominal pain or groin pain	Presence of mass with referred pain
Asymptomatic	Often presents as painless mass

Source: Created by author from References #1, #2, and #7.

Quickie tests and treatments

Tests:

- Palpation and transillumination with a special light: a mass will not transilluminate, so the light will not shine through to the other side of the scrotum in the presence of a mass.
- Testicular ultrasound, computed tomography (CT), magnetic resonance imaging (MRI): determines location and size of tumor.

Treatments:

- Orchiectomy: removal of the affected testicle.
- Radiation and chemotherapy with very close follow-up.
- Self-testicular exam: teach all male clients how to perform exam, it is just as important as the breast exam in women.

What can harm my client?

- Delayed diagnosis can result in decreased treatment efficacy due to advanced disease.
- Recurrence can occur within the first year.
- Treatment failure can result in death.
- Removal of a testicle may be emotionally disturbing to some men. Sensitivity to this issue must be considered when caring for these clients and may include the need for providing emotional support.

If I were your teacher, I would test you on . . .

- What is it, and what age group is most affected by it?
- Signs and symptoms and why.
- Prognosis.
- Teach testicular exams to the appropriate age group.
- Importance of providing emotional support.

✚ Prostate cancer

What is it?

Cancer of the prostate (Fig. 16-5) is the most common cause of cancer in males and is second to lung cancer as cause for cancer-related death in men.

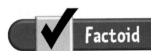

Factoid

The prognosis for testicular cancer is excellent when diagnosed early. Even with advanced disease, long term survival is possible due to advances in cancer research and treatments.

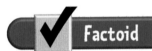

Factoid

Testicular prosthetics are now available to replace testes removed due to cancer, giving the scrotum a more normal appearance.

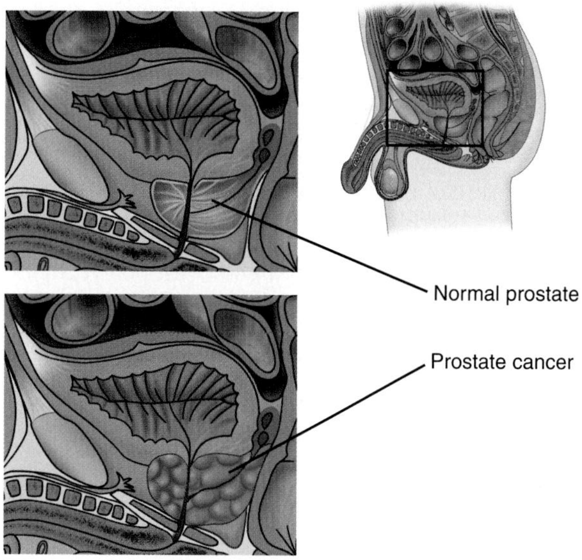

◀ Figure 16-5. Prostate cancer.

Normal prostate

Prostate cancer

What causes it and why

Table 16-17 explores the causes and reasons for prostate cancer.

Table 16-17

Cause	Why
Unknown	We don't know the exact cause of prostate cancer, but it is probably related to genetics and its effects on cell differentiation, cell growth, and male hormones
	Identified risk factors include: age (50 plus), race (African Americans with highest prevalence), heredity, dietary fat and meat consumption, and those who have had family members with prostate cancer

Source: Created by author from References #3, #6, and #9.

Signs and symptoms and why

Table 16-18 explores the signs and symptoms and background of prostate cancer.

Table 16-18

Signs and symptoms	Why
In the early stages, clients are usually asymptomatic	Symptoms usually suggest that the disease has metastasized or has become advanced
Voiding pattern changes such as frequency, urgency, nocturia, hesitancy, dysuria, hematuria, or blood in seminal fluid	Same as for BPH and prostatitis
Prostate is nodular and fixed	Due to mass
Bone metastasis usually presents with low back pain	Related to cancer having spread to the bones including the spine

Source: Created by author from References #3, #6, and #9.

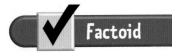

Factoid

PSA is a type of protein that lives in the cytoplasm of prostate cells. PSA is a marker and is not always reliable in the diagnosis of prostate cancer. For example, the patient can have cancer without an elevated PSA; however, 98% of clients with metastatic prostate cancer have elevated levels of PSA.

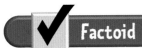

Factoid

Since prostate cancer is usually asymptomatic in the early stages, screening is important. Screening includes rectal exams and PSA starting at age 50. It usually starts at age 45 if African American or a strong family history.

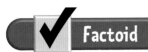

Factoid

Treatment is based on tumor grade and stage as well as age and health of the client.

Quickie tests and treatments

Tests:

- Biopsy of the prostate by transrectal ultrasound guidance: confirms diagnosis.
- Transrectal magnetic resonance imaging: detects the size and location of tumor.
- Blood test for prostate-specific antigen (PSA): tumor marker confirms diagnosis.
- Blood test for alkaline phosphatase and calcium: tumor marker; represents bone metastasis.
- Radionuclide bone scan for detecting bone metastasis.

Treatments:

- Radiation: to shrink the tumor.
- Prostatectomy: to remove the prostate.
- Monitoring: this alone may be appropriate for certain clients with localized prostate cancer.
- Cryosurgery: liquid nitrogen injected into prostate with ultrasound guidance.
- Androgen deprivation therapy: blocking androgen action on the prostate—prostate cancer is hormone dependent; this therapy is combined with radiation. Remember that testosterone is the major androgen.

What can harm my client?

- Metastasis to bone.
- Bone fractures if bone metastasis has occurred.
- Side effects of radiation and androgen deprivation therapy.
- Death.

FEMALE REPRODUCTIVE PATHOPHYSIOLOGY

The female reproductive system (Fig. 16-6) consists of internal organs: the uterus and vaginal passageway and a pair of fallopian tubes and ovaries. Externally, the lips (labia) cover the opening to the uterus (called the introitus). The clitoris is erectile tissue similar to the glans penis and is sensitive to sexual stimulation. Also external is the mons pubis, a fatty mound of tissue to pad the pubic bone. The breasts contain mammary glands, which secrete milk to provide infant nutrition. Hormones are necessary to initiate menstruation and ovulation, maintain pregnancy and initiate labor, and to produce lactation. Common nonmalignant tumors and cysts as well as acute and chronic infectious and inflammatory conditions can cause distress and impair reproductive function.

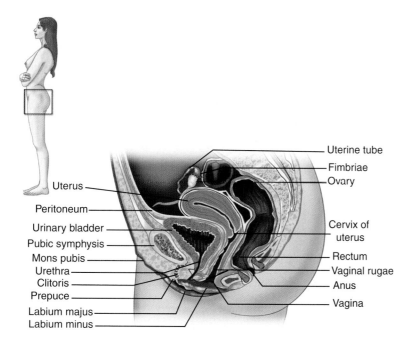

◄ Figure 16-6. Female reproductive system. (From Saladin K. *Anatomy and Physiology: The Unity of Form and Function*. 4th ed. New York: McGraw-Hill; 2007.)

✚ Endometriosis

The endometrium is the inside lining of the uterus that is shed each month in menstrual fluid and, under hormonal influence, grows anew to be ready for implantation of a fertilized ovum. It is great to have a brand new lining for your uterus every month, but it would be really nice if this stuff would stay where it belongs!

What is it?

In endometriosis (Fig. 16-7), small pieces of the endometrium lining that are shed migrate backward into the fallopian tubes and find a way out of the uterus. These pieces of tissue can start to grow in the tubes, or on the ovaries, or they may just take up residence in the intestines. They can live just about anywhere they can find a blood supply to support growth and oxygenation. Endometrial tissue has commonly been found growing abnormally in the cervix and vagina, but can travel to far away places like the lungs and the covering of the heart.

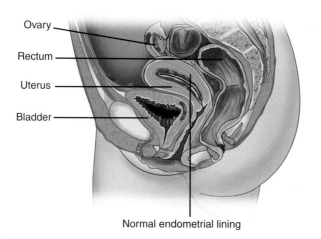

◄ Figure 16-7. Endometriosis. Common sites for endometrial growth are labeled.

What causes it and why

Endometriosis runs in families, and can affect menstruating women of all ages, even teenagers. It is more common in women who have delayed childbearing and women who have not given birth. Women of Asian descent and women with uterine abnormalities are also at greater risk for endometriosis. The endometrial tissue sheds and travels to sites outside of the uterus but never forgets what it is supposed to do each month: bleed! Yes, the tissue that is now attached to scar tissue in the abdomen from any previous surgery will still respond to hormone activation for "period time!" The actual cause of endometriosis is unknown.

Signs and symptoms and why

Table 16-19 explores the signs and symptoms and reasons for endometriosis.

Table 16-19

Signs and symptoms	Why
Pain can be mild, moderate, or very severe depending on the degree of the disease. Most common complaints are cramping pelvic pain with menses and constant pain in lower abdominal quadrants and low back	Blood vessels become engorged with blood and the swollen endometrial tissue irritates organs in surrounding areas; blood pockets can form in various locations where there is no outlet for blood flow, and any collection of blood will create local pressure
Menstrual irregularities may range from spotting to heavy bleeding	The displaced endometrial tissue responds to estrogen and progesterone, so bleeding can come from the cervix, vagina, fallopian tubes, ovaries, or any other affected location
Painful sexual intercourse (called dyspareunia = dis-pear-OON-e-ah)	Internal thrusting will precipitate pain when there is local congestion and tissue irritation from ectopic tissue in the cul-de sacs (little pockets on either side of the cervix)
Changes in bowel and bladder elimination	Endometrial tissue can attach to the intestine or bladder; adhesions can block the intestines causing bowel obstruction
Blood in stool	Endometrial tissue can invade the bowel and produce bloody stool during menstruation
Infertility	Masses of migrant endometrial tissue may block passageways, preventing the sperm from contact with the ovum
Abnormal (ectopic) implantation when pregnancy does occur	Strictures of the fallopian tubes from scarring may block the pathway to the uterus where implantation would normally occur

Source: Created by author from References #1 to #3.

Quickie tests and treatment

Tests:

- Endometriosis is suspected based on client menstrual history.

- Bimanual examination: very uncomfortable; the examiner can palpate painful masses of endometrial tissue on the ovaries or in the vagina or rectum.

- Blood tests: CA-125 and endometrial antibodies determine "serum markers," which are nonspecific but can be helpful in making a diagnosis.

- Open or laparoscopic surgery: visualizes the endometrial tissue and/or obtains tissue samples for biopsy.

- Ultrasound, computed tomography, magnetic resonance imaging.

Treatments:

- Treatment depends upon the woman's symptoms and extent of disease.

- NSAIDs: reduce pain and local inflammation.

- Bed rest with a heating pad on the lower abdomen or back: relief from painful menstrual cramps.

- Hormone therapy: suppresses hormonal activity and relieves symptoms. Hormone therapy: induces physiological amenorrhea; therefore, endometrial tissue is not under hormonal influence. Since it's not under hormonal influence, it won't bleed. Examples of these drugs are:

  1. Birth control pills containing estrogen and progestin.

  2. Progestins.

  3. Danazol (Cyclomen).

  4. Gonadotropin-releasing hormone agonists (GnRH agonists) turn off the ovarian production of estrogen and progesterone, creating a drug-induced menopause. Women taking such drugs are at risk for developing osteoporosis unless these drugs are given in combination with small doses of estrogen and progestin.

- Nothing short of menopause will totally eradicate the disease.

- Laser, electrocautery, and surgical excision of endometrial tissue: temporary measures that do not result in a cure, especially when there is widespread endometrial tissue throughout the abdominal cavity.

- Following surgery, women are given estrogen plus progestin for symptomatic relief, and if estrogen alone is used, it cannot be given for 6 months or any existing tissue in the affected area will become symptomatic again.

- Infertility may occur depending on where the endometrial implants occur and the extent of the disorder (e.g., may block the fallopian tubes or attach to ovaries). If fertility has not been affected and the client can become pregnant, it may actually help, because the endometrial tissue will not be under hormonal influence, which induces atrophy of the endometrial tissue.

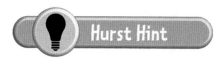

Pregnancy relieves many of the symptoms associated with endometriosis because the period and ovulation stop. The only problem is . . . it can be _very_ difficult to get pregnant if you have endometriosis.

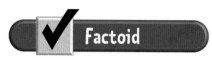

Menopause (through surgery or naturally) is the only "cure" for endometriosis.

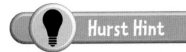

"Pan" means everything. For example, a pan-hysterectomy means the uterus, ovaries, oviducts, cervix and related lymph nodes have been removed. Sounds like "everything" to me.

What can harm my client?

- Endometriosis is not a life-threatening disease but, in its most severe form, can lead to pan-hysterectomy, making death a possibility due to a complication such as a postoperative pulmonary embolus or postoperative hemorrhage.

If I were your teacher, I would test you on . . .

- Times when the woman with endometriosis is the most symptomatic? The least? Remember the influence of hormones and menstruation!
- Signs and symptoms and why.
- Relief of symptoms through measures other than medications.
- The nurse's role in pregnancy counseling and fertility planning when the female client is advised to accomplish desired childbearing quickly before the disease becomes too advanced.

✛ Mastitis

The main parts of the female breasts are the milk-producing glands, called lobules, and ducts (milk passageways) that connect the lobules to the nipple (the exit portal). Fatty tissue surrounds the lobules and ducts, with a system of blood and lymph vessels. Mastitis (Fig. 16-8) is inflammation of the breast and can be acute or chronic.

▶ Figure 16-8. Mastitis.

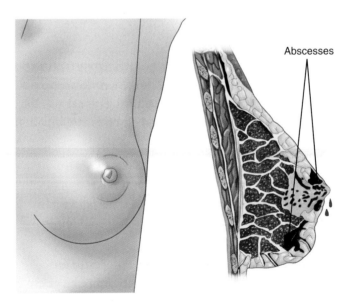

Abscesses

What is it?

Mastitis is inflammation of the breast.

What causes it and why

Table 16-20 shows the causes and explanations for mastitis.

Table 16-20

Causes	Why
Postpartum lactation	Staph or strep can invade the skin through cracks or fissures in the nipple from vigorous suckling by an infant during the early days of lactation. The source of the microorganism can be from the infant's nasopharynx or from normal flora on mom's hands or breast. Mastitis is not related to poor hygiene, and moms should not be made to feel guilty if they develop this infection!
Plugged milk duct	Sometimes, milk ducts can become blocked during breast-feeding because all of the milk may not be expressed with feedings (some moms produce lots of milk—more than others but this is great!). When ducts are blocked, milk can stagnate creating a breeding ground for invading bacteria. Solution for this? Encourage mom to pump the remainder of milk after the infant is finished to avoid engorgement, and to take excellent care of her nipples with emollients safe for baby
Hormone fluctuations	Adolescent period: cyclic periods of inflammation may occur due to fluctuating hormone levels
Trauma	Ductal blockage of trapped blood and cellular debris from the trauma
Tumor	Can invade the lymphatic system or the skin, causing tissue inflammation

Source: Created by author from References #1 and #5.

Signs and symptoms and why

Table 16-21 explores the signs and symptoms and causes of mastitis.

Table 16-21

Signs and symptoms	Why
Tenderness, pain, swelling, tight or distended breasts (engorgement), redness, warmth, fever	Infection with microorganism (usually staph or strep) causing local inflammatory or systemic response
Simple breast inflammation—less than previously mentioned	Inflammation related to hormone fluctuations during adolescence
Nipple retraction and change in the contour of the breast in menopausal women who have previously given birth	Called "comedo" mastitis due to caked secretions inside the lobules and ducts of the breast. Some of this matter can be discharged through the nipple
Fever and discharge of pus from the nipple	Local infection with possible abscess formation

Source: Created by author from References #1 and #5.

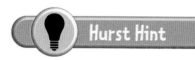

Hurst Hint

Good hand-washing should be encouraged—remind mom, as she is exhausted. Mom is busy changing diapers, nursing, pumping breasts, filling bottles, and possibly caring for other children as well.

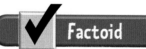

Factoid

It is scientifically proven that breast milk offered through breast-feeding is nutritionally superior to other forms of infant nutrition. Some of these benefits include higher IQs, improved immune system function resulting in less illness, and less chronic disease such as allergies and asthma. However, not all moms can or choose to breastfeed for various reasons and must be reassured that baby will be fine with infant formula! Remember, to completely support mom in whatever form of nutrition she chooses for her infant!

Quickie tests and treatments

Tests:

- History and physical examination: confirm diagnosis.
- Mammogram or ultrasound: visualize the breast tissue when masses are present.
- Biopsy: rules out cancer in the presence of solid or fluid-filled lumps.

Treatments:

- Breast-feeding: the affected breast is offered first to completely empty the inflamed breast. Yes, the infant will be exposed to the bacteria, but the breast milk is chock full of antibodies and is considered to be OK. The physician will decide if breastfeeding should be discontinued depending on the type of antibiotic given.
- Warm showers: promote comfort and vasodilation when milk ducts are clogged.
- A supportive bra should be worn at all times.
- Frequent nursing: empties the breasts.
- Penicillin or sulfonamides: treat infections.
- Surgical drainage of abscesses: incision and drainage (I&D) procedure to investigate any drainage from the nipple.

What can harm my client?

- Abscess formation.
- Sepsis.

If I were your teacher, I would test you on . . .

- What is it?
- Causes and why.
- Prevention: hand hygiene, nipple care, and complete emptying of breast.
- Proper breast-feeding technique.
- Client education for menopausal women regarding nipple discharge.
- Nonpharmacological measures to relieve the inflammatory symptoms of mastitis.

✚ Pelvic inflammatory disease (PID)

What is it?

Pelvic inflammatory disease (PID) is an infection caused by bacteria that enters the vagina during intercourse. PID is also caused by medical procedures such as dilation and curettage (D&C) or conization, where a portion of the cervix is excised. The infection spreads to the upper reproductive tract including the uterus (endometritis), ovaries (oophoritis), and fallopian tubes (salpingitis). Once in the fallopian tubes, the infection can travel to the abdominal cavity. The ovaries are not usually affected unless the infection is severe and widespread. The sexually transmitted diseases (STDs) gonorrhea and *Chlamydia* are commonly implicated in the development of PID. These infections tend to be recurrent and are currently the leading cause of preventable infertility due to scarring and closure of the fallopian tubes. Women who have a single healthy sex partner are at low risk for contracting PID because the risk of exposure to bacteria entering the vagina is minimal with the possible normal exceptions of childbirth and invasive vaginal medical exams. Normal vaginal flora and the alkaline pH of the vagina all serve to keep the reproductive tract healthy. Women who practice good hygiene, including front to back wiping, even further reduce their susceptibility to bacterial invasion. Women who engage in regular douching place themselves at risk for contamination and subsequent infection.

What causes it and why

Any bacteria can cause PID, but most commonly the sexually transmitted diseases (STDs) gonorrhea and *Chlamydia* are implicated. Younger women who are sexually active and who have unprotected sex with multiple partners are at the greatest risk. Women under the influence of drugs or alcohol are less likely to take usual precautions to prevent exposure to STDs.

Signs and symptoms and why

The onset of symptoms usually presents in cycles, beginning a few days before and persisting until the end of the menstrual cycle. Table 16-22 explores the signs and symptoms and rationales of PID.

Table 16-22

Signs and symptoms	Why
Mild to moderate pain initially. Severe pain occurs with spread into the abdominal cavity. Pelvic pain and pressure may be worse on one side or the other depending on the degree of involvement. Low abdominal pain is referred to the low back and inner thighs	The inflammatory response causes blood vessels to become engorged and swollen tissues irritate organs in surrounding areas. Pelvic congestion is responsible for much of the pain; however, pus pockets can form creating even more local pressure and stretching pain in fallopian tubes
Purulent vaginal discharge	Formation of pus (suppuration) is the body's response to invading organisms
Extremely tender cervix	Infection of cervix
Fever is initially low grade, but rises as the infection becomes more widespread. A spike in temperature is associated with increasingly severe symptoms	Fever is the body's response to infection, making the environment less friendly to bacteria
Infertility	Widespread and repeated scarring of the fallopian tubes prevents access of the sperm to the ovum
Nausea and vomiting	Severe pain stimulates the vomiting reflex in the brain
Abdominal guarding with sudden severe abdominal pain	Protective positioning is an effort to minimize pain as tense muscles provide support to internal organs

Source: Created by author from References #1 to #3.

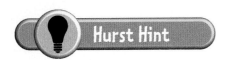

Hurst Hint

I know it can be embarrasing but never skip over a patient's sexual history when taking a health history. Be direct and nonjudgemental when questioning your patient.

Quickie tests and treatments

Tests:

- Client history and physical examination: confirm diagnosis.
- Culture and sensitivity: identify causative organism; determine which antibiotic therapy will be effective.
- Serum blood test: elevated white blood cells (WBCs).
- Ultrasound: visualizes pelvic mass and distended tubes.
- Abdominal laparoscopic exam: visualizes internal pelvic organs.

Treatments:

- Antibiotic therapy: for the client and all sexual partners to treat infection.
- If significant improvement is not made within 48 to 72 hours from start of treatment, or if peritonitis is suspected, the client is hospitalized for more aggressive therapy.

What can harm my client?

- Pelvic adhesions.
- Ectopic pregnancy.
- Infertility.
- Chronic abdominal pain.
- Abscesses on the tubes or ovaries.
- Peritonitis.
- Sepsis.

If I were your teacher, I would test you on . . .

- What is it?
- What causes it and why.
- Population most commonly affected (ages 16 to 24).
- Client education and prevention.
- Care of dependent minors with STDs (embarrassment, privacy issues, knowledge deficit).
- Risk factors including single status (not married), no children, multiple sex partners (or history of), past history of PID.

✚ Bartholin gland cysts and abscesses

The Bartholin glands are located on either side of the opening of the vagina (called the introitus). These glands have one function, and that is to secrete a thick lubricating fluid when stimulated. This glandular secretion provides lubrication for sexual intercourse. The gland can become inflamed when bacteria from the vagina enters the gland. A cyst occurs when there is enlargement without inflammation.

What are they?

A cyst forms when secretions cannot exit the Bartholin glands. When the cyst is noninfectious, the Bartholin gland enlarges but causes no pain, and the woman is asymptomatic. Inflammation of the gland (bartholinitis) can progress to a local infection with an abscess forming locally or pus forming in the Bartholin sac. When an infectious, pus-filled sac develops, the Bartholin gland becomes painful and enlarged. Swelling and pain also affects nearby tissue, such as the labia (external lips which cover the vagina). Abscesses can be caused by gonorrhea or *Chlamydia* as well as staph, strep, or *E. coli*.

What causes them and why

Bacteria from the vagina invade the gland, producing local infection, which leads to a cyst or an abscess. A noninfectious cyst develops when a duct from the gland becomes plugged. The cysts due to a plugged duct are not usually treated in women under the age of 40, but a biopsy may be indicated for older women due to concerns regarding possible cancer of the Bartholin gland—a rare cancer.

Signs and symptoms and why

Table 16-23 explores the signs and symptoms and explanations for Bartholin gland abscess and cyst.

Table 16-23

Signs and symptoms	Why
Swelling of the vulva without pain	Blocked duct or narrowing of the duct secondary to previous infection or trauma
Fever, malaise	Inflammatory response and toxins produced by infection
Swelling of the vulva with pain	Local distention with pressure on nerve endings; pain can prevent the client from participating in sports or having sex
Purulent exudates seen at the opening of the duct	Byproducts of infectious organisms
Redness of the local area surrounding the infected cyst	Increased congestion of blood and inflammatory response

Source: Created by author from References #1 and #4.

Quickie tests and treatments

Tests:

• Client history and physical examination: confirm diagnosis.

Treatments:

- Antibiotics: treat infection.
- Analgesics: relieve pain.
- Warm sitz baths: relieve pain.
- Incision and drainage (I&D): drains infective fluid from cyst or abscess using a specialized catheter.
- Culture and sensitivity of fluid: identify causative organism and guide antibiotic therapy.

What can harm my client?

A Bartholin cyst is not a life-threatening condition. The pain prompts women to seek immediate treatment, which responds well to antibiotic therapy or surgical intervention. Bartholin gland cysts tend to recur.

If I were your teacher, I would test you on . . .

- What causes cysts of the Bartholin glands?
- What causes infection or abscess?
- What treatments and interventions relieve symptomatic bartholinitis and Bartholin cysts?
- Patient education regarding infection prevention and management.

✚ Uterine fibroid tumors

The uterus is a hollow, muscular organ whose only function is to house the products of conception. This "baby-box" provides the ideal environment to support the growing fetus to term. The upper portion is called the fundus, which supplies the powerful uterine contractions for labor and childbirth. The body of the uterus (called the corpus) is lined with endometrium, which thickens each month in readiness for pregnancy, then sheds and starts over anew with the next month's reproductive cycle. The round and broad ligaments that hold the uterus in place and the uterine (myometrial) muscle can stretch to accommodate a large single fetus (a singleton) or a multiple gestation.

What are they?

Fibroids are benign, nonmalignant tumors that grow in the myometrial tissue (Fig. 16-9). These tumors are called by several different names, all ending with "omas" (fibromas, fibromyomas, myofibromas, leiomyomas, or just plain ol' myomas). Fibroids can be little bitty or HUGE, growing in the wall of the uterus, under the lining (endometrium), or outside of the uterus. Really large tumors can outgrow their blood supply and become necrotic.

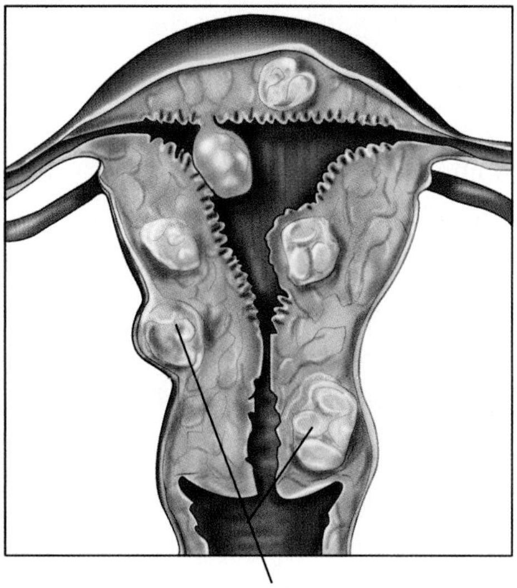

◀ Figure 16-9. Uterine fibroid tumors.

Fibroid tumors may occur in various regions of the uterus

What causes them and why

The actual cause of the growth is unknown, but it grows faster and larger when estrogen levels are high. Pregnancy makes fibroids larger and menopause makes them smaller.

Signs and symptoms and why

The location and degree of the signs and symptoms are dependent upon the number, size, and position of the tumors in the uterus. Table 16-24 explores the signs and symptoms and explanations for fibroids.

Table 16-24

Signs and symptoms	Why
Enlarged uterus	Increased epidermal growth factors and estrogen
Irregular or heavy menstrual bleeding	The inside surface area of the uterus increases in size with the mass of the tumors and thereby increases the surface area of endometrial lining to shed and bleed during each monthly reproductive cycle
Intrauterine crowding with pregnancy and spontaneous abortus, preterm births, and fetal malposition	Fibroid tumors occupy space and when the uterus reaches maximum capacity, the uterus (under the influence of oxytocin) contracts to evacuate the contents
Infertility	Masses of fibroid tissue can displace or compress the fallopian tubes
Pelvic pain and cramping	Pressure on structures near the uterus, blood vessel compression, and resultant local ischemia
Dragging backache	Multiple large fibroids increasing the size of the uterus can simulate the backache of pregnancy by changing the center of gravity and placing extra strain on uterosacral ligaments
Urinary frequency	The uterus is flexed forward and sits on top of the bladder. A heavy uterus filled with large fibroids can simulate the weight of a pregnant uterus, producing constant pressure on the bladder and a feeling of the need to void
Anemia	Excessive blood loss occurs with unusually long, heavy periods of menstrual bleeding (menorrhagia) and frequent irregular bleeding (metrorrhagia)

Source: Created by author from Reference #1.

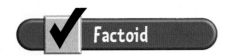

Fibroids are quite often asymptomatic and are found during routine pelvic exams.

Quickie tests and treatment

Tests:

- Bimanual examination: reveals enlarged nodular uterus that is nontender.
- Ultrasound and magnetic resonance imaging (MRI): determines size, location, and number of tumors in the uterus.
- Endometrial biopsy: rules out carcinoma due to excessive menstrual bleeding associated with cervical cancer.
- Hemoglobin and hematocrit: detects anemia.

Treatments:

- NSAIDs: relieve menstrual cramping and pelvic pain; begun 4 to 5 days before onset of menses and continued for several days afterward.
- GnRH agonists: shrink tumors preoperatively; induce menopause if menarche is approaching.
- Hysterectomy: if more conservative measures do not reduce symptoms.
- Myomectomy: if the woman wishes to preserve fertility, just the tumors can be removed from the uterine muscle (myomectomy).
- Out-patient laparoscopic procedure: destroys fibroids (myolysis) using electric current, cryoablation, or laser ablation.
- Iron supplements: treat mild anemia.
- Blood transfusions: treat severe anemia.

What can harm my client?

When abdominal surgery is performed, the client is always at risk for postoperative complications such as hemorrhage and pulmonary embolus, which can be deadly.

If I were your teacher, I would test you on . . .

- Definition of a uterine fibroid tumor.
- Causes and why.
- Signs and symptoms and why.
- Side effects of medication therapy.
- Care of the client undergoing surgery.
- Treatment options for the woman with symptomatic fibroids who desires to preserve fertility.

✚ Polycystic ovarian syndrome (PCOS)

At the birth of a female infant, the pair of ovaries contains millions of baby eggs (oocytes), which either degenerate or remain in a dormant state until puberty, at which time hormones initiate maturation of the ovum during each monthly reproductive cycle. The pituitary gland produces the follicle-stimulating hormone (FSH) and lutenizing hormone and the ovaries produce estrogen and progesterone. These hormones regulate the three phases of the menstrual cycle: follicular, ovulatory, and luteal. FSH stimulates the growth of numerous egg-containing follicles, but normally only the dominant one will continue to grow and produce estrogen as the others degenerate. A big bolus of lutenizing hormone causes the follicle to burst and spew the egg out into the peritoneal cavity, where the fingers on the fallopian tube pull the egg into the tube to await fertilization. The place on the ovary that ruptured to release the egg heals over to become the corpus luteum, which makes progesterone. If the egg is not fertilized, this place degenerates after about 2 weeks and the cycle starts all over again.

What is it?

"Poly" means many cysts on the ovary, and "syndrome" means that another set of symptoms (these particular ones are endocrine) accompany the ovarian problem. The result is that the ovaries get clogged (Fig. 16-10) with bunches of baby follicles, none of which mature to spew out a single egg and the hormones are all messed up. It happens mainly to young women (under age 30). In addition to not ovulating, these women are at risk for developing cardiac disease and diabetes.

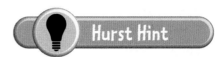

Hurst Hint

During a woman's childbearing years, approximately 400 eggs (oocytes) will mature.

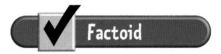

Factoid

Women with polycystic ovarian syndrome are at risk for developing cardiac disease and diabetes.

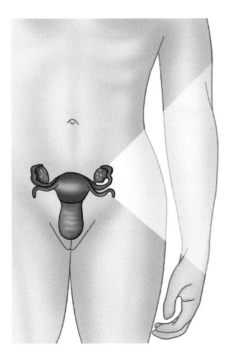

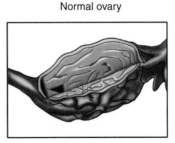

Normal ovary

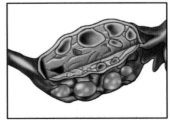

Polycystic ovary

◀ Figure 16-10 Polycystic ovarian syndrome.

What causes it and why

Table 16-25 explores the causes and reasons for PCOS.

Table 16-25

Causes	Why
Metabolic disorder	Exact cause of metabolic disorder unknown
Genetic endocrine abnormality	Enzyme triggers excessive androgen activity from the ovaries and adrenals
Cushing's syndrome, thyroid disease, androgen-producing tumors, metabolic syndrome	Excess male sex hormones from the adrenals and ovaries are triggered by high levels of lutenizing hormone
Steroids	Cause metabolic problems including insulin resistance and abnormal fat metabolism

Source: Created by author from References #1, #3, and #5.

Signs and symptoms and why

Table 16-26 explores the signs and symptoms and rationales for PCOS.

Table 16-26

Signs and symptoms	Why
Abnormal menstrual cycles	Scant, irregular or absent menses due to hormone imbalance, beginning with inappropriate gonadotropin secretion that triggers all the other imbalances, resulting in follicles that never mature or produce viable ova
Mild pain in one or both lower quadrants, low back pain	Pressure from multiple ovarian cysts
Dyspareunia (painful intercourse) especially with deep thrusting	Pressure from multiple ovarian cysts
Obesity	Impaired fat metabolism and insulin resistance
Abnormal hair growth (hirsutism) and male pattern scalp hair loss	Excessive levels of circulating androgens
Acne	Excessive steroids (androgens)
Infertility	Ovulatory failure occurs because no dominant follicle ever matures, ruptures, or releases an egg. The causes are lack of GnRH and abnormalities in ovarian and adrenal hormones. Insulin has a role in survival of follicles that should have disintegrated

Source: Created by author from References #1 to #3.

Quickie tests and treatment

Tests:

- Bimanual exam: enlarged ovaries are palpated.
- Urine specimen: 24-hour urine shows increase of 17-ketosteroids.
- Blood tests: elevated luteinizing hormone (LH); excess androgens (testosterone, androstenedione, dehydroepiandrosterone).

Treatments:

- Reduction of dietary carbohydrates: allows ovulation.
- Weight loss: allows ovulation.

- Hormonal contraceptives: suppress androgen production; not indicated for women who wish to become pregnant.
- Insulin sensitizers: allow for insulin uptake.
- Antiandrogen agents: decrease effects of androgens.
- Fertility drugs: clomiphene (Clomid) stimulates ovulation; medroxy-progesterone (Provera) for 10 consecutive days each month to simulate a normal ovarian pattern for the woman desiring pregnancy.

What can harm my client?

- Rupture of cyst.
- Peritonitis.
- Hemorrhage.
- Shock.
- Postoperative complications including pulmonary embolus.
- Cardiac disease.
- Diabetes.

If I were your teacher, I would test you on . . .

- Definition of polycystic ovarian syndrome.
- Signs and symptoms and why.
- Long-term complications associated with polycystic ovarian syndrome.
- Treatment modalities used to increase fertility.
- Possible complications and medical emergencies.

+ Breast mass

What is it?

A breast mass is characterized by lesions of the breast that are either benign or malignant. They are described as lumps, nodules, or masses that are different from surrounding tissue and are not like the other breast.

What causes it and why

Table 16-27 explores the causes and rationales for breast mass.

> **Deadly Dilemma**
>
> Take immediate action for a ruptured cyst! Monitor vital signs for fever, tachycardia, tachypnea (fast breathing), and hypotension. A rigid board-like abdomen can be caused by peritoneal inflammation and bleeding into the peritoneal cavity.

> **✔ Factoid**
>
> Early detection of breast cancer results in a better prognosis. All women should be taught breast self-examination regardless of age.

Table 16-27

Causes	Why
Fibrocystic changes (benign); used to be called fibrocystic breast disease	Most common lesion of the breast; characterized as "lumpy breasts." Restructuring of tissue related to hormone changes or imbalance. Can be difficult to differentiate this mass from a malignant one
Fibroadenoma (benign)	Round, rubbery, MOBILE lump that can be difficult to distinguish from cysts. May be brought on by pregnancy, then goes away with menopause
Cysts (benign)	Usually begin at age 40+ and around menopause; round, well-defined, smooth but firm and MOBILE mass
Breast cancer (malignant)	Malignant lesion of the breast occurring most commonly in upper outer quadrant, with a variety of presentations

Source: Created by author from References #1 and #5.

Signs and symptoms and why

Table 16-28 explores the signs and symptoms and explanations for breast mass.

Table 16-28

Signs and symptoms	Why
Fibrocystic changes	Thickened tissue changes that may feel rubbery without discreteness but blend into the surrounding breast tissue; no obvious mass is usually palpated
Fibroadenoma	Single, smooth, round, MOBILE, painless lump. May feel rubbery or firm and is most often located in the upper outer quadrant
Cyst	Round or oval in shape and distinguishable from surrounding tissue. Smooth, firm, and MOBILE
Cancer	Usually presents as painless, firm, and fixed (in other words, NONMOBILE) and does not change with menstruation. Appears most commonly in upper outer quadrant, but can appear anywhere

Source: Created by author from References #1 and #5.

Quickie tests and treatments

Tests:

- Client history and physical exam: clients under the age of 30 can opt to have the mass re-evaluated to see if it has changed in size in relationship to their menstrual cycle.
- Mammography: confirms mass.
- Ultrasound: complements mammography.
- Fine needle aspiration: fluid is sent for cytological evaluation.
- Excisional biopsy: determines if mass is malignant.

Treatments:

- Referral to specialist: if abnormal findings on diagnostic workup are found.
- If breast cancer: surgery, chemotherapy, radiation and hormone manipulation, and radical mastectomy (removal of entire breast).
- Aspiration of fluid: relieves pain in benign cysts.
- Supportive bra.
- Low-caffeine, low-sodium diet: relieves symptoms and fluid congestion.
- Hormone therapy: relieves severe pain.
- Oral contraceptives: relieve pain.
- NSAIDs: relieve pain.
- Excision: removes fibroadenomas.

What can harm my client?

- Death related to breast cancer.
- Infection related to procedures.

If I were your teacher, I would test you on . . .

- Causes and why.
- Signs and symptoms and why.
- Differences between breast lesions with physical characteristics.
- Diagnostic tests.
- Treatment and client education.

✚ Cervical cancer

What is it?

Cervical cancer occurs in the lower part of the uterus that extends into the vagina (Fig. 16-11).

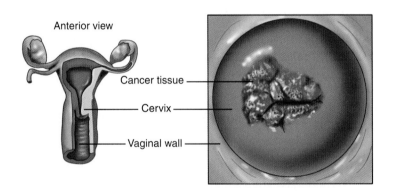

Anterior view

Cancer tissue

Cervix

Vaginal wall

◄ Figure 16-11. Cervical cancer.

What causes it and why

Table 16-29 shows the causes and background for cervical cancer.

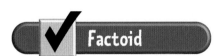
Factoid

A vaccine is now available to protect females against several strains of HPV. This vaccine has been shown to reduce the incidence of cervical cancer in young women.

Table 16-29

Cause	Why
Human papilloma virus (HPV): there are several high-risk strains	Virus that is transmitted during sexual intercourse. Also causes genital warts. Types include squamous cell, adeno-carcinoma, or adenosquamous cell

Source: Created by author from References #5 to #7.

Signs and symptoms and why

Table 16-30 shows the signs and symptoms and associated rationales for cervical cancer.

Table 16-30

Signs and symptoms	Why
Asymptomatic	Early stages
Spotting between periods	Slow, progressive change of normal cells, which is called dysplasia; dysplastic cells can eventually turn into cancer cells if not treated
Bleeding after intercourse	Cellular changes with disruption in the integrity of normal tissue
Heavy periods or hemorrhage	Extensive ulceration due to cancer
Foul-smelling discharge	Lesions, ulceration, necrotic tissue, infection
Low back pain	Suggests neurologic involvement
Swelling of the legs	Suggests vascular and lymphatic stasis related to presence of tumor

Source: Created by author from References #5 to #7.

Quickie tests and treatments

Tests:

- Papanicolaou (Pap) test: beginning with onset of becoming sexually active or by age 18 and yearly thereafter. If normal for 3 years in a row, may be tested every 2 to 3 years if there has been no change in sexual lifestyle (increased risk due to HPV).
- If dysplasia exists, will need to be tested again in 3 to 4 months.
- Biopsy (colposcopy) or cone biopsy.
- Cystoscopy, chest x-ray, intravenous urography, CT, MRI, barium enema, bone scan, liver scan, and sigmoidoscopy: determine extent of metastasis, if any.

Treatments:

- Depends on the stage of cancer.
- Removal of part of the cervix if only the cervix is involved.
- Hysterectomy.
- Radical hysterectomy: removal of surrounding tissues, ligaments, and lymph nodes if metastasis is within the pelvic area. Ovaries may or may not be removed.
- Radiation.
- Chemotherapy with extensive metastasis or recurrence.
- Prevention: Gardisil® vaccine prevents several strains of HPV.

What can harm my client?

- If not treated, the urinary tract could become obstructed, causing renal failure and eventual death.
- Extensive metastasis resulting in death.

If I were your teacher, I would test you on . . .

- What causes it and why?
- Signs and symptoms and why.
- Guidelines for pap test.
- Care of the client undergoing surgery, chemotherapy, radiation.

✚ Ovarian cancer

What is it?

Ovarian cancer is also known as ovarian carcinoma (Fig. 16-12). It may develop in women between the ages of 50 and 70. Ovarian cancer is correlated with a high-fat diet; previous cancers of the uterus, breast, or colon; and genetic predisposition (presence of BRCA1 gene).

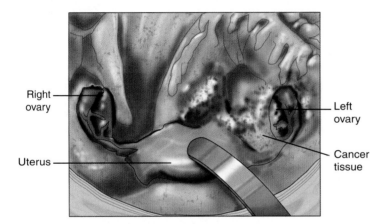

◀ Figure 16-12. Ovarian cancer.

What causes it and why

Table 16-31 lists the causes and explanations for ovarian cancer.

Table 16-31

Causes	Why
Strong family history	Strong history of breast or ovarian cancer is the most important risk factor. Exact cause unknown
Nulliparity (no pregnancies)	Constant stimulation of the ovarian epithelium without interruption (pregnancy) and ovulation without interruptions
Genetic tendency	Inherited mutation of two genes, BRCA1 and BRCA2

Source: Created by author from References #3 to #5.

Signs and symptoms and why

Table 16-32 explores the signs and symptoms and associated rationales of ovarian cancer.

Table 16-32

Signs and symptoms	Why
Asymptomatic	Symptoms may be absent until the disease is well advanced
Enlarged ovary	Tumor
Abdominal swelling and/or bloating with pain or distress, flatulence after ingesting food	Accumulation of fluid along with enlarged ovary leads to swelling, bloating, and pelvic pain. Other GI symptoms may be caused by biochemical changes in peritoneal fluids, which irritate the bowel. Pain originating in the ovary may be referred to the abdomen and interpreted as GI disturbances

Source: Created by author from References #3 to #5.

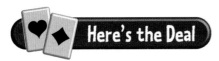

An enlarged ovary after menopause can be indicative of ovarian cancer. In young women, enlarged ovaries are usually related to cysts.

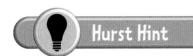

Ovarian cancer is a "silent killer" because there are no symptoms until the disease is advanced. Annual pelvic exams should be continued, even after menopause.

Quickie tests and treatments

Tests:

- Ultrasound: detects location and size of tumor.
- CT: detects location and size of tumor.
- MRI: detects location and size of tumor.
- Blood tests: detects tumor markers such as cancer antigen 125 (CA-125) to confirm diagnosis.

Treatments:

- Surgery: remove tumor and/or fallopian tubes and uterus.
- Prognosis is based on the stage of cancer.
- Chemotherapy: based on the stage of cancer.
- Radiation is rarely used.

What can harm my client?

- With treatment, 70% to 100% of clients with stage I cancer are still alive after 5 years of diagnosis.
- After 5 years of diagnosis, 50% to 70% of clients with stage II ovarian cancer are still living. It is important to note that 5% to 40% of clients with stage III or IV ovarian cancer are still living after 5 years.
- Cancer is usually advanced by the time signs and symptoms become evident, and diagnosing it in the early stages is difficult.

If I were your teacher, I would test you on . . .

- Signs and symptoms and why. Remember, GI symptoms can occur with ovarian cancer.
- Ovarian cancer is silent and clients may not even know they have it until the disease is advanced.
- Risk factors.
- Diagnostic tests.
- Care of the client undergoing chemotherapy and surgery.

✚ Premenstrual syndrome (PMS)

What is it?

Premenstrual syndrome refers to the physical and psychological manifestations marking the onset of menses each month. PMS can vary from mild to severe, and begins within hours or up to 2 weeks prior to the onset of menses. Symptoms are usually relieved with the onset of menses. This disorder was once thought to be psychosomatic, and only recently has been recognized as a valid disorder causing significant disturbances in the quality of lives of clients who suffer from it.

What causes it and why

Table 16-33 shows the cause and explanation for PMS.

Table 16-33

Cause	Why
Hormones	Estrogen and progesterone fluctuation during the menstrual cycle

Source: Created by author from References #5 to #7.

Signs and symptoms and why

Table 16-34 shows the signs and symptoms and associated rationales for PMS.

Table 16-34

Signs and symptoms	Why
Dysmenorrhea (painful period) with heavy crampy feeling in the lower abdomen	Signs and symptoms are considered to be hormone dependent. Same as above, and applies all the way down this column
Irritability, agitation, and emotional instability with crying spells, depression	
Difficulty concentrating	
Bloating and backache	
Breast tenderness	
More seizures in those who already have them	
Exacerbations of autoimmune disorders such as rheumatoid arthritis and lupus, as well as respiratory problems such as allergies, nasal congestion, asthma	
Palpitations	
Appetite changes and cravings with weight gain	
Dizziness and fainting	
Nausea and vomiting	
Acne	
Fluid retention with weight gain	

Source: Created by author from References #5 to #7.

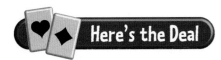

Here's the Deal

If PMS symptoms are bad enough to interfere with relationships, work, and quality of life, then the client may be diagnosed with premenstrual dysphoric disorder, but only after keeping a journal to track the onset of symptoms.

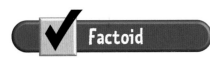

Factoid

Too much vitamin B₆ can be harmful, causing nerve damage with only as little as 200 milligrams per day.

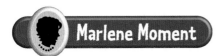

Marlene Moment

PMS causes enough "nerve" damage, don't you agree?!

Quickie tests and treatments

Tests:

- No diagnostic tests detect PMS.
- The primary care provider may ask the client to keep a journal of symptoms in order to diagnose and distinguish PMS and premenstrual dysphoric disorder from actual mood disorders (depression, bipolar, etc.).

Treatments:

- Treatment is aimed at providing relief of symptoms.
- Low-sodium diet and/or diuretics: relieve fluid retention and bloating.
- Exercise with meditation or other forms of relaxation: relieve anxiety.
- Caffeine reduction: relieves symptoms.
- Calcium supplementation at 1000 mg per day: relieves symptoms.
- Magnesium and vitamin B₆: may relieve symptoms.
- NSAIDs: relieve symptoms and reduce the flow of blood if taken 2 to 3 times per day the week prior to starting menses. This can dramatically improve the client's quality of life.
- Oral contraceptives that contain BOTH estrogen and progestin: pills that contain only the progestin component do not do any good.
- Antidepressants: relieve severe symptoms.
- Antianxiety medications: relieve severe symptoms.

What can harm my client?

- Decreased quality of life with strained relationships in and outside the home.
- Suicide.

If I were your teacher, I would test you on . . .

- Difference between premenstrual dysphoric disorder and PMS.
- Signs and symptoms and why.
- Pharmacological and nonpharmacological measures to relieve symptoms.
- Harm that can be brought to the client.
- This is a valid, medically accepted and recognized disorder that must be taken seriously.

✚ Dysmenorrhea

What is it?

Dysmenorrhea is pain experienced during menstruation that is categorized as primary or secondary. Primary dysmenorrhea is pain in the absence of abnormalities that occurs during the menstrual cycle. The pain can be mild to severe, with loss of work and school. Secondary dysmenorrhea is due to an abnormality.

What causes it and why

Table 16-35 explores the cause and background of dysmenorrhea.

Table 16-35

Cause	Why
Prostaglandin release during menstruation	Prostaglandins are hormone-like substances that cause the uterus to contract, decreasing blood supply; prostaglandins increase sensitivity of nerve endings in the uterus to pain sensations

Source: Created by author from Reference #4.

Signs and symptoms and why

Table 16-36 shows the signs and symptoms and associated rationales for dysmenorrhea.

Table 16-36

Signs and symptoms	Why
Pain in the lower abdomen extending to lower back or legs. Intermittent or constant dull ache starting shortly prior to onset of menses or during menses. Other symptoms include those for PMS	**Primary Dysmenorrhea** Prostaglandins are hormone-like substances that cause the uterus to contract, decreasing blood supply to it, with increased sensitivity of the nerve endings in the uterus to pain **Secondary Dysmenorrhea** Fibroids, pelvic adhesions, pelvic inflammatory disease, endometriosis, or adenomyosis (benign growth into the endometrium, which is the lining of the uterus). This type of dysmenorrhea usually occurs later in life rather than earlier, as with primary dysmenorrhea

Source: Created by author from Reference #4.

Quickie tests and treatments

Tests:

- Client history and physical exam: confirm diagnosis.
- Laparoscopy: rules out pelvic abnormalities by inserting a scope through an incision just below the navel; differentiates endometriosis from PID.
- Hysteroscopy: scope inserted through the vagina and cervix.
- Hysterosalpingography: radiopaque material to view the uterus, ovaries, tubes.

Treatments:

- NSAIDs: relieve pain.
- Oral contraceptives: suppress ovulation.
- Treatment of secondary dysmenorrhea involves treating the specific cause.
- Antiemetics: relieve nausea and vomiting.

Prevention:

- Adequate rest and sleep.
- Exercise on a regular basis.
- Oral contraceptives.
- NSAIDs: taken one week prior to onset of menses may decrease blood flow, bloating, and pain.
- Caffeine and alcohol avoidance.

What can harm my client?

- Does not pose a medical problem but interferes with quality of life.
- Complications can arise from secondary causes of dysmenorrheal: PID, endometriosis, adhesions.

If I were your teacher, I would test you on . . .

- Causes and why.
- Signs and symptoms and why.
- The difference between primary and secondary dysmenorrheal.
- Treatment and prevention.

✚ Amenorrhea

What is it?

Amenorrhea is the absence of a menstrual cycle. Amenorrhea should only be considered normal in the event of pregnancy, breast-feeding, after menopause, or before the onset of puberty. Amenorrhea is categorized as primary or secondary. Primary amenorrhea is failure of onset of menses by age 16 or failure to reach puberty by age 13. Amenorrhea may also occur in girls who have not started having periods within 5 years of starting puberty and who have short stature (under 5 feet at age 14). Secondary amenorrhea is the cessation of menses for 3 consecutive months in those who have already been menstruating.

What causes it and why

The number of causes for amenorrhea is many, but only the most common ones are presented in Table 16-37.

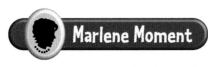

Marlene Moment

Have you ever noticed that the word amenorrhea begins with AMEN?! This is a trick to help you remember the term for NO PERIOD. But remember, there may be a serious problem going on if amenorrhea exists.

Table 16-37

Causes	Why
Pregnancy: the most common cause	Hormone suppression related to pregnancy induces amenorrhea so the baby can thrive inside the uterus
Hypothalamic repression	Emotional stress, depression, chronic disease, weight loss, obesity, severe dieting (anorexia nervosa), vigorous exercise, birth control pills, drugs
Central nervous system (CNS) lesion	Pituitary tumor, head injury with hypothalamic injury, and congenital syndromes
Ovary problems	Chromosomal abnormalities, ovarian injury due to autoimmunity, infection, polycystic ovarian disease, ovarian failure (premature or due to menopause)
Outflow problems	Absence of uterus or vagina, imperforate hymen, uterine lining defect
Defect in hormone synthesis or action	Adrenal hyperplasia, Cushing's disease, adrenal tumor, ovarian tumor (rare), and drugs such as steroids, antidepressants, or antipsychotics
Hypothyroidism	Can delay onset of adolescence

Source: Created by author from References #3 to #6.

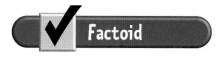

Factoid

The most common cause of amenorrhea is pregnancy.

Signs and symptoms and why

Amenorrhea may or may not be accompanied by other symptoms, depending on the cause. Table 16-38 shows the signs and symptoms and explanations for amenorrhea.

Table 16-38

Signs and symptoms	Why
No menstrual period for at least 3 months	Pituitary tumor; tumor of the ovaries or adrenal glands; delayed development: no signs of puberty by age 13 or no periods within 5 years of starting puberty

Source: Created by author from Reference #4.

Quickie tests and treatments

Tests:

- Pregnancy test: rules out pregnancy as cause of amenorrhea.
- Prolactin level (PRL), follicle stimulating hormone level (FSH), leuteinizing hormone (LH), thyroid stimulating hormone (TSH), testosterone level, and potassium: monitor status of ovaries.
- MRI: rules out pituitary tumor.
- Blood tests: monitor renal and hepatic (liver) function.

- Dexamethasone suppression test: used if client exhibits signs of hyper-cortisolism, as in Cushing's disease.
- Ultrasound: rules out mass or tumor.

Treatments:

- Nonpregnant women without abnormalities can be given progestin for about 10 days. When finished, the client should experience "withdrawal" menses. If not, there may be a lack of estrogen or a uterine abnormality.
- Estrogen replacement therapy for girls with hypogonadism and those with menopause.
- Treatment and prevention of osteoporosis with bisphosphonates.

What can harm my client?

What can harm your client depends on the cause of amenorrhea and includes the factors associated with the cause of amenorrhea:

- Tumor.
- Emotional distress.
- Depression.
- Severe dieting.
- Malnutrition.
- Pregnancy complications.
- Osteoporosis with fractures related to menopause.

If I were your teacher, I would test you on . . .

- Know that the hypothalamus, pituitary, and ovaries all work together and the ovaries are under the stimulation of hormones.
- Know that certain chromosomal abnormalities can cause primary amenorrhea.
- Know that anatomical abnormalities can result in amenorrhea such as absence of structures or obstructions to flow of blood.
- Know classification of primary versus secondary amenorrhea.

TERMS YOU SHOULD KNOW

Amenorrhea—absence of periods.

Dysmenorrhea—painful periods.

Hypomenorrhea—light period.

Menometrorrhagia—prolonged bleeding at irregular intervals.

Menorrhagia—long and heavy periods.

Metrorrhagia—frequent, irregular bleeding.

Oligomenorrhea—unusually infrequent periods.

Polymenorrhea—unusually frequent periods.

Postmenopausal bleeding—bleeding after menopause.

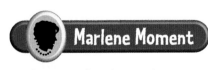
Marlene Moment

Isn't it enough to have only one type of period? But NO, we are burdened with the possibility of having up to 8 different versions of one?! Menopause . . . AMEN to amenorrhea!

✚ Menopause

What is it?

Menopause is the cessation of menstruation, usually between ages 48 and 55. If the client has not menstruated for a full year, she is considered to be menopausal.

What causes it and why

Table 16-39 shows the causes and explanations for menopause.

Table 16-39

Causes	Why
Ovaries stop responding to the effects of FSH	Gradual deterioration of ovaries as a normal part of aging
Surgically induced	Removal of ovaries (oophorectomy)

Source: Created by author from Reference #4.

Signs and symptoms and why

Table 16-40 shows the signs and symptoms and rationales for menopause.

Table 16-40

Signs and symptoms	Why
Cessation of menstruation	Ovarian failure
Decrease in breast tissue, body fat, body hair, skin elasticity	Loss of effects of estrogen
Vaginal dryness, stress incontinence, urgency, nocturia, vaginitis, UTI, painful intercourse	Urogenital atrophy due to loss of effects of estrogen
Hot flashes, palpitations, dizziness, headaches, insomnia, irritability, depression	Vasomotor instability related to decreased estrogen and increase in other hormones with resultant vasodilation; HORMONE IMBALANCE!

Source: Created by author from Reference #4.

Quickie tests and treatments

Tests:

- Blood test for follicle-stimulating hormone and leuteinizing hormone: elevated.

Treatments:

- Treat vasomotor symptoms with estrogen with the lowest dose possible for the least amount of time possible.
- Alternative treatment includes antiseizure medications such as gabapentin (Neurontin) or clonidine (Catapres).

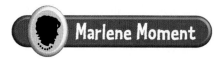

Marlene Moment

Why is it called menopause? Perhaps it should be called "menostop!" ("menocease?") A pause suggests that it might come back!

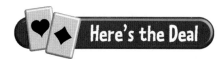

Here's the Deal

Surgically induced menopause usually results in more severe symptoms due to an abrupt decrease in estrogen.

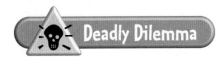

Deadly Dilemma

Clients should not be given estrogen-progestin replacement therapy for periods longer than 3 to 4 years due to increased risk for cardiovascular disease, cerebrovascular disease, and breast cancer.

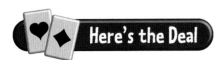

Here's the Deal

Teach clients to take calcium with food to help with absorption. Vitamin D is also necessary to enhance absorption.

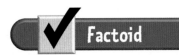

Factoid

Estrogen deprivation results in bone remodeling. Formation does not keep up with resorption. This results in decreased bone mass with eventual brittle bones.

- Osteoporosis treatment and prevention includes ingesting 800 mg of calcium through the diet in addition to 1000 mg of elemental calcium with vitamin D 400 units/day in the form of a supplement; walking and other forms of weight-bearing exercise to help maintain bone mass; medications to prevent and treat osteoporosis.

What can harm my client?

- Osteoporosis, resulting in fractures.
- Emotional instability related to hormone imbalance.
- Hot flashes are extremely bothersome.
- Effects of hormone replacement therapy, as mentioned earlier.

If I were your teacher, I would test you on . . .

- Definition of menopause.
- Signs and symptoms and why.
- Tests.
- Treatments.
- Osteoporosis prevention and complications.
- Therapeutic dosages of calcium and vitamin D.
- Importance of encouraging clients to exercise to maintain bone mass.

SUMMARY

The nurse's understanding of the male and female reproductive systems leads to improved outcomes for the client. The nurse's role in caring for clients with illnesses of the reproductive system includes providing a thorough assessment, establishing appropriate nursing goals, and maintaining client support.

PRACTICE QUESTIONS

1. A young male client is admitted to the emergency department with sudden, severe pain in the testicles. Which nursing action is priority?

   1. Elevate the hips with a pillow.

   2. Apply an ice pack to the scrotum.

   3. Prepare for emergency surgery.

   4. Monitor the color and temperature of the scrotum.

   Correct answer: 3. Testicular torsion must be relieved immediately to restore blood flow to the scrotum. Elevating the hips and applying an ice pack to the scrotum will further reduce arterial blood flow to the area. Monitoring the color and temperature of the scrotum delays treatment.

2. An elderly male client with a history of repeated urinary tract infections reports a small stream with urinary hesitancy and bothersome nocturnal voiding. Which statement by the nurse is most appropriate?

1. "Sit and lean forward on the toilet rather than standing for voiding."

2. "Do not stop taking your antibiotics even when the symptoms subside."

3. "Do not drink fluids with the evening meal or before bedtime."

4. "Keep your physician appointments for regular digital massage of the prostate."

Correct answer: 1. Compressing the bladder while sitting and leaning forward on the toilet will help empty the bladder. The question stem notes the client has a history of urinary tract infections, not symptoms of a current infection. Therefore, the client is most likely not on antibiotic therapy. Withholding fluids further complicates the client problem, since urinary stasis is compounded by withholding fluids. An enlarged prostate gland that is constricting the urethra will not benefit from massage through the rectum.

3. A client with a diagnosis of benign prostatic hypertrophy reports decreased urinary output and low pelvic pain. Which nursing action is priority?

1. Advise increased intake of fluids by mouth.

2. Assess the bladder for distention.

3. Ask if burning is experienced with voiding.

4. Administer pain medication.

Correct answer: 2. If the bladder is distended, back pressure in the kidney (hydronephrosis) can lead to postrenal failure. Increasing fluids will intensify the distention indicated by the complaint of low pelvic pain. Asking about burning with voiding incorrectly assumes that infection is the cause of the problem. Administering pain medication may mask the problem by further reducing bladder tonus.

4. A male client seeks treatment for erectile dysfunction. Which nursing intervention is priority?

1. A complete physical examination to determine current health status.

2. A psychological examination to rule out emotional disturbances and stress reactions.

3. Referral to a neurologist, since erection is dependent upon intact sacral nerves.

4. Obtain a patient history to assess medications that could interact with sildenifil (Viagra).

Correct answer: 1. Performing a complete physical examination to determine current health status is the most comprehensive and basic nursing action and must be completed before other measures are considered.

5. A woman is taking gonadotropin-releasing hormone agonists (GnRH agonists) to shrink fibroid tumors. Based on this data, which counseling by the nurse is priority for health maintenance of this client?

1. Monthly gonadotropin hormone levels must be drawn.

2. Yearly mammograms and Pap-smear tests are mandatory.

3. A bone density test should be a part of regular health screenings.

4. The GnRH agonists must be discontinued 1 year before conception.

Correct answer: 3. Decreasing bone density puts clients at high risk for osteoporosis and is an adverse effect of the GnRH agonists.

6. A client with a family history of endometriosis tells the nurse that, in addition to using tampons, a cleansing douche at the end of menses is recommended by her grandmother. Which health teaching by the nurse demonstrates the best understanding of the pathophysiology of endometriosis?

1. Tampons should be changed frequently.

2. Use only cool, isotonic, pH-balanced solutions for douching.

3. A low-pressure douche is needed to evacuate old menstrual blood and any remaining endometrial shed that could lodge in the cervix.

4. Douching is never recommended unless medically prescribed.

Correct answer: 4. Douching is implicated in the backward flow of endometrial tissue into the fallopian tubes and ovaries. This may allow passage of the migrant tissue into the abdominal cavity, where it can cause infection.

7. A 15-year-old client states pelvic pain and a foul greenish-yellow vaginal discharge. The client has only recently become sexually active and requests oral contraception. Which is the priority nursing intervention?

1. Obtain parental consent for treatment since the patient is a minor.

2. Provide information about the risks associated with oral contraceptives.

3. Give verbal support and factual information during the pelvic examination.

4. Insist that the boyfriend (her known sex partner) also receive STD treatment.

Correct answer: 3. Support and information is the client's most immediate need as she is facing a painful pelvic exam by a health care provider not known to her. Parental consent is not required of a sexually active minor, and treatment remains confidential as her legal status is that of an emancipated minor. After the exam, the nurse may discuss the risks of oral contraceptives with the client. The priority is to focus on the client being treated, not the boyfriend.

8. Following surgery for polycystic ovarian syndrome, a client complains of sudden sharp, stabbing chest pain with shortness of breath and cough. Which nursing intervention is priority?

1. Notify the physician of suspected pulmonary embolus.

2. Raise the head of the bed and apply oxygen per facial mask.

3. Notify respiratory therapy for an immediate respiratory treatment.

4. Encourage the client to cough vigorously and expectorate secretions.

Correct answer: 2. Raising the head of the bed and applying oxygen provides the most immediate help when pulmonary embolus is suspected.

9. A client diagnosed with fibroids experiences frequent, heavy menstrual cycles with fatigue and low energy. Which action by the nurse is of most benefit based on the client's symptoms?

1. Advise the client to balance periods of activity with rest.

2. Advise the client to consume dietary sources of iron on a daily basis.

3. Recommend an iron supplement be taken with orange juice.

4. Recommend a complete physical examination with a complete blood count (CBC).

Correct answer: 4. Signs of anemia must be evaluated and treated accordingly. All other options should be taken AFTER the severity of the anemia is evaluated, because if severe, a blood transfusion may be indicated. In that case, all other answer options delay treatment.

10. A client is being prepared for a hysterectomy due to large symptomatic fibroid tumors. The client expresses concern that hormone replacement will be necessary to avoid surgically induced menopausal symptoms. Which information given by the nurse would be most helpful to relieve this client's concern?

1. Provide factual information about surgically induced menopause.

2. Advise the woman that these symptoms will gradually disappear.

3. Explain that removal of the uterus does not induce menopause.

4. Explore alternatives to hormone replacement therapy.

Correct answer: 1. The nurse may relieve the client's anxiety by providing factual information about surgically induced menopause and postoperative care including the risks and the benefits of hormone replacement therapy.

References

1. Huether SE, McCance KL. *Understanding Pathophysiology*. 3rd ed. St. Louis: Mosby; 2004:889–905.

2. Springhouse. *Pathophysiology: A 2-in-1 Reference for Nurses*. Philadelphia: Lippincott Williams & Wilkins; 2004.

3. *Straight A's in Pathophysiology*. Philadelphia: Lippincott Williams & Wilkins; 2005.

4. Beers MH, ed. *Merck Manual of Medical Information*. 2nd home ed. Whitehouse Station, NJ: Pocket Books; 2003:1329–1337,1369–1379.

5. Merck CJ. *Handbook of Pathophysiology*. 2nd ed. Philadelphia: Lippincott Williams & Wilkins; 2005.

6. Uphold CR, Graham MV. *Clinical Guidelines in Family Practice*. 4th ed. Barmarrae Books; 2003.

7. Porth CM. *Essentials of Pathophysiology: Concepts of Altered Health States*. 2nd ed. Philadelphia: Lippincott Williams & Wilkins; 2006.

8. Tierney LM, McPhee S, Papadakis MA. *Current Medical Diagnosis and Treatment*. New York: McGraw-Hill; 2005.

9. Hay W, Levin M, Sondheimer J, et al. *Current Pediatric Diagnosis and Treatment*. 17th ed. New York: McGraw-Hill; 2005.

Bibliography

Hurst Review Services. www.hurstreview.com.

INDEX

Note: The page numbers with e indicate the pages in the CD.

A

abdominal aortic aneurysm, 197–199
abducens nerve (CN VI), 387
ABGs (arterial blood gases), 121
   metabolic acidosis, 57
   metabolic alkalosis, 60
   normal, 44–45
   respiratory acidosis, 51
   respiratory alkalosis, 54
abnormal electrolyte loss, 7–8
abnormal fluid loss, 4–5
ABO blood types, 284
absence seizure, 300
accommodation, 356
ACE (angiotensin-converting enzyme),
   158
ACE inhibitors, 583, 590
acetaminophen, 82
acetylcholine (ACh), 316
achalasia, 448–449
acid–base balance
   carbon dioxide (CO_2), 45–48
   metabolic acidosis, 46, 55–58
   metabolic alkalosis, 46, 58–61
   normal ABGs, 44–45
   respiratory acidosis, 46–52
   respiratory alkalosis, 46, 52–55
acidosis, 121. *See also* metabolic
   acidosis; respiratory acidosis
acne, e9–e12
acoustic nerve (CN VIII), 387
ACP (antivenom *Crotalidae* polyvalent),
   e53
acral-lentiginous melanoma, 108
ACS. *See* acute coronary syndrome
ACTH (adrenocorticotropin
   hormones), 533, 541–542, 564
acute bacterial prostatitis, 617
acute coronary syndrome (ACS),
   214–216
acute hemolytic reaction, 285
acute idiopathic polyneuropathy. *See*
   Guillain–Barré syndrome
acute pericarditis, 182–183
acute radiation syndrome, e81–83
acute renal failure, 588–591, 593
acute respiratory distress syndrome
   (ARDS), 122–123

acute tubular necrosis, 579
addisonian crisis, 538–540
Addison's disease, 536–540
adenocarcinoma
   breast cancer, 92
   lung cancer, 97
adenomas, 101, 452
ADH (antidiuretic hormone),
   11, 564–565
   cardiovascular system, 158
   decrease in secretion of, 566
   diabetes insipidus (DI), 566–570
   increase in secretion of, 565
   renal system, 580
   syndrome of inappropriate
      antidiuretic hormone (SIADH),
      570–573
adrenal cortex, 533–534
   Addison's disease, 536–541
   Cushing's syndrome and disease,
      541–545
   hormones of, 512
adrenal glands
   adrenal cortex, 533–534
   diagram, 511
   F & E homeostasis, 10–11
   glucocorticoids, 534–535
   hormones of, 512
   mineralcorticoids, 535–536
   sex hormones, 536
adrenal hypofunction. *See* Addison's
   disease
adrenal insufficiency. *See* Addison's
   disease
adrenal medulla, 533
   hormones of, 512
   pheochromocytoma, 547–549
adrenaline, 546
adrenocortical insufficiency. *See*
   Addison's disease
adrenocorticotropin hormones
   (ACTH), 533, 541–542, 564
advanced shock, 227–228
afterload, 157
agranulocytosis, 520
A-I (angiotensin I), 158, 578
A-II (angiotensin II), 158, 578
airborne precautions, e99

albumin, 13–14, 500, 580, 584
alcohol-based hand rubs, e97
aldosterone
   Addison's disease, 537
   adrenal cortex, 533
   functions of, 6, 10, 158
   nephrotic syndrome, 585
   secretion, 535
aligned fractures, 407–408
alkalosis, 121. *See also* metabolic
   alkalosis; respiratory alkalosis
alpha cells, 550
ALS. *See* amyotrophic lateral sclerosis
alveoli, 120, 133, 135
Alzheimer's disease, 306–308
amenorrhea, 654–656
American pit viper, e49
AMI (antibody-mediated immunity), 67
ammonia, 59, e79
amphetamines, 550
Amphotericin B, e141
amputation, 410–412
amyotrophic lateral sclerosis (ALS)
   (Lou Gehrig's disease),
   309–310
anaphylactic shock, 236–238
anaphylaxis, 70–71
   blood transfusion reactions, 285–286
   insect stings, e57–e59
anaplastic lung cancer, 98
anasarca, 585
androgens, 536, 544, 612. *See also* sex
   hormones
androstenedione, 612
anemia, 256–266
   heart failure, 500
   non-Hodgkin lymphoma (NHL), 107
   renal issues, 578
aneurysm
   abdominal aortic, 197–199
   headache, 300
   thoracic aortic, 199–201
angina, 214
angiotensin I (A-I), 158, 578
angiotensin II (A-II), 158, 578
angiotensin-converting enzyme (ACE),
   158
angle-closure glaucoma, 359